The Physiological Development
of the Fetus and Newborn

The Physiological Development of the Fetus and Newborn

edited by

C. T. JONES
The Nuffield Institute for Medical Research,
University of Oxford, Oxford, UK

P. W. NATHANIELSZ
Department of Reproductive Studies, New York State College of
Veterinary Medicine, Cornell University, Ithaca, New York, USA

WITHDRAWN

Rock Valley College
Educational Resources
Center

1985

ACADEMIC PRESS
HARCOURT BRACE JOVANOVICH, PUBLISHERS
LONDON   ORLANDO   SAN DIEGO   NEW YORK
TORONTO   MONTREAL   SYDNEY   TOKYO

ACADEMIC PRESS INC. (LONDON) LTD.
24/28 Oval Road,
London NW1 7DX

United States Edition published by
ACADEMIC PRESS INC.
Orlando, Florida 32887

Copyright © 1985 by
ACADEMIC PRESS INC. (LONDON) LTD.

All Rights Reserved
No part of this book may be reproduced in any form by photostat, microfilm, or any other
means, without permission from the publishers

British Library Cataloguing in Publication Data

The Physiological development of the fetus and
  newborn.
  1. Embryology
  I. Jones, C. T. II. Nathanielsz, P. W.
  599.03'34   QL951

  ISBN 0-12-389080-2

Phototypeset by Dobbie Typesetting Service, Plymouth, Devon
Printed by St Edmundsbury Press,
Bury St Edmunds, England

Contributors

Numbers in parentheses indicate the first page of each author's contribution.

Abramovich, D. R., *Department of Obstetrics & Gynaecology, University of Aberdeen, Forester Hill, Aberdeen AB9 2ZD, UK* (p. 659)

Abramovici, H., *Dept. of Obstetrics & Gynaecology, Carmel Hospital, Michal St., Haifa 34362, Israel* (p. 312)

Adelantado, J. M., *Nuffield Dept. of Obstetrics and Gynaecology, John Radcliffe Hospital, Headington, Oxford OX3 9DU, UK* (p. 489)

Ahmed, A. G., *Department of Obstetrics & Gynaecology, Royal Infirmary, Forester Hill, Aberdeen AB9 2ZB, UK* (p. 83)

Albersheim, S., *Dept. of Pediatrics, University of Manitoba, Winnipeg, Manitoba, USA* (p. 643)

Alexander, D. P., *Department of Physiology & Biophysics, St. Mary's Hospital Medical School, London W2 1PG, UK* (p. 479)

Allen, H. D., *University of Arizona, Health Sciences Center, Tucson, Arizona, USA* (p. 789)

Allotta, E., *Faculty of Medicine, University of Newcastle, Shortland, NSW 12308, Australia* (p. 33)

Althabe, O., *Las Heras 1877 12A, 1127 Buenos Aires, Argentina* (p. 801)

Amankwah, K. S., *Department of Obstetrics & Gynaecology, Southern Illinois University School of Medicine, P.O. Box 3926, Springfield, Illinois 62708, USA* (p. 611)

Anand, K. S., *Department of Paediatrics, John Radcliffe Hospital, Headley Way, Oxford, UK* (p. 811)

Anderson, D. F., *Dept. of Physiology and Medicine, School of Medicine, Oregon Health Sciences University, Portland, Oregon 97201, USA* (p. 371)

Andrews, D. C., *Nuffield Dept. of Obstetrics and Gynaecology, John Radcliffe Hospital, Headley Way, Oxford OX3 9DU, UK* (p. 795)

Arkinstall, S., *The Nuffield Institute for Medical Research, Oxford University, Headley Way, Oxford OX3 9DS, UK* (p. 511)

Aynsley-Green, A., *Department of Child Health, Royal Victoria Infirmary, Newcastle upon Tyne NE1 4LP, UK* (pp. 771,811)

Ayres, N. A., *Dept. of Pediatrics and the Cardiovascular Research Center, University of Iowa, Iowa City, Iowa 52242, USA* (p. 527)

Azancot, A., *Hôpital Bretonneau, Service des Exploration Functionnelles, 7 bis rue Carpeaux, 75018 Paris, France* (p. 789)

Baer, S., *Dept. of Obstetrics and Gynaecology, University Hospital, CH 8091 Zurich, Switzerland* (p. 747)

Bain, A. D., *Dept. of Child Life and Health, University of Edinburgh, Royal Infirmary, Edinburgh, UK* (p. 93)

Ballard, F. J., *Div. of Human Nutrition CSIRO, Kintore Av., Adelaide, S.A., Australia 5000* (p. 27)

Ballard, P. L., *C.V.R.I., University of California San Francisco, San Francisco, CA 94143, USA* (p. 229)

Bamford, O. S., *The Nuffield Institute for Medical Research, University of Oxford, Headley Way, Oxford OX3 9DS, UK* (pp. 439,605,653)

Barberis, C., *University of Southern California School of Medicine, Los Angeles, USA* (p. 211)

Bassett, J. M., *The Nuffield Institute for Medical Research, Oxford University, Headley Way, Oxford OX3 9DS, UK* (p. 71,123)

Batenburg, J. J., *Laboratory of Veterinary Biochemistry, State University of Utrecht, PO Box 80177, 3508 TD Utrecht, The Netherlands* (p 191)

Bell, R. J., *Department of Physiology, University of Melbourne, Parkville, Victoria, Australia 3052* (p. 537)

Berger, P. J., *Monash University Centre for Early Human Development, Queen Victoria Medical Centre, Lonsdale St., Melbourne 3000, Australia* (p. 287)

Bernal, A. L., *The Nuffield Department of Obstetrics & Gynaecology, John Radcliffe Hospital, Headley Way, Oxford, UK* (p. 489)

Bhutani, V. K., *Newborn Paediatrics, Pennsylvania Hospital, Eighth & Spruce Sts., Philadelphia, P.A. 19107, USA* (p. 337)

Birnholz, J. C., *Rush Presbyterian Hospital, 1753 West Congress Parkway, Chicago, USA* (p. 617)

Blanc, W. A., *Department of Pathology, College of Physicians & Surgeons, Columbia University, 630 West 168th St, New York, NY 10032, USA* (p. 293)

Blanco, C., *Department of Paediatrics, University of Maastricht, St. Annadal Zuikenhuis, St. Annadal 1, Maastricht, Netherlands* (pp. 595,639)

Bloom, S. R., *Hammersmith Hospital, London W12 0HS, UK* (pp. 417,771,811)

Bocking, A. D., *Dept. of Physiology, Monash University, Clayton, Melbourne, Victoria, Australia* (p. 247)

Boer, G. J., *Netherlands Institute for Brain Research, Z. IJdijk 28, 1095 KN Amsterdam, The Netherlands* (p. 89)

Bossina, K. K., *Dept. of Pediatric Cardiology & Obstetrics, University Hospital, Groningen, The Netherlands* (p. 749)

Boyd, R. D. H., *Department of Child Health, University of Manchester, Manchester, UK* (p. 519)

Brace, R. A., *Division of Perinatal Biology, Loma Linda University, Loma Linda, California 92350, USA* (p. 545)

Brigham, K. L., *Dept. of Pediatrics and Medicine, Vanderbilt University School of Medicine, Nashville, Tennessee, USA* (p. 331)

Britton, H. G., *Department of Physiology, St. Mary's Hospital Medical School, London W2 1PG, UK* (p. 479)

Brodecky, V., *Monash University Centre for Early Human Development, Queen Victoria Medical Centre, Melbourne, Australia* (p. 287)

Broughton-Pipkin, F., *Department of Obstetrics & Gynaecology, University Hospital, QMC, Nottingham, NG7 2UH, UK* (p. 699)

Brown, M. J., *Royal Post Graduate Medical School, Hammersmith Hospital, London, UK* (p. 811)

Bryan, C. A., *Respiratory Physiology, Hospital for Sick Children, 555 University Ave., Toronto, Canada* (p. 733)

Bryan, M. H., *Respiratory Physiology, Hospital for Sick Children, Toronto, Ontario, Canada* (p. 733)

Buckley, B., *Div. of Pediatric Cardiology, Schneider Children's Hospital, New Hyde Park, NY 11042, USA* (p. 599)

Burks, A. H., *Nuffield Institute for Medical Research, Headley Way, Headington, Oxford OX3 9DS, UK* (p. 71)

Buster, J. E., *Harbor UCLA, Medical Centre, 100 West Carson Street, Torrance, California 90509, USA* (p. 429)

Butler, J. H., *Developmental Physiology Laboratory, Dept. of Paediatrics, University of Auckland, Auckland, New Zealand* (p. 21)

Cabal, L. A., *University of Southern California School of Medicine, Los Angeles, USA* (p. 211)

Caces, R., *Dept. of Pediatrics, University of Manitoba, Winnipeg, Manitoba, USA* (p. 643)

Campbell, D., *University of California, San Francisco, CA 94143, USA* (p. 467)

Cannata, J. P., *Monash University for Early Human Development, Queen Victoria Medical Centre, Melbourne, Australia* (p. 395)

Caple, I., *Department of Animal Physiology & Nutrition, University of Leeds, Leeds LS2 9JT, UK* (p. 135)

Care, A. D., *Dept. of Animal Physiology and Nutrition, University of Leeds, Leeds LS2 9JT, UK* (p. 135)

Carter, A. M., *Department of Physiology, University of Odense, Campusvej 55, DK-5230 Odense M, Denmark* (p. 47)

Cassin, S., *Department of Physiology, College of Medicine, University of Florida, Gainesville, FLA 32610, USA* (pp. 253,299)

Castle, B. M., *Nuffield Department of Obstetrics and Gynaecology, John Radcliffe Hospital, Headington, Oxford OX3 9DU, UK* (p. 499)

Caudell, T., *Hôpital Bretonneau-Bichat, INSERM U 120, Paris, France* (p. 789)

Challis, J. R. G., *Research Institute, St. Joseph's Hospital, 268 Grosvenor St., London, Ontario, Canada* (pp. 241,363,493)

Chard, T., *St. Bartholomew's Hospital Medical School, 51–53 Bartholomew Close, London EC1, UK* (p. 691)

Charles, R., *Dept. of Anatomy & Embryology, University of Amsterdam, Meibergdreef 15, 1105 AZ Amsterdam, The Netherlands* (p. 41)

Chase, M. H., *Department of Physiology, UCLA School of Medicine, Center for Health Sciences, Los Angeles, CA 90024, USA* (p.581)

Cheek, D. B., *Dept. of Obstetrics and Gynaecology, University of Adelaide, South Australia, Australia* (p. 541)

Chernick, V., *Perinatal Physiology, Dept. of Pediatrics, University of Manitoba, Winnipeg, Manitoba, Canada* (p. 663)

Chrousos, G. P., *Dept. of Obstetrics & Gynecology, George Washington University, DC, USA* (p. 141)

Ciccimarra, F., *Viale Raffaello 24, 80129 Naples, Italy* (p. 807)

Cleave, J. P., *Dept. of Mathematics, Child Health & Physiology, University of Bristol, Bristol, UK* (p. 265)

Clyman, R., *1403 HSE — University of California San Francisco, San Francisco, CA 94143, USA* (p. 467)

Cohen, H. L., *Jewish Hillside Medical Center, New Hyde Park, New York, NY 11042, USA* (p. 223)

Collins, M. H., *College of Physicians & Surgeons, Columbia University, New York, NY 10032, USA* (p. 293)

Comline, R. S., *The Physiological Laboratory, Downing St., Cambridge CB2 3EG, UK* (p. 417)

Cook, M. J., *Dept. of Perinatal Physiology, Oregon Regional Primate Research Center, Beaverton, Oregon 97006, USA* (p. 423)

Cotton, W., *Dept. of Clincal Biochem., Central Pathology Lab., North Staffordshire Hospital Centre, Hartshill Rd., Hartshill, Stoke on Trent, UK* (p. 93)

Crequat, J., *Hôpital Bretonneau-Bichat, INSERM U 120, Paris, France* (p. 789)

Cuezva, J. M., *Dept. Bioquimica, Faculty Ciencias, U.A.M. Cantoblanco, Madrid-34, Spain* (p. 63)

Curzi-Dascalova, L., *Inserm U 29, Hôpital Port Royal, 123, Blvd. de Port Royal, 75014 Paris, France* (pp. 273,817)

Dalton, J. K., *Department of Obstetrics & Gynaecology, University of Cambridge, Cambridge CB2 2SW, UK* (p. 753)

Daniel, S. S., *Columbia University, 630 W 168th Street, New York, NY 10032, USA* (pp. 165,293,533)

Davidson, I. A., *Dept. of Obstetrics and Gynaecology, University of Aberdeen, UK* (p. 659)

Davis, B. A., *Dept. of Clincal Biochemistry, North Staffordshire Hospital Centre, Hartshill Rd., Hartshill, Stoke on Trent ST4 7P, UK* (p. 93)

Dawes, G. S., *The Nuffield Institute for Medical Research, Oxford, UK* (pp. 439,499, 595,605,633,695,821)

Dawson, A. J., *Dept. of Obstetrics and Gynaecology, Welsh National School of Medicine, Cardiff CF4 4XN, UK* (p. 752)

De Curtis, M., *Patologia Neonatale e Clinica Pediatrica, 2nd School of Medicine, University of Naples, Naples, Italy* (p. 807)

De Graaf, A., *Department of Anatomy and Embryology, University of Amsterdam, Meibergdreef 15, 1105 AZ Amsterdam, The Netherlands* (p. 41)

DeSmedt, M. C. H., *Department of Pediatrics, University Hospital, 59 Oostersinel, Groningen, The Netherlands* (p. 749)

DeVries, A. C. J., *Laboratory of Veterinary Biochemistry, State University of Utrecht, PO Box 80177, 3508 TD Utrecht, The Netherlands* (p. 191)

DiRusso, S. M., *Dept. of Physiology, Downstate Medical Center, State University of New York, Brooklyn, NY 11203, USA* (p. 445)

Ducsay, C. A., *505 N.W. 185th Avenue, Beaverton, Oregon, USA* (p. 423)

Durand, M., *Los Angeles County USC—Medical Center, Women's Hospital, 1240 North Mission Rd., Los Angeles, California 90033, USA* (p. 211)

Dutton, A., *Nuffield Institute for Medical Research, Headley, Way, Headington, Oxford OX3 9DS, UK* (p. 557)

Eberle, L. P., *Jewish Hillside Medical Center, New Hyde Park, New York, NY 11042, USA* (p. 223)

Edwards, D. A., *Dept. of Physiology, University of Sydney, Sydney, NSW, Australia* (p. 627)

Eitan, G. D., *Dept. of Biology, Technion-Israel Institute of Technology, Haifa, Israel* (p. 311)

El Badry, A., *State University of New York, Upstate Medical Center, Syracuse, New York 14853, USA* (p. 355)

Engelhardt, B., *Dept. of Pediatrics and Medicine, Vanderbilt School of Medicine, Nashville, TN 37232, USA* (p. 331)

Engelke, S., *Dept. of Pediatrics, East Carolina University School of Medicine, Greenville, NC 27834, USA* (p. 777)

England, S., *Respiratory Physiology, Hospital for Sick Children, Toronto, Ontario, Canada* (p. 733)

Evans, M. I., *Department of Obstetrics & Gynaecology, Hutzel Hospital, 4707 St. Antoine, Detroit, MI 48201, USA* (p. 141)

Faber, J. J., *Department of Physiology L334, Oregon Health Sciences University, Portland, Oregon 97201, USA* (p. 371)

Falconer, J., *Faculty of Medicine, University of Newcastle, Shortland, NSW 12308, Australia* (pp. 33,51)

Fallenstein, F., *Dept. of Obstetrics and Gynaecology, University Hospital, CH 8091 Zurich, Switzerland* (p. 747)

Farrell, E., *Rush Presbyterian Medical Center, 1753 West Congress Parkway, Chicago, USA* (p. 617)

Farrow, S. M., *Nuffield Department of Obstetrics & Gynaecology, John Radcliffe Hospital, Oxford, UK* (p. 77)

Fatone, M., *Department of Obstetrics and Gynecology, University of Parma, Parma, Italy* (p. 561)

Faulder, C. G., *Dept. of Clinical Biochem., Central Pathology Lab., North Staffordshire Hospital Centre, Hartshill Rd., Hartshill, Stoke on Trent, UK* (p. 93)

Fewell, J. E., *University of Arkansas for Medical Sciences, 4301 W. Markham, Department of Pediatrics, Little Rock, AR 72205, USA* (pp. 217, 293)

Figueroa, J. P., *NYS College of Veterinary Medicine, Cornell University, Ithaca, NY 14853, USA* (pp. 145,355,551)

Fisher, J., *Respiratory Physiology, Hospital for Sick Children, Toronto, Ontario, Canada* (p. 733)

Fleming, P. J., *Department of Child Health, Southmead Hospital, Bristol, UK* (p. 265)

Flohr, E., *Dept. of Clinical Chemistry, Carmel Hospital, Michal St., Haifa 34362, Israel* (p. 311)

Fontwit, K., *Reproductive Studies, State University of New York, College of Veterinary Medicine, Cornell University, Ithaca, NY 14853, USA* (p. 505)

Ford, F. A., *Department of Obstetrics and Gynaecology, University of Sheffield, Jessop Hospital for Women, Sheffield S3 7RE, UK* (p. 761)

Fore, I. M., *Nuffield Institute for Medical Research, Headley Way, Headington, Oxford OX3 9DS, UK* (p. 557)

Fowden, A., *Physiological Laboratory, Downing St., Cambridge, CB2 3EG, UK* (pp. 157,417)

Francis, G. L., *Div. of Human Nutrition, CSIRO, Kintore Ave., Adelaide, S.A., Australia 5000* (p. 27)

Frank, D. A., *NYS College of Veterinary Medicine, Cornell University, Ithaca, NY 14853, USA* (p. 355)

Fraser, M., *Developmental Physiological Laboratory, University of Auckland, Auckland, New Zealand* (p. 163)

Fraser, R. B., *University Department of Obstetrics & Gynaecology, Jessop Hospital for Women, Sheffield S3 7RE, UK* (p. 761)

Fredholm, B. B., *Nobel Institute for Neurophysiology & Dept. of Pharmacology, Karolinska Hospital, Box 60400, S-104 01 Stockholm, Sweden* (p. 767)

Garfield, R. E., *Dept. of Neurosciences, Obstetrics & Gynecology, McMaster University, Hamilton, Ontario, Canada* (pp. 411,473)

Georgie, S., *University of Southern California School of Medicine, Los Angeles, USA* (p. 211)

Gilfillan, C. A., *Dept. of Pediatrics, Case Western Reserve University School of Medicine, Cleveland Metropolitan General Hospital, Cleveland, Ohio, USA* (p. 739)

Glazier, J. D., *Dept. of Paediatrics, University of Manchester at St. Mary's Hospital, Manchester M13 0JH, UK* (p. 519)

Gluckman, P. D., *Department of Paediatrics, University of Auckland, Private Bag, Auckland, New Zealand* (pp. 21,103,145,163,551,621)

Gonzales, L. K., *Department of Pediatrics, University of California, San Francisco, CA 94143, USA* (p. 229)

Gonzalez, F., *University of Southern California School of Medicine, Los Angeles, USA* (p. 211)

Gootman, N., *Department of Paediatrics, Division of Pediatric Cardiology, Schneider's Children Hospital, New Hyde Park, NY 11042, USA* (p. 599)

Gootman, P. M., *State University of New York, Downstate Medical Center, Department of Physiology, Box 31, 450 Clarkson Ave., Brooklyn, NY 11203, USA* (pp. 223,445,599)

Greenough, A., *Department of Paediatrics, Level E3, New Addenbrooke's Hospital, Cambridge, UK* (pp. 259, 263)

Grogaard, J., *Department of Pediatrics, Central Hospital Karlstad, S-65185 Karlstad, Sweden* (pp. 283,331)

Gronlund, J., *Dept. of Physiology, University of Odense, Odense, Denmark* (p. 47)

Gruener, N., *Dept. of Clinical Chemistry, Carmel Hospital, Michal St., Haifa 34362, Israel* (p. 311)

Gu, W., *Nuffield Department of Obstetrics & Gynaecology, John Radcliffe Hospital, Oxford, UK* (pp. 11,59)

Gunn, T. R., *St. Helen's Hospital, Linwood Ave., Auckland, New Zealand* (p. 163)

Hall, K., *Dept. of Endocrinology, Karolinska Institute, Stockholm, Sweden* (p. 97)

Hanson, M. A., *Department of Physiology & Biochemistry, University of Reading, Whiteknights, Reading RG6 2AJ, UK* (pp. 277,595,639)

Harding, J. E., *Department of Paediatrics, University of Auckland Medical School, Auckland, New Zealand* (p. 11)

Harding, P. G. R., *Department of Obstetrics & Gynaecology, St. Joseph's Hospital, London, Ontario, Canada N6A 4V2* (pp. 235,241,325)

Harding, R., *Department of Physiology, Monash University, Melbourne, Australia 3168* (p. 247)

Harper, M. J. K., *Dept. of Obstetrics & Gynecology, University of Texas, San Antonio, Texas, USA* (p. 411)

Harper, R. A., *Department of Physiology, UCLA School of Medicine, Center for Health Sciences, Los Angeles, CA 90024, USA* (p. 571)

Harris, T. R., *Dept. of Pediatrics and Medicine, Vanderbilt University School of Medicine, Nashville, Tennessee, USA* (p. 331)

Haslam, R. R., *Queen Victoria Hospital, Fullarton Road, Rose Park, South Australia 5067, Australia* (p. 541)

Hayashi, R. H., *UCLA-Harbor General Hospital, Department of Obstetrics & Gynecology, 1000 West Carson St., Los Angeles, California, USA* (p. 411)

Henderson-Smart, D. J., *Perinatal Medicine, King George V Hospital, Camperdown, Sydney, NSW 2062, Australia* (p. 627)

Heyman, M. A., *1403 HSE, University of California, San Francisco, CA 94143, USA* (pp. 401,451,467,721)

Hobel, C. J., *Department of Obstetrics and Gynecology, University of California, Los Angeles, California, USA* (p. 757)

Hodgman, J. E., *University of Southern California School of Medicine, Los Angeles, USA* (p. 211)

Hofmeyr, G. J., *The Nuffield Institute for Medical Research, Oxford University, Oxford OX3 9DS, UK* (pp. 439,605,653)

Hohimer, A. R., *Obstetric Research, L 458, Oregon Health Sciences University, Portland, Oregon 97201, USA* (p. 711)

Hohmann, M., *Dept. of Obstetrics and Gynecology, University of Giessen, Giessen, West Germany* (p. 405)

Hokegard, K.-H., *Dept. of Obstetrics and Gynecology, University of Goteborg, Goteborg, Sweden* (p. 461)

Hoppenbrouwers, T., *University of Southern California School of Medicine, Los Angeles, USA* (p. 211)

Horne, R., *Monash University Centre for Early Human Development, Queen Victoria Medical Centre, Melbourne, Victoria, Australia* (p. 287)

Howlett, T., *Dept. of Chemical Endocrinology, St. Bartholomew's Hospital Medical College, London, UK* (p. 653)

Huch, A., *Dept. of Obstetrics and Gynecology, University Hospital CH 8091, Zurich, Switzerland* (p. 747)

Huch, R., *Dept. of Obstetrics and Gynaecology, University Hospital, CH 8091 Zurich, Switzerland* (p. 747)

Huisjes, H. J., *Dept. of Pediatric Cardiology & Obstetrics, University Hospital, Groningen, The Netherlands* (p. 749)

Hume, R., *Dept. of Child Life and Health, University of Edinburgh, Royal Infirmary, Edinburgh, UK* (p. 93)

Humphreys, J., *Nuffield Department of Obstetrics and Gynaecology, John Radcliffe Hospital, Headington, Oxford OX3 9DU, UK* (p. 489)

Hunt, A. N., *Child Health, Faculty of Medicine, Southampton General Hospital, Southampton, UK* (p. 305)

Ioffe, S., *Department of Paediatrics, Children's Hospital, 678 William Ave., Winnipeg, Manitoba, Canada RE3 OW1* (p. 663)

Iwamoto, H. S., *1403-HSE, University of California, San Francisco, California 94143, USA* (p. 37)

Jager, W., *Dept. of Pediatric Cardiology & Obstetrics, University Hospital, Groningen, The Netherlands* (p. 749)

James, D. K., *Southmead Hospital, Westbury on Trym, Bristol, UK* (p. 315)

James, L. S., *Babies Hospital, Box No. 34, 3959 Broadway, New York, NY 10032, USA* (pp. 165,293,533)

Jansen, A. H., *Perinatal Physiology Laboratory, Dept. of Pediatrics, University of Manitoba, Winnipeg, Manitoba, Canada* (p. 663)

Jenkin, G., *Department of Physiology, Monash University, Clayton, Victoria 3168, Australia* (p. 429)

Jenkins, P. A., *Dept. of Paediatrics, John Radcliffe Hospital, Headley Way, Headington, Oxford OX3 9DU, UK* (p. 771)

Jensen, A., *The Nuffield Institute for Medical Research, University of Oxford, Oxford OX3 9DS, UK* (pp. 405,605)

Johnson, P., *The Nuffield Department of Obstetrics & Gynaecology, John Radcliffe Hospital, Oxford, UK* (pp. 201,259,783,795)

Johnston, B. M., *Department of Paediatrics, University of Auckland, Auckland, New Zealand* (pp. 163, 620)

Jones, C. T., *The Nuffield Institute for Medical Research, Oxford University, Headley Way, Oxford OX3 9DS, UK* (pp. 11,59,77,97,106,151,173)

Jorgensen, G., *Dept. of Physiology, Monash University, Clayton, Melbourne, Victoria 3168, Australia* (p. 429)

Joubert, S. M., *Depts. of Chemical Pathology, Obstetrics & Gynecology, MRC Unit for Preclinical Diagnostic Research, University of Natal, Durban, South Africa* (p. 483)

Kalhan, S. C., *Cleveland Metropolitan General Hospital, 3395 Scranton Rd., Cleveland, OH 44109, USA* (p. 739)

Kaufmann, R. C., *Div. of Maternal/Fetal Medicine, Dept. of Obstetrics & Gynecology, Southern Illinois University School of Medicine, Springfield, Illinois, USA* (p. 611)

Kjellmer, I., *Dept. of Pediatrics, Children's Hospital, Ostra sjukhuset, 41685 Goteborg, Sweden* (p. 461)

Kleinerman, J., *Dept. of Pediatrics, Physiology and Pathology, College of Physicians and Surgeons, Columbia University, New York, NY, USA* (p. 293)

Klopper, A., *Dept. of Obstetrics and Gynaecology, University of Aberdeen, Royal Infirmary, Aberdeen, AB9 2ZB, UK*   (p. 83)

Knox, J., *Physiological Laboratory, Cambridge, UK*   (p. 417)

Kopelman, A. E., *Department of Neonatology, School of Medicine, East Carolina University, Grenville, NC 27834, USA*   (p. 777)

Korn, G., *Hôpital de Port Royal, 123 Bld. de Port Royal, 75014 Paris, France* (p. 273)

Kramer, D., *The Research Institute, St. Joseph's Hospital, University of Western Ontario, London, Ontario, Canada*   (p. 493)

Kunzel, W., *Universitats-Frauenklinik Giessen, Klinikstrasse 28, D-6300 Giessen, West Germany*   (p. 405)

Labarrere, C., *Department of Pathology, Gascon 450 (1181) Hospital Italiana, Buenos Aires, Argentina*   (p. 801)

Lafeber, H. N., *Department of Paediatrics, Sophia Children's Hospital, Rotterdam, The Netherlands*   (pp. 11,97)

Lagercrantz, H., *Department of Pediatrics, Karolinska Hospital, S-104 01 Stockholm, Sweden*   (p. 767)

Lamers, W. H., *Department of Anatomy & Embryology, University of Amsterdam, AMC, Meibergdreef, Amsterdam, The Netherlands*   (p. 41)

Lancu, T. C., *Departments of Paediatrics and Neonatal Intensive Care, Carmel Hospital, Michal St., Haifa 34362, Israel*   (p. 311)

Larsen, J. W., *Dept. of Obstetrics & Gynecology, George Washington University, DC, USA*   (p. 141)

Lawrence, G. F., *Dept. of Obstetrics and Gynaecology, University of Sheffield, Jessop Hospital for Women, Sheffield S3 7RE, UK*   (p. 761)

LeBlanc, R., *Department of Obstetrics & Gynaecology, University of Dusseldorf, D-4000 Dusseldorf, West Germany*   (p. 433)

Lee, D., *Dept. of Pediatrics, University of Manitoba, Winnipeg, Manitoba, USA*   (p. 643)

Levine, M. R., *Depts. of Mathematics, Child Health and Physiology, University of Bristol, Bristol, UK*   (p. 265)

Liggins, G. C., *Postgraduate School of Obstetrics & Gynaecology, National Women's Hospital, Claude Rd., Auckland, New Zealand*   (p. 179)

Lilja, H., *Dept. of Obstetrics and Gynecology, University of Goteborg, Goteborg, Sweden*   (p. 461)

Llanos, A. J., *Cardiovascular Research Institute, Depts. of Pediatrics, Obstetrics and Gynecology, University of California, San Francisco, California 94143, USA*   (p. 401)

Long, A. M., *Depts. of Mathematics, Child Health and Physiology, University of Bristol, Bristol, UK*   (p. 265)

Longo, L. D., *Division of Perinatal Biology, Loma Linda University, Loma Linda, CA 92350, USA*   (p. 1)

Longstaff, A., *Dept. of Obstetrics & Gynaecology, University of Aberdeen, Aberdeen, Scotland*   (p. 659)

Louis, T. M., *Department of Anatomy, ECU School of Medicine, 7N-100 Brody Building, Greenville, NC 27834, USA*   (p. 777)

Lowy, C., *Unit of Endocrinology & Diabetes, St. Thomas's Hospital, London SE1, UK*

Lye, S., *Research Institute, St. Joseph's Hospital, 268 Grosvenor St., London, Ontario, Canada N6A 4V2*   (pp. 241,363)

MacDonald, A. A., *Department of Anatomy, School of Veterinary Studies, Edinburgh EH19 1QH, UK*   (p. 401)

Mackenzie, I. Z., *Dept. of Obstetrics & Gynaecology, John Radcliffe Hospital, Headley Way, Headington, Oxford OX3 9DU, UK*   (p. 771)

MacKenzie, L. W., *Department of Neurosciences, McMaster University, Health Sciences Center, 1200 Main St. W., Hamilton, Ontario, Canada L8N 3Z5* (p. 473)

MacLennan, A. H., *Dept. of Obstetrics and Gynaecology, University of Adelaide, South Australia, Australia* (p. 541)

Maloney, J. E., *Department of Obstetrics & Gynaecology, University of Calgary, Health Sciences Center, 3330 Hospital Drive N.W., Calgary, Alberta, Canada* (pp. 287,395)

Marivate, M., *Dept. of Chemical Pathology and Obstetrics and Gynecology, MRC Unit for Preclinical Research, University of Natal, Durban, South Africa* (p. 483)

Markiewicz, A., *Department of Anatomy and Embryology, University of Amsterdam, Meibergdreef 15, 1105 AZ Amsterdam, The Netherlands* (p. 41)

Mauray, F., *University of California, San Francisco, CA 94143, USA* (p. 467)

McCooke, H. B., *Department of Physiology & Biochemistry, University of Reading, Whiteknights, Reading RG6 2AJ, UK* (pp. 277,595,639)

McDonald, T. J., *NYS College of Veterinary Medicine, Cornell University, Ithaca, NY 14853, USA* (pp. 145,551)

Medina, J. M., *Departmento de Bioquimica, Facultad de Farmacia, Universidad de Salamanca, Salamanca, Spain* (p. 63)

Meijboom, E. J., *Department of Pediatric Cardiology, University Hospital, Oostersingel 59, Groningen, The Netherlands* (p. 749)

Merialdi, A., *University Degli Studi Di Parma, Istituto di Clinica Obstetriece Ginecologica, Parma, Italy* (p. 561)

Metcalf, J., *Oregon Health Sciences University, 3181 S.W. Sam Jackson Park Rd., Portland, Oregon 97201, USA* (p. 711)

Mitchell, B. F., *Research Institute, St. Joseph's Hospital, 268 Grosvenor Rd., London, Ontario, Canada* (p. 363)

Mitchell, M. D., *Division of Biological Sciences, University of California, 225 Dickinson St., San Diego, CA 92103, USA* (p. 355,505)

Moessinger, A. C., *Babies Hospital, Box 34, 3975 Bivay, New York, NY 10032, USA* (p. 293)

Mohan, P., *Dept. of Pediatrics and Medicine, Vanderbilt University School of Medicine, Nashville, Tennessee, USA* (p. 331)

Moore, M., *Dept. of Pediatrics, University of Manitoba, Winnipeg, Manitoba, USA* (p. 643)

Mooren, P. G., *Dept. of Anatomy and Embryology, University of Amsterdam, Meibergdreef 15, 1105 AZ Amsterdam, The Netherlands* (p. 41)

Morgenstern, J., *Department of Obstetrics & Gynaecology, University of Dusseldorf, Moorenstrasse 5, D-4000 Dusseldorf, West Germany* (p. 433)

Mori, T., *Dept. of Gynecology & Obstetrics, Kyoto University, Faculty of Medicine, 54 Shogoin Kawaharacho Sakyoku, Kyoto, Japan* (p. 319)

Morley, C. J., *Dept. of Paediatrics, University of Cambridge, Cambridge, UK* (pp. 259,263)

Morton, M. J., *Dept. of Physiology and Medicine, School of Medicine, Oregon Health Sciences, University, Portland, Oregon 97201, USA* (pp. 371,711)

Mott, J. C., *The Nuffield Institute for Medical Research, Oxford University, Headley Way, Oxford OX3 9DS, UK* (pp. 113,557)

Muneshige, A., *Dept. of Gynecology and Obstetrics, Kyoto University, Faculty of Medicine, 54 Shogoin Kawaharacho Sakyoku, Kyoto, Japan* (p. 319)

Nakamura, K. T., *Dept. of Pediatrics & the Cardiovascular Research Center, University of Iowa, Iowa City, Iowa 52242, USA* (p. 527)

Nathanielsz, P. W., *NYS College of Veterinary Medicine, Cornell University, Ithaca, NY 14853, USA* (pp. 145,355,429,505,551)

Newcombe, R. G., *Dept. of Medical Computing Statistics, Welsh National School of Medicine, Cardiff CF4 4XN, UK* (p. 753)

Newman, C. B., *College of Physicians & Surgeons, Columbia University, 630 West 168th St, New York, NY 10032, USA* (p. 165)

Nisula, B. C., *Dept. of Obstetrics & Gynecology, Wayne State University, Detroit, Michigan, USA* (p. 141)

Norman, L., *Dept. of Obstetrics & Gynecology, St. Joseph's Hospital, University of Western Ontario, London, Ontario, Canada* (p. 363)

Norman, R. J., *Department of Reproductive Physiology, St. Bartholomew's Hospital, West Smithfield, London, UK* (pp. 483,691)

Normand, I. C. S., *Department of Child Health, Southampton General Hospital, Southampton SO9 4XY, UK* (p. 305)

Novy, M. J., *Dept. of Obstetrics and Gynecology, Oregon Health Sciences University, Portland, Oregon 97201, USA* (p. 423)

Oh, W., *Dept. of Pediatrics, Brown University, Providence, Rhode Island, USA* (p. 37)

Okazaki, T., *Department of Obstetrics & Gynecology, Faculty of Medicine, Kyoto University, 54-Kawahara-cho, Shogo-in, Sakyo-ku, Kyoto 606, Japan* (p. 319)

Olsen, G. D., *Department of Pharmacology, School of Medicine, Oregon Health Sciences University, Portland, OR 97201, USA* (p. 633)

Olson, D. M., *The Research Institute, St. Joseph's Hospital, London, Ontario, Canada, N6A 4V2* (pp. 363,493)

Oosterbaan, H. P., *Groot Ziekengasthuis, Department of Obstetrics & Gynecology, Nieuwstraat 34, 5211 NL's Hertogenbosch, The Netherlands* (p. 89)

Opavsky, A., *The Research Institute, St. Joseph's Hospital, University of Western Ontario, London, Ontario, Canada* (p. 493)

Ousey, J. C., *Beaufort Cottage Stables, High St., Newmarket, Suffolk CB8 8JS, UK* (p. 457)

Owens, J. A., *Room 510, Medical Sciences Building, University of Newcastle, Shortland, 2308 NSW, Australia* (pp. 33,51)

Paludetto, R., *Patologia Neonatale e Clinica Pediatrica, 2nd School of Medicine, University of Naples, Naples, Italy* (p. 807)

Parer, J. T., *Department of Obstetrics & Gynecology, HSE 1462, University of California, San Francisco, CA 94143, USA* (pp. 11,59,97)

Parkes, M. J., *The Nuffield Institute for Medical Research, Oxford University, Oxford OX3 9DS, UK* (pp. 55,439,605,653)

Parks, C. M., *Dept. of Physiology and Medicine, School of Medicine, Oregon Health Sciences University, Portland, Oregon 97201, USA* (p. 371)

Parsons, Y., *Developmental Physiology Laboratory, Dept. of Paediatrics, University of Auckland, Auckland, New Zealand* (pp. 145,621)

Patrick, J., *Department of Obstetrics & Gynaecology, St. Joseph's Hospital, London, Ontario, Canada N6A 4V2* (p. 669)

Pearson, C. K., *Dept. of Obstetrics and Gynaecology & Biochemistry, University of Aberdeen, Aberdeen, UK* (p. 659)

Peiran, P., *INSERM U-29, Hôpital Port Royal, Paris, France* (p. 817)

Perks, A. M., *Department of Zoology, University of British Columbia, Vancouver, BC., Canada V6T 2A9* (p. 253)

Pesonen, E., *Cardiovascular Research Inst., Depts. of Pediatrics, Obstetrics & Gynecology, University of San Francisco, California 94143, USA* (p. 401)

Pettigrew, A. G., *Dept. of Perinatal Medicine, King George V Memorial Hospital, Missenden Rd., Camperdown, NSW 2050, Australia* (p. 627)

Pickard, D. W., *Dept. of Animal Physiology and Nutrition, University of Leeds, Leeds LS2 9JT, UK* (p. 135)

Pierce, P., *Dept. of Physiology, Downstate Medical Center, State University of New York, Brooklyn, NY 11203, USA* (p. 445)

Pimentel, G., *NYS College of Veterinary Medicine, Cornell University, Ithaca, NY 14853, USA* (p. 355)

Pinches, R. A., *Nuffield Institute for Medical Research, Headley Way, Headington, Oxford OX3 9DS, UK* (p. 71)

Pinson, C. W., *Dept. of Physiology and Medicine, School of Medicine, Oregon Health Sciences University, Portland, Oregon 97201, USA* (p. 371)

Poore, E. R., *NYS College of Veterinary Medicine, Cornell University, Ithaca, NY 14853, USA* (pp. 355,505)

Possmeyer, F., *Department of Obstetrics & Gynecology, University of Western Ontario, London, Ontario, Canada N6A 5A5* (pp. 234,241,325)

Post, M., *Dept. of Pediatrics, Harvard Medical School, 75 Francis St., Boston, MA 02115, USA* (p. 191)

Postle, A. D., *Department of Child Health, Southampton General Hospital, Southampton, UK* (p. 305)

Power, S. G. A., *The Research Institute, St. Joseph's Hospital, 268 Grosvenor St., London, Ontario, Canada N6A 4V2* (p. 363)

Price, D. A., *Dept. of Child Health, University of Manchester, Manchester, UK* (p. 97)

Pucklavec, M., *William Dunn School of Pathology, South Parks Rd., Oxford, UK* (p. 151)

Ravina, J. H., *University of Arizona, Health Services Center, Tucson, Arizona, USA* (p. 789)

Read, L. C., *CSIRO, Division of Human Nutrition, Kintore Ave., Adelaide, S.A., Australia 5000* (p. 27)

Reimers, T., *Reproductive Studies, State University of New York, College of Veterinary Medicine, Cornell University, Ithaca, NY 14853, USA* (p. 551)

Richardson, B. S., *St. Joseph's Hospital, London, Ontario, Canada N6A 4V2* (p. 669)

Rigatto, H., *Room WS 108, Women's Hospital, 700 William Ave., Winnipeg, Manitoba, Canada R3E 0Z3* (p. 643)

Ritchie, B. C., *Monash University Centre for Early Human Development Queen Victoria Medical Centre, Melbourne, Australia* (p. 395)

Ritchie, J. W. K., *Department of Midwifery & Gynaecology, Institute of Clinical Science, Grosvenor Rd., Belfast, UK* (p. 151)

Robillard, J. E., *Department of Pediatrics, University of Iowa, Iowa City, Iowa 522420, USA* (p. 527)

Robinson, J. S., *Faculty of Medicine, University of Newcastle, Newcastle Hospital, Waratah 2298, Australia* (pp. 33,51,683)

Rodbard, D., *NIH, Bethesda, Maryland, USA* (p. 141)

Roebuck, M. M., *Nuffield Department of Obstetrics & Gynaecology, John Radcliffe Hospital, Oxford, UK* (p. 499)

Rojas, J., *Department of Pediatrics and Medicine, Vanderbilt University School of Medicine, Nashville, Tennessee, USA* (p. 331)

Rolfe, P., *The Bio-engineering Unit, Department of Paediatrics, John Radcliffe Hospital, Oxford, UK* (p. 795)

Rolph, T. P., *Glaxo Animal Health Laboratories, Brakespear Rd South, Harefield, Middx, UK* (p. 11)

Roman, C., *University of California, San Francisco, CA 94143, USA* (p. 451)

Romano, G., *Patologia Neonatale e Clinica Pediatrics, 2nd School of Medicine, University of Naples, Naples, Italy* (p. 807)

Rose, J. C., *Dept. of Physiology & Pharmacology, Bowman Gray School of Medicine, Wake Forest University, Winston Salem, NC 27103, USA* (p. 145)

Rosen, K. G., *Department of Pediatrics, Ostra Sjukhuset, S-41685 Goteborg, Sweden* (p. 461)
Rossdale, P. D., *Beaufort Cottage Stables, High St., Newmarket, Suffolk CB8 8JS, UK* (p. 457)
Rudolph, A. M., *1403-HSE, University of California, San Francisco, CA 94143, USA* (pp. 37,343,401)
Runold, M., *Nobel Institute for Neurophysiology & Dept. of Pharmacology, Karolinska Hospital, Box 60400, S-104 01 Stockholm, Sweden* (p. 767)
Sagawa, N., *Department of Obstetrics & Gynaecology, Faculty of Medicine, Kyoto University, 54-Kawahara-cho, Kyoto 606, Japan* (p. 319)
Saldanha, R., *Dept. of Epidemiology and Biostatistics, East Carolina University School of Medicine, Greenville, NC 27834, USA* (p. 777)
Salinas-Zeballos, M.-E., *Department of Physiology, State University of New York, Downstate Medical Center, Brooklyn, New York, USA* (p. 599)
Sara, V., *Dept. of Psychiatry, Karolinska Institute, Stockholm, Sweden* (p. 97)
Schellenberg, J.-C., *Postgraduate School of Obstetrics and Gynaecology, University of Auckland, Auckland, New Zealand* (p. 179)
Schreiber, M. D., *University of California, San Francisco, CA 94143, USA* (p. 451)
Schulman, J. D., *Dept. of Obstetrics & Gynecology, Wayne State University, Detroit, Michigan, USA* (p. 141)
Shafer, T. H., *Department of Physiology, Temple University School of Medicine, 3420 N. Broad St., Philadelphia, PA 19140, USA* (p. 337)
Sibley, C. P., *Dept. of Obstetrics and Gynaecology, University of Manchester at St. Mary's Hospital, Manchester M13 0JH, UK* (p. 519)
Siddiqi, J., *Dept. of Obstetrics & Gynecology, St. Joseph's Hospital, London, Ontario, Canada* (p. 363)
Sigger, J. N., *Dept. of Physiology, Monash University, Clayton, Melbourne, Victoria, Australia* (p. 247)
Silver, M., *Physiological Laboratory, Downing St., Cambridge CB2 3EG, UK* (pp. 157,417)
Singh, M., *Dept. of Pediatrics, Physiology and Pathology, College of Physicians and Surgeons, Columbia University, New York, NY 10032, USA* (p. 293)
Smeal, M. M., *College of Physicians & Surgeons, Columbia University, 630 West 168th St, New York, NY 10032, USA* (p. 165)
Smieja, Z., *The Research Institute, St. Joseph's Hospital, University of Western Ontario, London, Ontario, Canada* (p. 493)
Smith, B. T., *Dept. of Pediatrics, Harvard Medical School, 75 Francis St., Boston, MA 02115, USA* (p. 191)
Soifer, S. J., *650M, Department of Pediatrics, UCSF, San Francisco, CA 94143, USA* (p. 451)
Soltesz, G., *Dept. of Paediatrics, John Radcliffe Hospital, Headley Way, Headington, Oxford OX3 9DU, UK* (p. 771)
Somes, G., *Div. of Epidemiology and Biostatistics, East Carolina University School of Medicine, Greenville, NC 27834, USA* (p. 777)
Sorokin, Y., *Department of Obstetrics & Gynecology, Carmel Hospital, Michael St., Haifa 34362, Israel* (p. 311)
Spencer, J. A. D., *Nuffield Department of Obstetrics & Gynaecology, John Radcliffe Hospital, Oxford, UK* (pp. 783,795)
Sprague, C., *The Research Institute, St. Joseph's Hospital, University of Western Ontario, London, Ontario, Canada* (p. 363)
Stark, R. I., *College of Physicians & Surgeons, Columbia University, 630 W 168th St., NYC, NY 10032, USA* (pp. 165,293,533)

Staton, R. C., *Dept. of Obstetrics & Gynecology, George Washington University, Washington, DC, USA* (p. 141)

Steele, A. M., *Div. of Neonatology, Schneider Children's Hospital, Long Island, New York, USA* (p. 223)

Strange, R. C., *Department of Biochemistry, Central Path. Labs., North Staffs. Hospital, Hartshill Rd., Stoke-on-Trent, Staffs, UK* (p. 93)

Sundell, H., *Vanderbilt University, School of Medicine, Nashville, TN 37232, USA* (pp. 283,331)

Sunderji, S., *State University of New York, Upstate Medical Center, 750 East Adams St., Syracuse, NY, USA* (p. 355)

Swaab, D. F., *Netherlands Institute for Brain Research, Z. IJdijk 28, 1095 KN Amsterdam, The Netherlands, UK* (p. 89)

Szeto, H. H., *Department of Pharmacology, Cornell University Medical College, Ithaca, NY, USA* (p. 649)

TambyRaja, R. L., *University Department of Obstetrics & Gynaecology, Kandang Kerban Hospital, Singapore 0821* (p. 757)

Tan, C. B., *Department of Physiology & Biophysics, St. Mary's Hospital Medical School, London W2 1PG, UK* (p. 479)

Telenta, M., *Dept. of Pathology and Obstetrics, Gascon 450 (1181), Hospital Italiano, Buenos Aires, Argentina* (p. 801)

Thorburn, G. D., *Department of Physiology, Monash University, Clayton, Victoria, Australia 3168* (pp. 381,429)

Thornburg, K. L., *Oregon Health Sciences University, Portland, Oregon 97201, USA* (p. 371)

Tindell, D. J., *The Nuffield Department of Obstetrics & Gynaecology, John Radcliffe Hospital, Headley Way, Oxford, UK* (p. 173)

Tod, M. L., *Dept. of Physiology, College of Medicine, University of Florida, Gainesville, Fla. 32610, USA* (p. 299)

Toscani, G., *University of Arizona, Health Sciences Center, Tucson, Arizona, USA* (p. 789)

Troncone, R., *Patologia Neonatale e Clinica Pediatrica, 2nd School of Medicine, University of Naples, Naples, Italy* (p. 807)

Tropper, P. J., *College of Physicians & Surgeons, Div. of Perinatology, Columbia University, New York, NY, USA* (p. 533)

Turnbull, A. C., *Nuffield Department of Obstetrics and Gynaecology, John Radcliffe Hospital, Headington, Oxford OX3 9DU, UK* (pp. 489,499)

Umans, J. G., *Dept. of Pharmacology, Cornell University Medical School, New York, USA* (p. 649)

Valcarce, C., *Departmento de Bioquimica y Biologie Molecular, IUBM-CBM, Facultad de Ciencias, Universidad Autonoma Madrid, Cantoblanco, Madrid, Spain* (p. 63)

Valdes Cruz, L. M., *Nuffield Institute for Medical Research, Headley Way, Headington, Oxford OX3 9DS, UK* (p. 557)

Van den Abbeele, A., *Dept. of Pediatrics and Medicine, Vanderbilt University School of Medicine, Nashville, Tennessee, USA* (p. 331)

Van Golde, L. M. G., *Laboratory of Veterinary Biochemistry, P.O. Box 80177, 3508 TD Utrecht, The Netherlands* (p. 191)

Veille, J. C., *Dept. of Perinatal Physiology, Oregon Regional Primate Research Center, Beaverton, Oregon 90076, USA* (p. 423)

Vetter, K., *Universtaetsfrauenklinik Zurich, CH 8091 Zurich, Switzerland* (p. 747)

Vicente, G., *INSERM U-29, Hôpital de Port Royal, Paris, France* (p. 817)

Vilos, G. A., *St. Joseph's Hospital, London, Ontario, Canada N6A 4V2* (p. 241)

Visser, G. H. A., *Dept. of Pediatric Cardiology & Obstetrics, University Hospital, Groningen, The Netherlands* (p. 749)

Vojcek, L., *Dept. of Obstetrics and Gynaecology, University Medical School of Debrecen, Debrecen, Hungary* (p. 499)

Walker, A. M., *Monash University Centre for Early Human Development, Queen Victoria Medical Centre, Melbourne 3000, Australia* (pp. 287,395)

Walton, P., *Dept. of Obstetrics and Gynaecology, University of Western Ontario, London, Ontario, N6A 5A5, Canada* (p. 235)

Ward, B. S., *Dept. of Obstetrics and Gynaecology, University of Manchester at St. Mary's Hospital, Manchester, M13 0JH, UK* (p. 519)

Wardlaw, S. L., *College of Physicians & Surgeons, Columbia University, 630 West 168th St, New York, NY 10032, USA* (p. 165)

Weberg, A., *Div. of Maternal/Fetal Medicine, Dept. of Obstetrics & Gynecology, Southern Illinois University School of Medicine, Springfield, Illinois, USA* (p. 611)

Weingold, A., *George Washington University Medical Center, Washington DC, USA* (p. 499)

Weintraub, Z., *Dept. of Pediatrics and Neonatal Intensive Care, Carmel Hospital, Michal St., Haifa 34362, Israel* (p. 311)

Whitteridge, D., *Winterslow, Lincombe Lane, Boars Hill, Oxford OX1 5DZ, UK* (p. 565)

Wickham, P. J. D., *Dept. of Physiology, Monash University, Clayton, Melbourne, Victoria, Australia* (p. 247)

Wilkinson, M. H., *Monash University Centre for Early Human Development, Queen Victoria Medical Centre, Melbourne, Australia* (p. 287)

Willis, D. M., *Dept. of Physiology and Medicine, School of Medicine, Oregon Health Sciences University, Portland, Oregon 97201, USA* (p. 371)

Wilson, F., *Monash University Centre for Early Human Development, Queen Victoria Medical Centre, Melbourne, Australia* (p. 287)

Wimmer, J., *Dept. of Pediatrics, East Carolina University School of Medicine, Greenville, NC 27834, USA* (p. 777)

Wintour, E. M., *Dept. of Physiology, University of Melbourne, Parkville, Victoria 3052, Australia* (p. 537)

Wishart, J., *Dept. of Obstetrics and Gynaecology, University of Adelaide, South Australia, Australia* (p. 541)

Wlodek, M. E., *Dept. of Obstetrics & Gynecology, St. Joseph's Hospital, University of Western Ontario, London, Ontario, Canada* (p. 363)

Wolfson, M. R., *Department of Physiology, Temple University School of Medicine, 3420 N. Broad St., Philadelphia, PA 19140, USA* (p. 337)

Wollner, J. C., *Nuffield Dept. of Obstetrics and Gynaecology, John Radcliffe Hospital, Headley Way, Oxford, UK* (p. 795)

Wolton, R. S., *Bio-Engineering Unit, Dept. of Pediatrics, John Radcliffe Hospital, Headley Way, Oxford, UK* (p. 795)

Yao, A. C., *Downstate Medical Center, Department of Pediatrics, Box 49, 450 Clarkson Ave., Brooklyn, NY 11203, USA* (p. 445)

Yu, S.-H., *Department of Biochemistry, University of Western Ontario, London, Ontario, Canada N6A 5A5* (p. 325)

Zubrow, A. B., *Columbia University, College of Physicians & Surgeons, New York, NY, USA* (p. 533)

Preface

The King to Oxford send a troop of horse,
For Tories own no argument but force:
With equal skill to Cambridge books he sent;
For Whigs admit no force but argument.

Sir William Browne

In 1972 the Whigs met at St Catharine's College, Cambridge, to honour Sir Joseph Barcroft and extend his contributions to Fetal and Neonatal Physiology. So when twelve years later the Tories planned to meet at St Catherine's College, Oxford, to honour Geoffrey Dawes, and his continued inspiration to all with interests in the Physiology of Development, there was an understandable apprehension that the natural conservatism of the 'other' place might suppress progressive thought. Such unnecessary fears were expelled totally and the past six days have shown admirably that studies on pre- and postnatal development have 'come of age' through the major discoveries of the past twelve years. The observations, for instance, on the control of the developing lung, the processes of growth and maturation, the regulation of behaviour, and on the changes at birth are examples of exciting areas in which the admirable ground work of the past now indicate both important new directions and their manner of investigation. We hope that these proceedings will provide an appropriate tribute to the influence of Geoffrey Dawes and an inspiration to convince present and future generations of the challenge that studies on development provides.

The success of this conference owes much to the many who helped behind the scenes. In particular the staff of St Catherine's, and to Mr S. Arkinstall, Dr S. Farrow, Mrs D. Tindell, and Dr Gu Wei, but most of all to our secretary Mrs S. Mingos.

Popularity necessitated a tight programme, and while we have no regrets of our expectations of participants, it is appropriate that a distinguished Oxford man should have the last word:

A superfluity of lecturering causes ischial bursitis.

Sir William Osler

C. T. Jones
P. W. Nathanielsz

Oxford, July 1984

Contents

Part 2. The Endocrine Development of the Fetus

Part 3. The Development of Lung Function

Part 4. Causes and Consequences of Birth

Part 5. Fluid and Electrolyte Balance in Pregnancy

Part 6. Functional Development of the Central Nervous System

Part 7. Perinatal Physiology and Clinical Care

The Role of the Placenta in the Development in the Embryo and Fetus

Lawrence D. Longo

Division of Perinatal Biology, Departments of Physiology and Obstetrics and Gynecology, Loma Linda University, Loma Linda, California, USA

Placental Exchange and Fetal Development

In *De generatione* (1), in addition to enunciating the principle "ex ovo omnia" (everything from an egg), Harvey asked the fundamental question "How does it happen that the foetus continues in the mother's womb after the seventh month?" He correctly observed that if it is born at that time if may breathe and live, but if it remains *in utero* it lives in health and vigour without respiring and continues to grow. Harvey suggested the true nature of the placenta, proposing that its transfer of nutrients was vital to fetal existence. During the past several decades we have striven to understand the mechanisms by which various substrates exchange, to determine the factors which affect their exchange and their relative importance, and to define the kinetics and rate-limiting steps of these processes (2).

The placental and fetal circulations form during the early weeks of embryonic life, with both the placenta and fetus continuing to develop. Several workers have derived equations based on the assumption that if fetal linear growth is uniform with time, the cube root of mass is also linear (3). The coefficients which determine the slope for these relations differ for the several species for reasons as yet unknown. It has been observed empirically in humans (4), rhesus monkeys (5) and in all other species studied that during the latter half to two-thirds of gestation the weight of the fetus is a function of that of the placenta (3). However, as yet we are uncertain how placental nutrient exchange is matched to meet the requirements of fetal growth.

Several classes of nutrients cross the placenta by mechanisms ranging from passive diffusion to active transport and pinocytosis (2). These substances can be categorized into those for which exchange is limited by the rates of blood flow, and those the exchange of which is limited by diffusion or active transport. Oxygen

The Physiological Development of the Fetus and Newborn
ISBN 0 12 389080 2   *Copyright © 1985 by Academic Press, London.*
All rights of reproduction in any form reserved.

and other respiratory gases and probably glucose, free fatty acids, steroids, etc. are in the former category, while amino acids, monovalent and divalent ions, water soluble vitamins, and proteins are in the latter class (2).

Differential equations can be derived which describe the changes in concentration of any substance being studied (5). Using such equations, which can be applied to any flow-limited substance, one can predict the changes in oxygen partial pressure and content as uteroplacental and umbilical blood traverse the exchange vessels (6). Further, one can predict the critical levels of uteroplacental or umbilicoplacental oxygen flow below which fetal oxygen deliver, and, therefore, growth would be interfered with (6). In general, these theoretical predictions can be verified experimentally, for the effects of changes in maternal arterial O_2 tension or changes in uteroplacental blood flow (7).

For those molecules which exchange by energy-dependent processes, one also can calculate the kinetics of exchange, although we do not know their exact mechanisms of transfer or how the processes are regulated (2).

Placental Hormones and Fetal Development

In addition to its role in supplying nutrients to the embryo and fetus, the placenta has proved to be a complex endocrine organ synthesizing and metabolizing a number of protein and steroid hormones (8) (Fig. 1). The exact role of placental and fetal hormones and the manner in which they co-ordinate optimal growth and differentiation of embryonic, fetal and placental tissues is as yet unknown.

Chorionic gonadotropin (hCG) concentration in fetal blood is low compared to that in the mother, and its role in embryonic development is unknown. Several hormones produced by the fetus (as well as the mother) such as cortisol (9) can increase hCG synthesis. Progesterone and several of its metabolites suppress hCG secretion in term human placental explants (10). To complicate matters further, some fetal organs, such as the kidney and to a lesser extent the liver, synthesize and secrete hCG and the alpha subunit common to glycoprotein hormones, which in turn stimulate testosterone synthesis by Leydig cells (11).

Chorionic somatomammotropin (hCS) may be considered a growth-promoting hormone because of its effects on intermediary metabolism leading to the mobilization of free fatty acids, whereby glucose utilization in the maternal organism is blocked and fetal glucose supply is promoted. It may indirectly act as a fetal growth hormone, as it stimulates the secretion of insulin-like growth factors (12,13) which in turn stimulates further hCS secretion. Chorionic somatomammotropin is also stimulated by insulin and estrogens, and by progesterone in the 2-month placenta (14). The catecholamines dopamine, norepinephrine, and epinephrine inhibit hCS secretion (14). In turn, as reported in this volume by Graham et al., ovine somatomammotropin stimulates catecholamine release from fetal sheep adrenal medullary cells in vitro (15). Thus the fetus both of itself, and with the placenta, via hCG and hCS, appears to participate in its metabolic homeostasis.

Prolactin derived from the decidua and myometrium has been suggested to play several potential roles which relate to fetal development, including being

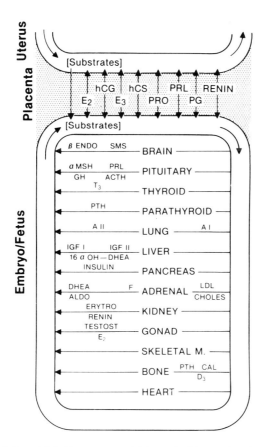

Figure 1. Placental and fetal hormones which probably are involved in embryonic and fetal growth. Several of the polypeptide and steroid hormones of the placenta either directly or indirectly stimulate fetal growth and differentiation and, in turn, several fetal hormones stimulate or inhibit placental hormone production (see text for details and abbreviations).

a fetal growth hormone *per se* (16) stabilization of uterine prostaglandin production (important not only in the prevention of premature labour, but in the regulation of umbilical and uteroplacental blood flows), and perhaps in the regulation of amniotic fluid volume (important in the regulation of fetal blood volume).

Evidence of placental synthesis has been obtained for other peptides such as pro-opiomelanocortin (the precursor molecule for ACTH), beta-lipoprotein, alpha-melanocyte-stimulating hormone (α-MSH), beta-endorphin, and other thus far uncharacterized peptides (17). Possible actions for the recently described peptides might include actions on maternal, fetal, or local (paracrine) effects on other placental hormones. For instance, α-MSH has been shown to play such a role in the rat fetus (18).

The steroid hormones produced by the placenta are also growth-promoting to those cells with appropriate receptors. The concentrations of both estradiol 17-β and progesterone are quite high in fetal blood, reflecting the elevated maternal concentrations (12). Actually the placental production of estrogens is to a great extent dependent upon the production of the precursor dehydroepiandosterone by the fetal adrenal glands. Estrogen and progesterone act on steroid responsive maternal cells and may be responsible for many of the maternal adaptations to pregnancy, such as the marked increase in blood volume, cardiac output, uteroplacental blood flow, etc. (19). The fetus and placenta may in fact play a key role in regulating the maternal adaptations to pregnancy, and thus in effect their own destiny (19).

An additional role of the placental hormones in fetal growth is that progesterone, and perhaps other hormones, probably promote growth of the fetus indirectly by protecting it from homograft rejection through a variety of mechanisms (20).

Cellular Growth Factors and Development of the Embryo, Fetus, and Placenta

Although classical endocrinological studies have established the importance of circulating hormones in the regulation of growth and differentiation, perhaps one of the most exciting areas of the biology of the fetus and newborn is the role of cellular growth factors in development. These polypeptides can stimulate *in vitro* cellular DNA replication and cell growth in a reversible and dose dependent manner. Since the discovery of polypeptide epidermal growth factor (EGF), a number of other extracellular signals have been found including insulin-like growth factors I and II (IGF-I and IGF-II), glial growth factor (GGF), fibroblast growth factor (FGF), nerve growth factor (NGF), platelet-derived growth factor (PDGF), skeletal growth factor (SGF), transforming growth factors (TGFs), and others. Most of the growth factors identified to date have been shown to operate locally in a paracrine or autocrine mode; however, some may function as classical endocrines operating at sites distant from where they are released into the circulation.

Growth Factors in the Embryo and Fetus

Almost all of the known growth factors have been shown to be synthesized and released by various embryonic and fetal cells (21). For instance, epidermal growth factor, which is mitogenic, stimulating the proliferation of the basal cell layer of various epithelia, has been postulated to play a key role in embryonic and fetal development (22). EGF is acquiring the status of a hormone in that it circulates in the blood of the fetus as well as the pregnant mother throughout gestation (23).

Nerve growth factor, which stimulates the development of sympathetic adrenergic neurons (24) and platelet-derived growth factor (25) also circulate, the latter substance having properties similar to the transforming growth factor found in the embryo.

Recent evidence suggests that insulin-like growth factor I (IGF-I; or somatomedin C) and perhaps IGF-II play an important role in fetal growth. These factors have been shown to be synthesized at multiple sites, including liver, lung, kidney, heart etc. (26). Although the absolute value of fetal IGF-I is lower than that of adults, its concentration has been shown to correlate with both gestational age and birth weight in humans (27) and sheep (28). In contrast, IGF-II concentration has been reported to be about the same in the fetus (male female) as in the adult, and does not change during the course of gestation (27). Following delivery in the lamb, IGF-I levels continued to rise until about day 7, then declined to adult values by day 60 (28) remaining relatively constant during the first year of life (29). In rats the concentration of multiplication-stimulatory activity (SA), related to IGF-II, is 20–100 times higher in fetal serum than in the mother, the levels gradually declining following birth (30).

Growth Factors in the Placenta

In addition, trophoblast cells *in vitro* have been shown to synthesize and release several of the growth factors and have receptors for several of these polypeptides. For instance amnion and chorion have both high and low affinity receptors with a high capacity to bind EGF 31-33 which may play an important role in "soaking-up" excessive EGFs from the fetus. EGF has been shown to stimulate and/or modulate the secretion of chorionic gonadotrophin (hCG) in normal trophoblast (34). It also may stimulate the active placental transport of ions, sugars, and amino acids (35). Preincubation of trophoblast cells with EGF downregulates the receptor population (36).

The placenta also is rich in nerve growth factor which has been isolated in high concentration from cotyledons and at lower levels from amnion (37). Both maternal and fetal blood contain biologically active NGF (37). At least in the fetus this may be of placental origin as the concentration in umbilical venous blood is almost 50% higher than in the umbilical artery (30.4 ± 3.2 *vs* 22.4 ± 3.3 pM ml) (24).

As early as the 6th week postconception IGF-I receptors appear on trophoblast cells (38). Receptors for insulin-like activity (54,61) and somatomedin-like activity (31) are also present.

Trophoblastic cells also contain transforming growth factors (TGF) and colony stimulating activity for bone marrow cells (39). Marrow cell colony formation activity is also derived from human umbilical vessels (40) and mitogenic angiogenic growth factor is also derived from human amnion and chorion (41), and these cells possess receptors for multiplication stimulatory activity (MSA) (31). Finally, inhibitors are also present, as evidenced by inhibition by boving placental tissue of ^{3}H-thymidine incorporation into DNA of a variety of tumour cells (42), and suppression of maternal lymphocyte mitogenic response (43).

In vivo Administration of Growth Factors or their Blockers

Several groups have explored the consequences of administering either growth factors or antibodies to such factors *in vivo*. Sundell *et al.* (44) infused EGF into

7 fetal and 2 neonatal lambs for 3–5 days. These treated lambs demonstrated "markedly stimulated epithelial growth in many sites" including the upper and lower airways. None of the animals developed respiratory distress syndrome. They also had "enlarged endocrine organs" without increased plasma cortisol, estradiol, or thyroxin concentrations. This group also injected EGF into 24-day rabbit fetuses, which at sacrifice on day 27 showed greater distensibility of the lung, stability on deflation, and a relative increase in Type II alveolar cells. EGF had no apparent effect on body or lung weight (45). Thorburn et al. (46) infused EGF for 3–14 days into fetal sheep at 110–125 days gestation. They observed striking hypertrophy of the skin and wool follicles, and increased weights of the thyroid, liver, and kidney. Adrenal cortical hypertrophy was associated with increased cortisol secretion, while thyroid hypertrophy was associated with increased colloid stores and decreased plasma T_4 concentration (46).

The role of nerve growth factor has been studied indirectly by injecting antiserum to NGF into fetal rats at 16–17 days gestation (47). The injected animals were significantly smaller at one week of age, 14.3% of the animals (18/126) died by the end of the first week and an additional 17.5% (22/126) by the end of the second week. Before they died, these animals, as well as most of the others, displayed decreased vitality, sluggishness, and apathetic behaviour. The pups showed irreversible destruction of sympathetic ganglia (47), as well as degeneration of chromaffin adrenal and extra-adrenal cells (48). In congenitally hypothyroid mice (hyt/hyt) Scott et al. demonstrated abnormally low concentrations of NGF which increased, but not to normal values, in response to treatment with thyroxine (49).

In vitro Administration of Growth Factors or their Blockers

Nerve growth factor demonstrates several effects in vitro, including stimulation of neurite outgrowth in clonal rat pheochromocytoma (PC-12) cells (a response inhibited with anti-NGF) (24), and inhibition of parathormone induced bone reabsorption (50). As suggested from the above, anti-NGF inhibited neurite outgrowth in PC-12 cells (24). Explanted superior cervical ganglia from 14-day mouse embryos exhibited neurite outgrowth with increased tyrosine hydroxylase activity in basal media without added NGF, even in the presence of anti-NGF (51). In contrast, absence of NGF prevented growth of superior cervical ganglia from 18-day mouse embryos (51). An antineuronal growth factor inhibited NGF stimulated neurite outgrowth from neonatal ganglia cells (52).

Epidermal growth factor stimulated cell growth and a 2-fold increase in secretion of huma chorionic gonadotropin in a JAr line of choriocarcinoma cells (34). It also stimulated hCG production and release in perfused human placentas (53). Fetal rabbit cartilage in vitro increased ^{35}S-sulphate uptake in response to IGF (54).

Platelet-derived growth factor stimulated 21-day fetal rat calvaria to increase ^{3}H-thymidine incorporation, increased bone DNA content, and increased ^{3}H-proline incorporation in noncollagen protein (55). Cortical bone extracts from adult rats stimulated DNA synthesis in calvarian osteoprogenitor cells from fetal rats (56).

In summary, the identification of these putative peptide regulatory substances has broadened our understanding of the regulation of growth and differentiation. The current repertoire of growth factors probably represents only a fraction of the ultimate spectrum of such peptides which regulate development, and which some day may be used therapeutically.

Communication between the Placenta and Embryo and Fetus

Unfortunately little is known of the function of these growth factors *in vivo*, much less the detailed molecular basis for their actions. As noted above, of particular concern to physiologists since the classic studies, is the manner in which development of the embryo and fetus is regulated. Figure 2 suggests how the individual embryonic and fetal organs and the placenta might communicate with one another, so that their growth and differentiation can proceed in an orderly and orchestrated manner. Substrate availability is an obvious requirement for the synthesis and release of hormones and growth factors. Hormones from the placenta and fetus probably stimulate or inhibit the elaboration of various growth factors, or may otherwise modulate their function. In addition, these hormones may influence transplacental nutrient flux. Finally, the several growth factors may, in addition to their local regulatory function, stimulate or inhibit not only the synthesis and release of various hormones, but substrate availability as well.

Thus one can postulate a hierarchical system (Fig. 2) of regulation by substrates — hormones — growth factors which in a sense is analogous to the neuroendocrine system. That is, chemical mediators produced locally can regulate the activities of neighbouring cells, and these messenger molecules may also act at more distant sites. That such a system is not totally unreasonable is suggested

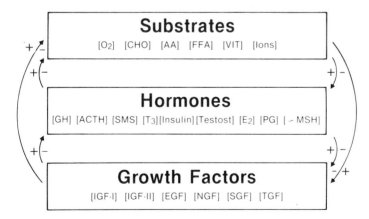

Figure 2. The regulatory mechanisms whereby various substrates exchange across the placenta, the various hormones are synthesized by the placenta and the embryo/fetus, and the cellular growth factors are released. These factors are probably interrelated by a complex set of positive and negative feedback loops (see text for details).

by the fact that many of the growth factors (IGFs, EGF, NGF, etc.) appear to be similar to classical hormone molecules in their structure and in their mechanism of actions at their target cells. In addition, as with the neuroendocrine system, these peptides may have differing specificities and biological actions depending upon their location.

References

1. Harvey, W. (1651). "Exercitationes de generatione animalium. Quibus accedunt quaedam de partu: de membranis ac humoribus uteri et de conceptione. . . ." Octaviani Pulleyn, Londini.
2. Hill, E. P. and Longo, L. D. (1980). *Fed. Proc.* **39**, 239–244.
3. Dawes, G. S. (1968). "Foetal and Neonal Physiology", Year Book, Chicago.
4. McKeown, T. and Record, R. G. (1953). *J. Endocrinol.* **9**, 418–426.
5. Hill, E. P., Power, G. G. and Longo, L. D. (1972). *Am. J. Physiol.* **222**, 721–729.
6. Longo, L. D., Hill, E. P. and Power, G. G. (1972). *Am. J. Physiol.* **222**, 730–739.
7. Power, G. G. and Jenkins, F. (1975). *Am. J. Physiol.* **229**, 1147–1153.
8. Simpson, E. R. and MacDonald, P. C. (1981). *Ann. Rev. Physiol.* **43**, 163–188.
9. Wilson, E. A. and Jawad, M. J. (1982). *Am. J. Obstet. Gynecol.* **142**, 344–349.
10. Wilson, E. A., Jawad, M. J. and Lesley, L. R. (1980). *Am. J. Obstet. Gynecol.* **138**, 708–713.
11. McGregor, W. G., Kuhn, R. W. and Jaffe, R. B. (1983). *Science* **220**, 306–308.
12. Porter, D. G. (1980). *Placenta* **1**, 259–274.
13. Robinson, J. S., Kingston, E. J. and Thorburn, G. D. (1978). *Postgrad. Med. J.* **54**, 51–61.
14. Hochberg, Z., Perlman, R., Brandes, J. M., and Benderli, A. (1983). *J. Clin. Endocrin. Metab.* **57**, 1311–1313.
15. Graham, A., Longo, L. D. and Cheung, C. Y. (1985). Unpublished work.
16. Sinha, Y. N. and Vanderlaan, W. P. (1982). *Endocrinology* **110**, 1871–1878.
17. Liotta, A. S. and Krieger, D. T. (1980). *Endocrinology* **106**, 1504–1511.
18. Honnebier, W. J. and Swaab, D. F. (1974). *J. Obstet. Gynaecol. Brit. Commonwealth* **81**, 439–447.
19. Longo, L. D. (1983). *Am. J. Physiol.* **245**, R720–R729.
20. Siiteri, P. K. and Stiles, D. P. (1982). *Biol. Reprod.* **26**, 15–27.
21. Gospodarowicz, D. (1981). *Ann. Rev. Physiol.* **43**, 251–263.
22. Patt, L. M. and Houck, J. C. (1983). *Kidney Internat.* **23**, 603–610.
23. Ances, I. G. (1973). *Am. J. Obstet. Gynecol.* **115**, 357–362.
24. Walker, P., Tarris, R. H., Weichsel, Jr., M. E., Scott, S. M. and Fisher, D. A. (1981). *J. Clin. Endocrin. Metab.* **53**, 218–220.
25. Childs, C., Proper, J. A., Tucker, F. and Moses, H. L. (1982). *Proc. Nat. Acad. Sci. USA* **79**, 5312–5316.
26. D'Ercole, A. J., Stiles, A. D., and Underwood, L. E. (1984). *Proc. Nat. Acad. Sci. USA* **81**, 935–939.
27. Gluckman, P. D., Johnson-Barrett, J. J., Butler, J. H., Edgar, B. W. and Gunn, T. R. (1983). *Clin. Endocrinol.* **19**, 405–413.
28. Gluckman, P. D. and Butler, J. H. (1983). *J. Endocrinol.* **99**, 223–232.
29. Kaplowitz, P. B., D'Ercole, A. J., Van Wyk, J. J., and Underwood, L. E. (1982). *J. Pediat.* **100**, 932–934.

30. Moses, A. C., Nissley, P. S., Short, P. A., Rechler, M. M., White, R. M., Knight, A. B. and Olga, Z. (1980). *Proc. Nat. Acad. Sci. USA* **77**, 3649–3653.
31. Brinsmead, M. W. and Liggins, G. C. (1978). *Aust. J. Exp. Biol. Med. Sci.* **56**, 527–544.
32. Deal, C. L., Guyda, H. J., Lai, W. H. and Posner, B. I. (1982). *Pediat. Res.* **16**, 820–825.
33. Carson, S. A., Chase, R., Ulep, E., Scommegna, A. and Benveniste, R. (1983). *Am. J. Obstet. Gynecol.* **147**, 932–939.
34. Huot, R. I., Foidart, J. M., Nardone, R. M. and Stromberg, K. (1981). *J. Clin. Endocrin. Metab.* **53**, 1059–1063.
35. Carpender, G. and Cohen, S. (1979). *Ann. Rev. Biochem.* **48**, 193–216.
36. Lai, W. H. and Guyda, H. J. (1984). *J. Clin. Endocrin. Metab.* **58**, 344–352.
37. Goldstein, L. D., Reynolds, C. P. and Perez-Polo, J. R. (1978). *Neurochem. Res.* **3**, 175–183.
38. Grizzard, J. D., D'Ercole, A. J., Wilkins, J. R., Moats-Staats, B. M. and Williams, R. W. (1984). *J. Clin. Endocrin. Metab.* **58**, 535–543.
39. Ruscetti, F. W., Chou, J. Y. and Gallo, R. C. (1982). *Blood* **59**, 86–90.
40. Knudtzon, S. and Mortensen, B. T. (1975). *Blood* **46**, 937–943.
41. Burgos, H. (1983). *Europ. J. Clin. Invest.* **13**, 289–296.
42. Letnansky, K. (1982). *Biosci. Rep.* **2**, 39–45.
43. Rubinstein, A., Koren, Z., and Murphy, R. A. (1982). *Am. J. Reprod. Immunol.* **2**, 260–264.
44. Sundell, H., Serenius, F. S., Barthe, P., Friedman, Z., Kanarek, K. S., Escabedo, M. B., Orth, D. N. and Stahlman, M. T. (1975). *Pediat. Res.* **9**, 371.
45. Catterton, W. Z., Escobedo, M. B., Sexson, W. R., Gray, M. E., Sundell, H. W. and Stahlman, M. T. (1979). *Pediat. Res.* **13**, 104–108.
46. Thorburn, G. D., Waters, M. J., Young, I. R., Dolling, M., Buntine, D. and Hopkins, P. S. (1981). "The Fetus and Independent Life", pp. 172–198. Pitman, London.
47. Aloe, L., Cozzari, C., Calissano, P., and Levi-Montalcini, R. (1981). *Nature* **291**, 413–415.
48. Aloe, L. and Levi-Montalcini, R. (1979). *Proc. Nat. Acad. Sci. USA* **76**, 1246–1250.
49. Scott, S. M., Chou, P. J. and Fisher, D. A. (1983). *J. Develop. Biol.* **5**, 413–418.
50. Teitelbaum, S. L., Andres, R. Y., Cooke, N. E., Hahn, T. J. and Kahn, A. J. (1978). *Calif. Tiss. Res.* **26**, 203–208.
51. Coughlin, M. D., Boyer, D. M., Black, I. B. (1977). *Proc. Nat. Acad. Sci. USA* **74**, 3438–3442.
52. Coughlin, M. D. and Kessler, J. A. (1982). *J. Neurosci. Res.* **8**, 289–302.
53. Takemori, M., Nishimura, R., Ashitaka, Y., and Tojo, S. (1981). *J. Clin. Endocrin. Metab.* **53**, 1059–1063.
54. Hill, D. J. and Milner, R. D. G. (1981). "The Fetus and Independent Life", pp. 124–151. Pitman, London.
55. Canalis, E. (1981). *Metabolism* **30**, 970–975.
56. Shimizu, N., Yoshikawa, H., Takaoka, K. and Ono, K. (1983). *Clin. Ortho. Rel. Res.* **178**, 252–257.

Experimental Studies on the Control of Fetal Growth

Colin T. Jones, Timothy P. Rolph,[1] Harrie N. Lafeber,[2]
W. Gu, J. E. Harding[3] and J. T. Parer[4]

The Nuffield Institute for Medical Research,
University of Oxford, Oxford, UK

Introduction

Major questions of the mechanisms of control of fetal growth are: (i) What determines growth at the cellular level and selects the preferential growth and maturation at a particular time of one tissue by comparison with another? (ii) How are high rates of growth maintained in prenatal tissues and what is the relationship of this to the control of nutrient supply and utilization? (iii) What is the role of the fetal endocrine system in determining the appropriate rate of fetal growth? (iv) How do fetus, mother and placenta interact to select satisfactory rates of prenatal growth and maturation? It is often supposed that for any one species growth and maturation are relatively predetermined immutable processes that, although altered by a pathological environment, are not subject to substantial variation under normal physiological conditions. A natural consequence of such an hypothesis is that there are critical phases of development and if these do not occur at the predetermined time a permanent impairment will occur (1–3). This appears to apply to postnatal development, at least for brain maturation, which if slowed by nutritional deprivation will not recover fully, but does not necessarily apply to skeletal development (1,2,4,5). For prenatal and possibly some of postnatal development these views have to be modified for at least two reasons. Whether

[1]Glaxo Animal Health Laboratories, Brakspear Rd South, Harefield, Middlesex, UK
[2]Department of Paediatrics, Sophia Children's Hospital, Rotterdam, The Netherlands
[3]Department of Paediatrics, University of Auckland Medical School, Auckland, New Zealand
[4]Department of Obstetrics and Gynaecology, HSE 1462, University of California, San Francisco, CA 94143, USA

The Physiological Development of the Fetus and Newborn
ISBN 0 12 389080 2
Copyright © 1985 by Academic Press, London.
All rights of reproduction in any form reserved.

caused by varying location in the uterus (6,7), by alteration of nutritional state (1,2,4,5,8–11) or by changes in general environment (12–14) important maturational events can be shifted (3,5,7,11,15,16). Secondly the movement of such events, usually to later in gestation, need not necessarily lead to long-term impairment. It is possible that such flexibility of prenatal development, which may not be entirely representative of postnatal maturation, is a response to slow growth and maturation before birth awaiting a more favourable extra-uterine environment, as is indicated by the rapid increase in growth observed after delivery (16,17). Such flexibility may be a fairly common feature of animal development, at least as applied to insects, amphibia and mammals (18–21). The mechanisms allowing flexibility of fetal maturation remain unclear. They must be able to sense and respond to changes in nutrient supply, hence the endocrine glands are an obvious candidate for involvement (7,11,15–17,21–23). Alternatively the placenta is the first intra-uterine site to sense changes in prenatal nutrition and attention is directed there by the observation that the most profound effects on fetal growth and development are caused by restriction of uterine blood flow (7,11,15–17,22,24–29). The results from such studies will be used to explore this hypothesis.

Approaches to investigating growth control fall naturally into three broad classes; the study of the normal physiological processes, such as placental function, under-lying fetal development; the study of the regulation of cell proliferation and maturation; and the use of various models for acceleration and slowing of prenatal growth to unravel physiological mechanisms of control. The latter approach will be considered. In addition to observing fetuses with large variations in natural growth rates arising from location (6) in the uterine horn, fetal growth rate has been modified by altering uterine and umbilical blood flow (7,11,15–17,22,24–30), or by changing maternal or fetal nutritional or endocrine state (4,5,8–10,14,31–35). Broadly, such studies illustrate that change in nutrient supply is a determinant of fetal growth rate and manipulates, in a highly selective way, the rate of maturation of tissues so that development is appropriate to substrate availability (36). Postnatal growth and maturation is largely under the regulatory influence of insulin and growth hormone with effects on maturation of steroids and thyroid hormones (37). Although insulin appears to play a pivotal role for the fetus (7,11,14–16,22,23,26,27,31,33,35,38–40) and there are important actions of thyroid and steroid hormones on development (41–45), growth hormone has a less central function (23) and this may be taken over by IGF-II (23,46,47). However, as discussed below, these alone do not explain growth regulation. Moreover if the proposal that the IGF-II is the fetal growth hormone is correct, the important question of where it comes from and what controls its production remains (23,48); its output is probably in part regulated by placental lactogen. One argument to develop is the concept that the placenta produces, dependent on its nutritional state, signals, some of which are inhibitory, that manipulate prenatal maturation (49,36).

Fetal Growth and Nutrient Supply

Glucose is a major substrate used by the fetus (50,51) and, although others make important contributions, it is therefore not surprising that growth rate and fetal availability of glucose can be related closely (7,11,14,16,27,29,33,36,38). Thus in small fetuses hypoglycaemia and hypoinsulinaemia are common and the converse is true for fetuses large for gestational age (14–17). Moreover, chronic glucose or insulin administration stimulates prenatal growth (31,33). These facts and the close relationship between maternal arterial glucose and fetal umbilical venous glucose and insulin concentrations have lead to the suggestion that prenatal growth is determined to a large extent by supply of glucose across the placenta. An important assumption in these conclusions is that uptake and plasma level of glucose should be closely related, implying that small fetuses have a low rate of consumption. In the mature sheep fetus this does not necessarily appear to be true, as hypoglycaemic fetuses with low plasma insulin concentrations have higher than normal rates of turnover and growth-retarded fetuses with a small placenta have a normal rate of glucose consumption despite being hypo-insulinaemic (Table 1). Although glucose supply is an important factor determining fetal growth, the above observations suggest that fetal responses to reduced supply are complex.

Table 1. Glucose metabolism in normal-size and retarded 125–135 days fetal sheep

	Normal		Growth retarded
	Normoglycaemic	Hypoglycaemic	
Weight (kg)	3.1 ± 1.2	2.9 ± 0.59	1.7 ± 0.45
Glucose (mmol)	1.06 ± 0.07	0.69 ± 0.09	0.63 ± 0.12
Turnover (μmol/min/kg)	29.4 ± 8.6	59.0 ± 17.2	29.6 ± 13.1
Insulin (units/ml)	19.6 ± 5.3	10.0 ± 3.1	7.3 ± 2.5

means ± SD; $n = 4$–6
Glucose turnover was measured in fetal sheep by constant infusion of ^{14}C-glucose (68). Growth retardation was produced as described previously (40).

This is amply illustrated by the fact that the maturation of tissues is considerably slowed in fetal growth retardation with liver, muscle, heart and even the brain being affected (8,11,14–17,22,24,30). Thus for instance hind-limb muscle of the growth-retarded late fetal or new-born guinea-pig is structurally similar to that of fetuses some 25–30 days younger (52, Fig. 1). The slowing of maturation coincides with the shift of phases of biosynthesis to later in development (36). Organs such as the brain are affected less than liver and skeletal muscle and this has led to the proposal that the restriction of growth and maturation, because it affects the insulin-sensitive tissues most, is brought about largely by hypoglycaemia and hypoinsulinaemia (7,11,14–17). There are, however, several reasons for considering that this, at most, only explains partly the mechanisms involved. For instance the genes whose expression appears to be inhibited, such as the gluconeogenic enzymes of the fetal liver (53), would be expected to be activated rather than repressed by hypoglycaemia. Moreover, daily injections of glucose into fetuses subjected to reduced uterine blood flow does not reverse

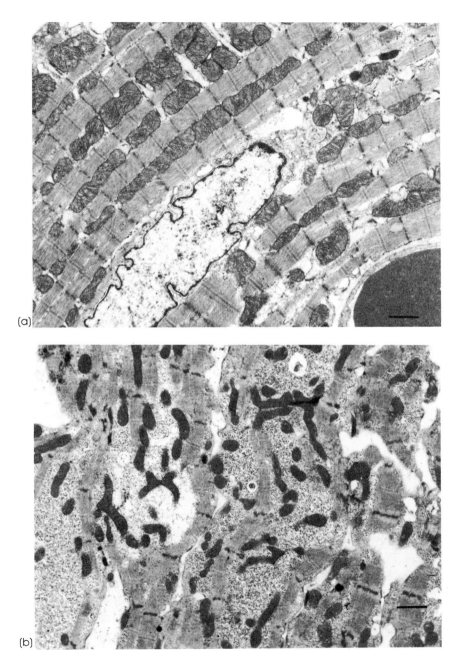

Figure 1. Electronmicrographs of hind-limb muscle of normal (a) and growth-retarded (b) fetal guinea-pigs. The body weights were respectively 81.4 g and 27.6 g at time of sacrifice which was day 60 of gestation.

Table 2. The effect of chronic glucose administration on the fetal effects of uterine artery ligation in the guinea-pig

	Control		Ligated	
	Saline	Glucose	Saline	Glucose
Body weight (g)	39.6±8.4	47.3±12.9	23.4±6.9	25.8±11.3
Plasma glucose (μmol/ml)	2.6±0.5	3.9±1.0	1.5±0.3	2.8±0.9
Hepatic PEPCK activity (units/g)	2.8±0.7	2.2±0.5	0.6±0.2	0.8±0.3

Uterine artery ligation was carried out at day 30 of pregnancy and twice daily intra-fetal injections (0.2 ml) of saline or 100 mg of glucose given. Samples were taken 2–3 h after the last injection. Fetuses were studied at days 50–52 of gestation.

completely the restriction of growth and maturation despite normal glucose and insulin concentrations (Table 2).

Thus whilst the low plasma glucose concentration in the fetus, and the attendant fall in insulin, is the background for slowed fetal development it does not provide the sole mechanism for growth manipulation nor is it associated even with a reduced glucose consumption per unit mass of fetus.

Information on the metabolism of other nutrients in states of altered fetal growth is much more limited. It is probable that there is a restricted supply of fatty acids across the placenta and this, together with the delay in appearance of the hepatic pathway for synthesis, could limit tissue growth (15,16). Amino acids are supplied to the fetus in excess of need of accretion and this is reflected in the relatively high rates of protein and amino acid turnover (51). Thus the increased plasma amino acid level and reduced tissue aminotransferase activity in intra-uterine growth retardation (15,16) is likely to reflect reduced rates of amino acid turnover. If amino acids are an important energy fuel for the fetus, which seems probable for the sheep (50,51) reduced metabolism may be another restriction on growth. This, however, would be secondary to limitations of other substrates as there is no direct evidence that placental transport of amino acids is limiting under these circumstances, although reduced fetal accumulation of labelled synthetic amino acids has been reported (54). Low capacity for transamination and hence provision of the amino group could restrict growth and provision of essential intermediates such as ornithine the precursor for polyamines.

Endocrine Involvement in Control of Fetal Growth

Early experiments on the effects of hypophysectomy on prenatal growth in rats and rabbits lead to the suggestion that pituitary hormones have a relatively minor role to play (23). Subsequent studies with primates and sheep have not confirmed entirely such views but the concept that hormones such as growth hormone have a comparatively minor role has persisted (23). By comparison destruction of the fetal pancreas or thyroidectomy have marked effects (41,42,55,56). The role of steroid hormones in growth control is less clear, but they are obviously involved in the maturation of a number of tissues such as the lung and liver (45). To what extent do studies on growth-retarded fetuses confirm such views? In addition to being hypoinsulinaemic small fetuses have high plasma glucagon, low corticosteroid, thyroid hormone and prolactin and normal plasma growth hormone concentrations (7,11,14–17,22,33,40,49,52). In most instances the developmentally related changes in plasma concentration appear to be slowed (22,36) and the results support the relatively minor prenatal role for growth hormone. As far as relating the manipulation of development to hormonal changes the best correlations are found with thyroid hormones. For instance the development of hepatic fatty acid synthesis correlates closely with plasma T_4 levels in both normal and retarded fetuses (7,36), which is consistent with the marked effects of hypothyroidism on postnatal growth and maturation (57). Some hormonal changes in growth retardation, such as the high plasma glucagon concentration, are surprising as the effects on hepatic enzyme development and glycogen deposition (7,16,17,22,52) are the opposite of what might be expected. The significance of the very low plasma prolactin concentrations has yet to be established. It is a hormone that rises late in gestation and has been suggested to have growth-promoting effects (58,59). The general lack of a close correlation between the developmental and plasma hormone changes in growth retardation has led to the search for other possible agents controlling maturation. The obvious candidate is the growth factors IGF-I and II which appear to be required for fetal growth (23,37,47,60–64). Thus intra-uterine growth retardation has been associated with lowered plasma levels of somatomedins (60,63,64). However somatomedin levels, when measured by radioimmunoassay, have been reported elevated in growth retardation despite lowered somatomedin activity as measured by bioassay (65). This has led to the suggestion that growth may be controlled also be inhibitory factors (36,49,65). Hence plasma from small fetuses has been found to be inhibitory to mitogenesis and gene expression in fetal isolated hepatocytes. Moreover the levels of such factors appears to rise in umbilical venous blood in response to short-term reductions of uterine blood flow indicating a potential placental origin (36).

The Placenta and Control of Fetal Growth

Close relationships between placental weight and uterine blood flow and fetal growth have been reported (28,29,66,67) which have been used to indicate that for much of prenatal life placental capacity may determine growth whilst at the same time retaining a significant reserve for transport until late in gestation (13,67,68). In growth retardation however this relationship breaks down and there is probably little reserve (11,29,68) and fetal glucose availability seems more sensitive than normal to reduced uterine blood flow (29,68). The fact that the placenta is responsible for the consumption of the major portion of glucose extracted from the uterine artery (50,51,68) means that the fetal needs are probably met after those of the placenta, and in some but not all instances of reduced uterine flow this appears to be so (69). Moreover to sustain such a high nutrient requirement, fetal provision of nutrient for the placenta is initiated in response

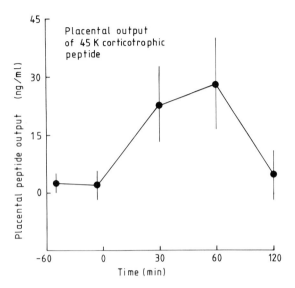

Figure 2. Placental production of a corticotrophic peptide in the 125–135 days fetal sheep. The peptide was extracted from umbilical vein plasma and separated by polyacrylamide gel electrophoresis, it cross-reacts with an antibody specific for the 4–12 region of the ACTH molecule. At time 0–60 min uterine blood flow was reduced by 35 $\pm$ 11% by an infusion of adrenaline (0.5 μg/min/kg) into the maternal circulation.

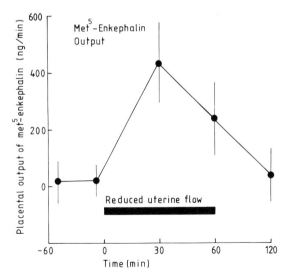

Figure 3. Placental output of a met-enkephaline-like peptide from the placenta of the 125–135 days fetal sheep. Peptide was measured by radioimmunoassay with an antibody specific for met-enkephalin. Other details as for Fig. 2.

to reduced uterine flow even when the reductions are insufficient to cause any obvious changes blood gas concentration (69). This indicates an inter-communication between the fetus and placenta designed to meet placental needs and consequently tailor fetal response. What may such a communication be? The fact that density of placental insulin receptors appears to correlate with fetal size suggests some functional intercommunication (70). The placenta is the sight of production of a wide range of hormones and protein factors mostly of unknown function (71,72) and may also produce inhibitory peptides, chalones (73). Moreover when uterine blood flow is reduced it is responsible for the production of a corticotrophic factor (Fig. 2) that inhibits adrenal steroidogenic responses (74,75), it produces enkephalin peptides (Fig. 3) that alter fetal physiological state, and is probably the site of production of protein factors inhibitory to cell growth and somatomedin action (36,49). However the strongest candidate for such a role, placental lactogen, that can stimulate somatomedin production, has not yet been shown to be correlated with fetal growth rate (76).

These observations point to a concept of the placenta being the first point at which maternal nutritional state, and in particular the state of uterine blood flow is sensed, partly because of its own dependence. Alterations in supply initiate short-term responses such as mobilization of fetal glucose and reduction in placental oxygen consumption (69) that require placental–fetal intercommunication, possibly using placentally derived peptides. In the long-term this communication system is likely to be an important regulator of fetal growth and this may be achieved by the production of factors inhibitory to fetal maturation as well as those that may stimulate the process.

Acknowledgements

This work has been supported by grants from the MRC, the Royal Society, Action Research for the Crippled Child and the Muscular Dystrophy Group.

References

1. Winick, M. and Noble, A. (1966). *J. Nutr.* **89**, 300–306.
2. Lau, M. C., Thye, F. W. and Ritchey, S. J. (1974). *Nutr. Rep. Int.* **10**, 249–260.
3. Widdowson, E. M. and McCance, R. A. (1963). *Proc. Roy. Soc. B.* **158**, 329–342.
4. Williams, J. P. G., Tanner, J. M. and Hughes, P. C. R. (1974). *Pediat. Res.* **8**, 149–156.
5. Toews, J. G. and Lee, M. (1975). *Nutr. Rep. Int.* **11**, 223–230.
6. McLaren, A. (1965). *J. Reprod. Fertil.* **9**, 79–98.
7. Jones, C. T., Lafeber, H. N., Rolph, T. P. and Fellows, G. F. (1980). *In:* "Fetal Medicine", (Salvadori, B. and Merialdi, A. eds) pp. 86–109. Borla, Rome.
8. Zamenhoff, S., Van Martens, E. and Gravel, L. (1971). *Science* **172**, 850–851.
9. Howarth, R. E. and Baldwin, R. L. (1971). *J. Nutr.* **101**, 477–484.
10. Chow, B. F. and Lee, C. J. (1964). *J. Nutr.* **82**, 10–18.
11. Jones, C. T., Harding, J. E., Robinson, J. S., Lafeber, H. N. and Rolph, T. P. (1981). *Adv. Anim. Comp. Physiol.* **20**, 53–60.
12. Gilbert, R. D., Cumming, C. A., Juchau, M. R. and Longo, L. D. (1979). *J. Appl. Physiol.* **46**, 828–834.

13. Alexander, G. and Williams, D. (1971). *J. Agric. Sci.* **76**, 53–72.
14. Fletcher, J. M. and Bassett, J. M. (1982). *Diabetol.* **23**, 124–130.
15. Jones, C. T. and Robinson, J. S. (1979). *In:* "Maternal Effects in Development", (Newth, D. R. and Balls, M. eds) pp. 395–409. Cambridge University Press, Cambridge.
16. Lafeber, H. N., Jones, C. T. and Rolph, T. P. (1979). *In:* "Nutrition and Metabolism of the Fetus and Infant", (Visser, H. K. A. ed.) pp. 43–62. Martinus Nijhoff Publishers B.V., The Hague.
17. Lafeber, H. N., Rolph, T. P. and Jones, C. T. (1984). *J. Develop. Physiol.* **6**, 441–459.
18. Lees, A. D. (1966). *Adv. Insect Physiol.* **3**, 207–240.
19. Johnson, C. G. (1974). *In:* "The Physiology of Insecta", (Rockstein, M. ed.) 2nd Edn, Vol. 3, pp. 279–334. Academic Press, New York and London.
20. Sprules, W. G. (1974). *Can. J. Zool.* **52**, 393–405.
21. Estes, R. D. (1974). *In:* "The Behaviour of Ungulates and its Relation to Management", (Geist, V. and Walther, F. eds) pp. 166–205. ICVN, Morges.
22. Jones, C. T., Lafeber, H. N. and Roebuck, M. M. (1984). *J. Develop. Physiol.* **6**, 461–472.
23. Gluckman, P. D. and Liggins, G. C. (1984). *In:* "Fetal Physiology Medicine", (Beard, R. W. and Nathanielsz, P. W. eds) 2nd Edn, pp. 511–557. Marcel Dekker, New York.
24. Wigglesworth, J. C. (1964). *J. Path. Bact.* **88**, 531–545.
25. Hohenauer, L. and Oh, W. (1969). *J. Nutr.* **99**, 23–26.
26. Myers, R. E., Hill, D. E., Holt, A. B., Scott, R. E., Mellits, E. D. and Cheek, D. B. (1971). *Biol. Neonate* **18**, 379–394.
27. Robinson, J. S., Kingston, E. J., Jones, C. T. and Thorburn, G. D. (1979). *J. Develop. Physiol.* **1**, 379–398.
28. Gilbert, M. and Leturque, A. (1982). *J. Develop. Physiol.* **4**, 134–143.
29. Jones, C. T. and Parer, J. T. (1984). *J. Physiol.* **343**, 525–537.
30. Emmanouilides, G. C., Townsend, D. E. and Bauer, R. A. (1968). *Pediat.* **42**, 919–927.
31. Picon, L. (1967). *Endocrinology* **81**, 1419–1421.
32. Parvez, H., Ismahan, G. and Parvez, S. (1976). *J. Endocrinol.* **71**, 159–160.
33. Susa, J. B., McCormick, K. L., Widness, J. A., Singer, D. B., Adamsons, K. and Schwartz, R. (1979). *Diabetes* **28**, 1058–1063.
34. Swaab, D. B., Boer, G. J. and Visser, M. (1978). *Postgrad. Med. J.* **54**, 63–69.
35. Pitkin, R. M. and Van Orden, O. A. (1974). *Endocrinology* **94**, 1247–1253.
36. Jones, C. T. (1985). *Biochem. Soc. Trans.* **13**, 89–91.
37. Phillips, L. S. (1981). *In:* "Endocrine Control of Growth", (Daughaday, W. H. ed.) pp. 121–173. Elsevier, New York.
38. Girard, J. R., Rieutort, M., Kervan, A. and Jost, A. (1976). *In:* "Proceedings of 5th European Congress of Perinatal Medicine", (Booth, G. and Bratteby, L. E. eds) pp. 197–202. Almqist & Wicksell, Stockholm.
39. Metzger, P. and Brachet, E. (1979). *Biol. Neonate* **33**, 297–303.
40. Robinson, J. S., Hart, I. C., Kingston, E. J., Jones, C. T. and Thorburn, G. D. (1980). *J. Develop. Physiol.* **2**, 239–248.
41. Kerr, G. R., Tyson, I. B., Allen, T. R., Wallace, J. H. and Scheffler, G. (1972). *Biol. Neonate* **21**, 285–295.
42. Thorburn, G. D. (1974). *CIBA Symp.* **27**, 185–200.
43. Hamburgh, M., Lynn, E. and Weiss, E. P. (1964). *Anat. Rec.* **150**, 147–156.
44. Pickering, D. E. and Fisher, D. A. (1953). *Am. J. Dis. Child.* **86**, 147–153.
45. Liggins, G. C., Kitterman, J. A. and Foster, C. S. (1979). *Anim. Reprod. Sci.* **2**, 193–207.
46. Moses, A. C. (1980). *Proc. Nat. Acad. Sci. USA* **77**, 3649–3653.

47. Gluckman, P. D. and Butler, J. H. (1983). *J. Endocrinol.* **99**, 223-232.
48. D'Ercole, A. J., Applewhite, G. T. and Underwood, L. E. (1980). *J. Develop. Biol.* **75**, 315-328.
49. Jones, C. T., Michael, E., Lafeber, H. N. and Band, G. C. (1984). *Proc. Nutr. Soc.* **43**, 179-188.
50. Battaglia, F. C. and Mechia, G. (1978). *Physiol. Rev.* **58**, 499-527.
51. Jones, C. T. and Rolph, T. P. (1985). *Physiol. Rev.* (in press).
52. Jones, C. T., Rolph, T. P., Band, G. C. and Michael, E. (1981). *In:* "Metabolic Adaptation to Extrauterine Life", (DeMeyer, R. ed.) pp. 55-78. Martinus Nijhoff Publishers BV, The Hague.
53. Rolph, T. P. and Jones, C. T. (1982). *J. Develop. Physiol.* **4**, 1-21.
54. Nitzan, M., Orlof, S. and Schulman, J. D. (1979). *Pediat. Res.* **13**, 100-103.
55. Hill, D. E., Holt, A. B., Reba, R. and Cheek, D. B. (1972). *Pediat. Res.* **6**, 336.
56. Lemons, J. A., Ridenow, R. and Orsini, E. N. (1979). *Pediat.* **64**, 255-257.
57. Mosier, H. D. (1981). *In:* "Endocrine Control of Growth", (Daughaday, W. H. ed.) pp. 25-66. Elsevier-North Holland, New York.
58. Gluckman, P. D. (1980). *In:* "Maternal-Fetal Endocrinology", (Tulchinsky, D. and Ryan, K. eds) pp. 196-232. W. B. Saunders, Philadelphia.
59. Nicoll, C. S. (1978). *In:* "Progress in Prolactin Physiology and Pathology", (Robyn, C. and Harter, M. eds) pp. 175-187. Elsevier-North Holland, Amsterdam.
60. Gluckman, P. D. and Brinsmead, M. W. (1976). *J. Clin. Endocrin.* **43**, 1378-1381.
61. Daughaday, W. H., Parker, K., Borowsky, S., Trivedi, B. and Kapadia, M. (1982). *Endocrinology* **110**, 575-581.
62. Clemmons, D. R. and Van Wyk, J. J. (1981). *In:* "Tissue Growth Factors", (Baserga, R. ed.) pp. 161-208. Springer-Verlag, Berlin.
63. D'Ercole, A. J., Foushee, D. B. and Underwood, L. E. (1976). *J. Clin. Endocrin. Metab.* **43**, 1069-1077.
64. Foley, T. P., DePhilip, R., Pericelli, A. and Miller, A. (1980). *J. Pediat.* **96**, 605-610.
65. Jones, C. T., Lafeber, H. N., Parer, J. T., Price, D. A., Hall, K. and Sara, V. (1985). *In:* "The Physiological Development of the Fetus and Newborn", (Jones, C. T. and Nathanielsz, P. W. eds) pp. 97-102. Academic Press, London and Orlando.
66. Duncan, S. L. B. and Lewis, B. V. (1969). *J. Physiol.* **202**, 471-481.
67. Rosenfeld, C. R., Morriss, F. H., Makowski, E. L., Meschia, G. and Battaglia, F. C. (1974). *Gynecol. Invest.* **5**, 252-268.
68. Harding, J. E. (1982). D. Phil. Thesis, Oxford.
69. Gu, W., Jones, C. T. and Parer, J. T. (1985). *In:* "The Physiological Development of the Fetus and Newborn", (Jones, C. T. and Nathanielsz, P. W. eds) pp. 59-62. Academic Press, London and Orlando.
70. Potau, N., Ridor, E. and Ballabriga, A. (1981). *Pediat. Res.* **15**, 798-802.
71. Buster, J. E. and Marshall, J. R. (1979). *In:* "Endocrinology", Vol. 3, (DeGroot, L. J. *et al.* eds) pp. 1595-1612. Grune & Stratton, New York and London.
72. Grudzinskas, J. G., Teisner, B. and Seppala, M. (1982). "Pregnancy Proteins", Academic Press, New York and London.
73. Baden, H. P. (1975). *J. Nat. Cancer Inst.* **50**, 43-48.
74. Krieger, D. T., Liotta, A. S., Brownstein, M. J. and Zimmerman, E. A. (1980). *Rec. Prog. Horm. Res.* **36**, 277-336.
75. Roebuck, M. M., Jones, C. T., Holland, D. and Silman, R. (1980). *Nature* **284**, 616-618.
76. Gluckman, P. D., Kaplan, S. L., Rudolph, A. M. and Grumbach, M. M. (1979). *Endocrinology* **104**, 1828-1833.

Insulin-like Growth Factors in the Fetus

Peter D. Gluckman and John H. Butler

Developmental Physiology Laboratory, Department of Paediatrics,
University of Auckland, Auckland, New Zealand

In the recent past, considerable progress has been made in defining the role of the insulin-like growth factors (IGFs) in postnatal growth. It is now apparent that there are two major forms of IGF in the postnatal circulation; IGF-I which is also known as somatomedin C and IGF-II. Multiplication stimulating activity (MSA) is the rat homologue of IGF-II. Both restore growth in hypophysectomized rats, stimulate mitosis in a large number of cell lines in culture and are believed to mediate the effects of growth hormone (GH) on postnatal growth. IGF-I and IGF-II bind to distinct receptor molecules. Interest in the possible role of the IGFs in the fetus arose from early observations that bioassayable IGF concentrations in human umbilical blood showed a statistical relationship to birth size (1).

More recently with the clarification of the identity of the IGF peptides and the development of specific radioligand assays for IGF-I and IGF-II this relationship has been reexamined. A statistically significant positive correlation between birth weight and umbilical cord IGF-I levels in term infants was found using a radioimmunoassay for IGF-I (2). No relationship was found between birth size and IGF-II concentrations measured by the rat placental membrane assay. However IGF-II concentrations measured by this assay system were similar to those in adult sera whereas when cord blood IGF-II levels were measured by an immunoassay specific for IGF-II, low levels, approximately 30% of adult values, were reported (3,4). The discrepancy between these two assay systems raises the possibility that there is a second peptide in fetal blood that binds to the IGF-II receptor with high affinity but which is immunologically distinct from IGF-II. The possibility of a distinct fetal form of IGF has been suggested previously (5).

In the sheep, IGF-I concentrations in the fetus are low, and rise markedly

The Physiological Development of the Fetus and Newborn
ISBN 0 12 389080 2

Copyright © 1985 by Academic Press, London.
All rights of reproduction in any form reserved.

between 4 and 6 days after birth. This postnatal surge is followed by a decrease to adult values between 30 and 40 days after birth (6). IGF-I concentrations in midgestation are not affected by either decapitation or median eminence destruction which leads to very low GH concentrations (Fig. 1). There is a report in abstract form of low IGF-I levels in hypophysectomized fetuses but these were examined after normal term (7). We postulate that the postnatal rise in IGF-I levels is due to the appearance of hepatic somatotropic receptors 3–6 days after birth (8). The subsequent fall in IGF levels is postulated to be a consequence of the impairment of nutrition associated with the switch from monogastric to ruminant nutrition. If older lambs are fed a high nutrient diet, IGF-I levels rise to levels comparable to those measured in the postnatal surge, suggesting nutrient limitation is the cause for the fall in IGF-I after 40 days (9). Circulating IGF-I levels in the fetus are low and this may reflect the likelihood that IGF-I has primarily a paracrine function in the fetus (10).

In contrast IGF-II levels measured by receptor assays are markedly elevated in the fetal circulation from as early as 50 days of gestation. They remain high until 3 days prior to birth when they fall to reach adult values within 12 h after parturition (6). Parenthetically these observations point out the lack of value

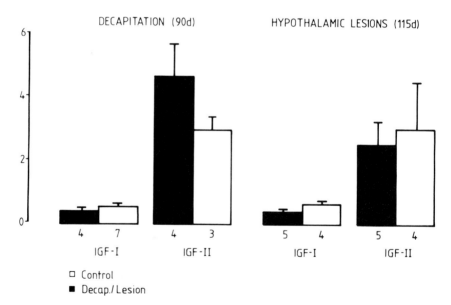

Figure 1. Left hand panels: Effect of fetal decapitation at 60 days of gestation. No significant effect was observed.

Right hand panels: The effect of median eminence destruction at 109 days of gestation on fetal IGF-I and IGF-II secretion at 115 days of gestation. The number of fetuses studied is shown under each bar. IGF-I concentrations are expressed in units/ml where 1 unit is equivalent to 31 ng of purified IGF-I (preparation I 3, Prof. R. Humbel). IGF-II concentrations are also expressed in units/ml where 1 unit is equivalent to 700 ng of purified IGF-II (preparation 16SPII, Prof. R. Humbel, Zurich).

of umbilical cord IGF-II measurement in assessing fetal IGF-II secretion. The very high levels of IGF-II-like activity in fetal sheep plasma (1932 ± 133 ng/ml, $n = 37$) argues against a purely paracrine role for the IGF-II like activity measured in fetal blood. Both *in vitro* and *in vivo* studies in the rat also support the concept that, in the fetus, IGF-II like peptides are the primary form of IGF secreted and that IGF-I becomes more important subsequently (11,12).

The high IGF-II levels in the fetal circulation falling prior to birth suggest that a pregnancy-related factor maintains fetal IGF-II secretion. While GH levels fall over a similar time course, fetal decapitation or median eminence lesions in midgestation do not affect fetal IGF-II levels (Fig. 1). Placental lactogen (PL) levels also fall with a similar time course (13) and there is a report that ovine PL stimulates fetal rat fibroblasts to secrete IGF-II *in vitro* whereas GH and prolactin do not (11). However, caution must be expressed when such a heterologous system is used. Recently we infused sheep fetuses with antiserum to oPL for periods of 72–144 h in late gestation. Excess antibody was present in the fetal circulation throughout the infusion but IGF-I and IGF-II levels were not affected (Gluckman, Butler and Waters unpublished observations). This suggests that oPL is not the factor maintaining IGF-II secretion *in utero* although further studies are warranted.

As fetal growth is, in contrast to postnatal growth, primarily determined by the supply of substrates, we have considered the possibility that substrate availability may directly or indirectly determine IGF-II secretion *in utero*. We studied 10 chronically instrumented fetuses at least 7 days postsurgery. The ewes were fasted totally, apart from access to water for 48 h, then administered intravenous glucose alone aiming to achieve a plasma glucose of 100 mg/100 ml for 4 h then returned to oral feeding. In the 3 fetuses less than 120 days of gestation, no significant effect of maternal starvation on fetal IGF-I or II was observed. However in the 7 older fetuses (126–135 days) maternal starvation led to a marked fall in IGF-II levels (Fig. 2). Four hours of intravenous glucose increased IGF-II levels to a value not different to the prestarvation value. There was no significant change in fetal or maternal oPL values during the experiment. The time course of the change in IGF-II values was paralleled by changed in fetal plasma insulin levels. Maternal glucose levels fell from 52.4 ± 3.2 mg/dl to 29.6 ± 2.4 mg/dl during the starvation and rose to 85.3 ± 8.9 mg/dl after 4 h of glucose infusion. These observations suggest that fetal IGF-II levels can be rapidly modulated by changes in maternal glucose concentrations. The mechanism of these changes remains to be resolved; they may be mediated by changes in fetal insulin although this requires direct evaluation. Fetal IGF-I levels did not fall during the period of starvation and did not rise during the period of fetal hyperglycaemia during the glucose infusion; however the duration of the hyperglycaemia was not long enough to evaluate this fully. There is previous evidence that chronic fetal hyperinsulinaemia in the pig increases bioassayable somatomedin levels (14) and this is a possible mechanism by which hyper-insulinaemia is associated with fetal overgrowth.

The major shifts in circulating fetal IGF-II concentrations in relation to changes in maternal nutrition argue for a role for IGF-II in mediating the effects of

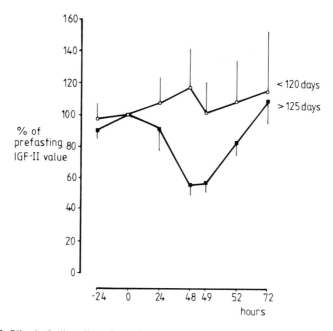

Figure 2. Effect of alterations in maternal nutrition on fetal IGF-II like activity. Ewes at least 7 days postsurgery were fasted for 48 h from 0 h. At 48 h the mother was infused with intravenous glucose (100 mg/min) for 24 h with oral feeding being introduced at 52 h. IGF-II concentrations are expressed as a percentage of the prefasting IGF-II concentrations. In fetuses less than 120 days of gestation ($n=3$) at the onset of the fast IGF-II values did not vary significantly during the experiment. In fetuses greater than 125 days of gestation ($n=7$), IGF-II levels were less ($P<0.01$) at the end of the fast but were restored to prefasting concentrations by 4 h of maternal glucose. Note that the scale on the abscissa is variable.

substrate availability on fetal growth. However there is as yet no direct evidence that IGF-II does affect fetal growth. It is of interest that the placenta is a rich source of IGF receptors, particularly IGF-II receptors (15), yet does not appear to synthesize IGFs (10). It is an intriguing possibility that fetal IGF-II secretion is altered directly or indirectly by changes in substrate availability and that a principal target organ is the placenta to alter either placental growth or function.

One further aspect of IGF secretion that merits consideration is that the molecular form of the IGF-binding protein complex differs in the fetus from that of the adult. In the adult, IGF-I and IGF-II circulate bound to large molecular proteins—this may provide a storage pool for the IGFs; it is not yet certain whether the IGF requires to be separated from the carrier proteins to be biologically active. In the postnatal sheep IGF-I circulates primarily as a 160 000 dalton complex. In the fetus, IGF-I circulates primarily as a 50 000 dalton complex, the 160 000 dalton complex not appearing until 3–6 days after birth. This may reflect the appearance of the hepatic GH receptor at this age (8) as the large molecular weight binding protein is known to be GH dependent in the adult (16). In the adult sheep IGF-II circulates primarily in a 50 000 dalton complex, and similarly in the fetus. However in the fetus we find a small percentage in a 200 000 dalton complex not seen in the adult. The significance of this is not clear, a similar finding is reported in the rat (17). The physiological significance of these changes in molecular form of circulating IGFs with development remains to be resolved—it is possible that they lead to altered bioavailability of IGFs to the tissues from the plasma pool.

Acknowledgements

These studies were supported by grants from the Medical Research Council of New Zealand and the National Children's Health Research Foundation.

References

1. Gluckman, P. D. and Brinsmead, M. W. (1976). *J. Clin. Endocrin. Metabn.* **43**, 1378-1381.
2. Gluckman, P. D., Johnson-Barrett, J. J., Butler, J. H., Edgar, B. W. and Gunn, T. R. (1983). *Clin. Endocrinol.* **19**, 405-413.
3. Bennett, A., Wilson, D. M., Liu, F., Nagashima, R., Rosenfeld, R. G. and Hintz, R. L. (1983). *J. Clin. Endocrin. Metab.* **57**, 609-612.
4. Zapf, J., Walter, H. and Froesch, E. R. (1981). *J. Clin. Invest.* **68**, 1321-1328.
5. Sara, V. R., Hall, K., Rodeck, C. H. and Wetterberg, L. (1981). *Proc. Nat. Acad. Sci. USA* **78**, 3175-3179.
6. Gluckman, P. D. and Butler, J. H. (1983). *J. Endocrinol.* **99**, 223-232.
7. Van Vliet, G., Styne, D. M., Kitterman, J. A., Rudolph, A. M., Kaplan, S. L. and Grumbach, M. M. (1982). *Endocrinology* **110**, 181A (Abstract).
8. Gluckman, P. D., Butler, J. H. and Elliott, T. B. (1983). *Endocrinology* **112**, 1607-1612.
9. Bass, J. J., Gluckman, P. D., Fairclough, R. I., Peterson, A. T. and Davis, S. R. (1983). *Proc. Endocrin. Soc. Aust.* **26** (Suppl. 2) **30**, (Abstract).
10. D'Ercole, A. J., Applewhite, S. T. and Underwood, L. (1980). *Develop. Biol.* **75**, 315-328.
11. Adams, S. O., Nissley, S. P., Kasuga, M., Foley, T. P. and Rechler, M. M. (1983). *Endocrinology* **112**, 971-978.
12. Daughaday, W. H., Parker, K. A., Borowsky, S., Trivedi, B. and Kapadia, M. (1982). *Endocrinology* **110**, 575-581.
13. Lowe, K. C., Gluckman, P. D., Jansen, A. M. and Nathanielsz, P. W. (1982). *J. Endocrinol.* **94**, 18P.
14. Spencer, G. S. G., Hill, D. J., Garssen, G. J., MacDonald, A. A. and Colenbrander, B. (1983). *J. Endocrinol.* **96**, 107-114.
15. Daughaday, W. H., Mariz, I. K. and Trivedi, B. (1981). *J. Clin. Endocrin. Metab.* **53**, 282-288.
16. Moses, A. C., Nissley, S. P., Cohlen, K. C. and Rechler, M. M. (1976). *Nature* **263**, 137-140.
17. White, R. M., Nissley, S. P., Short, P. A., Rechler, M. M. and Fennoy, I. (1982). *J. Clin. Invest.* **69**, 1239-1252.

Rock Valley College - ERC

Milk Growth Factors: Concentrations in Human Milk and Effects of Premature Birth

Leanna C. Read, Geoffrey L. Francis and F. John Ballard

Division of Human Nutrition, CSIRO (Australia),
Adelaide, South Australia, Australia

Abstract

We have measured EGF and insulin in milk from mothers of full-term and premature infants to determine whether the concentrations of these milk growth factors are changed following premature birth. Compared with women delivering at term, mothers of premature infants produced milk containing higher concentrations of EGF. This effect was probably maintained throughout lactation and may represent a maternal compensatory response to accelerate growth and development in the premature infant. In contrast, the insulin concentration in milk was transiently diminished during the early stages of lactation following premature birth, an effect which is unlikely to be related to neonatal development.

Introduction

Recent studies showing that human milk is a rich source of growth factors have led to the hypothesis that these factors play an important role in neonatal growth and tissue maturation (1,6). This role may be particularly important in premature infants where many tissues are immature at birth and gut closure is delayed (3).

In a previous study, we measured high concentrations of insulin and epidermal growth factor (EGF) in milk from mothers of full-term infants. Since the concentrations of several milk components are modified by premature delivery (1), possibly as a compensatory response, we have now measured the concentrations of insulin and EGF in milk from mothers of premature infants to determine whether these modifications include changes in milk growth factor

The Physiological Development of the Fetus and Newborn
ISBN 0 12 389080 2
Copyright © 1985 by Academic Press, London.
All rights of reproduction in any form reserved.

concentrations. EGF and insulin concentrations were also determined in commercial cow's milk-based formulae which are fed to premature infants.

Experimental

Milk samples were collected during the first 6 weeks of lactation from mothers of premature (26–36 weeks) and full-term infants (38–42 weeks) and treated to obtain the fat-free infranatants by procedures which have been described previously (6). Cow's milk-based formulae (Nan, Lactogen, De-Lact and S-26 brands) were prepared according to the manufacturers' directions and treated identically to milk samples. Methods for measurement of the concentrations of insulin (radioimmunoassay) and EGF (radioreceptor assay) in milk have been reported previously (6).

Results

Table 1 shows that human milk contained a very high concentration of EGF on day 1 of lactation. The concentration fell rapidly during the next few days and then stabilized at approximately 10–20% of that in day 1 milk. Throughout lactation, milk from mothers of premature infants contained a higher concentration of EGF than did milk from women delivering at term. Regression analysis showed that this effect was not significant on the first ($r = -0.26$, $P = 0.16$) or second day ($r = -0.26$, $P = 0.24$) of lactation but thereafter, gestational age correlated strongly with the EGF concentration in milk (days 5–8: $r = -0.53$, $P < 0.001$; days 21–42: $r = -0.67$, $P < 0.001$). The correlation was strongest in milk expressed on days 21–42, milk from mothers of very premature babies containing approximately 300% of the EGF in milk from mothers of term infants. This increased EGF concentration was not associated with a general enrichment of milk components since protein concentrations in milk infranatants were not affected by premature birth (results not shown) and insulin concentrations were depressed (see below).

Insulin concentrations were highest in day 1 milk, falling to a stable concentration during the first week of lactation (Table 1). In contrast to the effects on EGF, premature birth was associated with a pronounced diminution in the insulin content of milk during the first two days of lactation (day 1: $r = +0.40$, $P = 0.022$; day 2: $r = +0.53$, $P = 0.002$). Thereafter, the insulin concentration was similar in milk from mothers of term and premature infants (days 5–8: $r = +0.01$, $P = 0.53$; days 21–42: $r = +0.24$, $P = 0.19$).

Cow's milk-based formulae contained less than 5% of the insulin and EGF concentrations in human milk, with mean concentrations in the four brands of 0.015 ± 0.002 nmol insulin and 0.43 ± 0.04 nmol EGF ($n = 24$).

Discussion

The concentrations of insulin and EGF in human milk exceed those in adult serum (8) by many fold, indicating that the suckled infant ingests large amounts of growth factors. This suggests that milk-derived growth factors play an important

Table 1. Concentrations of EGF and insulin in human milk

	Day 1			Day 2			Day 5–8			Day 21–42		
	T	P	VP	T	P	VP	T	P	VP	T	P	VP
EGF												
nmol	53±7	71±15	79±13	28±6	30±5	35±6	10±3	14±1	22±5	5±0.4	9±2	16±6
n	17	9	6	12	9	9	9	17	10	17	8	6
sig.		ns			ns			*			*	
Insulin												
nmol	3.8±0.9	1.3±0.3	0.6±0.2	1.6±0.4	0.6±0.1	0.6±0.1	0.5±0.1	0.4±0.1	0.4±0.1	0.5±0.1	0.3±0.1	0.4±0.1
n	18	9	6	7	10	9	7	14	10	18	8	6
sig.		+			+			ns			ns	

Data are mean±SEM. T = birth at 38–42 weeks, P = 31–36 weeks, VP = 26–30 weeks.
Significance: significant ($P < 0.05$) negative (*) or positive (+) correlation with gestational age, using simple linear regressional analysis. ns = non-significant.
Correlation coefficients and probability values are given in the text.

role in neonatal development, particularly EGF which is present in human milk at 100 to 1000-fold the serum level. Such a role would require that sufficient amounts of growth factors survive digestion, cross the intestinal wall intact and reach responsive tissues in biologically active form. There is some evidence that these conditions apply for EGF. Milk probably provides the major source of EGF to the suckled human infant because endogenous production appears very low in the neonate (8). Thornburg *et al.* (10) have provided evidence that EGF reaches the small intestine intact in the newborn rat and biological activity has been observed following oral administration to neonatal mice (4). This suggests that a significant proportion can enter the newborn's circulation in biologically active form. Furthermore, EGF is known to stimulate the maturation of a number of crucial tissues such as gut, lung and liver (7,9). Taken together, this evidence suggests that milk-derived EGF may accelerate growth and maturation in the newborn. Although insulin probably also survives digestion and reaches the neonatal circulation intact, it seems unlikely that milk provides an important source of insulin to the infant because the concentration in serum is already high at birth (5). This may not exclude a role in intestinal maturation where insulin could act topically (7).

We have found that human milk contains significantly more EGF following premature birth, an effect that is probably sustained throughout lactation. Other evidence suggests that in premature infants, the intestine is permeable to whole proteins for longer periods and growth factor-responsive tissues such as the lung and intestine are very immature (7,9). Thus, milk-derived EGF may be particularly important to the pre-term infant due to the combined effects of an increased concentration in milk, enhanced uptake into the circulation and a greater sensitivity of target tissues. The lowered insulin content of milk may have less significance to the premature newborn because the effect is apparent only during the first 2 days of lactation when milk consumption is low. Furthermore, it is unlikely to affect concentrations of insulin in the serum of premature infants because endogenous production is already high at birth (5). It is possible that the insulin concentration in milk is depressed for reasons unrelated to neonatal growth. For example, it may reflect hormonal changes associated with a stressful birth since most of the premature infants were delivered by caesarian section.

Cow's milk-based formulae contained very low concentrations of both insulin and EGF. Furthermore, studies in cultured cells have suggested that these formulae also lack other growth factors present in human milk (results not shown). If milk-derived growth factors are able to stimulate neonatal development, our findings suggest that there are considerable advantages in feeding infants their own mother's milk rather than pooled human milk or formulae, particularly following premature birth.

Although the results of this and other studies support a role for milk-derived growth factors in neonatal development, verification of this hypothesis requires direct measurement of intestinal uptake and biological activities of orally administered growth factors in the newborn. We are currently testing this using neonatal rabbits.

Acknowledgements

This work was supported in part by the Rural Credits Development Fund. We wish to thank Jamie McNeil and Faye Upton for technical assistance.

References

1. Anderson, G. H. and Bryan, M. H. (1982). *J. Paediatr. Gastro. Nutr.* **1**, 157–159.
2. Beardmore, J. M., Lewis-Jones, D. I. and Richards, R. C. (1983). *Pediat. Res.* **17**, 825–828.
3. Blum, P. H., Phelps, D. L., Ank, B. J., Krantman, H. J. and Stiehm, E. R. (1981). *Pediat. Res.* **15**, 1256–1260.
4. Cohen, S. and Taylor, J. M. (1974). *Rec. Prog. Horm. Res.* **30**, 533–550.
5. Cowett, R. M., Oh, W. and Schwartz, R. (1983). *J. Clin. Invest.* **71**, 467–475.
6. Read, L. C., Upton, F. M., Francis, G. L., Wallace, J. C., Dahlenburg, G. W. and Ballard, F. J. (1984). *Pediat. Res.* **18**, 133–139.
7. Simon, P. M., Kedinger, M., Raul, F., Frenier, J. F. and Haffen, K. (1982). *In Vitro* **18**, 339–346.
8. Starkey, R. H. and Orth, D. N. (1977). *J. Clin. Endocrin. Metab.* **45**, 1144–1153.
9. Sundell, H. W., Gray, M. E., Serenius, F. S., Escobedo, M. B. and Stahlman, M. T. (1980). *Am. J. Pathol.* **100**, 707–726.
10. Thornburg, W., Matrisien, L., Magun, B. and Koldovsky, O. (1984). *Am. J. Physiol.* **246**, G80–G85.

Effect of Restricted Placental Growth upon Oxygen and Glucose Delivery to the Fetus

Julie A. Owens, Elizabeth Allotta,
John Falconer and Jeffrey S. Robinson

Faculty of Medicine, University of Newcastle,
Shortland, New South Wales, Australia

Summary

Endometrial caruncles was excised from sheep (caruncle sheep) before pregnancy. The effect of this on oxygen and glucose delivery to, and consumption by, the pregnant uterus and fetus in a subsequent pregnancy was examined. Eight caruncle and 5 control sheep with indwelling vascular catheters were studied at 121 and 130 days of pregnancy. Total uterine weight, fetal weight and placental weight were significantly lower in caruncle sheep than in controls. Both oxygen and glucose delivery to the pregnant uterus decreased with uterine weight. Fetal umbilical vein PO_2 and glucose concentration were significantly lower in the caruncle fetus as were oxygen and glucose delivery to the fetus when compared to controls. Fetal oxygen and glucose consumption were also significantly lower in caruncle sheep than in controls. However, fetal extraction of oxygen and glucose was significantly higher in caruncle sheep.

It is concluded that intra-uterine growth retardation (IUGR) following restriction of placental growth is associated with a reduced supply of oxygen and glucose to both the pregnant uterus and fetus. In addition, the greater fetal extraction of oxygen, and in particular glucose, suggests a smaller margin of safety exists between supply and consumption in IUGR.

Introduction

Intra-uterine growth retardation (IUGR) in man and other species is characterized by hypoglycaemia, hypoxaemia and polycythaemia (1,2). This implicates altered

The Physiological Development of the Fetus and Newborn
ISBN 0 12 389080 2
Copyright © 1985 by Academic Press, London.
All rights of reproduction in any form reserved.

placental exchange of substances, particularly of oxygen and the major fetal substrate, glucose, in the development of IUGR. Restriction of placental growth resulting in IUGR can be produced in sheep by the excision of endometrial caruncles before pregnancy. The aim of the present study was to assess the effect of this upon delivery of oxygen and glucose to, and consumption by the pregnant uterus and fetus.

Materials and Methods

Thirteen Border Leicester-Merino cross-bred sheep were used. Eight ewes were operated on before pregnancy and endometrial caruncles removed as previously described (2). All surgical procedures were carried out with strict aseptic and antiseptic procedures. In 5 control and 6 caruncle ewes, the fetal femoral artery, common umbilical and tarsal vein and in the remainder, the fetal jugular vein and carotid artery were catheterized (2,3). Maternal jugular vein, carotid and femoral arteries and utero-ovarian vein were also catheterized (2). A minimum of 10 days after surgery was allowed for recovery. Experiments were carried out at 120.6 (SD 1.7) and 130.1 (SD 1.9) days gestation. One day after the second experiment, at 131.1 (SD 3.6) days, ewes were sacrificed and fetal, placental and uterine weights recorded. Umbilical and/or uterine blood flows were measured simultaneously by the steady transplacental diffusion technique (4) 6 times during each experiment and the mean values calculated. Blood pH, PCO_2 and PO_2 were measured using a Corning 168 pH/Blood gas system with automatic corrections for temperature (to $39°C$). Oxygen saturation and haemoglobin concentration were measured using a Radiometer OSM2 Hemoximeter and and used to calculate blood oxygen contents. Haematocrits were measured in duplicate for each sample. Plasma glucose concentrations were assayed in triplicate for each sample using glucose oxidase. Arterial or venous concentrations together with uterine or umbilical blood flow rates were used to calculate delivery rates to the pregnant uterus or fetus. Arteriovenous concentration differences together with uterine or umbilical blood flow rates were used to calculate consumption rates by the pregnant uterus or fetus.

Results and Discussion

Total uterine weight ($P < 0.001$), fetal weight ($P < 0.025$) and placental weight ($P < 0.005$) were significantly lower in caruncle sheep compared to controls, as previously reported (5). Both oxygen ($r = 0.70$, $P < 0.025$, $n = 10$) and glucose ($r = 0.65$, $P < 0.025$, $n = 7$) consumption by the uterus at 121 days decreased with uterine weight.

As shown in Tables 1 and 2, fetal umbilical vein PO_2 and glucose concentration were significantly lower in the caruncle fetus at both gestational ages. Similarly, both fetal oxygen and glucose delivery to the caruncle fetus were markedly decreased compared to that in controls. Fetal oxygen and glucose consumption were also significantly lower in caruncle sheep compared to controls. However, fetal extraction of oxygen and glucose was significantly higher in

Table 1. Oxygen delivery to and consumption by the fetus in control and caruncle sheep[1-3]

	Control (n)	Caruncle (n)	
Umbilical vein PO$_2$ (mmHg)			
121 days	39.5±4.0(5)	29.8±2.7(6)	P<0.0005
130 days	36.8±2.8(3)	31.4±8.1(6)	P<0.025
Oxygen delivery (mmol/min)			
121 days	3.561±0.983(5)	1.813±0.383(6)	P<0.0025
130 days	4.547±0.2392(3)	1.894±0.665(6)	P<0.025
Oxygen consumption (mmol/min)			
121 days	0.944±0.275(5)	0.643±0.119(6)	P<0.025
130 days	1.208±0.488(3)	0.748±0.215(6)	P<0.05
Oxygen extraction			
121 days	0.296±0.138(5)	0.356±0.062(6)	P<0.025
130 days	0.280±0.037(3)	0.438±0.113(6)	P<0.05

[1]Mean ± standard deviation
[2]Caruncle, carunclectomized sheep
[3]Controls compared to caruncles, unpaired t test

Table 2. Glucose delivery to and consumption by the fetus in control and caruncle sheep[1-3]

	Control (n)	Caruncle (n)	
Umbilical vein [glucose] (μmol/ml)			
121 days	1.057±0.071(3)	0.742±0.248(5)	P<0.05
130 days	1.192±0.203(3)	0.822±0.63(5)	P<0.05
Glucose delivery (mmol/min)			
121 days	0.753±0.079(3)	0.290±0.129(5)	P<0.001
130 days	1.000±0.298(3)	0.347±0.154(5)	P<0.005
Glucose consumption (mmol/min)			
121 days	0.0902±0.007(3)	0.0614±0.024(5)	P<0.05
130 days	0.102±0.015(3)	0.0616±0.024(5)	P<0.025
Glucose extraction			
121 days	0.133±0.016(3)	0.234±0.107(5)	P<0.05
130 days	0.124±0.032(3)	0.208±0.115(5)	P<0.05

[1]Mean ± standard deviation
[2]Caruncle, carunclectomized sheep
[3]Controls compared to caruncles, unpaired t test

caruncle sheep. This study has demonstrated that fetal growth retardation following restriction of placental growth, characterized by chronic fetal hypoxaemia and hypoglycaemia, is associated with a reduced delivery of oxygen and glucose to both the pregnant uterus and fetus. Moreover, fetal extraction of oxygen and particularly glucose is increased, suggesting a smaller margin of safety exists between supply and consumption in IUGR.

References

1. Robinson, J. S. (1979). *Br. Med. Bull.* **35**, 137–144.
2. Robinson, J. S., Kingston, E. J., Jones, C. T. and Thorburn, G. D. (1979). *J. Develop. Physiol.* **1**, 379–398.
3. Young, W. G., Creasy, D. R. and Rudolph, A. M. (1974). *J. Appl. Physiol.* **37**, 620–621.
4. Meschia, G., Cotter, J. R., Meakowski, E. L. and Barron, D. H. (1966). *Q. J. Exp. Physiol.* **52**, 1–18.
5. Owens, J. A., Alotta, E., Falconer, J. and Robinson, J. S. (1985). *In:* "The Physiological Development of the Fetus and Newborn" (Jones, C. T. and Nathanielsz, P. W. eds) pp. 51–54, Academic Press, London and Orlando.

Renal Metabolism in Fetal and Newborn Sheep

Harriet S. Iwamoto, William Oh and Abraham M. Rudolph

Departments of Pediatrics, Physiology, and Obstetrics, Gynecology,
and Reproductive Sciences, and the Cardiovascular Research Institute,
University of California, San Francisco, California
and Department of Pediatrics, Brown University,
Providence Rhode Island, USA

Introduction

The transition from pre- to postnatal life is associated with an increase in metabolic requirements such as an increase in total body and myocardial oxygen consumption (1,2). Following the removal of the placenta from circulation, the kidney must assume fluid regulatory and excretory functions. It might be expected that renal consumption of oxygen and substrates increases after birth. To examine renal metabolism and oxygen consumption we have developed a method of sampling renal venous blood from chronically maintained preparations of sheep (3) and we have used this method to measure arteriovenous concentration differences of oxygen and various potential substrates of renal metabolism in fetal and newborn sheep.

Methods

A total of 11 fetal sheep (123–133 days gestation) and 8 newborn lambs (5–6 days old) were used in these studies. Aseptic procedures were used to place polyvinyl catheters in the descending aorta, inferior vena cava, left renal vein and urinary bladder as previously described (3). At least 4 days were allowed for recovery from the surgical procedures. Blood samples from the descending aorta and renal vein were obtained simultaneously for the determination of pH, blood gases, oxygen content, glucose and lactate, and in newborn lambs of β-hydroxybutyrate and α-amino nitrogen. Renal blood flow was determined in the

The Physiological Development of the Fetus and Newborn
ISBN 0 12 389080 2

Copyright © 1985 by Academic Press, London.
All rights of reproduction in any form reserved.

fetal sheep by the radionuclide-labelled microsphere technique, and in the newborn lambs, by measuring renal extraction of ^{14}C-inulin and applying the Fick principle using Wolf's equation (4).

Results

All animals included in these studies were in good health and had total body and kidney weights, arterial pH and blood gas values within the range previously reported (1,2,5). Renal blood flow and arterial oxygen content were greater in newborn lambs than in the fetal sheep (Table 1). Oxygen delivery to the newborn kidney, calculated as arterial oxygen content times renal blood flow, was 5–7 times that to the fetal kidney. Despite this greater oxygen delivery rate to the newborn kidney, it extracted a larger amount of oxygen. Consequently, the amount of oxygen consumed by the newborn kidney was much greater than the amount consumed by the fetal kidney.

Table 1. Renal blood flow, oxygen delivery and oxygen consumption in fetal and newborn sheep

	Fetus	Newborn
Renal blood flow		
ml/min	44±3	162±12
ml/min/100 g	154±9	406±32
Oxygen content mmol		
Descending aorta	2.71±0.18	5.48±0.14
Renal vein	2.04±0.17	3.61±0.19
Oxygen delivery		
μmol/min	121±12	881±47
μmol/min/100 g	418±38	2231±127
Oxygen extraction (%)	25±2	35±3
Oxygen consumption		
μmol/min	30±3	312±31
μmol/min/100 g	104±10	785±79

Values are expressed as mean±SEM

Arterial glucose concentrations were greater and lactate concentrations were lower in newborn lambs than in the fetal sheep (Table 2). In 9 of 11 fetuses and in 4 of 8 newborn lambs there was a net negative arteriovenous concentration difference for glucose across the kidney indicating glucose production by the kidney. There was a consistent positive arteriovenous difference for lactate across the fetal renal circulation indicating net lactate consumption. The lactate–oxygen quotient, an indication of the maximum amount of oxygen consumed to oxidize lactate to carbon dioxide and water, was 54±11% in the fetuses. There was no significant net flux of lactate or α-amino nitrogen across the kidney of the newborn lamb but there was net consumption of β-hydroxybutyrate by the newborn

Table 2. Glucose and lactate fluxes across the kidney in fetal and newborn sheep

	Fetus	Newborn
Glucose mmol		
Descending aorta	0.960 ± 0.090	6.00 ± 0.175
Renal vein	0.984 ± 0.098	6.10 ± 0.207
A-V	-0.024 ± 0.011	-0.10 ± 0.07
Flux μmol/min	$-0.947 \pm 0.420^{*}$	-27 ± 16
μmol/min/100 g	$-3.67 \pm 1.57^{*}$	-65 ± 41
Lactate mmol		
Descending aorta	1.42 ± 0.12	0.866 ± 0.037
Renal vein	1.31 ± 0.11	0.807 ± 0.035
A-V	$0.12 \pm 0.024^{*}$	0.059 ± 0.027
Flux μmol/min	$5.35 \pm 1.46^{*}$	8.375 ± 4.99
μmol/min/100 g	$18.1 \pm 4.1^{*}$	19.94 ± 13.07

Values are expressed as Mean $\pm$ SEM.
Flux represents the arteriovenous concentration difference times renal blood flow.
$^{*}P < 0.05$ significantly different from zero as assessed by paired t test.

kidney. The amount of β-hydroxybutyrate consumed, 7.7 ± 1.1 μmol/min or 19.6 ± 2.8 μmol/min/100 g could account for $13 \pm 1.8\%$ of the oxidative metabolic rate.

Discussion

Among the important changes that occur at birth are the removal of the placenta from the circulation and the assumption by the kidney of fluid regulatory and excretory functions. The increase in blood flow coupled with an increase in arterial oxygen content resulted in an increase in oxygen delivery to the kidney after birth. Renal oxygen extraction was greater in the newborn kidney and there was a marked increase in oxygen consumption by the newborn kidney relative to the fetal kidney. This increase in oxygen consumption after birth probably reflects the increase in renal function after birth. Using data reported previously by others (5,6) the amount of sodium filtered by the fetal kidney at 120–130 days gestation is approximately 250 μEq/min. Of this sodium 93–95% or 230–240 μEq/min is reabsorbed. In the newborn lambs in the present study, sodium reabsorption was 99.8% and 2300 μEq of sodium was reabsorbed per min. Since sodium reabsorption represents a major portion of renal tubular activity, this difference in sodium reabsorption could account for the difference in oxygen consumption rates at the different stages of development. A similar correlation between sodium reabsorption and oxygen consumption has been previously reported (7). The increase in renal oxygen consumption may be due to changes in regional distribution of blood flow. At birth blood flow to the outer cortex increases markedly while blood flow to the juxtamedullary cortex remains the same (8). Since there are regional differences in renal metabolism (10), these changes in regional blood flow and filtration may alter overall renal metabolism.

At most, half of the oxygen consumption rate of the fetal kidney can be accounted for by the oxidation of lactate to carbon dioxide and water. Other possible substrates are amino acids, which provide the fetus with 25% of its total fuel requirement (11), as well as glycerol, pyruvate or ketone bodies, none of which were measured in these studies.

The newborn kidney consumed β-hydroxybutyrate at a rate which could account for 13% of the oxygen consumption rate. This finding contrasts with the results of Levitsky *et al.* (12) in their studies of neonatal baboons; however species differences relative to ketone body metabolism could account for this discrepancy.

We have presented evidence that the kidney of the fetal and newborn lamb can produce glucose under basal conditions. The source of the glucose could be a result of either glycogen breakdown or gluconeogenesis. The kidneys of developing lambs do store glycogen (13) but the amount stored is probably inadequate to account for the amount of glucose released under basal conditions. Gluconeogenesis is a more likely source of glucose since the enzymes necessary for gluconeogenesis are present during the last trimester of gestation (14). Although significant gluconeogenesis from either lactate or alanine has not been unequivocally determined, it is possible that measurements of total glucose turnover in previous studies would not have demonstrated the small amount of glucose produced by the kidneys. Gluconeogenesis has been reported to occur in the neonatal baboon kidney and in adult sheep (11,15) and in preliminary studies we have demonstrated gluconeogenesis from ^{14}C-lactate in late gestation fetal sheep. The glucose formed may be used by the rest of the body or may be used by the kidney itself.

References

1. Fisher, D. J., Heymann, M. A. and Rudolph, A. M. (1981). *Pediat. Res.* **15**, 843–846.
2. Fisher, D. J., Heymann, M. A. and Rudolph, A. M. (1980). *Am. J. Physiol.* **238**, H399–H405.
3. Iwamoto, H. S. and Rudolph, A. M. (1983). *Am. J. Physiol.* **245**, H524–H527.
4. Wolf, A. V. (1941). *Am. J. Physiol.* **133**, 496–497.
5. Robillard, J. E., Sessions, C., Kennedy, R. L., Hamel-Robillard, L. and Smith, F. G. Jr. (1977). *Am. J. Obstet. Gynecol.* **128**, 727–734.
6. Lumbers, E. R. (1983). *J. Develop. Physiol.* **6**, 1–10.
7. Elinder, G. and Aperia, A. (1982). *Pediat. Res.* **16**, 351–353.
8. Aperia, A., Broberger, O., Herin, P. and Joelsson, I. (1977). *Acta Physiol. Scand.* **99**, 261–269.
9. Aperia, A., Broberger, O. and Herin, P. (1974). *Pediat. Res.* **8**, 758–765.
10. McCann, W. P. (1962). *Am. J. Physiol.* **203**, 572–576.
11. Gresham, E. L., James, E. J., Raye, J. R., Battaglia, F. C., Makowski, E. L. and Meschia, G. (1972). *Pediatrics* **50**, 372–379.
12. Levitsky, L. L., Paton, J. B., Fisher, D. E. and Delannoy, C. W. (1980). *Pediat. Res.* **14**, 926–932.
13. Shelley, H. J. (1961). *Br. Med. J.* **17**, 137–143.
14. Stevenson, R. E., Morriss, F. J., Adcock, E. W. III and Howell, R. R. (1976). *Develop. Biol.* **52**, 167–172.
15. Kaufman, C. F. and Bergman, E. N. (1971). *Am. J. Physiol.* **221**, 967–972.

Perinatal Organ Development in Rat and Spiny Mouse: its Relation to Altricial and Precocial Timing of Birth

W. H. Lamers, P. G. Mooren, A. de Graaf,
A. Markiewicz and R. Charles

Department of Anatomy and Embryology,
University of Amsterdam, Amsterdam, The Netherlands

The enzymic development of organs in the rat that are derived from the embryonic gut is characterized by a so-called perinatal cluster of enzymes with elevated activities in the perinatal period and by a so called (pre)weaning cluster of enzymes that show steeply rising activities in the 3rd and 4th postnatal week (1). The common developmental profiles that are defined by clusters point to a common control mechanism.

Experiments that were aimed at the elucidation of these control mechanisms have generally involved the manipulation of the hormonal or nutritional status of the animals or the explanation of organ segments, and have identified glucocorticosteroid hormone, cyclic AMP and to a lesser extent thyroid hormone as the main modulating factors of organotypic gene expression (2). However, these modulating effects of hormones are probably superimposed upon an inherent developmental program (3,4).

Rat fetuses start to prepare for birth biochemically and physiologically as soon as organogenesis is completed (day 16 *post coitum*), thus providing a clear example of an altricial mode of development. In contrast, a precocial mode of development is characterized by a relatively long interval between the completion of organogenesis and the moment of birth. In order to be able to further elucidate and analyse the factors that control the level and extent of organotypic gene expression in the fetal and neonatal period, it could be very advantageous to complement the altricial "rat model" with a model exhibiting the characteristics of precocial mode of development. Ideally this "model" species should be closely related to the rat and differ in the developmental timing of birth only.

The Physiological Development of the Fetus and Newborn
ISBN 0 12 389080 2
Copyright © 1985 by Academic Press, London.
All rights of reproduction in any form reserved.

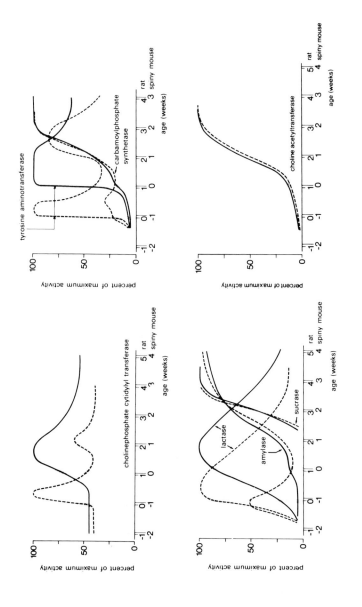

Figure 1. Developmental profiles of rat (– – –) and spiny mouse (———) organotypic enzymes in lung (a), liver (b), small intestine and pancreas (c) and cerebrum (d). On the horizontal axis, the ages for both species have been aligned so that the developmental stages match (6). 0 indicates birth.

The spiny mouse, *Acomys cahirinus*, seems to meet this requirement, having a long gestation period (39 days), associated with small (2-4) litter size. Organogenesis proceeds somewhat slower in this species than in the rat, requiring 1 additional week to be completed (5). The neonates shows an advanced stage of development, having a fur coat, open eyes and ears and are capable of locomotion and thermoregulation. Self-feeding begins a few days after birth.

The rat has developed to a comparable extent in the middle of the 2nd and 3rd postnatal week respectively. The late intra-uterine developmental stages of the spiny mouse therefore seem comparable to the early extra-uterine developmental stages of the rat (5,6). Comparison of the developmental profiles of the rat and spiny mouse organotypic enzymes may therefore answer the question to what extent the developmental profiles are related to the developmental timing of birth. Furthermore, the assessment of the effects of hormonal treatment on enzyme levels in the late fetal period may show whether the incomplete induction of organotypic gene expression by hormones that is seen in fetal rats (2) has a developmental or an environmental basis. To address these questions we have studied the development of surfactant synthesis in the lung, gluconeogenesis and ureagenesis in the liver, carbohydrate hydrolysis in the small intestine and pancreas and neurotransmittor synthesis in the brain. The examples shown in Fig. 1 were selected because they most clearly demonstrate the spectrum of developmental behaviour that was observed.

Inspection of Fig. 1 shows that all organ-specific enzyme activities become detectable by the standard enzyme assays at approximately 12 days before birth in the spiny mouse and approximately 4 days before birth in the rat, i.e. at the same developmental timepoint shortly after the completion of organogenesis. This developmental landmark was coined the secondary transition, i.e. from the protodifferentiated to the differentiated, mature state in which enzyme synthesis can be modulated by hormones (7). Subsequently 2 types of developmental profiles were seen in both rat and spiny mouse (cf: 1): those of enzymes that attain their developmental maximum shortly after birth (cholinephosphate cytidylyl transferase, tyrosine aminotransferase and lactase) and those of enzymes that attain their developmental maximum at weaning (carbamoylphosphate synthetase, amylase, sucrase, choline acetyltransferase). While the maximum of the perinatal phase of enzymic profiles is dictated by the developmental timing of birth (and associated hormonal adaptation) and therefore lies 7-8 developmental days apart in rat and spiny mouse, the surge of the weaning phase of enzymic profiles may again express an inherent biological program (with additional, superimposed hormonal modulation) because the developmental profiles of organotypic enzyme coincide during this period in both species. The main difference between rat and spiny mouse therefore resides in the different developmental timing of birth, resulting in well-separated perinatal and weaning phases of enzymic profiles in the rat and merged perinatal and weaning phases in the spiny mouse due to a "delayed" occurrence of birth.

The observation that the development of the microscopic anatomy of the organs that were studied (e.g. the development of alveolar septa, crypts of Lieberkühn and biliary tree) proceeds independent of the process of birth and reflects the altricial or precocial condition at birth, suggests that morphogenesis and functional maturation are not tightly coupled. However, closer observation of Fig. 1 shows that there are no birth-associated changes in the developmental profile of choline acetyltransferase in the brain. This, and in fact the mere presence of recognizable altricial and precocial modes of development, show that the co-ordination between morphogenesis and functional maturation in the neurectoderm is much tighter than in the endoderm from which lung, liver, small intestine and pancreas are derived.

The previous discussion raises the question of the regulatory factors involved in establishment of the respective enzymic profiles. As far as tested no difference in the hormonal regulation of the rate of gene expression was found between rat and spiny mouse. However, despite the more advanced state of morphological development of organs in the spiny mouse at birth, it was found that the inducibility of organotypic gene expression by hormones was as limited as in rat fetuses (up to approximately 30% of the maximally attainable levels immediately after birth). This observation suggests that the conditions of the intra-uterine milieu rather than the more or less advanced state of development of the respective parenchymal cells are responsible for the relative failure of this "hormone therapy".

The simultaneous presence within one taxonomic group of altricial and precocial patterns of development is extremely rare, and offers a good opportunity for a comparative approach of the analysis of regulatory factors of perinatal adaptation. In particular, this comparison may shed more light on the human condition that exhibits an altricial (rat-like) mode of development for the neurectoderm-derived organs and a precocial (spiny mouse-like) mode of development for the endoderm-derived organs. As mentioned above the evidence points to exogenous factors that control perinatal adaptation. The blood insulin/glucagon ratio, that determines the cyclic AMP content of many organs, decreases around birth in both species but the change is far less pronounced in the spiny mouse. Triiodothyronine levels that increase only in the 2nd postnatal week in the rat, show a surge immediately after birth in the spiny mouse. In both cases the developmental profiles of the spiny mouse much more reflects the human condition than those of the rat, stressing its importance as a relevant model system. This is further underlined by the fact that cortisol has been identified as the circulating glucocorticosteroid hormone. A developmental profile of this hormone in the spiny mouse is currently being determined.

References

1. Greengard, O. (1970). *In:* "Biochemical Action of Hormones", Vol. 1 (Litwack, G., ed.) pp. 53–87. Academic Press, New York and London.
2. Lamers, W. H. and Mooren, P. G. (1981). *Mech. Ageing Dev.* **15**, 93–118.
3. Lamers, W. H. and Mooren, P. G. (1981). *Mech. Ageing Dev.* **15**, 77–92.
4. Lee, P. C. and Lenthal, E. (1983). *Pediat. Res.* **17**, 645–650.

5. Lamers, W. H., Mooren, P. G., Oosterhuis, W. P., Lunstroo, H. de Graaf, A. and Charles, R. (1982). *Adv. Exp. Med. Biol.* **153**, 229–240.
6. Oosterhuis, W. P., Mooren, P. G., Charles, R. and Lamers, W. H. (1984). *Biol. Neonate* **45**, 236–243.
7. Rutter, W. J., Kemp, J. D., Bradshaw, W. S., Clark, W. R., Ronzio R. A. and Sanders, T. G. (1968). *J. Cell Physiol.* **72** (suppl. 1) 1–18.

Influence of 2,3-Diphosphoglycerate (DPG) Concentration in Maternal Red Cells on the Transplacental Exchange of Respiratory Gases

Anthony M. Carter and Jørgen Grønlund

Department of Physiology, University of Odense, Denmark

One of the principal factors determining blood oxygen affinity is the intra-erythrocytic concentration of 2,3-diphosphoglycerate (DPG). Rigorous analysis of the part played by DPG in regulating placental gas exchange in late pregnancy is difficult, however, since human fetal blood contains 2 haemoglobins with different affinities for DPG, and the ratio between them is continuously changing. Ovine red cells lack DPG and the sheep is therefore unsuitable for experimental or theoretical studies. In contrast, the guinea-pig offers a well-defined system: mother and fetus share the same haemoglobin and differences in the oxygen affinity and co-operativity of the haemoglobin molecule are largely due to the lower DPG concentration of fetal blood.

We have developed a model of placental gas exchange in the guinea-pig that is able to predict the pH, PCO_2, PO_2 and SO_2 of umbilical venous blood, and the oxygen and carbon dioxide fluxes across the placenta, from a set of input variables that readily can be obtained experimentally (2). To investigate the influence of varying maternal DPG levels on fetal oxygenation, we used this model to simulate a progressive reduction from the normal value of 7 mmol to 2 mmol. The model requires a value for the intra-erythrocytic DPG concentration of fetal guinea-pig blood. This was obtained experimentally, as there was a large discrepancy between previously published values (1,4).

Determination of DPG

One ml blood samples were obtained by umbilical venous puncture from 13 guinea-pig fetuses near term of pregnancy (mean weight $\pm SD = 87.9 \pm 12.3$ g).

The Physiological Development of the Fetus and Newborn
ISBN 0 12 389080 2

Copyright © 1985 by Academic Press, London.
All rights of reproduction in any form reserved.

A blood sample was also taken from each of the 5 dams. Haemoglobin was measured as cyanmethaemoglobin. Haematocrit was determined with a microhaematocrit centrifuge, applying a correction of 2% for trapped plasma. An 0.5 ml aliquot of blood was deproteinized with ice-cooled perchloracetic acid and centrifuged. The supernatant was neutralized and centrifuged and the new supernatant was stored at $-80°C$ until analysed. DPG concentrations were measured in triplicate using a commercial kit (Boehringer Mannheim). The results are given in Table 1.

Table 1. Haemoglobin, haematocrit and intra-erythrocytic DPG concentrations in guinea-pig dams and their fetuses

	Fetal blood	Maternal blood
No. samples	13	5
Haemoglobin mmol/l	2.20 ± 0.12	1.98 ± 0.09
Haematocrit	0.41 ± 0.02	0.38 ± 0.02
DPG mol/mol Hb	0.26 ± 0.05	1.28 ± 0.10

Values are means $\pm$ SD

The mean fetal intra-erythrocytic DPG concentration of 0.26 ± 0.05 mol/mol haemoglobin (tetramere) is in good agreement with the value of 0.33 ± 0.12 mol/mol obtained by Bard and Shapiro (1). The lower value of 0.14 ± 0.06 mol/mol reported by Jelkmann and Bauer (4) has therefore been disregarded.

Model Considerations

The blood chemistry of the guinea-pig resembles that of man in important respects, including the standard haemoglobin oxygen dissociation curve, the ratio of intracellular to extracellular pH, the Bohr coefficient, and other interaction coefficients of the haemoglobin ligands (5,6). It is therefore possible to describe a mathematical model of placental gas exchange in the guinea-pig that builds upon the extensive information presently available on the binding of respiratory gases in adult human blood. The model requires the assumption that the uterine and umbilical venous blood reach common PO_2 and PCO_2 values (3). It uses an iterative procedure involving the following steps:

1) A preliminary guess is made at the common PCO_2 value in the umbilical and uterine veins and at the oxygen saturation in the uterine vein.

2) The oxygen saturation in the umbilical vein is calculated on the assumption that the amount of oxygen delivered by the maternal blood, less the amount consumed by the placenta, is equal to the amount received by the fetus.

3) The pH in each of the two veins is calculated by utilizing the conservation equations for the buffer bases in the maternal and fetal arterial blood. Account is taken of changes in the charge on the haemoglobin molecule due to variations in pH, PCO_2, DPG concentration and SO_2. Allowance is also made for changes

in the charge of plasma protein due to variations in pH and for alterations in the amount of bicarbonate and its distribution across the red cell membrane.

4) The oxygen tensions in the umbilical and uterine veins are calculated from the standard oxygen dissociation curve of haemoglobin and data on the interaction coefficients is then used to correct the calculated oxygen tensions to the actual values of pH, PCO_2 and DPG. If the oxygen tensions in the umbilical and uterine veins are not identical, a new oxygen saturation is calculated for the uterine vein and a return is made to step 2.

5) The amount of carbon dioxide delivered by the fetal blood and the amount received by the maternal blood is calculated. This is done by determining the arteriovenous differences in intracellular and extracellular bicarbonate concentrations and in the haemaglobin-linked carbamate concentration. The difference between the amounts of carbon dioxide delivered and received should be equal to the amount of carbon dioxide produced by the placenta. If this is not the case, a new common PCO_2 value is calculated for the uterine and umbilical veins and a return is made to step 3.

6) Otherwise the last set of values for $\bar{p}H$, PCO_2, PO_2 and SO_2 in the umbilical and uterine venous blood is accepted.

This model has been used to investigate the influence of the maternal intra-erythrocytic DPG concentration on PCO_2, PO_2 and SO_2 in the umbilical vein and on the placental transfer of oxygen and carbon dioxide (Fig. 1). The

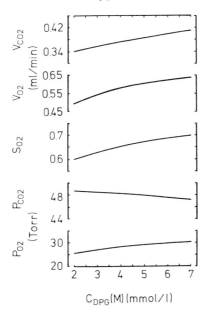

Figure 1. Effect of varying the maternal intra-erythrocytic DPG concentration on placental transfer of respiratory gases, on the oxygen saturation in the umbilical vein, and on the calculated common values for PO_2 and PCO_2 in uterine and umbilical venous blood.

intra-erythrocytic DPG concentration was varied between 2.0 and 7.0 mmol/l, corresponding to an increase in the P_{50} value of maternal blood from 21 to 31 torr. The observed increase in umbilical venous PO_2 and SO_2 is dependent upon the reduced oxygen affinity of the maternal blood. The fall in PCO_2 is caused by an increase in the Haldane effect which aids carbon dioxide transport and is due to the liberation of protons and carbon dioxide from the haemoglobin molecule as it binds oxygen. The amount of carbon dioxide liberated is proportional to the numerical value of the corresponding interaction coefficient ($\delta \log PO_2 / \delta \log PCO_2$) and the number of protons liberated is proportional to the Bohr coefficient ($\delta \log PO_2 / \delta$ pH). The first coefficient falls considerably when the DPG concentration is increased but the Bohr effect increases and, since this effect is quantitatively dominant, the carbon dioxide flux due to the Haldane effect increases.

Acknowledgements

This work was supported by a grant from the Danish Medical Research Council.

References

1. Bard, H. and Shapiro, M. (1979). *Pediat. Res.* **13**, 167–169.
2. Carter, A. M. and Grønlund, J. (1982). *J. Develop. Physiol.* **4**, 257–263.
3. Fischer, W. M. (1968). *Verh. Anat. Ges.* **62**, 241–248.
4. Jelkmann, W. and Bauer, C. (1981). *Acta Biol. Med. Germ.* **40**, 661–664.
5. Messier, A. A. and Schaefer, K. E. (1973). *Resp. Physiol.* **19**, 26–34.
6. Schaefer, K. E., Messier, A. A. and Morgan, C. C. (1970). *Resp. Physiol.* **10**, 299–310.

Effect of Restricted Placental Growth upon Umbilical and Uterine Blood Flows

Julie A. Owens, E. Allotta, J. Falconer and J. S. Robinson

Faculty of Medicine, University of Newcastle,
Shortland, New South Wales, Australia

Summary

Endometrial caruncles were excised from sheep (caruncle sheep) before pregnancy. The effect of this on umbilical and uterine blood flows in a subsequent pregnancy was examined. Eight caruncle and 7 control sheep with indwelling vascular catheters were studied at 121 and 130 days of pregnancy. Fetal weight, placental weight, umbilical blood flow, uterine blood flow and placental transfer of antipyrine were significantly lower in the caruncle sheep compared to controls. Umbilical blood flow, uterine blood flow and antipyrine clearance at both times correlated with placental weight. However, umbilical blood flow per 100 g placenta but not uterine blood flow per 100 g placenta correlated inversely with placental weight in a curvilinear fashion. Fetal weight correlated linearly with placental weight but in a curvilinear fashion with umbilical blood flow, uterine blood flow and antipyrine clearance such that fetal weight did not decrease greatly until these variables were restricted to about 60% of control values. It is concluded that restriction of placental growth limits umbilical and uterine blood flow and flow-limited placental transfer and so limits fetal growth.

Introduction

In many species, a significant correlation between fetal weight and placental weight is observed at specific gestational ages, particularly in late gestation (1). Moreover, if placental growth is restricted experimentally, substantial fetal growth retardation occurs (1–3). The mechanisms which mediate this relationship between fetal and

The Physiological Development of the Fetus and Newborn
ISBN 0 12 389080 2

Copyright © 1985 by Academic Press, London.
All rights of reproduction in any form reserved.

placental growth are unknown. The aim of the present study was to assess the contribution, if any, of reduced rates of placental blood flow to the fetal growth retardation observed when placental growth is restricted. The effect of restriction of placental growth, following removal of endometrial caruncles from sheep prior to pregnancy, on umbilical and uterine blood flows and their correlation with placental and fetal weight was therefore determined.

Materials and Methods

Fifteen Border Leicester-Merino cross-bred sheep were used. Eight ewes were operated on before pregnancy and endometrial caruncles removed as previously described (3). All surgical procedures were carried out with strict aseptic and antiseptic precautions. In 5 control and 6 caruncle ewes, the fetal femoral artery common umbilical and tarsal vein and in the remainder, the fetal jugular vein and carotid artery were catheterized (3,4). Maternal jugular vein, carotid and femoral arteries and utero-ovarian vein were also catheterized (3). A minimum of 10 days recovery from surgery was allowed before experimentation. Experiments were then carried out at 120.5 (SD 2.1) and 129.7 (SD 1.7) days gestation. One day after the second experiment, at 131.2 (SD 4.8) days, ewes were sacrificed and fetal, placental and uterine weights recorded. Umbilical and/or uterine blood flows were measured simultaneously by the steady state trans-placental diffusion technique (5), 6 times during each experiment and the mean values calculated.

Results and Discussion

Morphometric data were obtained after the second experiment at 131 days in control and caruncle ewes and are shown in Table 1. Removal of endometrial caruncles prior to conception reduced placental weight and to a lesser extent, as indicated by the increase in fetal weight to placental weight ratio. The weight of the uterus alone as well as of total uterine contents was also lower in the caruncle ewes.

The blood flows observed in control and caruncle ewes at 121 and 130 days gestation are shown in Table 2. In caruncle fetuses, umbilical blood flow was

Table 1. Morphometric variables in control and caruncle sheep[1-3]

	Control (*n*)	Caruncle (*n*)	
Fetal weight (kg)	3.72±0.807 (7)	2.198±0.653 (8)	$P<0.002$
Placental weight (kg)	0.485±0.105 (7)	0.197±0.091 (8)	$P<0.001$
Fetal weight/Placental weight	7.8±1.3 (7)	12.6±3.9 (8)	$P<0.02$
Uterine weight	1.486±0.578 (6)	0.85±0.255 (8)	$P<0.02$
Total uterine contents weight (kg)	6.766±0.869 (6)	3.175±0.867 (8)	$P<0.001$

[1]Data obtained at 131 days gestation.
[2]Mean±standard deviation.
[3]Caruncle, carunclectomized sheep.

Table 2. Umbilical and uterine blood flows in control and carunclectomized sheep[1-3]

	Control (n)	Caruncle (n)	
Umbilical flow			
(ml/min)			
121 days	845±105 (5)	462±103 (6)	P<0.001
130 days	990±345 (3)	503±137 (6)	P<0.02
(ml/min/kg fetus)			
121 days	329±63 (5)	261±52 (6)	P>0.05
130 days	268±34 (3)	217±46 (6)	P>0.1
Uterine blood flow			
(ml/min)			
121 days	2417±770 (5)	877±633 (7)	P<0.005
130 days	2026±892 (5)	1111±793 (3)	P>0.1
(ml/min/kg total ut. contents)			
121 days	370±147 (5)	265±138 (7)	P>0.2
130 days	293±123 (5)	303±165 (3)	P>0.5
Antipyrine clearance			
(ml/min)			
121 days	441±146 (5)	186±81 (7)	P<0.005
130 days	570±106 (5)	237±121 (4)	P<0.005

[1]Data obtained at 120.5 (SD2.1) and 129.7 (SD1.7) days gestation.
[2]Mean±standard deviation.
[3]Caruncle, carunclectomized sheep.

lower than that in control fetuses at both gestational ages. Uterine blood flow was also lower in caruncle ewes than in control ewes at 120 days gestation. Placental clearance of antipyrine at both gestational ages was lower in caruncle ewes than in controls.

Umbilical blood flow at both gestational ages correlated with placental weight ($r=0.88$, $P<0.001$, $n=11$; $r=0.90$, $P<0.001$, $n=9$ respectively). Umbilical blood flow, calculated per 100 g placental mass, correlated inversely with placental weight ($r=0.81$, $P<0.005$, $n=11$; $r=0.67$, $P<0.05$, $n=9$ respectively) in a curvilinear fashion. Uterine blood flow at 121 days also correlated with placental weight ($r=0.73$, $P<0.01$, $n=12$). However, there was no significant correlation between uterine blood flow per 100 g placenta at either gestational age and placental weight. Antipyrine clearance by the placenta at both gestational ages was linearly correlated with placental weight ($r=0.76$, $P<0.005$, $n=12$ and $r=0.80$, $P<0.01$, $n=9$ respectively).

Fetal weight correlated with placental weight ($r=0.90$, $P<0.001$, $n=15$). Fetal weight was significantly correlated with umbilical blood flow at 121 ($r=0.78$, $P<0.005$, $n=11$) and 130 ($r=0.91$, $P<0.001$, $n=9$) days gestation in a curvilinear fashion. From this it was evident that fetal weight is reduced as umbilical blood flow declines, particularly after it reaches about 600 ml/min when a more rapid decrease in fetal weight with umbilical blood flow is seen.

Fetal weight was also significantly correlated with uterine blood flow at 121

($r=0.76$, $P<0.01$, $n=12$) and 130 ($r=0.79$, $P<0.02$, $n=8$) days in a curvilinear fashion. Little change in fetal weight is observed however, until uterine blood flow is restricted to about 1500 ml/min, after which a precipitate decline in fetal weight occurs. Similarly, fetal weight was found to correlate closely with antipyrine clearance at both 121 ($r=0.87$, $P<0.001$, $n=12$) and 130 ($r=0.80$, $P<0.01$, $n=9$) days gestation in a curvilinear fashion.

The present study has demonstrated that restriction of placental growth after removal of endometrial caruncles before pregnancy in sheep is associated with reduced umbilical and uterine blood flows in a manner which closely correlates with the decrease observed in fetal weight. It is suggested that restriction of placental growth limits umbilical and uterine blood flow and flow-limited placental transfer and so limits fetal growth.

References

1. Alexander, G. (1974). Birthweight of lambs: influences and consequences. *CIBA* Symp. **27**, 215–239.
2. Myers, R. E., Hill, D. E., Hole, A. B., Scott, R. E., Mellits, E. O. and Cheek, D. B. (1971). *Biol. Neonate* **18**, 379–394.
3. Robinson, J. S., Kinston, E. J., Jones, C. T. and Thorburn, G. D. (1979). *J. Develop. Physiol.* **1**, 379–398.
4. Young, W. G., Creasy, R. K. and Rudolph, A. M. (1974). *J. Appl. Physiol.* **37**, 620–621.
5. Meschia, G., Cotter, J. R., Makowski, E. L. and Barron, D. H. (1966). *Q. J. Exp. Physiol.* **52**, 1–18.

The Transition between Growth-hormone Independent and Growth-hormone Dependent Growth

M. J. Parkes

The Nuffield Institute for Medical Research,
University of Oxford, Oxford, UK

In postnatal life, growth requires the presence of growth hormone; hypophysectomy completely stops body weight and length gain and growth is restored only by treatment with growth hormone (and not with prolactin, adrenocorticotrophin, thyroid-stimulating hormone or insulin). As growth hormone is not present in the early embryo it is of interest to consider at what stage does growth become growth-hormone dependent.

Growth hormone is present in fetal plasma in late gestation (4) and both the levels in plasma and body growth rates (8) are higher than those seen in postnatal life. This circumstantial evidence would suggest that growth hormone might stimulate growth as soon as it appears in plasma. This has therefore prompted experiments designed to test such a causal relationship by observing whether hypophysectomy stops growth in the fetus. Hypophysectomy of the fetus is technically more difficult than in postnatal life, the fetus being smaller, relatively inaccessible and sensitive to placental damage. In many species fetal hypophysectomy is achieved only by decapitation. Another major problem is the difficulty in making serial measurements of growth in individual fetuses. Instead a compromise is achieved by comparing the body weights at term of intact fetuses with the term body weights of fetuses which had previously been hypophysectomized. In spite of these limitations, if allowance is made for the removal of the head, the decapitated fetal rat (6), mouse (3), rabbit (5) or pig (2) has almost the same body weight as its intact littermates. It is remarkable that even without a head (and therefore without swallowing or brain stimulated muscle activity) such fetuses continue to grow. It has been claimed that hypophysectomized fetal lambs are lighter than intact twins (7) and this claim

The Physiological Development of the Fetus and Newborn
ISBN 0 12 389080 2

Copyright © 1985 by Academic Press, London.
All rights of reproduction in any form reserved.

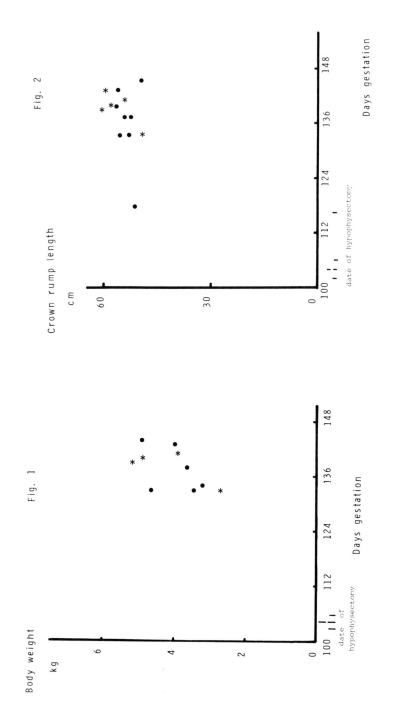

Figures 1 and 2. Body weights (singletons only) and crown rump lengths (including twins) of intact (●) and hypophysectomized (∗) fetal lambs plotted against days gestation.

has been used to argue that hypophysectomy retards fetal growth (10). However, in claiming that weight differences of 8 and 42% between intact and hypophysectomized twins were caused by fetal hypophysectomy, there was a failure to take into account the normal variation (of up to 33%) in body weight between term fetal lambs (1). My own larger study (9) has failed to demonstrate any difference in body weight between intact and hypophysectomized singleton fetal lambs (Figs 1 and 2).

Such debate also exposes a major weakness introduced by this type of cross-sectional study. The fundamental question is not what difference in weight is there between intact and hypophysectomized fetuses at term so much as *has the fetus continued to grow since hypophysectomy?* To answer this, what should be compared is the weight of the hypophysectomized fetus at term with the weight when hypophysectomy was performed. Between 100 days gestation and term the fetal lamb trebles its body weight and doubles its length (1). Figures 1 and 2 show that at term fetuses hypophysectomized at about 100 days are not one-third of the weight or one-half of the length of intact fetuses. There is no obvious weight or length deficit, and, even if a small deficit does exist and could be quantified with a larger study, it seems pointless to do so, since the fundamental conclusion remains the same. Unlike hypophysectomy in postnatal life, fetal hypophysectomy, even in lambs, does not stop growth. Hence growth hormone does not regulate fetal growth.

There still remains the question of at what stage does growth become growth-hormone dependent. Conceptually, since fetal growth is growth-hormone independent and postnatal growth is not, the obvious point for the transition is at parturition. Yet the transition does not occur here. In the rat, hypophysectomy does not stop further growth until the 25th day after birth (12), and in the rabbit growth may not be stopped until the 100th day (11). It is of considerable importance to establish the point of transition in other species and to find out why growth in all mammals is organized in such a way that progression beyond a certain point requires stimulation from the brain.

References

1. Barcroft, J. (1946). *In* "Researches on Prenatal Life", Blackwell, Oxford.
2. Colenbrander, B., Van Rossum-Kok, C. M. J. E., Van Straaten, H. W. M. and Wensing, C. J. G. (1979). *Biol. Neonate* **20**, 198–204.
3. Eguchi, P. (1961). *Endocrinology* **68**, 716–719.
4. Gluckman, P. D., Grumbach, M. M. and Kaplan, S. L. (1981). *Endocr. Rev.* **2**, 363–395.
5. Jack, P. M. B. and Milner, R. D. G. (1975). *Biol. Neonate* **26**, 195–204.
6. Jost, A. (1977). *J. Physiol. (Paris)* **73**, 877–890.
7. Liggins, G. C. and Kennedy, P. C. (1968). *J. Endocrinol.* **40**, 371–381.
8. Needham, J. (1931). *Chem. Embryol.* **1**, 368–558.
9. Parkes, M. J. (1983). D. Phil. Thesis, Oxford University.

10. Robinson, J. S., Kingston, E. J. and Thorburn, G. D. (1978). *Postgrad. Med. J.* **54**, suppl. 1, 43–50.
11. Vezinhet, A. (1968). *C. R. Sci. D.* **266**, 2348–2351.
12. Walker, D. G., Simpson, M. E., Asling, C. W. and Evans, H. M. (1950). *Anat. Rec.* **106**, 539–554.

Fetal Sheep and Placental O_2 Consumption in Reduction of Uterine Flow by Cuff-occluder and by Adrenaline

W. Gu, C. T. Jones and J. T. Parer

The Nuffield Institute for Medical Research,
University of Oxford, Oxford, UK

Knowledge of the effect of change in the maternal uteroplacental circulation is important in understanding normal or pathological fetal responses during and before labour. Spontaneous variations of uterine blood flow have only small effect upon the whole uterine and fetal O_2 consumption (1), and the O_2 supply to the gravid uterus normally well exceeds the fetal minimum requirements have been demonstrated (2). Therefore, it can be assumed that a significant limitation of uterine flow is necessary to impair the fetal O_2 uptake. To investigate that the experiments presented were designed to decrease uterine flow by two different methods: either with a cuff-occluder or maternal adrenaline infusion.

Material and Methods

Under general anaesthesia, late pregnant sheep were prepared. An inflatable cuff-occluder was put around the common uterine artery, an electromagnetic flow transducer was applied to one branch of the common artery (the one supplied to the pregnant horn in singleton, or to the bigger fetus in twins). Maternal carotid artery and uterine vein were catheterized for sampling blood which represent the uterine circulation, and fetal femoral artery and umbilical vein were used for sampling in the umbilical circulation. Also, maternal jugular vein and fetal femoral vein were catheterized for infusion.

Animals were given 3 days for recovery. Antipyrine solution was infused as described by Meschia et al. (3). During 60 min of control period 2 sets of blood

The Physiological Development of the Fetus and Newborn
ISBN 0 12 389080 2

Copyright © 1985 by Academic Press, London.
All rights of reproduction in any form reserved.

samples were collected, after that uterine blood flow was reduced either with the cuff-occluder or by maternal adrenaline infusion at 35 μg/min (approximately 0.5 μg/min/kg) for 60 min. During this period blood samples were taken at 30 and 60 min. Blood flow was estimated by flowmeter or by antipyrine infusion (3).

Blood gases, pH, O_2 saturation and Hgb in each sample were measured as soon as possible. Oxygen content was calculated as $1.34 \times Hgb \times O_2$ saturation. Oxygen consumption was calculated according to Meschia *et al.* (3).

Results

Fetal arterial blood pH and gases did not change significantly until the uterine blood flow was reduced to less than 70% of normal (range 34–67%) by the cuff-occluder. Below that, the fetal PO_2 fell from a mean of 20 mmHg to 12–14 mmHg, umbilical flow unchanged, but the veno-arterial O_2 content difference and hence fetal O_2 uptake was depressed. In contrast, the placental O_2 uptake was not affected (Table 1). Although the grouped mean fetal O_2 uptake fell, when its relation with the umbilical venous PO_2 was compared, only those whose $PO_2 < 15$ mmHg showed a significant decrease of O_2 uptake (Fig. 1).

Infusion of adrenaline reduced the uterine blood flow to 65% of normal (range 34–78%). However, this reduced flow had no effect in any instance the PO_2 and O_2 content of the umbilical circulation and fetal O_2 uptake unchanged. In contrast to the effect of physical occlusion the placental O_2 uptake fell in each case ($P < 0.001$).

Table 1. The effects of reduction of uterine flow on uterine uteroplacental and fetal oxygen consumption

	Reduction of uterine flow with cuff-occluder (n=6)		Reduction of uterine flow with maternal adrenaline infusion (35 μg/min) (n=5)	
	Control	Experimental	Control	Experimental
Uterine flow	1273±110	596±109 (ml/min)	324±50	189±24 (ml/min/kg of fetus)
Umbilical flow (ml/min/kg of fetus)	204±10	207±9	232±14	219±15
Umbilical v-a [O_2] different (μmol/ml)	1.60±0.15	0.85±0.1*	1.04±0.11	1.30±0.1
O_2 consumption				
Fetal (μmol/min/kg of fetus)	32.7±28.6	205±32.5 **	280±43	276±30
Uteroplacental	595±90	608±120 (μmol/min)	951±181	534±56 (μmol/min/kg)
Changes in uteroplacental consumption		−18±107		−420±71***

*$P < 0.01$ **$P < 0.05$ ***$P < 0.001$

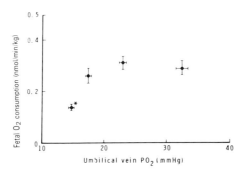

Figure 1. Relation between fetal O$_2$ consumption and umbilical venous PO$_2$. Vertical and horizontal bar represent SD. *$P<0.005$ by comparison with the mean consumption over a range of 15–37 mmHg PO$_2$.

Discussion

When uterine blood flow was reduced with a "cuff-catheter" the uteroplacenta remained with its O$_2$ uptake but the fetus did not. This is likely to reflect placental position and that its high O$_2$ consumption (4) is met before the needs of the fetus. However, this explanation is too simple. A similar reduction in uterine blood flow was achieved by adrenaline, but in contrast, uteroplacental O$_2$ uptake was reduced rather than that of the fetus, which was maintained.

It is well known that the uteroplacental vasculature has sympathetic control (5,6). Localized effects of α- and β-adrenergic agents on the introvillous spurts of rhesus monkey have been demonstrated by angiography (7). Sheep placenta is epitheliochrial, and cotyledon contains maternal and fetal capillaries. Maternal arteries go from the periphery to the central depression of cotyledon, giving off branches to supply the capillary network. There are no clear-cut studies on the control or distribution of adrenergic receptors on such network. It is tempting to speculate that the difference between the cuff-catheter and maternal adrenaline infusion could relate to selective restriction of flow through part of the capillaries network as a result of α-adrenergic alteration. Thus when uterine flow is reduced by external influence one might presume that the distribution of cotyledons perfusion could remain relatively constant, while produced by adrenaline a significant redistribution of cotyledon flow could be caused.

Whatever the mechanism of such changes the experiments showed clearly that reduction of uterine blood flow does not produce uniform response in placenta and fetus. This is dependent upon the manner in which the depression is caused.

References

1. Clapp, J. F. (1978). *Am. J. Obstet. Gynecol.* **132**, 410–413.
2. Wilkening, R. B. and Meschia, G. (1983). *Am. J. Physiol.* **244**, H749–H755.

3. Meschia, G. *et al.* (1966). *J. Exp. Physiol.* **52**, 1–18.
4. Meschia, G. *et al.* (1980). *Fed. Proc.* **39**, 245–249.
5. Bell, C. (1969). *J. Obstet. Gyneaecol. Brit. Commonwealth* **16**, 1123–1125.
6. Carter, A. M. and Olin, T. (1972). *J. Reproduc. Fertil.* **29**, 251–260.
7. Wallenberg, H. C. S. and Hutchinson, D. C. (1979). *J. Med. Primatol.* **8**, 57–65.

Substrates Availability for Maintenance of Energy Homeostasis in the Immediate Postnatal Period of the Fasted Newborn Rat

José M. Cuezva, Carmen Valcarce and José M. Medina*

Departamento de Bioquímica y Biología Molecular, I.U.B.M.-C.B.M., Facultad de Ciencias, Universidad Autónoma Madrid, Cantoblanco, Madrid, Spain and *Departamento de Bioquímica, Facultad de Farmacia, Universidad de Salamanca, Salamanca, Spain

Introduction

In the tissues of rat fetuses, the last days of intra-uterine life are characterized by the accumulation of energy substrate reserves. These reserves will enable the neonate to withstand the immediate postnatal period until maternal feeding is established. The main energy reserve stored by the rat fetuses is glycogen, since they are born with practically no white adipose tissue. The two main glycogen reserves in the fetal rat are liver and muscle glycogen. Both reserves differ considerably in their metabolism. Liver glycogen supplies the neonatal tissues with glucose residues because of the presence of hepatic glucose-6-phosphatase activity. However, muscle glycogen can only be exported as lactate residues, due to the absence of the former enzyme activity. The metabolic fate of lactate and its relevance during the immediate postnatal period depends upon the presence of other energy substrates and the operation of the gluconeogenic pathway. In this report, we will present a detailed time-course of the main energy substrates of neonatal metabolism during the first twelve postnatal hours. In addition, the appearance of postnatal gluconeogenesis and the metabolism of lactate through this pathway will be discussed.

The Physiological Development of the Fetus and Newborn
ISBN 0 12 389080 2

Copyright © 1985 by Academic Press, London.
All rights of reproduction in any form reserved.

Postnatal Hypoglycaemia and Lactate Oxidation

Immediately after birth, until suckling begins and adaptation to a high fat diet is established, the newborn rat must depend on the oxidation of endogenous fuels. As a metabolic consequence of the cessation in the maternal substrate supply, postnatal hypoglycaemia develops (Fig. 1) due to the high rates of glucose utilization (1,2) and low rates of glucose production (1,3). Although hypoglycaemia prevails during the first two postnatal hours, no net glycogenolysis was observed (Fig. 2), which contributes to the low rates of glucose production observed at this time. Similarly, gluconeogenesis, the other metabolic pathway involved in the glucose supply to the newborn rat, develops after birth (4,5). The development of gluconeogenesis in the newborn rat is necessarily preceded by *de novo* synthesis of cytosolic phosphoenolpyruvate carboxykinase (5). The emergence of this enzyme in the liver of newborn rats is a cAMP-dependent process (5), most probably brought about by the postnatal decrease in the insulin/glucagon ratio. Although significant amounts of the enzyme are already present in the liver and kidney of 2 h old neonates, the rates of gluconeogenesis from lactate are negligible (3,4,6). However, during the first two postnatal hours, blood lactate concentrations showed a sharp decrease (Fig. 1), indicating that it is being actively metabolized, although not being converted into glucose. Concurrently with the rapid utilization of blood lactate, there is a significant reduction in carcass glycogen (Fig. 2) that will presumably enhance the lactate supply to the newborn rat tissues. The main metabolic fate of lactate during the first two postnatal hours is CO_2 by its oxidation in the tricarboxylic acid cycle (6), with its utilization considerably increased by the availability of oxygen in these circumstances (7). Lactate has recently been shown to be actively oxidized by the fetal and neonatal rat brain *in vitro* (8). In the perinatal dog brain, its utilization is highly increased by hypoglycaemia (9). More recently, lactate has been proved to be the glucose alternative energy substrate for the brain of children with hepatic glucose-6-phosphatase deficiency (10). These results emphasize i) the importance of muscle glycogen mobilization after birth as a source of lactate and ii) the lactate oxidation in the immediate postnatal period as an alternative energy substrate before glucose derived from liver glycogenolysis and gluconeogenesis becomes available.

Liver Glycogenolysis and Gluconeogenesis

Reversal of postnatal hypoglycaemia occurs by the third postnatal hour (Fig. 1), due to the onset of liver glycogenolysis (Fig. 2) and a significant contribution of gluconeogenesis (Fig. 3). In addition, there is a concurrent carcass glycogenolysis (Fig. 2) that contributes to the observed high rates of lactate turnover (Fig. 4). However, at this postnatal hour 50% of the lactate being turned-over (Fig. 4) is being utilized in gluconeogenesis (Fig. 3). The induction of liver glycogenolysis seems to be mediated by the increase in plasma catecholamine concentrations secreted after delivery (11) as a result of postnatal hypoglycaemia (12).

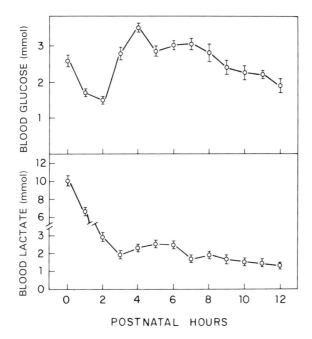

Figure 1. Blood glucose and lactate concentrations during the first 12 postnatal hours of the newborn rat. Each point is the mean ± SEM of 10-20 observations.

Nevertheless, other hormonal factors such as the postnatal decrease in the insulin/glucagon ratio (11,13,14) may be involved in the initiation of the process. In fact, the observed two hour delay in net liver glycogen mobilization (Fig. 2) could be partially explained by the antagonistic effects of insulin on liver glycogenolysis (15). Actually, after birth plasma insulin concentrations are very high (11,13,14) and the immediate administration of guinea-pig insulin anti-serum to the newborn rat produced a significant reduction of liver glycogen concentration during the first hour (16).

During the third six-hour period, blood glucose concentrations are maintained fairly constant (Fig. 1), due to the contribution of liver glycogenolysis (Fig. 2) and gluconeogenesis (Fig. 3). Carcass glycogen (Fig. 2) showed no significant changes after the fourth postnatal hour. At the sixth postnatal hour, although blood lactate concentrations (Fig. 1) are lower than at delivery, its metabolic turnover is still very high compared to later periods (Fig. 4), and is mainly metabolized by gluconeogenesis (Fig. 3). At this point, the contribution of gluconeogenesis to the glucose available is almost twice that of glycogenolysis, most probably because of (i) the sharp increase in phosphoenolpyruvate carboxykinase activity observed in the neonatal liver and (ii) the high availability of lactate for gluconeogenesis (Fig. 4).

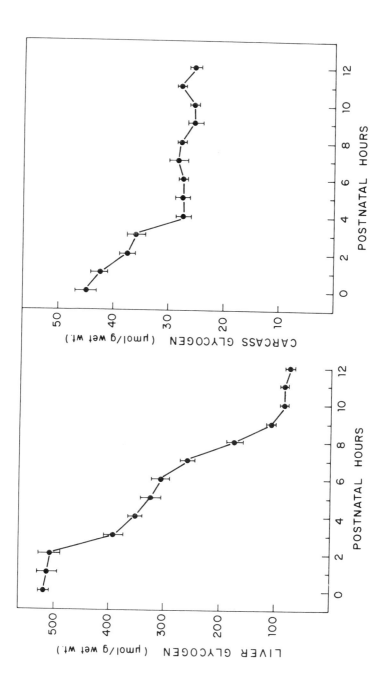

Figure 2. Liver and carcass glycogen concentrations during the first 12 postnatal hours of the newborn rat. Carcass glycogen was determined in decapitated and eviscerated neonates. Each point is the mean ± SEM of 10–20 observations.

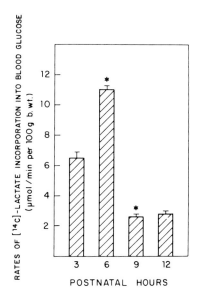

Figure 3. Gluconeogenesis from lactate during the first 12 postnatal hours. The rates of ^{14}C-lactate incorporation into blood glucose were measured after the intraperitoneal administration of 2 μCi of L-(U-^{14}C) lactate to the neonates (3,18). *$P<0.0005$ when compared to the previous time period. Data taken, in part, from (3).

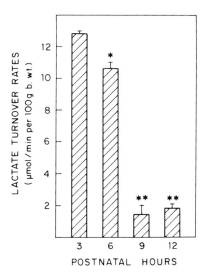

Figure 4. Lactate turnover rates during the first 12 postnatal hours. The fractional turnover rates were measured as indicated in Fig. 3 and (3). The lactate space was assumed to equal the total body water, i.e. 80 ml/100 g body wt. (19). *$P<0.0025$ and **$P<0.0005$ when compared 3 h vs 6 h and 6 h vs 9 h and 12 h, respectively. Data recalculated and taken, in part, from (3).

Fasting and the Inhibition of Gluconeogenesis

After the sixth postnatal hour, the fasted newborn rat enters into a new metabolic situation. An increase in the rates of liver glycogenolysis is observed during the 6-9 h period (Fig. 2), but the glucose made available cannot prevent the continuous decline in blood glucose concentrations observed at the same time (Fig. 1). After this, no net liver glycogen mobilization occurs (Fig. 2). In addition, the rates of gluconeogenesis at 9 and 12 hours after birth showed a sharp reduction compared to the sixth postnatal hour (Fig. 4). This four fold decrease in the rates of gluconeogenesis are surprisingly accompanied by a sharp increase in liver and kidney phosphoenolpyruvate carboxykinase activity. Therefore, this hypoglycaemic episode is due to a defective supply of glucose caused by glycogenolysis and gluconeogenesis.

The reduction in the rates of gluconeogenesis at the ninth and twelfth postnatal hour is accompanied by a sharp and similar reduction in the rates of lactate turnover (Fig. 4), indicating that gluconeogenesis at this time is limited mainly by the availability of gluconeogenic substrate. Another factor that may reduce the gluconeogenic flux during this time is the liver ATP concentration. In fact, the liver ATP/ADP ratio drops after the sixth postnatal hour in fasted newborn rats (17,18), and a positive linear correlation has been observed between this ratio and gluconeogenesis in these circumstances (17).

In conclusion, the first twelve postnatal hours of the full-term newborn rat can be divided into three different metabolic periods a) the first two postnatal hours, when hypoglycaemia develops, and carcass glycogenolysis supplies the neonatal tissues with lactate as a glucose alternative energy substrate, with an oxidizable metabolic fate, b) the 3-8 h period, in which liver glycogenolysis and gluconeogenesis from lactate supports the energy requirements of the neonate and, c) the last four hours, in which the liver glycogen reserve is exhausted and gluconeogenesis inhibited due to the limited availability of lactate and the poor energy state of the liver. Therefore another hypoglycaemic episode develops.

Acknowledgments

We are grateful to Mr. E. Fernández, Mrs. M. Chamorro and Miss A. M. Luis for their contributions to the present study. This work was supported by a grant from the "Comisión Asesora de Investigación Científica y Técnica", Spain.

References

1. Snell, K. and Walker, D. G. (1973). *Biochem. J.* **132**, 739–752.
2. Snell, K. (1981). *In* "Metabolic Adaptation to Extrauterine Life" (De Meyer, R. ed) pp. 81–105, Martinus Nijhoff Publishers, The Hague, Boston and London.
3. Fernández, E., Valcarce, C., Cuezva, J. M. and Medina, J. M. (1983). *Biochem. J.* **214**, 525–532.
4. Ballard, F. J. (1971). *Biochem. J.* **124**, 265–274.

5. Hanson, R. W., Reshef, L. and Ballard, F. J. (1975). *Fed. Proc.* **34**, 166-171.
6. Medina, J. M., Cuezva, J. M. and Mayor, F. (1980). *FEBS Lett.* **114**, 132-134.
7. Cuezva, J. M. and Medina, J. M. (1981). *Biol. Neonate* **39**, 70-77.
8. Arizmendi, C. and Medina, J. M. (1983). *Biochem. J.* **214**, 633-635.
9. Hellman, J., Vannucci, R. C. and Nardis, E. E. (1982). *Pediat. Res.* **16**, 40-44.
10. Fernándes, J., Berger, R. and Smit, G. P. A. (1984). *Pediat. Res.* **18**, 335-339.
11. Cuezva, J. M., Burkett, E. S., Kerr, D. S., Rodman, H. M. and Patel, M. S. (1982). *Pediat. Res.* **16**, 632-637.
12. Cuezva, J. M. and Patel, M. S. (1982). *Biochem. Soc. Trans.* **10**, 521.
13. Girard, J. R., Cuendet, G. S., Marliss, E. B., Kervran, A., Rieutort, M. and Assan, R. (1973). *J. Clin. Invest.* **52**, 3190-3200.
14. Di Marco, P. N., Ghisalberti, A. V., Martin, C. E. and Oliver, I. T. (1978). *Eur. J. Biochem.* **87**, 243-247.
15. Whitton, P. D. (1981). *In:* "Short-term Regulation of Liver Metabolism" (Hue, L. and Van de Werve, G. eds) pp. 45-62, Elsevier/North-Holland Biomedical Press, Amsterdam, New York and Oxford.
16. Snell, K. and Walker, D. G. (1978). *Diabetol.* **14**, 59-64.
17. Cuezva, J. M., Fernández, E., Valcarce, C. and Medina, J. M. (1983). *Biochim. Biophys. Acta* **759**, 292-295.
18. Cuezva, J. M., Chitra, C. I. and Patel, M. S. (1982). *Pediat. Res.* **16**, 638-643.
19. Ferre, P., Pegorier, J. P., Marliss, E. B. and Girard, J. R. (1978). *Am. J. Physiol.* **234**, E129-E136.

Glucose Metabolism in the Ovine Conceptus

J. M. Bassett, Anne H. Burks and R. A. Pinches

The Nuffield Institute for Medical Research,
University of Oxford, Oxford, UK

During pregnancy, alterations in glucose metabolism are of two kinds: 1. those due directly to metabolism of the developing conceptus(es); 2. adaptation of maternal tissue metabolism to the demands of pregnancy.

Radiotracer methods are ideally suited to quantitative analysis of these alterations. The mother and genetically different conceptus developing *in utero* can be represented as distinct, but interacting pool systems (Fig. 1). However, basic assumptions underlying the various models used for analysis of maternal and fetal glucose kinetics (1–3), have not been examined. In particular, it is not clear whether the placenta, an important site of glucose metabolism (4,5), uses glucose from the maternal pool, or whether maternal and fetal portions use glucose delivered by their own arterial vasculature. Both lactate and fructose are important products of ovine placental glucose metabolism, but unlike glucose, neither is transported across the placenta from conceptus to mother at very significant rates (4,6–8). Consequently, during dual-label 6-[^{3}H] and U-[^{14}C] glucose infusions to mother and fetus, [^{14}C]:[^{3}H] ratios in these metabolites within the fetal circulation should, under steady-state conditions, reflect those of the glucose used for their synthesis and thus its source, provided direct pathways of synthesis are the major ones.

Experimental Methods

Surgical and experimental procedures used were generally similar to those reported earlier (9) or described by others (10). During labelled infusion experiments the ewes (120–140 days pregnant) received a primed infusion of 6-[^{3}H] glucose and one fetus a similar infusion of U-[^{14}C] glucose.

The Physiological Development of the Fetus and Newborn
ISBN 0 12 389080 2

Copyright © 1985 by Academic Press, London.
All rights of reproduction in any form reserved.

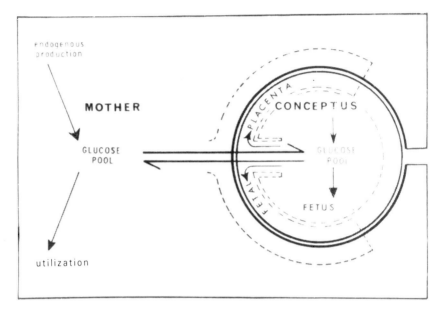

Figure 1. Schematic representation of the conceptus and mother, emphasizing integration of glucose metabolism within all tissues of the conceptus and its isolation from maternal metabolism.

Concentrations of metabolites in plasma samples were determined as described earlier (9). Glucose was isolated as the pentaacetate (11), after preliminary chromatography on Dowex 1 (acetate form) to remove lactate. Without this step, 5% of added lactate radioactivity may appear in the pentaacetate. Negligible added fructose radioactivity ($<1\%$) was recovered in glucose pentaacetate. Lactate was eluted from the Dowex column with 0.5M formic acid (12). Fructose concentration (13) and radioactivity were determined after conversion of glucose to gluconic acid (3), and isolation by ion exchange chromatography on Dowex. Statistical significance of differences was assessed by the paired *t* test.

Results

Plasma glucose levels of the ewes (7 with twins) in 14 experiments, when fed, were 2.57 ± 0.48 mmol/l (mean $\pm$ SD) during the steady-state period and in their fetuses were 0.71 ± 0.18 mmol/l ($n = 22$). Feeding on hay alone for 3 days, followed by 48 h maternal fasting, caused glucose levels to decrease to 1.34 ± 0.47 (6) and 0.41 ± 0.11 (11) mmol/l in mother and fetus. Fetal plasma fructose levels were also much lower after maternal fasting (3.79 ± 1.49 (22) and 1.73 ± 0.48 (11) mmol/l in fed and fasted experiments), but fetal lactate levels changed little (1.45±0.46 and 1.32±0.30 mmol/l in fed and fasted studies), though they were consistently higher than maternal levels (0.45±0.20 and 0.65±0.18 mmol/l).

Although fructose specific activities had not plateaued during the first 240 min infusion, substantial amounts of radioactivity were incorporated into both fructose and lactate, with lactate and fructose specific activities *ca* 32% and *ca* 47% those in glucose. [^{14}C]:[^{3}H] ratios in both these metabolites were stable and statistically indistinguishable from that in plasma glucose from the same fetus, in both fed and fasted sheep, whereas values for each in the U-[^{14}C] glucose-infused fetus differed greatly from those in the mother and uninfused co-twin (Table 1).

Table 1. Mean (±SD) steady-state* [^{14}C]:[^{3}H] ratios in maternal plasma glucose and in fetal plasma glucose, lactate and fructose during iv infusion of 6-[^{3}H] glucose into the ewe and U-[^{14}C] glucose into one fetus

	Glucose	Lactate	Fructose
a) Fed ewes 14 experiments			
Maternal plasma	0.146 ±0.052	—	—
Fetal plasma			
I. U-[^{14}C] glucose-infused	1.302 ±0.465	1.182 (9) ±0.565	1.236 ±0.430
II. uninfused twin (8)	0.120 ±0.047	0.109 ±0.059	0.160 ±0.111
b) Fasted ewes 6 experiments			
Maternal plasma	0.142 ±0.065		
Fetal plasma			
I. U-[^{14}C] glucose infused	1.082 ±0.530	0.828 (5) ±0.272	0.983 ±0.527
II. uninfused twin (5)	0.151 ±0.075	0.170 ±0.095	0.154 ±0.055

*The value for each experiment was the mean of 6 samples 90–240 min after start of the primed infusions.

Infusion of glucose into the mother after 240 min in 9 experiments on fed or fasted ewes, although altering glucose levels, had only a minor effect on the maternal/fetal concentration gradient. Lactate and fructose [^{14}C]:[^{3}H] ratios (0.82±0.27 and 0.78±0.25 respectively) remained statistically indistinguishable from that of glucose (0.83±0.24) in the same fetus. This was also so in 11 other experiments during infusion of insulin (0.05 or 0.1 U/h/kg) or glucagon (1.0 μg/h/kg) to the fetus and where there were larger changes in the maternal/fetal concentration gradient.

Discussion

These observations provide no evidence for any significant direct contribution of glucose from the maternal pool to synthesis of either fructose or lactate within tissues of the conceptus perfused by the fetal cardiovascular system. This result implies that the extracorporeal tissues of the conceptus, including the fetal placenta, as well as the fetal body use glucose from its own central pool and not, to any significant extent, glucose "in-transit" from the mother. This glucose appears to mix with that in the central vascular compartment of the conceptus before being utilized.

Glucose metabolism within extracorporeal tissues of the conceptus is therefore closely integrated with that in the body of the fetus as might be expected from the very high fraction (*ca* 50%) of combined ventricular output delivered to the umbilical circulation (14). The high rate of partial metabolism of glucose within the placenta and transfer of large quantities of lactate for oxidation elsewhere in the fetus must be viewed as reflecting interorgan metabolite cycling within the conceptus and not delivery to the fetus of an exogenous supply of lactate as frequently stated (4,5,7).

For purposes of modelling glucose kinetics, it is clear that the entire conceptus can be regarded as a separate and isolable subsystem interconnected with that of the mother (Fig. 1). Use of two pool models, or derivatives, allow quantitation of glucose utilization by both conceptus and mother, and glucose transfer between them, without blood flow measurements (1,2). Glucose metabolism in the fetal placenta and membranes, as well as the fetal body, contribute to the total rate of glucose utilization in the conceptus. Measurements of umbilical blood flow and concentration differences will be necessary to calculate the contribution of these organs to total glucose metabolism in the system (3). Provided other criteria can be satisfied, dual-label infusion procedures and the use of a two pool model can yield valid estimates of glucose utilization in the conceptus. Unfortunately, use of the term fetus instead of conceptus in many publications, together with calculation of glucose utilization relative to fetal body weight (1,2,9,15,16), has caused confusion in comparisons among studies (3,17).

Interposition of a third uteroplacental compartment between mother and fetus (3) can have no valid basis. The placenta, containing, as it does, elements of both maternal and fetal systems, does not behave as a homogeneous unit. Metabolism of the fetal placenta *in vivo* is separable from that of maternal placenta and other uterine tissues by radiotracer methods. Recognition of this should permit greater definition of the tissues contributing to the high rate of glucose utilization within the uteroplacenta.

Acknowledgements

These investigations were supported by the British Diabetic Association and the Medical Research Fund, Oxford University. Valued technical assistance was provided by Louise Wyatt, Ray Borrett, Mark Thomas and Cliff Hanson.

References

1. Anand, R. S., Sperling, M. A., Ganguli, S. and Nathanielsz, P. W. (1979). *Pediat. Res.* **13**, 783–787.
2. Hodgson, J. C., Mellor, D. J. and Field, A. C. (1980). *Biochem. J.* **1186**, 739–747.
3. Hay, W. W., Sparks, J. W., Quissell, B. J., Battaglia, F. C. and Meschia, G. (1981). *Am. J. Physiol.* **240**, E662–E668.
4. Meschia, G., Battaglia, F. C., Hay, W. W. and Sparks, J. W. (1980). *Fed. Proc.* **39**, 245–249.
5. Simmons, M. A., Battaglia, F. C. and Meschia, G. (1979). *J. Develop. Physiol.* **1**, 227–243.
6. Battaglia, F. C. (1984). *Am. J. Obstet. Gynecol.* **148**, 850–858.
7. Sparks, J. W., Hay, W. W., Bonds, D., Meschia, G. and Battaglia, F. C. (1982). *J. Clin. Invest.* **70**, 179–192.
8. Huggett, A. St G. (1961). *Br. Med. Bull.* **17**, 122–126.
9. Bassett, J. M., Burks, A. H. and Pinches, R. A. (1983). *J. Develop. Physiol.* **5**, 51–61.
10. Anand, R. S., Ganguli, S. and Sperling, M. A. (1980). *Am. J. Physiol.* **238**, E524–E532.
11. Jones, G. B. (1965). *Anal. Biochem.* **12**, 249–258.
12. Foster, D. M., Hetenyi, G. and Berman, M. (1980). *Am. J. Physiol.* **239**, E30–E38.
13. Bernt, E. and Bergmeyer, H. U. (1974). *In:* "Methods of Enzymatic Analysis", (Bergmeyer, H. U. eds) pp. 1304–1307, Academic Press, London and New York.
14. Mott, J. C. and Walker, D. W. (1983). *In:* "Handbook of Physiology, The Cardiovascular system III", (Shepherd, J. T. and Abboud, F. M. eds) pp. 837–883, American Physiological Society, Bethesda, MD.
15. Setchell, B. P., Bassett, J. M., Hinks, N. T. and Graham, N. McC. (1972). *Q. J. Exp. Physiol.* **57**, 257–266.
16. Kitts, D. D. and Krishnamurti, C. R. (1982). *Can. J. Anim. Sci.* **62**, 397–408.
17. Sparks, J. W., Hay, W. W., Meschia, G. and Battaglia, F. C. (1983). *Europ. J. Obstet. Gynec. Reprod. Biol.* **14**, 331–340.

Microsomal Glycolysis—A Potential Pathway in Fetal Guinea-pig Liver

Sheelagh M. Farrow and Colin T. Jones

The Nuffield Institute for Medical Research,
University of Oxford, Oxford, UK

Introduction

Although membrane-bound enzyme systems exist such as oxidative phosphorylation, glycolysis has been considered as located entirely in the cytosol (1,2,3). However, there are reports of particulate-bound glycolytic enzymes in skeletal muscle (4,5,6), erythrocytes (7,8,9,10), liver (11,12,13) and brain (14,15,16). As yet no separate function has been shown for these enzymes although ATP and GTP production for localized utilization within the membrane has been postulated in erythrocytes (7,8) and squid retinal axons (17).

Subcellular fractionation of fetal guinea-pig liver revealed a high proportion of glycolytic enzyme activities associated with the microsomal membrane fraction. This was not found in adult liver. To prove conclusively the existence of membrane-associated glycolysis and gain an insight into a possible function in the fetus, chromatographic and kinetic studies were done on microsomal pyruvate kinase.

Methods

Livers were homogenized in 9 volumes of 0.2 M sucrose-50 mmol Tris-HCl pH 7.5 containing 1 mmol EDTA, 0.1 mmol dithiothreitol, 5 mmol $MgCl_2$ and 1 mmol phenylmethylsulphonylfluoride. Subcellular fractions of the homogenate were prepared as described by De Duve et al. (18). A sample of microsomal pyruvate kinase for chromatography was obtained by resuspending the microsomal pellet in 0.2 M sucrose-50 mmol Tris-HCl buffer containing 0.25% (v/v) Triton X-100 and 1 mg/ml bovine serum albumin (BSA), sonicating for 3 s at 150 W,

The Physiological Development of the Fetus and Newborn
ISBN 0 12 389080 2
Copyright © 1985 by Academic Press, London.
All rights of reproduction in any form reserved.

recentrifuging at 74 000 g for 60 min and collecting the supernatant containing the solubilized enzyme activity.

All enzyme assays were carried out at 25°C in a Pye-Unicam SP1800 spectrophotometer and were as described by Faulkner and Jones (19).

Pyruvate kinase isoenzymes were eluted from DEAE-cellulose (Whatman DE52) with a linear concentration gradient of 0–0.5 M KCl according to Faulkner and Jones (20). Isoelectrofocussing columns containing a sucrose density gradient (5–50%, w/v) were prepared according to LKB, pre-equilibrated with 1% ampholine of the required pH range for 24 h, the sample added and run for a further 26 h at 5°C at 350 V and 1.0 mA.

Results

Subcellular localization of glycolytic enzymes

An example of the subcellular distribution of some glycolytic enzymes in fetal liver is given in Table 1. Approximately 20% of the total pyruvate kinase and phosphofructokinase activities were found in the microsomal fraction. In adult liver this fraction contained only 1–2% of the total cell pyruvate kinase activity.

Table 1. Subcellular distribution of glycolytic enzymes in one preparation of 50-days fetal liver

Enzyme	Percentage of total activity			
	nuclear	mitochondrial	microsomal	cytosolic
Pyruvate kinase	8.2	6.9	21.2	63.7
Phosphofructokinase	—	—	22.2	77.8
Aldolase	12.5	—	8.9	78.6
Lactate dehydrogenase	6.4	7.4	19.3	66.9
Enolase	14.0	—	8.6	77.4
Glyceraldehyde 3-phosphate dehydrogenase	—	14.8	6.7	78.5
Phosphoglyceromutase	24.1	8.4	7.8	59.7
Phosphoglucoseisomerase	18.7	4.9	5.8	70.6
Phosphoglucomutase	—	—	—	100

Sonication of the microsomal fraction increased the recovery of pyruvate kinase by 50% whilst treatment with 0.25% (v/v) Triton X-100 released latent activity more than doubling the recovery. After correction has been made for this latent activity, pyruvate kinase which is firmly bound to, possibly being part of the microsomal membrane, represents approximately 25–30% of total cell activity. This figure is an underestimate since even this high concentration of detergent failed to completely solubilize and expose the membrane-bound enzyme activity. However, 0.5% (v/v) Triton X-100 caused inactivation of the microsomal pyruvate kinase. This did not occur with the cytosolic activity suggesting that the particulate enzyme was structurally different. In subsequent studies on microsomal pyruvate kinase, 1 mg/ml BSA was added to prevent inactivation by "free" detergent.

Separation of pyruvate kinase isoenzymes

Elution of cytosolic extracts of adult and fetal liver from DEAE-cellulose columns resulted in a peak of activity which was not bound (PK4) and one which eluted at approximately 150 mmol KCl. A sample of microsomal pyruvate kinase showed a major part of the activity to elute in the same regions as PK1 and PK4 although there were several other smaller, unidentified peaks. Kinetic studies on the major peaks gave K_m and $S_{0.5}$ values for phosphoenolpyruvate which were not significantly different to those obtained for cytosolic PK1 and PK4.

Table 2. pI values of cytosolic and microsomal pyruvate kinase isoenzymes in a preparation of fetal liver (51 days gestational age)

Isoenzyme	pI
Cytosolic	
PK1	5.60
PK2	5.22
PK3	>7.5
PK4	6.21
Microsomal	
Range	4.25–4.70

Isoelectrofocussing gave better resolution of the pyruvate kinase activity. Table 2 gives an example of the pI values of cytosolic and microsomal isoenzymes. The microsomal pyruvate kinase activity had very different pI values to the cytosolic isoenzymes. It is possible that the microsomal enzyme runs as a BSA-PK complex. Since there was no such interaction between BSA and cytosolic isoenzymes, this supports the possibility that the membrane-bound isoenzyme(s) is structurally different. Kinetic studies of the isoenzymes separated by isoelectrofocussing (unlike DEAE-cellulose chromatography) suggested that the microsomal isoenzymes were unlike PK1 and PK4 for instance, in the absence of fructose-1,6-bisphosphate both cytosolic forms were inhibited by L-alanine and L-phenylalanine (5 mmol) whilst the microsomal isoenzymes were unaffected.

Discussion

The present experiments show a large proportion (at least 27%) of the total glycolytic enzyme activities in fetal liver are firmly associated with the microsomes possibly being an integral membrane protein. For pyruvate kinase the electrophoretic and kinetic properties of the membrane-bound enzyme are unlike those of the cytosolic isoenzymes indicating significant structural differences and hence separate membrane isoenzymes.

The presence of this particulate activity in the fetus and not the adult raises the question of its significance. Possibly it is a storage form or may represent a separate and independent pathway. Membrane-bound glycolysis has been reported in erythrocytes (8) and squid retinal axons (17).

Fetal guinea-pig liver tolerates longer periods of anoxia than adult liver before changes in metabolite concentrations are seen (21). A separate membrane-associated glycolytic pathway could be a contributing factor. The close proximity and possible sequential arrangement of glycolytic enzymes would provide a situation for "substrate channelling" (22) with the associated local high concentrations of intermediates, short response times and decreased transient times (23,24,25,26). Directing substrate down a tightly-coupled pathway should cause little perturbation of the surrounding environment. For example, if the enzymes were arranged so that lactate and thus hydrogen ions were released into the lumen of the endoplasmic reticulum, as has been suggested in the sarcoplasmic reticulum (26), this could minimize changes in cell pH and maintain glycolytic ATP production during anoxia. Limited studies in the present system have provided some evidence for selective coupling between membrane-associated glycolytic enzymes.

Acknowledgements

This work was supported by a grant from the Medical Research Council.

References

1. Le Page, P. A. and Schneider, W. C. (1948). *J. Biol. Chem.* **242**, 163–172.
2. De Duve, C., Wattiaux, R. and Baudhuin, P. (1962). *Adv. Enz.* **24**, 292–345.
3. Paigen, K. and Wenner, C. E. (1962). *J. Lab. Clin. Med.* **97**, 213–218.
4. Amberson, H. R., Roisen, F. J. and Bauer, A. C. (1965). *J. Cell. Comp. Physiol.* **66**, 71–90.
5. Sigel, P. and Pette, D. (1969). *J. Histochem. Cytochem.* **17**, 225–237.
6. Clarke, F. M. and Masters, C. J. (1975). *Biochem. Biophys. Acta* **381**, 37–46.
7. Schrier, S. L., Ben-Bassat, I., Junga, I., Seeger, M. and Grumet, F. C. (1975). *J. Lab. Clin. Med.* **85**, 797–810.
8. Green, D. E., Murer, E., Hultin, H. O., Richardson, S. H., Salmon, B., Brierly, G. P. and Baum, H. (1965). *Arch. Biochem. Biophys.* **112**, 635–647.
9. Duchon, G. and Collier, H. B. (1971). *J. Memb. Biol.* **6**, 138–157.
10. Tillman, W., Cordua, A. and Schroter, W. (1965). *Biochem. Biophys. Acta* **382**, 157–171.
11. Agostini, A., Vergani, C. and Villa, L. (1966). *Nature* **209**, 1024–1025.
12. Foemmel, R. S., Gray, R. H. and Bernstein, I. A. (1975). *J. Biol. Chem.* **250**, 1892–1897.
13. Weiss, T. L., Zieske, J. D. and Bernstein, I. A. (1981). *Biochem. Biophys. Acta* **661**, 221–229.
14. Crane, R. K. and Sols, A. (1953). *J. Biol. Chem.* **203**, 273–292.
15. Clarke, F. M., Masters, C. J. and Winzor, D. J. (1970). *Biochem. J.* **118**, 325–327.
16. Clarke, F. M. and Masters, C. J. (1972). *Arch. Biochem. Biophys.* **153**, 258–265.

17. Cecchi, X., Canessa-Fischer, M., Maturana, A. and Fischer, S. (1971). *Arch. Biochem. Biophys.* **145**, 240–247.
18. De Duve, C., Pressman, B. C., Gianetto, R., Wattiaux, R. and Appelmans, F. (1955). *Biochem. J.* **60**, 604–617.
19. Faulkner, A. and Jones, C. T. (1975). *Int. J. Biochem.* **6**, 789–792.
20. Faulkner, A. and Jones, C. T. (1975). *Arch. Biochem. Biophys.* **170**, 228–241.
21. Faulkner, A. and Jones, C. T. (1978). *Biochem. Biophys. Acta* **538**, 106–109.
22. Davis, R. H. (1967). *In:* "Organisational Biosynthesis", (Vogel, H. J., Lampen, J. O. and Bryson, V. eds) p. 303. Academic Press, London and New York.
23. Welch, G. R. and Gaertner, F. H. (1975). *Proc. Natl. Acad. Sci.* **72**, 4218–4222.
24. Mally, M. I., Grayson, D. R. and Evans, D. R. (1980). *J. Biol. Chem.* **255**, 113772–113780.
25. Christopherson, R. I. and Jones, M. E. (1980). *J. Biol. Chem.* **255**, 11381–11395.
26. Fahimi, H. D. and Karnovsky, M. J. (1966). *J. Cell. Biol.* **29**, 113–128.

Early Fetal Signals: Schwangerschaftsprotein 1 and Human Chorionic Gonadotrophin

A. G. Ahmed and A. Klopper

Department of Obstetrics and Gynaecology, University of Aberdeen, Royal Infirmary, Aberdeen, Scotland

Introduction

In conceptual cycles there are many biological changes essential for implantation of the conceptus and for maintenance of the pregnancy. The endometrium has to be prepared for the reception of the fertilized ovum, the corpus luteum has to continue its hormonal production and the immunological forces of the mother have to be held in abeyance. The mechanisms responsible for inducing these changes are very poorly understood.

In recent years substances specifically produced by the conceptus have been found in the maternal blood circulation as early as a week after fertilization. Human chorionic gonadotrophin (hCG) is the best known of these substances. Concomitant with hCG the embryo produces another newly described protein, Schwangerschaftsprotein 1 (SP_1). Our previous investigations showed that both hCG and SP_1 (1) appear in the maternal blood stream 6–14 days after ovulation. These findings led to the suggestion that the fertilized ovum signals its presence to the mother from the earliest days of pregnancy; probably before the blastocyst stage. It is likely that these signals might induce the histological, the hormonal and the immunological changes essential for implantation and the continuation of the pregnancy. There is some evidence that hCG is the signal which rescues the corpus luteum (2). An immunosuppressive function has been suggested for SP_1 (3).

If any of the trophoblastic proteins are essential for continuation of the pregnancy, their pattern in normal pregnancy must be different from that in early pregnancy failure.

The Physiological Development of the Fetus and Newborn
ISBN 0 12 389080 2
Copyright © 1985 by Academic Press, London.
All rights of reproduction in any form reserved.

In the course of some studies on endocrine changes in early pregnancy, we had a unique chance to contrast the pregnancy specific proteins pattern in normal pregnancy and in subclinical abortion.

Materials and Methods

Fifteen menstrual cycles in 15 patients who were attempting to get pregnant were examined. In 7 of these 15 women, ovulation occurred spontaneously, while in the remaining 8 subjects, it followed treatment with clomiphene citrate and/or bromocriptine. All the cycles were ovulatory; progesterone concentration exceeding 40 nmol/l 4–6 days after ovulation. All the patients were keeping records of their periods, noting their basal body temperature and were having assays of serum estradiol and progesterone at 1–2 day intervals during the follicular phase of their cycles. Venous blood samples were taken daily during the luteal phase from ovulation onwards. The serum was separated and divided into 2 aliquots. One was analysed for estradiol and progesterone on the same day and the other stored at $-20°C$ until assayed for hCG and SP_1 within 2 weeks. hCG was measured by radioimmunoassay using a commercial kit (Amersham, UK). All values below 10 IU/l were taken as negative findings. SP_1 was measured by enzyme immunoassay using the Enzygnost-SP_1 kit (Behringwerke, AG), the

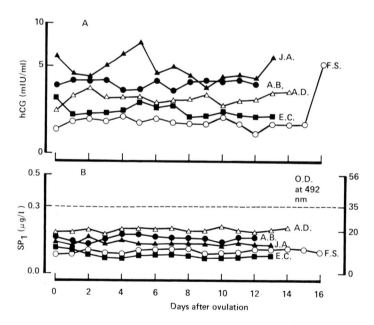

Figure 1. Serial hCG measurements (a) and serial SP_1 measurements (b) during the luteal phase in 5 nonpregnant women. Day of ovulation designated 0. Dotted horizontal line in Fig. 1(b) indicates the lower sensitivity limit of SP_1 assay.

lower sensitivity limit of which is 0.3 μg/l. All values of 0.5 μg/l or higher were taken as positive findings.

Results

In each of these 15 cycles ovulation occurred 11–14 days after the last menstrual period. The day of ovulation, designated day 0, was determined by basal body temperature, by the rise in plasma progesterone and by the preovulatory estradiol peak. On analysis of SP_1 and hCG findings during the luteal phase in these 15 patients, it was found that they fell into three clearly defined categories: non-pregnant, subclinical abortion and normal pregnancy. Figure 1 shows serial SP_1 and hCG measurements during the luteal phase in 5 patients with normal ovulatory, nonconceptual cycles. Neither SP_1 nor hCG could be detected and there were no clinical findings to suggest that the patients might have conceived. The subclinical abortions showed a transient positive SP_1 and hCG as illustrated in Fig. 2. These positives occurred between day 3 and 9 after ovulation. To our surprise these proteins could be detected on only one day; only in 1 of these 5 patients was SP_1 found on two consecutive days. In 3 of these patients with subclinical abortion, the period was delayed by 1–2 days and the patients had heavy periods with some blood clots and abdominal pain.

SP_1 and hCG findings in normal pregnancies are shown in Fig. 3. Both SP_1

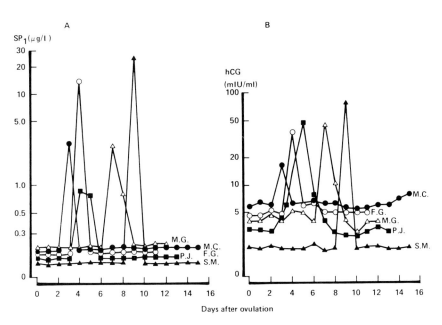

Figure 2. Serial SP_1 measurements (a) and serial hCG measurements (b) during the luteal phase in 5 women with a subclinical abortion pattern.

A. G. Ahmed and A. Klopper

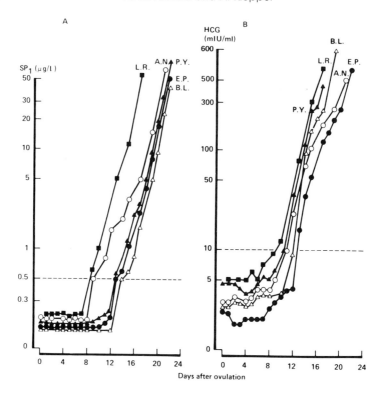

Figure 3. Serial SP₁ measurements (a) and serial hCG measurements (b) during the luteal phase in the conceptual cycle in 5 normal pregnant women. Dotted horizontal lines in Fig. 3 (a) and (b) indicate lowest level of placental protein regarded as positive for pregnancy.

and hCG were first detected 8–13 days postovulatory and rose steeply after the first positive findings. Pregnancy was later confirmed by ultrasonic scan and the patients went on to deliver a normal full-term baby.

Discussion

No SP_1 or hCG could be detected in nonconceptual menstrual cycles. This fact supports the trophoblastic origin of these proteins. In conceptual cycles, however, these two proteins are found in the maternal blood circulation but their pattern in normal pregnancy are different from those in whom the pregnancy fails to continue and is lost silently in the very early days of gestation even before the patients are aware that they were pregnant, i.e. subclinical abortion. Normal pregnancy positives occur late in the luteal phase, persist once they appear and rise briskly. In subclinical abortion positive findings occur earlier in the luteal phase and are transient, being present only a day or two. When they persist for more than a day, they show a decline from the initial value, unlike the sharp rise of a normal pregnancy.

The occurrence of hCG and SP_1 together in the conceptual cycle strengthens the view that they are coming from the fertilized ovum. It also suggests that assays of either or both proteins are useful for the diagnosis of subclinical abortion as they are for the diagnosis of pregnancy. It seems reasonable to suggest that both SP_1 and hCG are signals from the early conceptus and they may play an important role in the continuation of the pregnancy. In subclinical abortion, the signal pattern is unlike the normal one. It might be a result of the effect of pregnancy failure; the fertilized ovum might be forced to strengthen its signals in order to overcome some adverse reactions.

Acknowledgements

We are grateful to Dr F. Dati for the gift of SP_1 kits. This study is supported by a grant from the World Health Organization. We thank Miss Elaine Dalgarno for secretarial assistance.

References

1. Ahmed, A. G. and Klopper, A. (1983). *Br. J. Obstet. Gynaec.* **90**, 604–611.
2. Lenton, E. A., Salaiman, R., Sobowale, O. and Cooke, I. D. (1982). *J. Reprod. Fertil.* **65**, 131–139.
3. Cerni, C., Tatra, G. and Bohn, H. (1977). *Arch. Gynecol.* **223**, 1–7.

The Origin of Amniotic Oxytocin and Vasopressin and their Relationship to Intra-uterine Growth Retardation

H. P. Oosterbaan,* D. F. Swaab and G. J. Boer

*Groot Ziekengasthuis, Department of Obstetrics and Gynaecology,
5211 NL 's-Hertogenbosch, The Netherlands and
Netherlands Institute for Brain Research,
Amsterdam, The Netherlands

Apart from the well-known functions of oxytocin (OXT) and vasopressin (VP) as hormones in labour, lactation and osmoregulation, these peptides seem to be involved in central processes as well (1). Since smaller brains have been demonstrated in the Brattleboro rat strain, which in its homozygous form completely lacks VP (2), additionally VP is supposed to play a role in fetal brain development. In reproduction, moreover, a role for VP has been suggested in the regulation of the amount of amniotic fluid (3) and in the redistribution of the fetal blood flow in fetal stress (4).

Since OXT as well as VP are detectable in the amniotic fluid of both rat and man (5,6) we are currently trying to unfold possible relationships between the amniotic peptide levels and fetal brain development and the process of labour. Therefore it was essential to investigate the origin of the amniotic fluid peptides.

In order to investigate the contribution of the fetal brain to the amniotic peptide levels, two groups of human anencephalics were studied. In the first group ($n = 8$) maternal plasma, mixed umbilical cord blood and amniotic fluid were collected, while the second group ($n = 8$) consisted of amniotic fluid that had been stored for a longer time. Control values were obtained from normal pregnancies ($n = 31$, ranging from 33–41 weeks gestation, data not shown) for the first, and the amniotic fluid of normal pregnancies matched for gestation length and storage time for the second group. In addition, amniotic fluid of rat anencephalics was studied. They were experimentally obtained by aspirating the fetal brains on day 19 of gestation (see (7) for details). Decapitation of the mothers took place on day 21.

The Physiological Development of the Fetus and Newborn
ISBN 0 12 389080 2

Copyright © 1985 by Academic Press, London.
All rights of reproduction in any form reserved.

As control groups, normal pregnant rats of day 19, 20 and 21 were used, together with a sham-operated group. On all samples in this and the following studies a highly sensitive radioimmunoassay was performed (see (8) for details). For statistical analysis the Mann-Whitney-U test and Spearman-rank test were used for peptide levels and Student t test (two-tailed) for fetal measures. $P < 0.05$ was considered significant.

In human as well as rat anencephalics the maternal OXT levels were not different from control groups, while the VP levels were too often below detection level to allow any conclusions. In human anencephalics normal amniotic OXT levels were found, while normal umbilical OXT levels were found in 3 out of 5 cases. No VP could be demonstrated in the umbilical cord blood, which in normal pregnancies is extremely high, while levels of amniotic VP were always below the RIA detection level.

The amniotic fluid volume of all operated groups was lower than in day-21 controls. Six times more amniotic fluid was retrieved from the aspirated groups as compared with sham-operated fetuses.

Again amniotic VP levels were often below detection level. Amniotic OXT levels in sham-operated animals proved to be 8 times higher than in day-21 controls. Although in brain-aspirated rats these levels were significantly decreased compared with sham-operated levels, they still remained 2.5 times higher than day-21 control levels. When these results were corrected for the extreme differences in amount of amniotic fluid, and the absolute amount of OXT per litter was calculated, no differences existed between sham-operated, brain-aspirated, or day-21 control rats.

From these data we may conclude that the fetal brain does not substantially contribute to maternal or amniotic OXT levels in rat and human pregnancy (5).

Since no conclusions could be drawn from this material for amniotic VP we studied the Brattleboro rat. Homozygous (HOM) males were cross-bred with heterozygous (HET) females, leading to mixed litters of HOM and HET fetuses. Amniotic fluid was obtained on day 20 of gestation.

No differences existed for amniotic OXT between HOM and HET fetuses. However, a significant difference existed for amniotic VP, which was always detectable in HET and never, with one exception, in HOM fetuses ($P = 0.002$). Since in this situation VP is produced on the maternal side and by the HET littermates, amniotic VP seems to be mainly of fetal origin (9).

Finally we investigated the possible contribution of the mother to the amniotic OXT and VP levels in Wistar rats by applying a continuous peptide suppletion by means of an Accurel-collodion implant (10,11), to mothers on day 14 of gestation, with dosages for OXT of 600 μg/tube, VP 200 μg/tube, or with aq. dest. loaded devices as controls. Median maternal OXT levels increased 6–7 times and 5-fold for VP (OXT then decreased significantly, possibly as a result of an inhibition of endogenous peptide secretion). No differences were measured for amniotic OXT which points to an absence of effective passage. Consequently amniotic OXT does not seem to be derived from the mother, nor from the fetal brain, but from alternative fetal sources.

Amniotic VP levels in VP treated rats were elevated compared with control levels, which suggested a passage from the maternal side. However, in the VP treated group a significantly stunted growth was found in some litters, and the amniotic VP elevation was restricted to these litters. Highly significant inverse correlations were found between amniotic VP and fetal body, brain and placental weight, while in addition a positive correlation existed between amniotic OXT and placental weight. In the Accurel control group a negative relation existed between amniotic VP and fetal brain weight.

Furthermore it was found that the elevation of maternal VP in the normally developing litters was even more pronounced than in the growth retarded animals, also pointing to an ineffective passage of this peptide. So amniotic VP seems to be mainly derived from the fetus.

In order to investigate if indeed the above-mentioned VP enhancement resulted from fetal growth retardation two additional techniques were used to brint about stunted fetal growth: (a) intraperitoneal injections of methylazoxymethanol (MAM) to Wistar rats on days 14, 15 and 16 of gestation (20 mg/kg, cf. (12)), or physiological saline as control, and (b) undernutrition of Wistar rats from day 6 of gestation (50% of their normal daily dietary intake, cf. (13)), and normally fed dams as controls. All experimental procedures resulted in a significant stunted growth.

Maternal peptide levels were not influenced by any of the experimental procedures. In both MAM and undernourished groups amniotic VP levels were significantly elevated over control levels. After correction for the changes in total

Table 1. Relationship between fetal body, brain and placental weights and VP and OXT levels in the different experimental and control groups[1]

	VP		OXT	
	r	P	r	P
VP accurel				
Body weight	−0.6833	0.001 (21)[2]	—	—
Brain weight	−0.7059	0.001 (17)	—	—
Placenta weight	−0.4853	0.024 (17)	0.8810	0.002 (8)
Control accurel				
Brain weight	−0.4439	0.049 (15)	—	—
MAM				
Body weight	−0.5035	0.048 (12)	—	—
Brain weight	−0.1506	0.091 (12)	—	—
Control				
Body weight	—	—	0.4130	0.031 (21)
Undernutrit.				
Body weight	−0.3824	0.048 (20)	—	—
Brain weight	−0.3711	0.054 (20)	—	—
Control				
Body weight	—	—	0.5416	0.015 (16)
Brain weight	−0.4351	0.046 (16)	—	—

[1]Only correlations are shown where significance was (almost) reached.
[2]Number of correlated groups is given in parenthesis.

amount of amniotic fluid, this elevation remained significant in the undernourished rats. In the normally nourished group a negative correlation was found between amniotic VP and fetal brain weight. In the MAM-control and normally nourished groups a positive correlation was seen between amniotic OXT and fetal body weight (Table 1).

Moreover, in both experimental groups significant inverse correlations existed between amniotic VP and fetal body weight, while a same trend was observed for fetal brain weight (14).

From these results we may conclude that enhanced levels of amniotic VP reflect fetal growth retardation. VP might play a favourable role under stressful conditions, e.g. by redistributing the fetal blood flow to vital organs (15).

References

1. Swaab, D. F. (1982). *Progr. Brain Res.* **55**, 97–122.
2. Boer, G. J., Van Rheenen-Verberg, C. H. M. and Uylings, H. B. M. (1982). *Develop. Brain Res.* **3**, 557–575.
3. Perks, A. M. and Vizsolyi, E. (1973). *In:* "Foetal and Neonatal Physiology", (R. S. Comline *et al.*, eds) pp. 430–438. Cambridge University Press.
4. Pohjavuori, M. and Fyhrquist, F. (1980). *J. Pediat.* **97**, 462–465.
5. Swaab, D. F. and Oosterbaan, H. P. (1983). *Br. J. Obstet. Gynaecol.* **90**, 1160–1167.
6. Dawood, M. Y., Wang, C. F., Gupta, R. and Fuchs, F. (1978). *Obstet. Gynecol.* **52**, 205–209.
7. Swaab, D. F. and Honnebier, W. J. (1973). *J. Obstet. Gynaecol. Brit. Commonwealth* **80**, 589–597.
8. Dogterom, J., Snijdewint, F. G. M., Pevet, P. and Swaab, D. F. (1980). *J. Endocrinol.* **84**, 115–123.
9. Oosterbaan, H. P., Swaab, D. F. and Boer, G. J. (1984a). *J. Develop. Physiol.* (accepted for publication).
10. Boer, G. J. and Kruisbrink, J. (1984). *J. Endocrinol.* (in press).
11. Kruisbrink, J. and Boer, G. J. (1984). *J. Pharmacol. Sci.* (in press).
12. Haddad, R. K., Rabe, A., Laqueur, G. L., Spatz, M. and Valsamis, M. P. (1969). *Science* **163**, 88–90.
13. Patel, A. J., Balasz, R. and Johnson, A. L. (1973). *J. Neurochem.* **20**, 1151–1165.
14. Oosterbaan, H. P., Swaab, D. F. and Boer, G. J. (1984b). *J. Develop. Physiol.* (submitted for publication).
15. Iwamoto, H. S., Rudolph, A. M., Keil, L. C. and Heymann, M. A. (1979). *Circulat. Res.* **44**, 430–436.
16. Abramovich, D. R. (1978). *In:* "Amniotic Fluid — Research and Clinical Application" (D. V. I. Fairweather and T. K. A. B. Eskes, eds) pp. 31–49, Excerpta Medica, Amsterdam.
17. Cohn, H. E., Sacks, E. J., Heymann, M. A. and Rudolph, A. M. (1974). *Am. J. Obstet. Gynaecol.* **120**, 817–824.

The Human Glutathione S-transferases: Developmental Aspects of the GST1 and GST3 Loci

Brian A. Davis, Charles G. Faulder, William Cotton, A. D. Bain,* Robert Hume* and Richard C. Strange

Department of Clinical Biochemistry, Central Pathology Laboratory, North Staffordshire Hospital Centre, Staffordshire, UK
*Department of Child Life and Health, University of Edinburgh, Royal Infirmary, Edinburgh, Scotland

The glutathione S-transferases (GST; EC 2.5.1.18) are a group of ubiquitous, dimeric detoxicating enzymes that in humans are the products of three autosomal loci, GST1, GST2 and GST3 (1). The products of all three loci exhibit variability, but only in the case of *GST1* does this appear to be genetically determined (2). Although GST activity has been detected in various human fetal tissues, no systematic study of the development of these loci has been described and little is known of the details of their expression during and after pregnancy. We describe experiments using starch gel electrophoresis and chromatofocussing, to investigate the development of the isoenzymes of these different gene loci in fetal and neonatal liver cytosol.

Cytosol was prepared from samples of tissues obtained with the permission of the Ethics Committee of the Simpson Memorial Maternity Pavilion, Royal Infirmary, Edinburgh. Starch gel electrophoresis was performed using a continuous Tris-citrate buffer system and the GST isoenzymes detected by staining with an agarose overlay containing the substrates, reduced glutathione and 1-chloro-2,4-dinitrobenzene (2). Chromatofocussing was performed at 4°C using columns containing Polybuffer exchanger 94 (Pharmacia Fine Chemicals, Hounslow, Middlesex, TW3 1NE) previously equilibrated with start buffer (25 mM imidazole buffer, pH 7.4). The pH gradient was formed using Polybuffer 74 adjusted to pH 4.0 with HCl (5M). Fractions were analysed for enzyme activity and pH. In initial experiments each peak of activity was examined by starch-gel electrophoresis to determine which gene products were present.

The Physiological Development of the Fetus and Newborn
ISBN 0 12 389080 2
Copyright © 1985 by Academic Press, London.
All rights of reproduction in any form reserved.

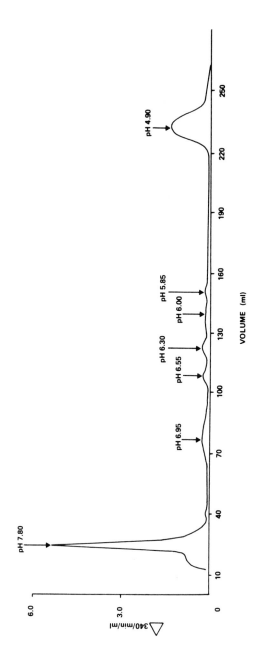

Figure 1. Chromatofocussing of liver cytosol from an 18-week human fetus.

Starch gel electrophoresis allowed resolution of the GST isoenzymes in tissue cytosols. GST3 isoenzymes exhibited fast, anodal mobility, GST1 isoenzymes slower anodal mobility and the GST2 isoenzymes cathodal mobility. There were changes in the expression of the GST loci both during and after pregnancy. For example, the GST1 isoenzymes were generally not detected, using starch gel electrophoresis, in cytosol obtained before 30 weeks gestation. Thereafter the distribution of observed phenotypes was as expected if the GST1 isoenzymes result from combinations of three alleles, GST1*0, GST1*1 and GST1*2 (1). As expected the GST1 phenotype was a constant individual characteristic in liver, spleen, adrenal, and kidney but not in diaphragm (2).

Changes in the expression of the GST2 locus were also detected in kidney. In adults this locus is strongly expressed in liver, adrenal and kidney but not in most other tissues. In kidney, GST2 isoenzymes were weakly expressed during intra-uterine life and did not appear to be fully expressed until about 1 year after birth. The GST3 locus codes for the most acidic isoenzymes. The expression of this locus was constant both during and after fetal life in all tissues except liver. In this tissue the GST3 locus was present until about 25 weeks gestation. Thereafter its expression appeared to decline.

Chromatofocussing resulted in the separation of the different GST isoenzymes. The GST2 isoenzymes eluted first, usually as two peaks of activity. The first was not retained and corresponded to the isoenzyme with fast cathodal mobility, the second peak where present (eluted between pH 6.70 and 6.95) to the isoenzyme with slower cathodal mobility. The GST1 isoenzymes eluted between pH 6.25 and 6.50 (GST1 2 phenotype) or between pH 5.90 and 5.95 (GST1 1 phenotype). The GST3 isoenzymes were not resolved and they eluted as a broad peak between pH 4.75 and 4.90.

Since GST activity in cytosols obtained before 20 weeks resulted almost entirely from the GST2 and GST3 isoenzymes, the elution profiles were relatively simple. However, even at this stage of gestation there was evidence of weak expression of the GST1 locus (Fig. 1). The elution profile of cytosol obtained after 24 weeks gestation was similar with several enzyme forms eluting between pH 6.65 and 5.75. It appears therefore that although the GST1 isoenzymes are not utually detected by starch gel electrophoresis the GST1 locus is weakly expressed in liver cytosol before 30 weeks gestation.

We conclude that the development of the GST is similar, in many respects, to that of other enzymes (3). The proportion of basic (GST2) to acidic (GST3) isoenzymes increased during gestation. Further, the change in the expression of isoenzymes was gradual and the patterns in tissues obtained early in gestation were simpler than those found later. The complexity of patterns increased after 20 weeks gestation and continued to do so into early infancy with adult-type patterns appearing almost 1 year after birth.

References

1. Board, P. G. (1981). *Am. J. Hum. Genet.* **33**, 36–43.

2. Strange, R. C., Faulder, C. G., Davis, B. A., Hume, R., Brown, J. A. H., Cotton, W. and Hopkinson, D. A. (1984). *Ann. Hum. Genet.* **48**, 11–20.
3. Edwards, Y. H. and Hopkinson, D. A. (1977). Isoenzymes: *Curr. Top. Biol. Med. Res.* **1**, 19–78.

Growth Factors and Intra-uterine Growth Retardation in the Guinea-pig

C. T. Jones, H. N. Lafeber* and J. T. Parer**

The Nuffield Institute for Medical Research,
University of Oxford, Oxford, UK

D. A. Price

Department of Child Health,
University of Manchester, Manchester, UK

K. Hall and V. Sara

Karolinska Institute, Sweden

Introduction

The natural and experimentally enforced variations in prenatal growth rate are associated with marked alterations in the maturation rates of liver, muscle, heart and possibly the brain (1–3). Some of this can be ascribed to the low plasma insulin concentrations common in this condition (1,4–6), but this alone is unlikely to explain satisfactorily problems such as delay in ossification of cartilage (1,7,8). Somatomedins have been implicated as related to different states of growth (9,10,15), but the relationship is not always particularly close. Thus raised, although not very high, prenatal somatomedin levels have been reported in some but not all studies (11–13). The decline in the relationship between plasma somatomedin concentration and the ability of plasma to stimulate cartilage growth

*Present address: Department of Paediatrics, Sophia Children's Hospital, Rotterdam, The Netherlands.
**Present address: Department of Obstetrics and Gynaecology, HSE 1462, University of California, San Francisco, CA 94143, USA

The Physiological Development of the Fetus and Newborn
ISBN 0 12 389080 2

Copyright © 1985 by Academic Press, London.
All rights of reproduction in any form reserved.

in states of undernutrition has been instrumental in initiating a search for inhibitors of somatomedin action and some have been proposed as being proteins of 20–30K (14,15). Such factors, if present in the fetal circulation in relatively large quantities, could potentially explain why prebirth plasma somatomedin concentrations could be considered to be low for the growth rates. To investigate this problem, somatomedin concentration in fetal plasma, with a very much reduced rate of growth, has been compared with the potency of that plasma to stimulate cartilage growth.

Methods

Pregnant guinea-pigs were subjected to uterine artery ligation at day 30 as outlined elsewhere (1,16). At day 50–52 of gestation the fetuses were delivered under nembutal anaesthesia (30 mg/kg) and up to 0.5 ml of umbilical venous blood collected in heparinized syringes. After separation the plasma was stored at $-20°C$ until assay. Sulphation-promoting activity was determined in the pig coastal cartilage assay as described by Van den Brande and Du Caju (17). Somatomedin A activity was measured by radioreceptor assay (18). IGF-I was measured by radioimmunoassay (12) with an antibody kindly provided by the National Hormone and Pituitary Agency. IGF-II was measured by radioreceptor assay using guinea-pig placental membranes prepared by a modification of the method for rat described by Daughaday *et al.* (19). In each case the interassay variation was < 19%. The cross-reactivity of IGF-I in the IGF-II assay was < 2% and *vice versa* < 10%.

Measurement of the insulin-like growth factors was made after acid-ethanol plasma extraction (20).

Results

In the sulphation assay setting adult male guinea-pig plasma, equivalent to 1 unit/ml, plasma from an hypophysectomized 500 g guinea-pig, had an activity of 0.23 ± 0.14 units/ml. The value for the 50 days pregnant female was 0.49 ± 0.28 units/ml. At 50–52 days gestation the fetal plasma sulphation-promoting activity was marginally below that of the adult male (Fig. 1) and by 60–63 days it had fallen to $41.4 \pm 18.7\%$. Plasma from growth-retarded fetuses, whose weight was 18.1 ± 3.2 g by comparison with 43.9 ± 4.8 g for controls, inhibited sulphate incorporation into cartilage (Fig. 1). Adding plasma from growth-retarded fetuses to that from normal fetuses also led to a plasma preparation that inhibited sulphate incorporation.

These results were all the more striking as although the somatomedin A activity in normal fetuses was comparable with that reported for other species and fell during gestation, the values in growth-retarded fetal guinea-pigs were 3–4 fold higher than normal (Fig. 2). Consistent with this, plasma IGF-II (probably identical to somatomedin A) concentrations were also dramatically raised in the growth-retarded fetuses (Fig. 3) as were the levels of IGF-I, although they did not show the same developmental pattern (Fig. 4).

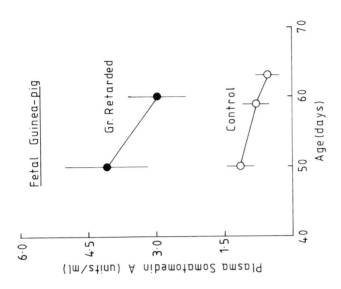

Figure 2. Plasma somatomedin A concentrations from normal and growth-retarded fetal guinea-pigs. Normal 50–52 day fetuses were 43.4±6.3 g (5) compared with 18.4±3.2 g (5) for the retarded ones and at 60–63 days the values were 87.1±9.3 g (5) and 30.5±4.8 g (5) respectively.

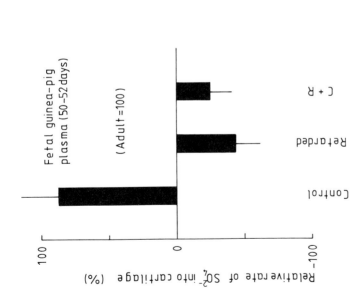

Figure 1. Relative rates of sulphate-incorporation into pig cartilage incubated with plasma, at 20% dilution, from normal and growth-retarded 50–52 day fetal guinea-pigs. The effects of adding plasma, at a combined dilution of 20%, from both sets of fetuses is also shown.

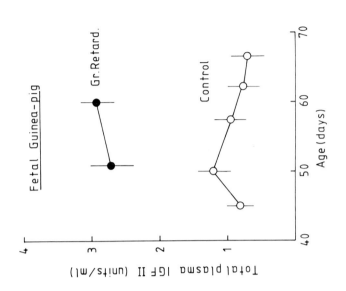

Figure 4. Changes in plasma IGF-II concentrations in normal and growth-retarded fetal guinea-pigs. Other details as for Fig. 2.

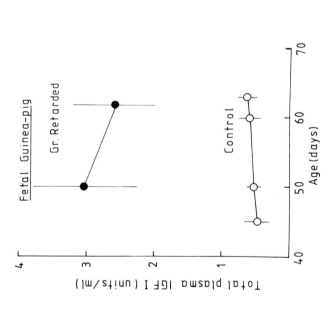

Figure 3. Changes in plasma IGF-I concentrations in normal and growth-retarded fetal guinea-pigs. Other details as for Fig. 2.

Discussion

There are a variety of studies in which plasma somatomedin concentrations have been measured in the fetal circulation. Those on extracted or unextracted plasma and measurement by radioimmuno- or radioreceptor assay report slightly higher prenatal than adult values (13–15). Those for the newborn tend to be somewhat higher. Measurement by sulphation assay often leads to similar levels (13), or as reported here lower fetal values. Somatomedin levels have been correlated with fetal growth rate (21) and growth-retarded fetal sheep have depressed plasma sulphation-promoting activity (13). However for obvious reasons most of the studies on the effect of undernutrition on plasma somatomedin concentration have been directed at postnatal life. Thus in the rat, fasting causes a decrease in cartilage growth preceded by a fall in plasma somatomedin activity (14). Similar changes are observed in hypoinsulinaemic states (14). In both of these conditions, and during their correction, the relationship between somatomedin concentration and bio-activity changes, with higher somatomedin concentrations than might be expected being detected. This led originally to the proposal of endogenous inhibitors of somatomedin action and subsequently semi-purified preparations have been reported with a wide range of molecular weights (14). The depression of somatomedin activity is most apparent with low protein intact and this is potentiated if caloric intake is also reduced (14). In none of these states of altered growth has a depression of somatomedin activity of the degree reported here been observed. The other hormones such as insulin, cortisol and thyroid hormones that have potentially direct effect on cartilage, although all somewhat depressed (6), are unlikely to account for the inhibitory effect on cartilage of plasma from growth-retarded fetuses. The observations are most consistent with the proposal from studies on the adult that endogenous inhibitors are present in plasma and during growth retardation there is an enhanced production. Such factors would explain the ability of this plasma to suppress sulphation-promoting activity of plasma from normal fetuses. Evidence has been presented elsewhere that such factors are probably proteins, at least one being 40K, and they may affect the growth and maturation of other tissues as well as that of cartilage (22). The growth-retarded fetuses behave as though they are subjected to both protein and calorie malnutrition (14).

References

1. Lafeber, H. N., Jones, C. T. and Rolph, T. P. (1979). *In:* "Nutrition and Metabolism of the Fetus and Infant". (H. K. A. Visser, ed.) pp. 43–62. Martinus Nijhoff, The Hague.
2. Jones, C. T. and Robinson, J. S. (1979). *In* "Maternal Effects in Development". (D. R. Newth and M. Balls, eds) pp. 395–409. Cambridge University Press.
3. Jones, C. T. and Rolph, T. P. (1981). *CIBA Symp.* **86**, 214–228.
4. Jones, C. T., Harding, J. E., Robinson, J. S., Lafeber, H. N. and Rolph, T. P. (1980). *Adv. Anim. Comp. Physiol.* **20**, 53–60.
5. Robinson, J. S., Hart, I. C., Kingston, E. J., Jones, C. T. and Thorburn, G. D. (1980). *J. Develop. Physiol.* **2**, 239–248.

6. Jones, C. T., Lafeber, H. N. and Roebuck, M. M. (1984). *J. Develop. Physiol.* **6** 461-472.
7. Robinson, J. S., Kingston, E. J., Jones, C. T. and Thorburn, G. D. (1979). *J. Develop. Physiol.* **1**, 379-398.
8. Scott, K. E. and Usher, R. (1966). *Am. J. Obstet. Gynecol.* **94**, 951-963.
9. Daughaday, W. H. (1981). *In:* "Endocrine Control of Growth" (Daughaday, W. H., ed.) pp. 1-24. Elsevier, New York.
10. Van Wyk, J. J. and Underwood, L. E. (1978). *Biochem. Act. Horm.* **5**, 101-148.
11. Falconer, J., Forbes, J. M., Hart, I. C., Robinson, J. S. and Thorburn, G. D. (1979). *J. Endocrinol.* **83**, 119-127.
12. Daughaday, W. H., Parker, K., Borowsky, S., Trivedi, B. and Kapadia, M. (1982). *Endocrinology* **110**, 575-581.
13. Gluckman, P. D. and Butler, J. H. (1983). *J. Endocrinol.* **99**, 223-232.
14. Phillips, L. S. (1981). *In:* "Endocrine Control of Growth" (Daughaday, W. H., ed.) pp. 121-173. Elsevier, New York.
15. Phillips, L. S., Belosky, D. C., Young, H. S. and Reichard, L. A. (1979). *Endocrinology* **104**, 1519-1524.
16. Jones, C. T. and Parer, J. T. (1984). *J. Physiol.* **343**, 525-537.
17. Van den Brande, J. L. and DuCaju, M. V. L. (1974). *Acta Endocrinol.* **75**, 233-242.
18. Hall, K., Brandt, J., Engerg, G. and Fyklund, L. (1979). *J. Clin. Endocrinol. Metab.* **48**, 271-278.
19. Daughaday, W. H., Trivedi, B. and Kapadia, M. (1981). *J. Clin. Endocrinol. Metab.* **53**, 289-294.
20. Daughaday, W. H., Mariz, I. K. and Blethen, S. C. (1980). *J. Clin. Endocrinol. Metab.* **51**, 781-788.
21. Gluckman, P. D. and Brinsmead, M. W. (1976). *J. Clin. Endocrinol. Metab.* **43**, 1378-1381.
22. Jones, C. T. (1985). *Biochem. Soc. Trans.* **13**, 89-91.

The Onset and Organization of Hypothalamic Control in the Fetus

P. D. Gluckman

Developmental Physiology Laboratory, Department of Paediatrics,
University of Auckland, Auckland, New Zealand

Introduction

Control of anterior pituitary hormone release by the hypothalamus develops as a gradual process within which several distinct phases are apparent. *In vitro* studies have suggested that Rathkes pouch will differentiate into the various classes of adenohypophysial secretory cells in the absence of hypothalamic influences even though hypothalamic neurohormones are detectable in the primitive neuraxis at this stage. However, these *in vitro* studies do suggest that hypothalamic factors with our observations of GH secretion in the fetus. The cell bodies for SRIF lie in the supraoptic region of the anterior hypothalamus and in 2 fetuses that by the time that the primitive primary plexus of the portal system has differentiated on the surface of the developing infundibulum, axons staining for corticotropin releasing factor (CRF) (3), luteinizing hormone releasing factor (LRF) (4) and somatostatin (SRIF) (5) are terminating in apposition to these capillaries. This stage (10–15 weeks in the human fetus, less than 60 days in the fetal sheep, 20 days postconception — 5 days postnatal in the rat) remains largely beyond *in vivo* investigation except for postnatal studies in altricial species.

However, the chronically catheterized fetal lamb offers an experimental approach to the maturation of the neuroendocrine axis at stages subsequent to this. The recent development of a stereotaxic approach to the fetal sheep diencephalon (6) extends the range of experiments possible. Recent studies in the ovine fetus suggest parallels in the manner in which neuroendocrine function develops in the second half of gestation with respect to the control of several adenohypophysial hormones.

The Physiological Development of the Fetus and Newborn
ISBN 0 12 389080 2   *Copyright © 1985 by Academic Press, London.*
All rights of reproduction in any form reserved.

Studies of Growth Hormone (GH) in the Perinatal Lamb

Growth hormone (GH) concentrations in the fetuses of nonaltricial species are markedly higher than in the postnatal animal (2). Despite this, GH does not play a significant role in the regulation of perinatal growth because of an immaturity of somatotropic receptors in the liver which is the primary target tissue for the effect of GH on growth. While this observation does not exclude other functions for GH in the fetus via its weaker affinity for the lactogenic receptor or in other tissues, it is clear that GH is not essential for fetal development (2). It has therefore been postulated that the basis for the high concentrations of GH in the fetal circulation is the immature state of hypothalamic control of GH secretion. Thus studies of GH secretion in the fetus may offer insights into the maturation of hypothalamic function.

Previous studies of GH concentrations in the fetus have been primarily restricted to longitudinal or cross-sectional measurements on samples taken at infrequent intervals, generally no more than once daily. One feature of these studies has been the large scatter of fetal GH concentrations which raises the possibility of short-term changes in GH secretion being masked by infrequent single point estimations. We have therefore re-examined the secretion of GH in the sheep fetus using frequent sampling at 20-min intervals for several hours. These studies demonstrate that GH secretion in the fetus from 70 days is characterized by markedly exaggerated pulsatile release. The mean amplitude of the GH pulse in the fetus is $92 \pm$ (SEM) 21 ng/ml ($n = 18$) compared to 23.7 ± 6.4 ng/ml ($n = 7$) in the infant lamb. The interpulse nadir can be considered as an index of basal secretion by the pituitary. In the fetal lamb the interpulse nadir is 102 ± 12 ng/ml which is much greater than in the neonatal lamb (5.8 ± 1.3 ng/ml) or adult sheep.

A preliminary analysis of 26 fetal studies between 85 days and term shows no change in the interpulse nadir with advancing maturation although at birth it falls markedly. The pulse height falls ($P < 0.05$) from 94.5 ± 16.4 ng/ml prior to 120 days to 53.5 ± 6.1 ng/ml after 120 days and further ($P < 0.05$) after birth. There is a significant negative correlation between pulse height and gestational age ($r = 0.61$, $P < 0.01$). These pulse studies therefore present a different picture of fetal GH release from that derived from single point sampling. They suggest that prior to birth, there is a progressive reduction in the height of GH pulses and in relationship to birth there is a fall in the interpulse nadir. The pulse frequency shows a trend to be higher ($P < 0.1$) in fetuses less than 120 days (0.80 ± 0.06 pulses/h) than in older fetuses (0.65 ± 0.05 pulses/h) or lambs (0.69 ± 0.06 pulses/h). While pulsatile GH release is characteristic of GH secretion postnatally, the distinct feature of GH secretion in the fetus is this markedly exaggerated pulsatility and high interpulse nadir.

These studies have been extended to fetuses in which electrolytic lesions were placed stereotaxically in the fetal hypothalamus at 110 days of gestation (6) and the pattern of GH secretion was evaluated 4–7 days later (7). Lesions of the median eminence abolished pulsatile GH release (Fig. 1) and basal GH concentrations were comparable to those of the neonatal lamb (Fig. 2). This demonstrates that in midgestation, GH release is entirely dependent on hypothalamic stimulation;

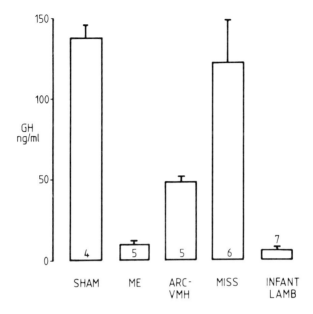

Figure 1. Basal growth hormone (GH) concentrations (mean ± SEM) in 4 groups of fetuses subject to stereotaxic surgery of the hypothalamus and in the infant lamb. The fetuses were operated on at 110 days of gestation and were considered in 4 groups; sham operated controls, those with complete destruction of the median eminence (ME), those with destruction of the arcuate-ventromedial region without destruction of the median eminence (ARC-VMH) and those with lesions outside the endocrine hypotalamus (Miss). Fetuses were studied 4-7 days after surgery and intact lambs were studied 3-20 days after birth. The number of animals studied in each group is shown. The basal GH was defined as the lowest GH value of 10 arterial samples collected over 3 h. The lambs and ME lesioned fetus had lower ($P < 0.01$) basal GH concentrations than all other groups. The ARC-VMH group had lower ($P < 0.05$) basal GH values than the sham or the Miss groups.

there is not evidence for autonomy of pituitary GH release or for direct extrahypothalamic stimulation of the somatotrope. These latter possibilities have been previously advanced as possible explanations of the high concentrations of GH in the fetal circulation. Lesions of the arcuate-ventromedial region of the hypothalamus that did not involve the median eminence also largely abolished pulsatility and lowered the interpulse nadir. This area of the hypothalamus is where cell bodies for growth hormone releasing factor (GRF) are located (8). This together with the observation that exogenous GRF has been demonstrated to stimulate fetal GH release from 72 days of gestation (9,10) suggests that fetal GH release is determined by pulsatile GRF release. This is supported by the observations that the height of spontaneous GH pulses decreases with advancing gestation in parallel with the decrease in responsiveness to exogenous GRF (10).

Current concepts of the neuroendocrine control of GH secretion in the postnatal mammal suggest that GH secretion is determined by pulsatile GRF release and

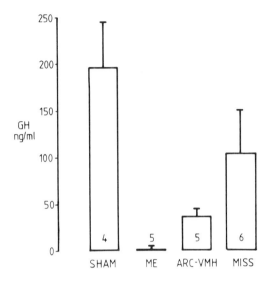

Figure 2. The amplitude of group hormone pulses in 4 groups of fetuses subject to stereotaxic surgery of the hypothalamus. The pulse height was calculated as the difference between the highest and lowest growth hormone estimations on 10 samples collected over 3 h, 4–7 days after surgery. The grouping of the fetuses is described in the legend to Fig. 1. The ME group had lesser pulsatility ($P < 0.01$) than all other groups and the ARC-VMH group had reduced ($P < 0.05$) pulsatility compared to the sham and Miss groups.

that SRIF non-competitively inhibits the action of GRF and thus determines the amplitude of the GH pulse (11). In addition, tonic SRIF secretion may determine the basal secretion of GH by the somatotrope although this is less certain. A deficiency of SRIF release or action would therefore be compatible with our observations of GH secretion in the fetus. The cell bodies for SRIF lie in the supraoptic region of the anterior hypothalamus and in 2 fetuses electrolytically lesioned in this region no change in the pattern of GH secretion was apparent. Although SRIF is present in the fetal hypothalamus (12) and exogenous SRIF can inhibit fetal GH release (13), there is no evidence for hypothalamic SRIF secretion *in utero*. Further studies using passive immunization against SRIF are indicated.

Recent studies have demonstrated that GH secretion in mature animals is regulated in part by a negative feedback loop by which GH and/or insulin-like growth factors (IGFs) stimulate hypothalamic SRIF release (14,15). An immaturity of this short feedback loop could thus explain fetal GH release in the late gestation sheep fetus. The recent observations that somatotropic receptors cannot be demonstrated in ovine hepatic tissue until 3–6 days postpartum (7) provides a basis for the lack of a major effect of GH on somatic growth *in utero*. It also demonstrates that differentiation of hormone receptors may occur independently from and much later than the onset of the secretion of a hormone and that this can determine hormone action at different stages of development. A similar late development of central GH receptors provides one possible explanation of the high GH concentrations in the fetal circulation. This process may be gradual; the decrease in both the responsiveness to GRF and of the height of spontaneous GH pulses with advancing gestation (9,10) suggests that there may be a gradual imposition of inhibitory control in late gestation. Alternatively these observations may reflect changing responsiveness of the somatotrope. The apparent sudden changes in GH secretion in the days around birth requires further evaluation taking cognisance of the pulsatility of GH release. It may represent a marked increase in the amount of SRIF released, a change in pituitary responsiveness or a marked decrease in GRF release. The potential role of the glucocorticoid surge or progesterone withdrawal in inducing this change remains to be resolved. Recent observations in the adult dog raise the possibility that progesterone alters the neuroendocrine axis to increase GH release (16). The possibility of extrahypothalamic factors (e.g. placental factors) indirectly affecting hypothalamic function has not yet been excluded.

Several issues remain to be resolved with respect to the control of GH release in the fetus. It is noteworthy that in all the neuropharmacological studies of fetal GH release reported to date including those where high doses of exogenous SRIF were administered, fetal GH secretion was not reduced by more than 50% (13,17–20). Relative autonomy of fetal pituitary GH release is excluded by the observations on fetuses with lesions of the median eminence discussed above and it seems more likely that the failure to completely inhibit fetal GH release by the infusion of SRIF may be a consequence of the short period of infusion used in these experiments. By analogy to other endocrine systems, it would not be surprising if a relatively long exposure to SRIF is necessary for maximal effect. It is possible that glucocorticoids induce changes in the somatotrope allowing greater responsiveness.

The basis for the generation of the GH pulses *in utero* remains to be elucidated. They are not synchronous to those of luteinizing hormone (LH) or thyrotropin (TSH). Presumably the pulse generator lies within the endocrine hypothalamus.

The maturation of the control of GH release via neurotransmitters modulating hypothalamic neurohormone release has been reviewed recently (1). These studies have used systematically not centrally administered agents and thus must be interpreted with caution. They demonstrate that although the potential for the neurohormonal control of GH release has differentiated by midgestation (9,10), the potential for specific classes of neurotransmitters to influence GH release develops over a broad gestational range. Some agents such as β-adrenergic (19) and GABA-ergic agonists (20) do not affect GH release until after 110 days of gestation after completion of the rapid phase of brain growth. In the case of GABA-ergic agonists, it seems probable that this late differentiation of a response is dependent on the appearance of the GABA-benzodiazepine receptor complex in the fetal hypothalamus (20). These observations serve to demonstrate the complexity of the maturation of hypothalamic function and show that well after morphological differentiation is complete, synaptogensis is continuing which leads to functional changes in the control of hormone release.

P. D. Gluckman

The hypothesis, thus presented, which suggests that GH secretion *in utero* is characterized by exaggerated pulsatility due to pulsatile-release factor release associated with immaturity of inhibitory control has parallels in recent observations of TSH and LH secretion in the fetus.

Studies of Thyrotropin (TSH) in the Perinatal Lamb

Despite the extensive studies of the maturation of the thyroid axis, relatively little is known of the maturation of the control of TSH release *in utero*. A number of studies in the sheep and simian fetus have demonstrated a fetal TSH response to thyrotropin releasing factor (TRF) and this response in late gestation is generally greater than that of the postnatal animal (21). Two studies have suggested that exogenous thyroid hormones fail to completely suppress the fetal TSH response to TRF (21–23). These studies together with clinical observations suggest relative immaturity of the negative feedback loop in the late gestation fetus.

We have re-evaluated the secretion of TSH in the ovine fetus and lamb using frequent sampling every 20 min for periods of 3–4 h. We observed markedly pulsatile TSH release in the fetus. The characteristics of the pulsatile release are summarized in Table 1. The fetal pusles were more frequent and significantly greater amplitude than after birth where there were only a few pulses of low amplitude observed (24). The TSH pulses were not synchronous with GH pulses. Further the interpulse nadir, an index of basal TSH secretion, was greater in fetuses less than 120 days than in older fetuses and was always undetectable in the postnatal studies (Table 1). This marked pulsatility of TSH release appears to be unique to the fetus and is postulated to be a consequence of a relative immaturity of inhibitory feedback control.

Table 1. The ontogeny of pulsatile TSH release

	pulse height (μU/ml)	interpulse nadir (μU/ml)	pulse frequency (pulses/h)
Fetuses <120 days (8)	7.4±9.6	3.4±4.8	0.76±0.40
>120 days (7)	3.0±1.4	0.4±0.5**	0.64±0.24
Lambs (5)	2.1±1.1*	<0.1	0.33±0.14*
Nonpregnant ewes (13)	1.5±0.5*	<0.1	0.28±0.11*

*$P<0.5$ compared to all fetuses
**$P<0.05$ compared to younger fetuses
mean±SD

The maturational changes in the secretion of TSH commence before birth but are accentuated following delivery. The marked change in TSH secretion at birth is presumably related to the increase in circulating triiodothyronine (T_3) concentrations firstly as a result of the parturition-related rise in fetal glucocorticoids leading to the induction of the outer-ring deiodinase in the fetal liver (25) and secondly due to the separation from the placenta. The placenta is rich in the inner-ring deiodinase which will convert thyroxine to inactive reverse

T_3 (26) and following cord separation, T_3 levels rise. However the reduction in basal TSH secretion and the trend for the TSH pulse amplitude and frequency to decrease after 120 days of gestation suggests that the sensitivity of the negative feedback control of TSH release increases after 120 days. Negative feedback by thyroid hormones is believed to be mediated by both circulating T_3 and particularly the intrapituitary conversion of thyroxine to T_3 followed by the induction of the synthesis of an intrapituitary peptide which inhibits TSH release. The changing sensitivity of thyroid-hormone mediated negative feedback may involve either of these processes. Immaturity of SRIF release could also contribute to the hypersecretion of TSH *in utero* as SRIF plays a role in the inhibition of postnatal TSH release (27).

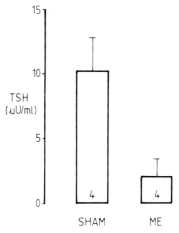

Figure 3. The amplitude of thyrotropin (TSH) pulses in sheep fetuses at 115 days of gestation following electrolytic destruction of the median eminence (ME) at 109 days of gestation and in sham operated controls. The ME fetus had a significantly reduced ($P<0.05$) amplitude which was calculated as the difference between the highest and lowest TSH value on 10 arterial samples collected over 3 h.

Fetal TSH release in the late gestation sheep fetus is dependent on hypothalamic stimulation. Following ME lesions, the amplitude of TSH pulses is reduced significantly (Fig. 3). As reported elsewhere in this volume (28), fetal TSH levels rise rapidly following cooling of the amniotic fluid demonstrating that the hypothalamic mechanisms by which cold induces TRF release have differentiated by 106 days of gestation. Studies in altricial species such as the rat demonstrate that at an earlier stage of neuroendocrine maturation, TSH secretion is independent of neural influences (29). It may be that TRF receptor development determines the onset of TSH release at an earlier stage than is possible to examine in the sheep fetus.

Studies of Gonadotropin Secretion in the Ovine Fetus

Cross-sectional studies in the ovine fetus demonstrate that circulating LH concentrations are highest in midgestation and fall after 120 days (30). Again frequent sampling experiments have demonstrated that fetal LH release in midgestation is pulsatile in nature (31). Pulsatile LH release has generally been considered to be a feature of pubertal control of gonadotropin release and the fetus in midgestation shows many of the features of puberty including active folliculogenesis or spermatogenesis. Late in gestation gonadotropin secretion and gonadal activity diminishes and this is associated with a decrease in responsiveness to exogenous LH releasing factor (LRF) (32). As responsiveness to exogenous LRF is generally considered to be an index of endogenous LRF release, this suggests a decrease in hypothalamic LRF release late in gestation. Exogenous estradiol -17B inhibits LH release at 110 days of gestation but not at 90 days (33). The decrease in activity of the gonadotropic axis late in gestation may therefore reflect the development of negative feedback. From studies in the fetal rat and mouse this may be due to the appearance of estrogen receptors in the hypothalamus at this stage (34). Thus the changing pattern of LH secretion *in utero* shows some similarities to GH and TSH in that, in midgestation, there is marked pulsatility of LH release, reducing in late gestation at least in part due to an increase in sensitivity of the negative feedback mechanism.

Concluding Comments

The marked pulsatility of GH, LH, TSH and possibly ACTH (35) in the sheep fetus has not been previously appreciated. This unique pattern of pituitary hormone release is a result of immaturity of hypothalamic control. In each case stimulatory influences are exerted in a pulsatile fashion by the hypothalamus from apparently independent pulse generators, subsequently to be modulated by the development of inhibitory feedback control. This marked pulsatility needs to be considered by investigators in the design of experiments in fetal endocrinology—in general single time point estimations of pituitary hormone concentrations will be of limited value.

Acknowledgements

This work was supported by grants from the Medical Research Council of New Zealand. I wish to thank those who have contributed to these studies; Mrs Y. Parsons, Ms M. Fraser, Miss V. Smith and Mr J. Butler.

References

1. Gluckman, P. D. (1983). *Curr. Top. Exp. Endocrinol.* **5**, 1–42.
2. Gluckman, P. D., Grumbach, M. M. and Kaplan, S. L. (1981). *Endocr. Rev.* **2**, 363–395.
3. Bugnon, C., Fellmann, D., Bresson, J. L. and Clavequin, M. L. (1982). *C.R. Acad. Sci. Paris* **294** (Series III), 491–496.
4. Bugnon, C., Bloch, B. and Fellman, D. (1977). *Brain Res.* **128**, 249–262.
5. Bugnon, C., Fellmann, D. and Bloch, B. (1978). *Metabolism* **27** (suppl. 1), 1161.
6. Gluckman, P. D. and Parsons, Y. (1983). *J. Develop. Physiol.* **5**, 101–128.

7. Gluckman, P. D. and Parsons, Y. (1985). *J. Develop. Physiol.* (submitted).
8. Bloch, B., Brazeau, P., Ling, N., Bohlen, P., Esch, F., Wehrenberg, W. B., Benoit, R., Bloom, F. and Guillemin, R. (1983). *Nature* **301**, 607–608.
9. Ohmura, E., Janson, A., Chernick, V., Winter, J., Friesen, H. G., Rivier, J. and Vale, W. (1984). *Endocrinology* **114**, 299–301.
10. Gluckman, P. D. (1984). *J. Develop. Physiol.* (in press).
11. Vale, W., Vaughan, J., Yamamoto, G., Spiess, J. and Rivier, J. (1983). *Endocrinology* **112**, 1553–1555.
12. Fisher, D. A., Dussault, J. M., Sack, J. and Chopra, I. J. (1977). *Rec. Prog. Horm. Res.* **33**, 59–116.
13. Gluckman, P. D., Mueller, P. L., Kaplan, S. L., Rudolph, A. M. and Grumbach, M. M. (1979). *Endocrinology* **104**, 974–978.
14. Berlowitz, M., Firestone, S. L. and Frohman, L. A. (1981). *Endocrinology* **109**, 714–719.
15. Tannenbaum, G. S., Guyda, H. J. and Posner, B. I. (1983). *Science* **229**, 77–79.
16. Eigenmann, J. E. and Rijnberk, A. (1981). *Acta Endocrinol.* **98**, 599–602.
17. Bassett, J. M., Thorburn, G. D. and Wallace, A. L. L. (1970). *J. Endocrinol.* **48**, 251–263.
18. McMillen, K., Jenkin, G., Thorburn, G. D. and Robinson, J. S. (1978). *J. Endocrinol.* **78**, 453–454.
19. Gluckman, P. D. (1982). *J. Develop. Physiol.* **4**, 207–214.
20. Gluckman, P. D. (1982). *J. Develop. Physiol.* **4**, 227–236.
21. Azukizawa, M., Maraka, Y., Idenoye, T., Martin, C. B. and Hershman, J. M. (1976). *J. Clin. Endocrin. Metab.* **43**, 1020–1028.
22. Melmed, S., Harada, A., Murata, Y., Socol, M., Reed, A., Carlson, H. E., Azukizawa, M., Martin, C., Jorgensen, E. and Hershman, J. M. (1979). *Endocrinology* **105**, 335–341.
23. Klein, A. H. and Fisher, P. A. (1980). *Endocrinology* **108**, 697–701.
24. Fraser, M., Gunn, T. R., Butler, J. H., Johnson, B. M., Gluckman, P. D. (1984). *Pediat. Res.* (submitted).
25. Thomas, A. L., Krane, E. T. and Nathanielsz, P. W. (1978). *Endocrinology* **103**, 17–23.
26. Roti, E., Gnudi, A., Braverman, E. E. (1982). *Endocr. Rev.* **4**, 131–149.
27. Tanjasiri, P., Kozbur, X., Florsheim, W. H. (1976). *Life Sci.* **19**, 657–660.
28. Gluckman, P. D., Gunn, T. R., Johnston, B. M. and Fraser, M. (1985). *In*: "The Physiological Development of the Fetus and Newborn" (Jones, C. T. and Nathanielsz, P. W., eds) pp. 163–166. Academic Press, London and Orlando.
29. Strbak, V. and Greer, M. A. (1979). *Endocrinology* **105**, 488–492.
30. Sklar, L. A., Mueller, P. L., Gluckman, P. D., Kaplan, S. L., Rudolph, A. M. and Grumbach, M. M. (1981). *Endocrinology* **108**, 874–880.
31. Clark, S. T., Ellis, N., Styne, D. M., Gluckman, P. D., Kaplan, S. L. and Grumbach, M. M. (1984). *Endocrinology* (in press).
32. Mueller, P. L., Sklar, L. A., Gluckman, P. D., Kaplan, S. L. and Grumbach, M. M. (1981). *Endocrinology* **108**, 881–886.
33. Gluckman, P. D., Marti-Henniberg, C., Kaplan, S. L. and Grumbach, M. M. (1983). *Endocrinology* **112**, 1618–1623.
34. Maclusky, N. T., Leiberbug, I., McEwan, B. S. (1975). *Brain Res.* **178**, 129–142.
35. Jones, C. T. (1979). *Horm. Metab. Res.* **11**, 237–241.

Humoral Control of
the Fetal Circulation

J. C. Mott

The Nuffield Institute for Medical Research,
University of Oxford, Oxford, UK

Vasoactive substances reach the general circulation from a variety of sources:

a) from specific tissues, e.g. vasopressin from the posterior pituitary or adrenaline from the adrenal medulla;

b) from overflow of neurotransmitters, e.g. noradrenaline from α-terminals;

c) by secretion of an enzyme, e.g. renal renin which initiates within vascular beds an enzymic cascade with production of angiotensins;

d) the so-called tissue hormones exemplified by the fatty acid derivatives collectively termed prostanoids. Many of these are rapidly metabolized *in vivo*. Nevertheless fetal plasma levels of some prostaglandins exceed maternal levels so that their actions may not be confined to the tissues where they are produced (1).

In considering the hormonal control of the fetal circulation we are faced with a tangle of interacting networks. We can attack each network separately by removal or inactivation of the hormone concerned. We can also attempt to measure its circulating levels. In the whole animal, not only may a single stimulus have more than one effect or a different set of effects under different conditions but any responses induced may themselves have secondary actions. Furthermore, secretion of an individual hormone may be effected by more than one mechanism.

The maintenance of the hormonal environment in circulating blood depends not only on production of vasoactive compounds but also on the mechanisms of their inactivation. In this the placenta plays an important role (2,3).

A great deal of painstaking work has been done in the last few years to

The Physiological Development of the Fetus and Newborn
ISBN 0 12 389080 2
Copyright © 1985 by Academic Press, London.
All rights of reproduction in any form reserved.

analyse the actions of exogenous hormones in both intact fetal lambs and in those subjected to anatomical or pharmacological interference. Much of this work has been reviewed fairly recently (4,5,6). This paper will concentrate on work published since 1981. Unless otherwise stated the information refers to unanaesthetized lambs in the last third of gestation. Some general points about the fetal circulation will be summarized first and the partition of the cardiac output between systemic and umbilical circuits in various circumstances discussed.

The Structural Background

The outstanding differences between fetal and adult circulations are firstly that fetal blood is, by adult standards, at asphyxial levels and secondly that the systemic circulation lies in parallel with the umbilical. While the systemic circulation is fuelling metabolic activity the umbilical subserves gas and metabolite exchange and much fetal excretion.

Estimates of cardiac (combined ventricular) output (CVO) in fetal lambs *in utero* in the last third of gestation are close to 0.5 l/kg body wt/min. In absolute terms this is between 1 and 3 l/min for lambs between 2 and 6 kg body weight. About 40% of this considerable flow perfuses the umbilical circuit.

There is no indication that fetal cardiac output can vary on the scale found in adult man where a 5-fold increase occurs during exercise. The considerable hypertension which sometimes follows bilateral nephrectomy in fetal lambs is not associated with raised cardiac output (7). Changes of blood volume have only small effects (8) but 40% increase has been reported following uterine ischaemia (9) or placental embolization (10).

It is convenient to consider conductance (flow/pressure), rather than resistance, of vascular beds in any attempt to assess the distribution of hormonal effects on the fetal circulation. The application of radioactive microsphere techniques in recent years has produced a substantial body of information as to the partition of cardiac output between different tissues (4,11). If we consider control measurements made before any experimental intervention an important point emerges concerning systemic blood flow assessed from the distribution of microspheres in organs and tissues. Organs that are easily defineable and in many cases of peculiar physiological interest and importance (e.g. heart and brain) in fact claim only a minor proportion of systemic flow. Categorization of tissues not surprisingly varies between investigators but any not otherwise accounted for are designated "carcass". This renders detailed comparison between different papers impracticable but taking Fore's (7) figures as an example it is clear that "carcass" and skin together account for about one-third of the cardiac output and two-thirds of the systemic flow. Thus the responses of the muscle vasculature in particular must constitute a large element in the overall response of the systemic circulation to circulating vasoactive substances.

Administration of a stimulus to the fetal vasculature may not only affect the calibre of vessels but also cardiac output and hence arterial pressure and the pressure drop across individual vascular beds. However central venous pressure

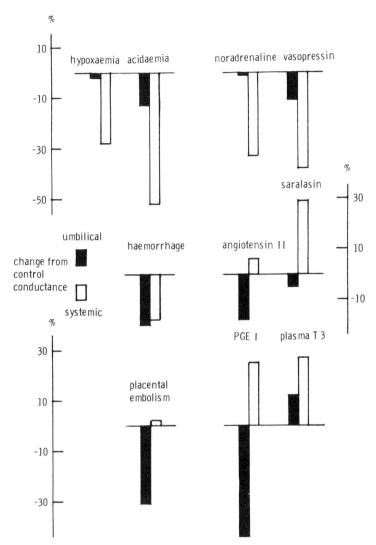

Figure 1. Per cent changes of conductance (flow/pressure drop) produced by the stimuli indicated in the umbilical (filled blocks) and systemic (open blocks) circulations in fetal lambs. Data from (4,11).

is usually very low and can in most circumstances be disregarded. Calculation from microsphere data in the literature of the change of conductance caused by different stimuli reveals a variety of patterns of change (Fig. 1; 4,11). Conductance does not always change in the same direction in both umbilical and systemic vascular beds. Comparison between the various investigations illustrated in

Fig. 1 is somewhat hazardous since each conductance represents only a single point on a flow/pressure curve. Nevertheless it is interesting to note that hypoxaemia, acidaemia, noradrenaline and vasopressin all produce larger falls of conductance in systemic vessels than in the umbilical circuit. These four agents all cause some fall of cardiac output. More substantial increase of umbilical resistance accompanies haemorrhage and placental embolism or administration of angiotensin II and prostaglandin E1. Angiotensin II caused 17% increase of cardiac output but PGE1 only 2%. Saralasin (a competitive inhibitor of angiotensin II) increases systemic conductance despite a small fall of arterial pressure. Triiodothyronine causes 20% increase of cardiac output reflected in increases in conductance in both systemic and umbilical circuits. Individually, relatively uncomplicated experimental stimuli (which may however themselves have secondary effects) can thus cause a variety of patterns of change of distribution of blood flow between umbilical and systemic circuits.

The wealth of possibilities of combinations of mechanisms underlying the usually remarkably stable control of fetal blood pressure also underlines the desirability of simultaneous measurement of as many vasoactive substances as possible.

Peptides

Renin-angiotensin-aldosterone system

Bilateral nephrectomy of the fetus abolishes secretion of renal renin and hence the fission of angiotensin I from plasma renin substrate. In these circumstances plasma renin activity and angiotensin II levels are extremely low. However, subnormal levels of fetal arterial pressure only develop in some anephric fetal lambs and are associated with high levels of protein intake by the ewe (12). Plasma renin activity starts to rise at about 105–110 days gestation (13). Using proportionately equivalent degrees of haemorrhage, Gomez and Robillard (1983) have distinguished in lambs of < 120 days gestation a significant fall of arterial pressure from 42 ± 1 to 37 ± 1 mmHg with no change of heart rate from an increase of heart rate and no change of arterial pressure in lambs of > 130 days gestation (14). At the peak of fetal haemorrhage, plasma renin activity and AII were significantly higher in near term than in younger fetal lambs. Both groups of lambs shewed significant increases of plasma adrenaline, noradrenaline, and vasopressin (15).

The younger lambs showed small falls of arterial pressure in response to progressive haemorrhage whether or not converting enzyme inhibitor (which prevents formation of angiotensin II) was administered. In near-term lambs however, inhibition by captopril of the normal rise of angiotensin II evoked by haemorrhage was accompanied by a 12% fall of blood pressure. Plasma vasopressin and catecholamines increased to a somewhat greater extent during haemorrhage in captopril treated fetal lambs than intact ones (14).

Aldosterone

This mineralocorticoid can be secreted by the adrenal cortex in response to angiotensin II (following conversion to angiotensin III) but also by raised plasma

K^+ and *in vitro* at least by ACTH (16). It is therefore interesting that the normal rise of aldosterone following haemorrhage in both young and near-term lambs was unaffected by captopril treatment (14). While aldosterone may well be of importance in the response to haemorrhage in virtue of its sodium-retaining action which would be expected to promote maintenance of plasma volume, renin activity is not essential to its provision. However arterial pressure fell in 4 bilaterally nephrectomized lambs subjected to a standard blood-letting regime in spite of a significant rise in aldosterone levels (17).

Aldosterone (mol. wt. 361) has been shown to cross the human placenta (16) and may do likewise in sheep (18). Neither captopril nor bilateral nephrectomy seem to affect control fetal plasma aldosterone concentration (14,18). However increased maternal sodium intake is associated with over 90% reduction of maternal plasma aldosterone but only about 50% reduction of fetal levels. This reverses a 3-fold maternal–fetal gradient to a 2-fold fetal–maternal gradient (18). Fetal plasma aldosterone has been observed to be correlated with fetal plasma K^+ (17,18).

Vasopressin

Although plasma levels of vasopressin are similar in ewes and fetal lambs it is cleared more rapidly by the fetus (presumably largely in the placenta) so that it seems reasonable to suppose that production is higher in fetus than adult (2). The hypertensive effect of exogenous vasopressin is proportionately greater in fetal lambs than in adult sheep; the rise of pressure is accompanied by bradycardia which is not however abolished by atropine. In contrast to most of the systemic circulation, during infusion of physiological amounts of vasopressin, renal blood flow is unchanged but that to the spleen doubles (4).

Rurak and Gruber (19) found that infusion of vasopressin 1.4–3.5 mU/min/kg fetal weight caused an increase in umbilical blood flow proportionate to the rise of arterial pressure in lambs 113–137 days gestation age. The calculated umbilical conductance is about 50% higher than found with measurements with labelled microspheres (20). Umbilical veno-arterial O_2 difference fell but fetal O_2 consumption remained constant. O_2 delivery to the fetus increased on average ~ 22% and fractional O_2 extraction fell correspondingly. These observations are consistent with the view that release of vasopressin promotes survival by maintenance of PO_2 levels at least in the short term.

Both hypoxaemia and haemorrhage increase plasma vasopressin to concentrations of the order of 100 pg/ml. The extent and duration of hypotension following controlled haemorrhage have been shown to be increased by prior administration of a vasopressin antagonist $(d(CH_2)_5Tyr(Me)AVP)$ (21). This group have further shown that a specific antagonist of the vasoconstrictor actions of arginine vasopressin, 1(β-mercapto-β, β-cyclopentamethylene proprionic acid), 2-0 methyl tyrosine Arg^8 vasopressin, inhibits the rise of both noradrenaline and adrenaline caused by haemorrhage. This raises the possibility that in addition to its peripheral action vasopressin may have an indirect action in the fetal response to haemorrhage by alteration of the sympathetic response to volume depletion (22).

Catecholamines

Exogenous noradrenaline infused at 1 μg/kg/min greatly reduced systemic though not umbilical conductance (Fig. 1). Parallel observations with adrenaline seem not yet to have been made. Plasma levels of catecholamines are very low (<1 ng/ml) in unanaesthetized fetal lambs but rise somewhat in the last few days before term. They are increased by hypoxaemia, insulin, hypoglycaemia and haemorrhage. It has been calculated that the placenta is responsible for about half of the total metabolic clearance of plasma catecholamines (23).

Noradrenaline is the predominant catecholamine in plasma but the adrenaline content increases as term approaches, presumably reflecting the increasing proportion of adrenaline in the adrenal medulla. In the fetus, in addition to the adrenal medulla, high concentrations of catecholamines especially of noradrenaline have been found in the paraganglia (4). Plasma noradrenaline will also be augmented by any overflow from sympathetic α-terminals in the vasculature.

Both noradrenaline and adrenaline when infused at rates which produce plasma levels comparable with those found during hypoxaemia cause 8–10 mmHg rise of arterial pressure, unaffected by propranolol but abolished by phentolamine. Phentolamine also blocked an initial small fall of heart rate seen during adrenaline infusion and augmented the later tachycardia produced by adrenaline alone. Noradrenaline caused a small rise of heart rate which was reversed when propranolol was infused simultaneously. Simultaneous phentolamine infusion however, augmented the tachycardia produced by noradrenaline (24).

It is therefore not surprising that the vascular responses to a mixture of endogenous catecholamines are complex. Inhalation by the ewe of 9% O_2 and 3% CO_2 in N_2 produces isocapnic hypoxaemia in the fetus and causes in lambs of 124–135 days gestation a small sustained rise of arterial pressure and pronounced bradycardia which diminishes substantially during 60 min exposure. Plasma catecholamine levels rise into the low (<10 ng/ml) range with noradrenaline levels roughly double adrenaline levels (26). These considerably exceed the range of values reported for the catecholamine responses to a 30% reduction of blood volume (15). Administration of the α-blocker phentolamine (100 μg/min) concurrently with isocapnic hypoxaemia reduced the rise of blood pressure seen in hypoxaemic controls; transient minimal bradycardia was followed after 15 min hypoxaemia by a progressive increase of heart rate. When the β-blocker propranolol (44 μg/min) was given during hypoxaemia, the rise of pressure was similar to that of controls but the bradycardia did not show the tendency to abate found in controls. During the hours following hypoxaemia arterial pressure remained above control levels particularly in the phentolamine experiments where high noradrenaline levels persisted (25).

Adrenal demedullation by bilateral injection of acid formalin did not affect basal plasma noradrenaline levels but reduced adrenaline levels significantly. It considerably increased the responses of arterial pressure and heart rate to exogenous adrenaline and noradrenaline. It was concluded that the adrenal medullary secretion in fetal sheep enhanced peripheral sensitivity to plasma catecholamines. Peripheral sympathectomy produced by administration of guanethidine to fetal lambs following adrenal medullectomy did not abolish plasma noradrenaline which may have originated from the enlarged paraganglia (26).

Prostaglandins

A wide range of fetal tissues have been shown to synthesize prostaglandins *in vitro* (1,4,5). The high concentration of PGE and PGF in fetal urine (27) compared with plasma or tracheal fluid, suggests that the kidney produces significant amounts of prostaglandins *in vivo*. These fatty acid derivatives are well known to have short half-lives and are often termed tissue hormones. The A series prostaglandins are mainly smooth muscle stimulants and the E series relaxants. Actions of endogenous prostaglandins arise from stimulation of their synthesis and are not due to activation of a storage form of prostaglandins.

The relation of prostaglandins to the prenatal and perinatal behaviour of that phylogenetic survivor, the ductus arteriosus, are well known and will not be recapitulated here (6). Their great interest and applicability to clinical problems may understandably have diverted attention from their other actions in various fetal tissues.

There is general agreement that in the fetal lamb prostaglandin E has an atypical action since it causes umbilical vasoconstriction. Infusion of PGE 1 reduced umbilical conductance by 44% and increased systemic conductance by 25% (11, Fig. 1). In another investigation, administration of 100 μg/kg PGE_2 increased fetal placental vascular resistance by up to 10-fold but the same dose of $PGE_{2\alpha}$ only caused 25% increase of placental resistance (28).

The effects of PGE1 and indomethacin on the constrictor response of isolated fetal or newborn mesenteric arteries to noradrenaline exemplifies the likelihood of variation of endogenous prostaglandin production modifying a wide range of response to other humoral agents. PGE1 (1.5 μmol) reduced vasoconstriction but indomethacin potentiated it. PGE1 prevented the potentiating effect of indomethacin. However, since neither PGE1 nor indomethacin altered basal muscle tension the authors (29) viewed this as a tissue effect.

The fetal pulmonary circulation normally receives only a small fraction of cardiac output but infusion of PGE1 11 μg/kg during 1 min produced a dramatic increase in conductance (30). However, exogenous arachidonic acid does not promote fetal pulmonary vasodilatation but results in increased pulmonary resistance and decreased systemic resistance. In this case, the end products of the prostanoid cascade produced in the pulmonary and systemic beds are different and the balance of production of different PGs from precursor seems to be very labile (31).

Renal blood flow is reduced by hypoxaemia though proportionately less than mesenteric and iliac flow. Administration of the prostaglandin synthetase inhibitor, meclofenamate, increased the renal circulatory response to hypoxaemia to a level similar to that in iliac and mesenteric beds (32). Thus here prostaglandin production may preferentially preserve renal blood flow.

Summary

In normal development several endocrine systems act in concert to maintain remarkable stability of fetal arterial pressure and hence perfusion of the placenta and systemic tissues. It is now possible to measure plasma levels of many circulating vasoactive hormones. This makes it clear that any vascular response to realistic fetal hazards may well involve more than one class of agent. The renin angiotensin system which seems to be little affected by hypoxaemia is extremely sensitive to volume reduction; vasopressin release is stimulated by hypoxaemia as well as by volume reduction. During isocapnic hypoxaemia catecholamine levels reach the low ng/ml range in the plasma, considerably above the corresponding vasopressin levels even without conversion to an equimolar basis.

The relative shifts of cardiac output indicated in Fig. 1 illustrate various extremes between overall decrease of conductance in both systemic and umbilical circuits during haemorrhage, acidaemia or vasopressin infusion; a predominantly systemic decrease during hypoxaemia and noradrenaline infusion or a decrease of umbilical conductance may even as with PGE, be accompanied by an increase of systemic conductance.

These gross sytemic changes must of course, be the sum of a host of variations of geometry in individual vascular beds, conditioned perhaps, by the lcoal states of various prostanoid enzymatic cascades in response to the vasoactive peptides and catecholamines reaching them in the blood.

There is now an outline available from investigation of a single species in the last third of gestation on which to build. Many aspects merit further investigation particularly perhaps afferent and central neural mechanisms.

References

1. Mitchell, M. D. (1982). *In:* "Biochemical Development of the Fetus and Neonate" (C. T. Jones, ed.) Elsevier, Amsterdam.
2. Jones, C. T. and Rurak, D. (1976). *Q. J. Exp. Physiol.* **61**, 287–295.
3. Lumbers, E. R. and Reid, G. C. (1978). *Aust. J. Exp. Biol. Med. Sci.* **56**, 11–24.
4. Mott, J. C. and Walker, D. W. (1983). *In:* "Handbook of Physiology" Section 2. The cardiovascular system Vol. III Peripheral circulation and organ blood flow Part 2 (Shepherd, J. T. and Abboud, F. M. eds) pp. 837–883, American Physiological Society, Bethesda, Md, USA.
5. Harris, W. H. (1982). *Pharmac. Ther.* **16**, 221–246.
6. Rudolph, A. M. and Heymann, M. A. (1981). *J. Perinat. Med.* **9** suppl. 1, 91–92.
7. Fore, I. M. (1981). *J. Physiol.* **324**, 72P.
8. Gilbert, R. D. (1980). *Am. J. Physiol.* **238**, H80–86.
9. Yaffe, H., Parer, J. T., Llanos, A. and Block, B. (1982). 29th Annual Meeting of the Society of Gynecological Investigation.
10. Creasy, R. K., De Swiet, M., Kahanpaa, K. V., Young, W. P. and Rudolph, A. M. (1973). *In:* "Foetal and Neonatal Physiology" (Comline, R. S., Cross, K. W., Dawes, G. S. and Nathanielsz, P. W. eds) Cambridge University Press, London.

11. Tripp, M., Heymann, M. A. and Rudolph, A. M. (1978). *In:* "Advances in Prostaglandin and Thromboxane Research" (Coceani, F. and Olley, P. M. eds) **4**, 221–230, Raven Press, New York.
12. Mott, J. C., Fore, I. M., Dutton, A. and Valdes Cruz, L. M. (1985). *In:* "The Physiological Development of the Fetus and the Newborn" (Jones, C. T. and Nathanielsz, P. W., eds) pp. 557–560. Academic Press, London and Orlando.
13. Carver, J. G. and Mott, J. C. (1974). *J. Physiol.* **245**, 73–75P.
14. Gomez, R. A. and Robillard, J. E. (1983). *Circulat. Res.* **54**, 301–312.
15. Gomez, R. A., Meernik, J. G., Kuehl, W. D. and Robillard, J. E. (1984). *Pediat. Res.* **18**, 40–46.
16. Mott, J. C. (1979). *In:* "The Influence of Maternal Hormones on the Fetus and Newborn" (Nitzen, M. ed.) Volume 5 "Pediatric and Adolescent Endocrinology". pp. 126–145, Karger Basel.
17. Robillard, J. E., Gomez, R. A., Meernik, J. G., Kuehl, W. D. and Van Orden, Dianna (1982). *Circulat. Res.* **50**, 645–650.
18. Dutton, A. and Mott, J. C. (1983). *J. Physiol.* **345**, 113P.
19. Rurak, D. W. and Gruber, N. C. (1984). *Can. J. Physiol. Pharmacol.* **62**, 27–30.
20. Iwamot, H. S., Rudolph, A. M., Keil, L. C. and Heymann, M. A. (1979). *Circulat. Res.* **44**, 430–436.
21. Kelly, R. T., Rose, J. C., Meis, P. J., Hargrave, B. Y. and Morris, M. (1983). *Am. J. Obstet. Gynecol.* **146**(7), 807–812.
22. Rose, J. C., Jones, C. M., Kelly, R. T., Hargrave, B. Y. and Meis, P. J. (1983). *Endocrinology* **113**, 2314–2317.
23. Jones, C. T. (1980). *In:* "Biogenic Amines in Development" (Parvez, H. and Parvez, S. eds) pp. 63–86. Elsevier Biomedical Press, Amsterdam, Holland.
24. Jones, C. T. and Ritchie, J. W. K. (1978). *J. Physiol.* **285**, 381–393.
25. Jones, C. T. and Ritchie, J. W. K. (1983). *J. Develop. Physiol.* **5**, 211–222.
26. Johnston, B. M., Jones, C. T., Lagercrantz, H., Roebuck, M. M. and Walker, D. W. (1983). *J. Physiol.* **348**, 68P.
27. Walker, D. W. and Mitchell, M. D. (1978). *Nature* **271**, 161–162.
28. McLaughlin, M. K., Brenner, S. C. and Chez, R. A. (1978). *Am. J. Obstet. Gynec.* **130**, 408–413.
29. Yabek, S. M. and Avner, B. P. (1979). *Prostaglandins* **17**, 227–233.
30. Cassin, S., Tyler, T. and Wallis, R. (1975). *Proc. Soc. Exp. Biol. Med.* **148**, 584–587.
31. Tyler, T. L., Leffler, C. W. and Cassin, S. (1977). *Chest* **71**, 271–273.
32. Millard, R. W., Baig, H. and Vatner, S. (1977). *Pediat. Res.* **11**, 395, (abstract 144).

Integration of Pancreatic and Gastrointestinal Endocrine Control of Metabolic Homeostasis during the Perinatal Period

J. M. Bassett

The Nuffield Institute for Medical Research,
University of Oxford, Oxford, UK

Birth represents a watershed in the development and function of many body systems. For metabolic homeostasis the change is as dramatic as any, with the requirement suddenly to maintain homeothermy, yet also switch from continuous parenteral nutrient inflow to intermittent enteral inputs of food. Despite enormous differences among species in their developmental maturity at birth, the success with which infants adapt to this new environment and to enteral feeding, attests to the early maturation of physiological and behavioural mechanisms involved.

It is tempting to believe that the first feed of colostrum may be the first exposure of the tract to food, but it must be borne in mind that the fetus ingests large volumes of amniotic fluid for much of gestation. Amniotic fluid has been detected in the stomach of human fetuses early in gestation (1) and in late gestation. Both sheep and human fetuses may swallow up to 500 ml fluid daily (1,2). Birth should, therefore, be more properly regarded as denoting a change in the nature and nutrient density of materials entering the tract, rather than the initiation of ingestive processes themselves.

There is considerable evidence that the establishment of enteral feeding itself is responsible for rapid and major alterations in the growth and functional maturation of the tract. In both pigs (3) and dogs (4) the jejunal mucosal mass of suckled infants virtually doubles during the first 24 h of life, whereas no similar change occurs in fasted or formula-fed infants. Recent

The Physiological Development of the Fetus and Newborn
ISBN 0 12 389080 2

Copyright © 1985 by Academic Press, London.
All rights of reproduction in any form reserved.

observations that colostrum and milk contain growth factors, including both
somatomedin C (5) and epidermal growth factor (6), suggest a possible mechanism
for this, although it is clear that there are also major alterations in the secretion
of the gastrointestinal neuropeptides (7), several of which have trophic effects
on the growth of the tract itself.

Regulation of Metabolic Homeostasis

Although insulin and glucagon, together with the catecholamines, continue to
be regarded as the principal effector agents involved in short-term regulation of
glucose homeostasis (8), major advances in peptide hormone methodology have
altered views about the regulation of pancreatic hormone release and metabolic
homeostasis. It is now recognized that a large number of peptides, functioning
as neurotransmitters, paracrine and/or endocrine effectors, are produced within
the tissues of the gastrointestinal tract and its associated organs. Besides regulating
digestion and absorption, they also modulate secretion of hormones governing
the subsequent utilization of absorbed metabolites and promote growth of the
tract itself (9,10).

The pancreatic islet has come to be recognized as a complex micro-organ,
containing at least 4 different peptide hormone producing cells secreting
insulin, glucagon, somatostatin and pancreatic polypeptide, with a structural
arrangement and rich innervation suggestive of complex neural and paracrine
control of hormone secretion. Changing concepts in the organization and
control of pancreatic islet function have been the subject of several reviews
(8,11–13).

Integrated functioning of these systems permits far more precise control of
metabolic homeostasis than envisaged earlier. Glucose concentration in the central
blood compartment provides important signals to the regulatory systems, but
it is increasingly evident that its main significance is as the regulated parameter
and that direct regulation of insulin and glucagon release by changes in the blood
glucose level is relatively inefficient. Glucose stimulation of insulin release and
inhibition of glucagon release have important places as "fail-safe" mechanisms
to prevent major disturbance of glucose levels, so protecting neural metabolism,
but under normal circumstances it is likely that alterations in humoral and
autonomic neural inputs to the islets play the major role in regulating islet insulin
and glucagon release. Such a mechanism permits large changes in the flux of
glucose and other metabolites through the system with minimal disturbance to
glucose levels in the blood, or glucose availability for oxidative metabolism in
the brain.

Meal consumption generates a complex sequence of signals to the pancreatic
islets, whose principal function, broadly speaking, is to maximize the efficiency
with which glucose can be utilized in the body. Initially this involves neural reflex
stimulation of pancreatic and gastrointestinal hormone secretion and subsequently
includes marked potentiation of pancreatic hormone secretion by gut hormones
and neuropeptides released by nutrients passing along the tract. The hormone
currently considered most likely to modulate luminal glucose effects on pancreatic

hormone release is GIP (14), but others which may be released by glucose or other luminal nutrients, including bombesin, CCK, enteroglucagon, neurotensin and VIP, stimulate insulin and glucagon secretion, while SRIF inhibits the release of both. Intrinsic enteral and autonomic neural mechanisms are also involved in co-ordinating and modulating responses to luminal nutrients, but their detailed elucidation is still far from complete.

The extent to which this system is functional at the time of birth remains largely a matter of conjecture. Before this, much of the homeostatic regulation is achieved by the mother and there is little evidence for independent regulation of glucose levels by the fetus, although it is clear that fetal glucose utilization is under the control of insulin (15,16). However, there is sufficient evidence to indicate that developmental changes in the secretion of the gastrointestinal tract hormones and their regulatory systems may play an important role in adaptation to extra-uterine life.

Ontogenesis of the Endocrine Pancreas

Studies of pancreatic islet ontogenesis demonstrate the presence of all the 4 principal endocrine cell types from an early stage of development. Cells staining for insulin, glucagon, somatostatin and pancreatic polypeptide by immuno-fluorescent techniques are present for approximately 75–80% of gestation in the longer gestation species such as man (17–19), pig (20) and sheep (21). In short-gestation species, such as the rat, the proportion is less and patterns of development are different (22,23).

Most workers report marked alterations with development in the proportions of the cell types within the islets, but because of the differing methods used to assess cell populations in the various reports it is difficult to determine a complete developmental profile for each cell type with any certainty. What is really necessary is an assessment of the total cell population for each endocrine cell during development so their rates of progress towards maturity can be determined. Nevertheless, it is evident from the very approximate and highly speculative growth curves, plotted from Rahier's data (15), and from other data on islet cell proportions in fetal life (17) (Fig. 1), that the developmental profile of the somatostatin-producing D cells in the human pancreas differs markedly from those of the other cell types. It represents a far higher fraction of islet cell mass throughout fetal life than in the adult and at birth has reached a far higher proportion of its adult cell mass than have any of the other cell types (Fig. 1). Nevertheless, development of all the islet endocrine cells in the human fetus is more rapid than that of the body as a whole and it has been calculated (1,5) that there may be about 4 times as much pancreatic endocrine tissue present at birth relative to bodyweight as there is in the adult.

Interestingly, while there may be an increased amount of pancreatic endocrine tissue in infants of diabetic mothers, there is no evidence for alterations in the proportions of the various endocrine cell types (24). On the other hand, there does appear to be an absolute deficiency of D cells and reduced somatostatin content in pancreatic tissue of infants suffering from nesidioblastosis (25).

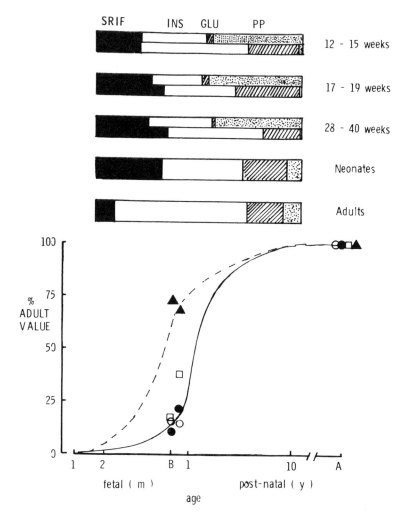

Figure 1. Proportions of pancreatic islet endocrine cells types (upper) and mass of pancreatic endocrine tissue (lower) in the human fetal pancreas during development (data from 17,19): (●) insulin, (○) glucagon, (□) pancreatic polypeptide, (▲) somatostatin.

Function of Pancreatic Islets

Studies of fetal endocrine pancreas tissue *in vitro* and *in vivo* have shown it is capable of responding to alterations in the metabolic state of the fetus (16,26) even though its responsiveness may differ from that of postnatal tissue. In the case of the B cell there is substantial evidence to indicate that its regulated release plays an important role in regulating glucose utilization and in modulating fetal growth (15). Observations in our own laboratory have shown that glucose is capable of stimulating insulin release from the fetal lamb pancreas *in vitro* as early as 50 days gestation (0.34 gestation) (26), though *in vivo* insulin responses of fetal lambs are generally less than those of postnatal lambs. Amino acids also stimulate glucagon release *in vitro* at the same early stage of pregnancy (26) and are effective *in vivo* later on (27,28). In addition, comparable perifusion studies have demonstrated opposing stimulatory and inhbitory effects of acetylcholine and adrenaline on insulin and glucagon release from 55 days gestation onwards (Fig. 2), indicating the early development of receptor mechanisms for response to neural stimuli. However, although comparable adrenergic effects on pancreatic hormone release have been observed during hypoxia in fetal lambs during late gestation (29) these could be consequent on adrenal catecholamine production rather than on direct neural stimulation of the pancreatic islets as in postnatal calves (30). The developmental timetable for functional innervation of the islets remains unknown. This may be of greater significance in maturation of islet responsiveness to metabolic stimuli than has been appreciated, for blockade of the parasympathetic with atropine greatly reduces the responsiveness of insulin release to stimulation by glucose (31). Regulation of the other endocrine cells in the pancreatic islets before birth remains largely a matter of conjecture. Plasma pancreatic polypeptide levels in the fetal lamb are only 4% of maternal levels at 100 days gestation. After this, they increase at an accelerating rate with a steep increase during the last week before delivery, consistent with increasing vagal

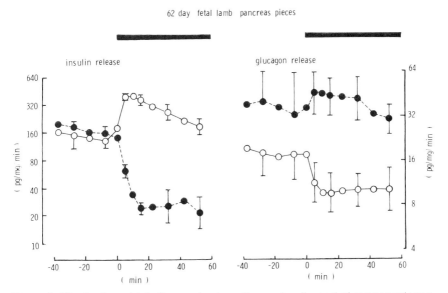

Figure 2. Effects of acetylcholine and adrenaline on insulin and glucagon release from fetal lamb pancreas pieces perifused *in vitro* in a bicarbonate medium containing glucose (5 mmol), Alanine (5 mmol) and caffeine (5 mmol): (○) 10 μmol acetylcholine (6). (●) 10 μmol adrenaline (6).

activity, although the response of pancreatic polypeptide levels to atropine at 125–135 days gestation was much less than that observed in adult sheep (32).

Even though there is suc a large population of D cells in the fetal pancreas and tissue concentrations of SRIF may be high in the long-gestation species, little is known of their functional status or regulation before birth. In the fetal lamb, SRIF infusion inhibits pancreatic polypeptide and gastrin release (33). In the newborn, infusion of somatostatin inhibits insulin and glucagon release as in adults (16,34), but the contribution of islet D cells to intra-islet regulation of insulin and glucagon release *in utero* is unknown. Further study of endocrine pancreatic function in infants suffering from nesidioblastosis, where there is a deficiency of SRIF-producing D cells (25), may give additional insight into the intra-uterine role of the pancreatic D cell.

Autonomic regulatory mechanisms play a major role in determining alterations in pancreatic hormone secretion after birth, when they are essential for adaptation to the new environment (16). However, studies in calves indicate that maturation of autonomic mechanisms is far from uniform, with differential maturation of mechanisms regulating insulin, glucagon and pancreatic polypeptide release in the early postnatal period (35,36). They raise the possibility that lack of functional cholinergic innervation explains some of the deficiencies in metabolite-stimulated insulin release *in utero* and suggest perinatal glucagon release may be regulated mainly by adrenaline from the adrenal medulla.

Ontogenesis of Gastrointestinal Hormones Influencing Endocrine Pancreas Function

Review of the vast and ever increasing literature on gastrointestinal endocrinology is beyond the scope of the present communication. Co-ordination of function by the gastrointestinal hormones extends well beyond digestion and absorption, to include modulation of pancreatic hormone secretion and thereby nutrient utilization. However, the functional integrity of these systems at birth remains uncertain.

Endocrine peptide cells appear in the gastrointestinal tract at a very early stage of development (20,37), so in the long-gestation species are present for a large fraction of intra-uterine life. Their distribution and developmental programmes have been characterized to some extent. Distribution patterns for the endocrine cells within the gut of human fetuses are very diverse (Fig. 3) and each cell type appears to follow its own developmental programme. As in the pancreas, SRIF-containing D cells appear to develop more rapidly than other cell types, whereas gastrin cells clearly develop more slowly. Developmental programmes for all these endocrine cell types, like those of the pancreas and that of the brain itself, are markedly accelerated by comparison with that of the rest of the gastrointestinal tract and body as a whole. Developmental patterns for each species will have to be defined, as marked differences among them are already evident. Enteroglucagon accumulation in the terminal ileum of the sheep is mainly prenatal, with large amounts present before birth (26), whereas the main increase in the rabbit intestine occurs during the early postnatal period. The development

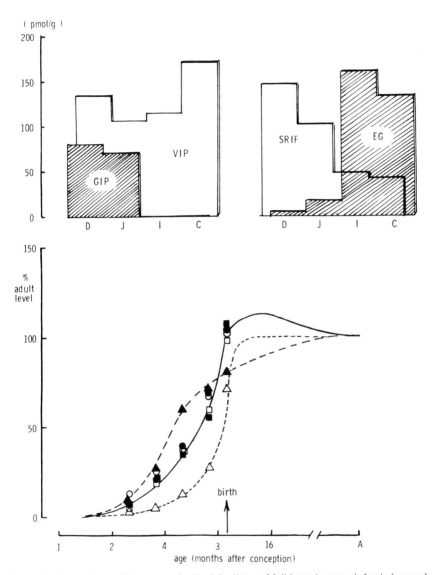

Figure 3. Distribution of hormones in the intestines of full-term human infants (upper) and changes in their concentration during intra-uterine life (lower) (data from ref 37): (●) enteroglucagon, (○) VIP, (■) GIP, (□) motilin, (▵) gastrin, (▲) somatostatin.

of SRIF concentrations in neonatal rat intestinal tissues also appears to differ markedly from the pattern seen in human intestines (38,39). However it is difficult to assess the extent to which tissue concentrations reflect the total amount of SRIF present or changes in the amounts of other tissue components.

Gastrointestinal Hormone Release in the Perinatal Period

While there is information about postnatal plasma levels for most of the hormones which may be involved in the enteral regulation of pancreatic islet function (7), there is little information about the prenatal release of any. Plasma enteroglucagon levels in fetal lambs are substantially above maternal concentrations (40,41) and can be increased by intra-abomasal or duodenal infusion of glucose or fructose in conscious animals (40), but the secretion of enteroglucagon in the fetus has not been investigated in detail. Plasma and tissue gastrin levels in fetal lambs increase steadily during the last third of gestation and from 110–120 days gestation are higher than maternal levels (32,42). Plasma levels remain high for 10–30 days after birth before declining. While plasma gastrin levels are high during the neonatal period in all species studied, gastrin is only detectable late in gestation in rodents (43).

There is only fragmentary evidence about the prenatal development of secretory activity for any of the hormones likely to be involved in regulation of endocrine pancreas function. Blood levels of GIP were reported to increase in exteriorized fetal pigs after intraduodenal infusion of glucose (44), but subsequent studies failed to show any comparable rise after triglyceride infusion (45). In neither case was there any effect on the fetal plasma insulin level. There was also no evidence for the existence of an active enteroinsular axis in neonatal pigs. In human infants, there is little or no change in GIP levels following milk feeding until 3 weeks after birth and insulin responses to the feed were less than those observed in the older infants, despite comparable glycaemic changes (46). The evidence, though scanty, therefore tends to suggest that the enteroinsular axis may play little direct role during the early neonatal period.

Aynsley-Green and associates (7,47) have, in addition, provided much valuable information about the plasma levels of many other gastrointestinal hormones in both normal and preterm human infants. Since marked prematurity is uncommon in other species for which information is available, information on premature infants is especially valuable from a developmental point of view as it should give an opportunity to determine how development of these tissues is influenced by the initiation of enteral feeding. They have demonstrated active secretion at birth for all the hormones studied and showed that alterations in the intra-uterine environment affected their release. In particular, fetal distress resulted in marked increases in the concentrations of glucagon, pancreatic polypeptide, GIP, VIP and motilin, thus possibly explaining the meconium-staining characteristic of the condition. Following birth there were major changes in the levels of most hormones which appeared to depend on the establishment of enteral feeding. Furthermore, there were marked differences between breast and formula-fed infants in the magnitude of changes in pre- and postprandial hormone levels. It was particularly notable that plasma levels of gastrin, enteroglucagon and neurotensin were substantially higher than normal adult values. Both gastrin and enteroglucagon have important trophic effects on gastrointestinal tissue growth (48). High concentrations of these hormones consequent on the establishment of enteral feeding may explain the very rapid growth of mucosal tissues during the first days of postnatal life in enterally fed infants. Aynsley-Green has postulated that this is an important component of the adaptive process following birth (7). These findings, and the observation of such marked differences between feeds and feeding programmes in the gastrointestinal hormone changes induced, indicate that this subject merits considerable attention in the future if the clinical nutritional care of newborn infants is to be optimized.

Reflex Neural Regulation of Pancreatic Hormone Release

Although alterations in gut hormone release may be important, functional integration of all the changes after a meal will depend on maturity of the intrinsic enteral and autonomic neural systems controlling gut function (49). Differences from adults in neonatal gastrointestinal hormone levels may relate to immaturity of neural regulatory pathways, even though gastrointestinal innervation appears early in development (50).

Neural responses to feeding may also influence function of the endocrine pancreas more directly. Anticipatory reflex responses to food ingestion, mediated via the vagus, include stimulation of insulin, glucagon and pancreatic polypeptide release from the islets (51,52). Studies in recent years have re-emphasized the importance of these changes in minimizing the disturbance to glucose homeostasis after a meal (53,54).

Lambs accustomed to drink milk from a bottle, show very large reflex-stimulated increases in insulin levels after a feed (51). Although the reflex was present at 5 days of age it could not be demonstrated during the first 24 h of life (55). Maternal interference makes studies of natural suckling in newborn lambs impractical. However, reflex release of insulin was observed in naturally suckled newborn rabbits after their first feed, despite the relative immaturity of the rabbit at birth (55). Limited observations on lambs and rabbits suggest glucagon release is also stimulated at the same time. In the calf, reflex responses to feeding include stimulation of glucagon release (52), but insulin release can be explained by rapid absorption of glucose. Sham feeding studies indicate this is not so in the lamb (55). Increases in blood glucose levels 30–240 min after the feed were far greater in lambs where the reflex was absent, despite the fact that insulin levels at this time were higher (55). Reflex release of pancreatic hormones at the time of feeding clearly minimizes the disturbance to glucose homeostasis after the meal. Reflex pancreatic hormone release in breast or bottle-fed human infants has not been reported, but such a mechanism may contribute to the different hormone response patterns seen by Aynsley-Green in breast-fed infants and in infants fed human milk or formulas by nasogastric tube (7,47).

Concluding Comment

Clearly, large gaps remain in our knowledge of the part played by gastrointestinal and pancreatic hormones in maintenance of metabolic homeostasis during the perinatal period and in adaptation to postnatal life.

Developmental profiles for gastrointestinal and pancreatic hormones indicate rates of development like those of neural tissues, emphasizing their close relationship and early maturation relative to other tissues. Within the endocrine cell population, rates of development of individual cell types seem to differ greatly, but more detailed information is required before developmental significance can be attached to these differences. In particular it is essential to obtain information about the growth of each cell population, independent of alterations in the development of other components in the tissue as a whole.

In view of the great significance of neural control for secretory regulation of many gastrointestinal and pancreatic hormones, progress in understanding their contribution to homeostatic regulation will be limited till detailed development of functional autonomic innervation has been elucidated. There is, however, already evidence to suggest considerable differences between species in these developmental programmes, so caution should be exercised in extrapolating from one to another.

Despite evident immaturity in many of the regulatory systems involved, it remains impressive how readily newborn infants cope with the transition to enteral nutrition. The gastrointestinal tract at birth, even in the premature baby, is "primed and ready to go". The consumption of food appears to be one component of the maturation process, so clearly should be utilized wherever possible.

References

1. Pritchard, J. A. (1965). *Obstet. Gynecol.* **25**, 289–297.
2. Bradley, R. M. and Mistretta, C. M. (1973). *Science* **72**, 248–254.
3. Widdowson, E. M. (1984). *Proc. Nutr. Soc.* **43**, 87–100.
4. Heird, W. C., Schwarz, S. M. and Hansen, I. H. (1984). *Pediat. Res.* **18**, 512–515.
5. Baxter, R. C., Zaltsman, Z. and Turtle, J. R. (1984). *J. Clin. Endocrinol. Metab.* **58**, 955–959.
6. Carpenter, G. (1980). *Science* **210**, 198–199.
7. Aynsley-Green, A. (1982). *Monogr. Paediatr.* **16**, 59–87.
8. Unger, R. H. (1981). *Diabetologia* **20**, 1–11.
9. Mutt, V. (1982). *Scand. J. Gastroenterol.* **17**, suppl. 77, 133–152.
10. Creutzfeldt, W. (1982). *Scand. J. Gastroenterol.* **17** suppl. 77, 7–20.
11. Orci, L. (1982). *Diabetes* **31**, 538–565.
12. Unger, R. H. and Dobbs, R. E. (1978). *Ann. Rev. Physiol.* **40**, 307–343.
13. Unger, R. H. (1983). *Diabetes* **32**, 575–583.
14. Brown, J. C. and Otte, S. C. (1979). *Clin. Endocrinol. Metab.* **8**, 365–377.
15. Bassett, J. M. and Fletcher, J. M. (1982). *In:* "Biochemical Development of the Fetus and Neonate" (Jones, C. T. ed.) pp. 393–423, Elsevier Biomedical, Amsterdam.
16. Sperling, M. A. (1982). *Monogr. Paediatr.* **16**, 39–58.
17. Rahier, J., Wallon, J. and Henquin, J. C. (1981). *Diabetologia* **20**, 540–546.
18. Clark, A. and Grant, A. M. (1983). *Diabetologia* **25**, 31–35.
19. Stefan, Y., Grasso, S., Perrelet, A. and Orci, L. (1983). *Diabetes* **32**, 293–301.
20. Alumets, J., Hakanson, R. and Sundler, F. (1983). *Gastroenterology* **85**, 1359–1372.
21. Willes, R. F., Boda, J. M. and Stokes, H. (1969). *Endocrinology* **84**, 671–675.
22. Pictet, R. L., Clark, W. R., Williams, R. H. and Rutter, W. J. (1972). *Develop. Biol.* **29**, 436–467.

23. McEvoy, R. C. and Madson, K. L. (1980). *Biol. Neonate* **38**, 248-254.
24. Milner, R. D. G., Wirdnam, P. K. and Tsanakas, J. (1981). *Diabetes* **30**, 271-274.
25. Bishop, A. E., Polak, J. M., Garin Chesa, P., Timson, C. M., Bryant, M. G. and Bloom, S. R. (1981). *Diabetes* **30**, 122-126.
26. Bassett, J. M. (1977). *Ann. Vet. Rech.* **8**, 362-373.
27. Bassett, J. M., Madill, D., Burks, A. H. and Pinches, R. A. (1982). *J. Develop. Physiol.* **4**, 379-389.
28. Bassett, J. M., Burks, A. H. and Pinches, R. A. (1982). *J. Develop. Physiol.* **5**, 51-61.
29. Jones, C. T., Ritchie, J. W. K. and Walker, D. (1983). *J. Develop. Physiol.* **5**, 223-235.
30. Bloom, S. R., Edwards, A. V. and Hardy, R. N. (1978). *J. Physiol.* **280**, 9-23.
31. Bloom, S. R. and Edwards, A. V. (1981). *J. Physiol.* **314**, 37-46.
32. Shulkes, A. and Hardy, K. J. (1982). *Acta Endocrinol.* **100**, 565-572.
33. Shulkes, A. and Hardy, K. J. (1982). *Biol. Neonate* **42**, 249-256.
34. Bloom, S. R., Edwards, A. V. and Jarhult, J. (1980). *J. Physiol.* **308**, 29-38.
35. Bloom, S. R. and Edwards, A. V. (1981). *J. Physiol.* **314**, 23-35.
36. Bloom, S. R., Edwards, A. V. and Vaughan, N. J. A. (1973). *J. Physiol.* **233**, 457-466.
37. Bryant, M. G., Buchan, A. M. J., Gregor, M., Ghatei, M. A., Polak, J. M. and Bloom, S. R. (1982). *Gastroenterology* **83**, 47-54.
38. McIntosh, N., Pictet, R. L., Kaplan, S. L. and Grumbach, M. M. (1977). *Endocrinology* **101**, 825-829.
39. Koshimizu, T. (1983). *Endocrinology* **112**, 911-916.
40. Bassett, J. M. and Madill, D. (1978). *J. Physiol.* **278**, 22-23P.
41. Bell, A. W., Bassett, J. M., Chandler, K. D. and Boston, R. C. (1983). *J. Develop. Physiol.* **5**, 129-141.
42. Lichtenberger, L. M., Crandell, S. S., Palma, P. A. and Morriss, F. H. (1981). *Am. J. Physiol.* **241**, G235-G241.
43. Braaten, J. T., Greider, M. H., McGuigan, J. E. and Mintz, D. H. (1976). *Endocrinology* **77**, 684-691.
44. Kuhl, C., Hornnes, P. J., Jensen, S. L. and Lauritsen, K. B. (1980). *Endocrinology* **107**, 1446-1450.
45. Kuhl, C., Hornnes, P. J., Jensen, S. L. and Lauritsen, K. B. (1982). *Diabetologia* **23**, 41-44.
46. Lucas, A., Sarson, D. L., Bloom, S. R. and Aynsley-Green, A. (1980). *Acta Paediat. Scand.* **69**, 321-325.
47. Aynsley-Green, A. (1983). *J. Pediat. Gastroenterol. Nutr.* **2**, 418-427.
48. Bloom, S. R. and Polak, J. M. (1982). *Scand. J. Gastroenterol.* **17**, suppl. 74, 93-103.
49. Holst, J. J., Knuhtsen, S., Jensen, S. L., Fahrenkrug, J., Larsson, L. I. and Nielsen, O. V. (1983). *Scand. J. Gastroenterol.* **18**, suppl. 82, 85-99.
50. Cochard, P. and LeDouarin, N. M. (1983). *Scand. J. Gastroenterol.* **18**, suppl. 82, 85-99.
51. Bassett, J. M. (1974). *Aust. J. Biol. Sci.* **27**, 157-166.
52. Bloom, S. R., Edwards, A. V. and Hardy, R. N. (1978). *J. Physiol.* **280**, 37-53.
53. Siegel, E. G., Trimble, E. R., Renold, A. E. and Berthoud, H. R. (1980). *Gut* **21**, 1002-1009.
54. Kraegen, E. W., Chisholm, D. J. and McNamara, M. E. (1981). *Horm. Metab. Res.* **13**, 365-367.
55. Porter, R. J. and Bassett, J. M. (1979). *Diabetologia* **16**, 201-206.

The Roles of the Parathyroid and Thyroid Glands on Calcium Homeostasis in the Ovine Fetus

A. D. Care, I. W. Caple and D. W. Pickard

Department of Animal Physiology and Nutrition,
University of Leeds, Leeds, UK

Introduction

Calcium homeostasis in the fetus involves the control of net transfer of calcium across the placenta and the distribution of that calcium between the extracellular fluid and the fetal skeleton. The concentrations of both total and ionized plasma calcium concentrations are maintained higher in the fetus than in its mother during the latter part of gestation (1), and appear to be relatively independent of maternal levels (2). Several factors, including parathyroid hormone (PTH) and 1,25-dihydroxyvitamin D_3 ($1,25(OH)_2D_3$) (3), involving the placenta, fetal kidney and bone may contribute to the maintenance of the placental calcium gradient and the largely unidirectional nature of the calcium transport to the fetal lamb (4). Thyroparathyroidectomy (TXPTX) of the fetal lamb results in a rapid decrease in fetal plasma calcium concentration and loss of the placental calcium gradient within one day (3). This observation is consistent with the view that fetal PTH is involved in the maintenance of hypercalcaemia in the fetus, e.g. the rat (5), but it is not known whether fetal TXPTX leads to a reduction in placental calcium transport or to redistribution of calcium between extracellular fluid and bone. Some studies have indicated that bone resorption is negligible in the intact fetal lamb (6), and the role of PTH in this process is unclear.

In a preliminary experiment it was observed that fetal TXPTX in the sheep resulted in a fall in the fetal plasma concentration of $1,25(OH)_2D_3$ in addition to the decline in calcium ions (3). Alterations in fetal plasma $1,25(OH)_2D_3$ concentrations have been associated with changes in the placental calcium

The Physiological Development of the Fetus and Newborn
ISBN 0 12 389080 2

Copyright © 1985 by Academic Press, London.
All rights of reproduction in any form reserved.

gradient. For example, intravenous infusion to the fetal lamb of a specific antibody to $1,25(OH)_2D_3$ resulted in a rapid loss of the calcium gradient (7) and fetal nephrectomy resulted in a marked reduction in the circulating concentrating of $1,25(OH)_2D_3$ and a gradual fall in fetal calcium concentration (8). These observations have led to the hypothesis that the action of PTH in the maintenance of fetal hypercalcaemia may involve the stimulation of production of $1,25(OH)_2D_3$ by the fetal kidney (3), and consequent stimulation of the placental calcium pump. Studies have now been conducted to test this hypothesis.

Materials and Methods

Ewes and fetal lambs

The fetal lambs in 12 cross-bred ewes were operated on during the last month of gestation. Only one fetal lamb was used when twins were present, and the carotid artery was catheterized to enable subsequent collection of fetal blood samples. In 6 fetal lambs, the superior parathyroid (PT) glands and thyroid glands with their internal PT glands were removed (TXPTX). In 4 lambs the thyroid and internal PT glands were removed (TX), and 2 lambs were kept as controls with only the carotid artery catheterized. The patency of the carotid catheters was maintained by means of a continuous infusion of 0.037 ml/h of heparinized physiological saline (100 units/ml).

Blood samples were collected from ewes and fetal lambs for measurement of PH, pCO_2 and PO_2, ionized calcium (Nova -2 Ionized Calcium Analyser, Nova Biomedical), and plasma total calcium concentration (Technicon Autoanalyser System, Technicon Instruments Limited). In 9 ewes, the placental calcium gradients and circulating levels of $1,25(OH)_2D_3$ in maternal and fetal blood were monitored during the last 20 days of gestation using an antiserum which discriminates against metabolites of vitamin D_2 in favour of those of vitamin D_3 (9).

The effects of administering exogenous thyroxine (10–25 µg/day, Sigma Chemical Co.) to TX and TXPTX fetuses, and intra-arterial (i.a.) infusions of $1,25(OH)_2D_3$ or pure bovine parathyroid hormone (b-PTH) to the fetuses were examined.

Placental perfusion studies

Acute experiments were performed on 3 ewes with twin lambs to determine if placental calcium transport was reduced 3 days after fetal TXPTX. By this time the placental calcium gradient had been reversed in two of the three TXPTX fetuses, the third being a chimaera. In each ewe, the placenta of each fetus was perfused with autologous fetal blood after cannulation of the umbilical arteries and veins (10) and the increase in calcium concentration was measured over 120 min of the perfusion. At the end of each perfusion the placentas were examined, numbers of cotyledons recorded, and the fetuses were weighed.

Results and Discussion

Effects of fetal TPTX and TX on placental calcium gradient

The mean ($\pm$ SEM) concentrations of plasma total and ionized calcium concentrations in 6 fetal lambs at surgery prior to TXPTX were 3.11 ± 0.25 mmol/l and 1.70 ± 0.08 mmol/l, respectively, and those in the ewes were 2.03 ± 0.19 mmol/l and 1.01 ± 0.06 mmol/l, respectively. The calcium concentrations in 5 of the 6 TXPTX fetal lambs decreased rapidly following surgery, and within 48 hours were less than those in the ewes. The mean ionized blood calcium concentrations in 3 TXPTX lambs and their mothers were 0.72 ± 0.02 and 1.1 ± 0.02 mmol/l, respectively, during the last 20 days of gestation.

The effects of TXPTX and TX on the placental calcium gradient were compared in chronically catheterized fetal lambs sampled during the last 20 days of gestation. Both TXPTX and TX reduced the concentrations of blood ionized calcium and plasma total calcium in fetal lambs. The fetal to maternal calcium concentration ratio in TX (hemiparathyroidectomized) lambs was intermediate between those in intact and TXPTX lambs (Table 1).

Table 1. Plasma calcium concentrations in ewes and intact, thyroid-ectomized and thyroparathyroidectomized (TXPTX) fetal lambs during the last 20 days of gestation

Lambs (n)	Observations	Plasma calcium concentration (mmol/l)		F/M[†] Ratio
		Maternal	Fetal	
Intact (2)	18	2.28 ± 0.10*	2.93 ± 0.02	1.29
Thyroidectomized (4)	59	2.53 ± 0.07	2.59 ± 0.08	1.02
TXPTX (3)	44	2.48 ± 0.04	1.95 ± 0.05	0.79

*Mean $\pm$ SEM
[†]Fetal/maternal plasma calcium concentration

Replacement of thyroxine i.a. at the rate of 10–25 μg/day was without significant effect on the ionized plasma concentration of the TXPTX fetuses. The infusion of pure b-PTH (2500 units/mg) at the rate of 24 units/h for 2 h to a TXPTX fetus resulted in only a small rise (0.08 mmol/l) in ionized calcium. Into a second TXPTX fetus 100 units b-PTH was injected i.a. followed by an infusion of b-PTH at the rate of 36.6 units/h for 6.25 h. This treatment was associated with a small rise in fetal plasma ionized calcium of 0.14 mmol/l. A third TXPTX fetus was injected i.a. with 28 units b-PTH and then infused at the rate of 2.31 units/h/3.1 kg fetus for 46.25 h. This caused no significant change in the fetal plasma ionized calcium concentration. At the end of the infusion an i.a. injection of 56 units b-PTH was given which was followed by an infusion of 4.62 units/h for 34.5 h. This also failed to increase the fetal ionized calcium significantly. The doses of b-PTH used are of the same order as the 150 units b-PTH infused over 0.5 h by Barlet *et al.* (11) into intact ovine fetuses of a similar age. They demonstrated a fetal phosphaturia in response to this b-PTH and a small rise (0.18 mmol/l) in plasma total calcium concentration which was only observed at 0.5–1.0 h after the end of the infusion.

Effects of fetal TXPTX on placental calcium transfer

In two of three ewes with twin lambs the total and ionized calcium concentrations of TXPTX lambs were less than those in their mother within 3 days after surgery, and were also less than those in their intact twin. Within 10 minutes after removal of the TXPTX fetus from the placental circulation for perfusion of the placenta, the concentrations of ionized and total calcium concentrations had increased above those in the ewe (Fig. 1). The calcium concentrations in the placental perfusate rose steadily throughout the perfusions which were continued for 120 min for each placenta. The rates of increase in calcium concentration in the placental perfusates were similar for placentas of intact and twin siblings and also between pairs of twins.

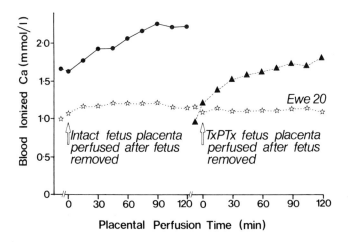

Figure 1. Changes in plasma ionized calcium concentration during perfusions of the placenta of a thyroparathyroidectomized (TXPTX) fetal lamb (▲ ------ ▲) and that of its intact twin (●———●) with autologous fetal blood, and compared with maternal levels (✿······✿).

The average net transfer of calcium into the placental perfusate reservoir (100 ml) during the 120 min was 6 mg. This represents about 17% of the rate of transfer of calcium into intact fetuses as measured by administration of labelled calcium to conscious ewes (4,6). Examination of the placenta of the TXPTX lamb which showed no decrease in plasma calcium concentration following surgery indicated that the placental blood supply was shared with its intact twin. The weights and crown-rump lengths of the twin lambs in each of the 3 ewes were similar. The mean (±SEM) weights of the 6 lambs was 2.35±0.10 kg. In the

2 ewes where separate placentas were present for each twin the numbers of cotyledons were similar.

The placental perfusion studies indicated that placental calcium transfer was not significantly affected by fetal TXPTX after a new steady hypocalcaemic state had been established in the fetus. However, the transfer rate tended to be reduced when the fetal plasma calcium concentration had been restored to the hypercalcaemic level appropriate for an intact fetus.

The relationship between plasma concentrations of $1,25(OH)_2D_3$ and ionized calcium in the TXPTX fetus

Although fetal TXPTX resulted in marked hypocalcaemia (Table 1) there was no associated fall in the plasma concentrations of $1,25(OH)_2D_3$ in contrast to that observed in lactating goats after TXPTX (12) and in a preliminary experiment on a fetal lamb (3). Concentrations of $1,25(OH)_2D_3$ ranged from 30 to 120 ng/l in maternal plasma and from 27 to 130 ng/l in fetal plasma. At the time of the placental perfusion the plasma concentration of $1,25(OH)_2D_3$ in the blood perfusing the placentas of the TXPTX fetuses was either the same or a little higher than that in the blood perfusing the placentas of the intact fetuses. This is in keeping with the similar rates of calcium flux from the mother observed during the placental perfusion (Fig. 1). Fetal TX and hemi PTX was also not associated wtih a significant change in the plasma concentration of $1,25(OH)_2D_3$ during the last 20 days of gestation.

Two TXPTX fetuses were maintained euthyroid with 20 μg thyroxine daily and were injected with 20 ng $1,25(OH)_2D_3$ followed by an i.a. infusion of 4 ng $1,25(OH)_2D_3$/h for 50 h. This produced no significant change in fetal plasma ionized calcium concentration despite a 10-fold increase in the fetal plasma concentration of $1,25(OH)_2D_3$ (up to 0.9 μg/l). A third TXPTX fetus was injected i.a. with 100 ng $1,25(OH)_2D_3$ which almost trebled the plasma concentration of $1,25(OH)_2D_3$ (from 87 to 230 ng/ml) within 4 h but only raised the plasma ionized calcium concentration by 0.02 mmol/l.

It is concluded that although in the parathyroid-intact ovine fetus the circulating level of $1,25(OH)_2D_3$ plays an important role in the maintenance of the placental calcium gradient (7,8), the parathyroid glands must also play an important part. It is not yet clear if PTH is the only parathyroid factor responsible, since the gradient was not restored in TXPTX fetuses by infusion of pure b-PTH over three days.

Acknowledgements

The skilled technical assistance of Dr Doreen Illingworth is gratefully acknowledged.

References

1. Care, A. D., Ross, R., Pickard, D. W., Weatherley, A. J. and Robinson, J. S. (1981). *In:* "Advances in Physiological Sciences" (Pethes, G. and Frengo, V. L., eds) Vol. 20, pp. 45–51, Pergamon Press, Oxford.

2. Care, A. D., Pickard, D. W., Garel, J. M., Barlet, J. P., Tomlinson, S. and O'Riordan, J. L. H. (1975). *Horm. Metab. Res.* **7**, 103-104.
3. Care, A. D. and Ross, R. (1984). *J. Develop. Physiol.* **6**, 59-66.
4. Symonds, H. W., Sansom, B. F. and Twardock, A. R. (1972). *Res. Vet. Sci.* **13**, 272-275.
5. Garel, J. M. (1983). *In:* "Perinatal Calcium and Phosphorus Metabolism" (Holick, M. F., Gray, T. K. and Anast, C. S., eds) pp. 71-104, Elsevier, Amsterdam.
6. Braithwaite, G. D., Glascock, R. F. and Riazuddin, S. (1972). *Br. J. Nutr.* **27**, 417-424.
7. Ross, R., Care, A. D., Robinson, J. S., Pickard, D. W. and Weatherley, A. J. (1980). *J. Endocrinol.* **87**, 17-18.
8. Care, A. D., Dutton, A., Mott, J. C., Robinson, J. S. and Ross, R. (1979). *J. Physiol.* **290**, 19-20.
9. Clemens, T. L., Hendy, G. N., Papapoulos, S. E., Fraher, L. J., Care, A. D. and O'Riordan, J. L. H. (1979). *Clin. Endocrinol.* **11**, 225-234.
10. Weatherley, A. J., Ross, R., Pickard, D. W. and Care, A. D. (1983). *Placenta* **4**, 271-278.
11. Barlet, J. P., Davicco, M. J. and Lefaivre, J. (1982-83). *J. Physiol. Paris* **78**, 809-813.
12. Hove, K., Horst, R. L., Littledike, E. T. and Beitz, D. C. (1984). *Endocrinology* **114**, 897-903.

Fetal Sex Developmental Differences are not Manifested by Steroid Hormone Binding Protein Interactions in Mid-trimester Amniotic Fluid

Mark I. Evans, George P. Chrousos, David Rodbard,
John W. Larsen, Jr., Richard C. Staton,
Joseph D. Schulman, and Bruce C. Nisula

Medical Genetics, CC, DEB, LTPD, NICHD, NIH, Bethesda, MD,
Depts of Obstetrics and Gynecology, George Washington University, DC
and Wayne State University, Detroit, Michigan, USA

Introduction

In the adult, steroid hormones circulate in complex with 3 major plasma proteins, testosterone-estradiol binding globulin (TeBG), corticosteroid binding globulin (CBG), and albumin (1). Despite voluminous data accumulated concerning the interactions of many steroid hormones and their binding proteins, only recently has progress been made in characterizing endogenous steroid binding protein interactions for the above mentioned binding proteins (2). Similarly, the presence of steroid hormones and binding proteins in amniotic fluid has been documented in several studies (3,4). However, attempts to elucidate the overall interaction of hormones, their binding proteins, and implications for fetal development have been somewhat limited. Using a mathematical model previously applied to describe the transport of steroid hormones in adult plasma (2), we have measured concentrations of estrone (E1), estradiol (E2), estriol (E3), progesterone (Prog), 17-hydroxyprogesterone 17-OHP, 11-deoxycortisol (S), cortisol (F), TeBG, CBG, and albumin. Using this model, we have been able to predict concentrations of each hormone bound to the particular binding proteins, unbound concentrations, and the unbound fractions.

The Physiological Development of the Fetus and Newborn
ISBN 0 12 389080 2

Copyright © 1985 by Academic Press, London.
All rights of reproduction in any form reserved.

Materials and Methods

Aliquots of amniotic fluid (2–3 ml) were obtained from specimens drawn for cytogenetic analysis at 17–18 weeks of gestation.

Analysis of E1, E2, E3, progesterone, 17-OHP, S, and F were measured by radioimmunoassay as previously described (2). TeBG and CBG were measured by Concanavolin A-Sepharose precipitation with Scatchard plot analysis.

Sex differences for each of the steroids were determined by two tailed *t*-tests using appropriate variance models as indicated. Estimations of free steroid concentrations were derived from our transport program previously published (2).

Calculations

The association constants (K) of each unlabelled steroid for binding TeBG and CBG were calculated from each steroid's respective relative binding activity (RBA) using the following equation:

$$K = K^* / [(1/RBA)\ (1+R) - R\ ],$$

where K^* is the association constant of the ^{3}H-labelled ligand (cortisol for binding CBG or testosterone for binding TeBG), RBA is the RBA of the unlabelled competing ligand, and R is the bound to free ratio of ^{3}H-labelled ligand at 50% displacement ($R = 0.3$ for testosterone and 0.2 for cortisol).

Results for the binding activities represent the mean $\pm$ SEM of at least 3 separate experimental determinations.

Computer simulation

The model assumes that equilibrium exists between each of the 7 steroids (m) and 3 binding proteins (n), as defined by the association constants previously published, with no co-operative or allosteric effects. The solution of this model must satisfy not only the $m \times n = 21$ but nonlinear equations defined by these association constants, but also the $m + n = 10$ equations for the conservation of mass. A straightforward solution would thus require the simultaneous solution of 33 equations. Feldman's technique reduces this to the simultaneous solution of 3 equations using an iterative technique (2). This is achieved using a computer program written in BASIC for the DEC-10 computer. We simply define the association constants for all possible reactions and the total molar concentrations for each steroid and each binding protein (literature values). The program then calculates the equilibrium composition of the system and provides the molar concentrations of each of the 21 steroid-protein complexes.

Results

Hormone levels were measured in 419 amniocentesis specimens selected randomly from excess fluid drawn for clinical cytogenetic analysis. Total concentrations of amniotic fluid binding proteins and their affinities for the corresponding tritiated ligands are shown in Table 1. No differences were observed in total concentrations or affinities between the two fetal sexes.

Table 1. Amniotic fluid binding proteins (pg/ml ± SEM)

	TeBG Capacity	TeBG (Kd^*)	CBG	Albumin
Total binding protein (M)	2292 ±123	7.90 ±0.43	37,400 ±2,158	2.83×10^9 ±0.87×10^8
(n)	(48)	(47)	(56)	(62)
Total binding protein (F)	2313 ±157	8.18 ±0.54	38,700 ±2,856	2.99×10^9 ±1.07×10^8
(n)	(48)	(48)	(46)	(46)
t-tests	ns	ns	ns	ns
Unbound binding protein (M)	1551		9688	2.83×10^9
Unbound binding protein (F)	1551		10,027	2.99×10^9
t-tests	ns		ns	ns
% Unbound binding protein (M)	67.7		25.9	100
% Unbound binding protein (F)	67.1		26.5	100

*nM

Table 2. Steroid hormone binding protein interactions*

Ligand (n)	Total concentration	TEBG Bound	CBG Bound	ALB Bound	Unbound concentration	% Unbound
E1 (M) (53)	383.4	89.68	0.178	182.4	111.2	28.99
E1 (F) (52)	386.5	88.02	0.186	189.2	109.1	28.24
E2 (M) (53)	53.67	27.57	0.0121	18.55	7.538	14.05
E2 (F) (50)	54.40	27.40	0.0127	19.49	7.495	13.78
E3 (M) (53)	1905	23.77	1.66	847.0	1033	54.20
E3 (F) (52)	2092	25.57	1.88	958.4	1106	52.87
Prog (M) (50)	43,330	493.9	6693	25,680	10,430	24.10
Prog (F) (54)	46,700	510.6	7338	28,060	10.790	23.11
170HP (M) (50)	1360	17.39	400.1	535.9	326.6	24.02
170HP (F) (54)	1341	16.43	480.9	535.0	308.7	23.02
S (M) (47)	534	13.03	307.5	62.09	151.4	28.35
S (F) (52)	566	13.26	331.8	66.78	154.1	27.23
F (M) (49)	31,500	85.7	20,230	1225	9959	31.62
F (F) (54)	31,000	81.02	20,280	1224	9418	30.38

*All measurements reported as pg/ml
All tests between male and female fetuses: not significant

Analysis of hormone concentrations in regard to the sex of the fetus and binding of individual steroids to each of the bonding proteins, their unbound concentration, and per cent unbound fractions are shown in Table 2. There were no statistical differences between the fetal sexes. From the above, using the transport program (2) the binding constants can be derived, and also showed no differences between the sexes.

Discussion

In the present study, we have used a computer model based on the law of mass action to characterize steroid hormone transport in mid-trimester amniotic fluid. Computer analysis is the only method available for solving the complex equilibrium interaction of multiple ligand-binding systems which most closely approximates the *in vivo* situation. The present model simulates the transport of steroids on 3 transport proteins in mid-trimester amniotic fluid.

Several studies have measured amniotic fluid steroid hormones—some in an attempt to determine fetal sex. Similarly, steroid binding hormones have been assayed. In this report we have attempted to expand these studies and with the use of computer simulations of binding to determine the relative contributions to binding of each of the proteins and ligands.

Analysis of the data fail to reveal any pattern of sex differences in amniotic fluid. Such results are consistent with there being in all cases excess binding protein available to buffer the fetus from modulation in sex steroid levels which could interfere with normal development. However, while concentrations of ligand and binding proteins are lower than in maternal plasma, the relative concentrations of unbound and measurably active hormones is greater than in plasma. Such observations are consistent with the ability of the female fetus to withstand mild elevations of maternally derived androgens without virilization. Similarly the data are consistent with sensitivity to higher doses of maternal or fetally derived androgens such as from 21 hydroxylase deficiency congenital adrenal hyperplasia which can produce external genital masculinization (5).

References

1. Dunn, J. F. (1984). Computer simulation of steroid transport in human plasma. *In:* "Computers in Endocrinology", (Rodbard and Forti, eds) pp. 277–285, Raven Press, New York.
2. Dunn, J. F., Nisula, B. C. and Rodbard (1981). *J. Clin. Endocrinn. Metab.* **53**, 58–68.
3. Bremme, K., Eneroth, P. and Nilsson, B. (1982). *Gynecol. Obstet. Invest.* **14**, 245–262.
4. Fenci, M. D., Koos, B. and Tulchinsky, D. (1980). *J. Clin. Endocrin. Metab.* **50**, 431–436.
5. Evans, M. I., Chrousos, G. P. and Mann, D. L. (1985). *J. Am. Med. Ass.* (in press).

ACTH Release following Electrolytic Lesions of the Fetal Hypothalamus in the Sheep

T. J. McDonald, Y. Parsons,* J. C. Rose,**
J. P. Figueroa, P. W. Nathanielsz and P. D. Gluckman*

Department of Reproductive Studies, New York State College of
Veterinary Medicine, Cornell University, Ithaca, New York, USA

*Developmental Physiology Laboratory, Department of Paediatrics,
University of Auckland, Auckland, New Zealand

**Department of Physiology and Pharmacology, Bowman Gray School of
Medicine, Wake Forest University, Winston-Salem, North Carolina, USA

Studies with mature animals have demonstrated that corticotropin releasing factor (CRF) is primarily located in neurons whose cell bodies lie in the paraventricular nucleus (PVN) of the hypothalamus (1,2,3,4). Recently lesions of the PVN have been demonstrated to greatly reduce adrenocorticotropin (ACTH) release following ether stress in adult rats (5).

In this study we have investigated ACTH release in the chronically instrumented fetal lamb, following bilateral electrolytic lesioning of the PVN. ACTH release in response to fetal hypotension and hypoxaemia has been measured in control and lesioned fetuses to evaluate the extent to which the hypothalamus regulates the fetal ACTH response to these stimuli.

Surgical Procedures

Under ketamine anaesthesia the fetuses of 13 Rambouillet-Columbia ewes were cannulated with polyvinyl catheters via the carotid artery and jugular vein as previously described (6). Surgery was performed at 108–110 days of gestation. Using the stereotaxic method and atlas of Gluckman and Parsons (7), electrodes were placed in the PVN (co-ordinates: AP 24 mm, lat. 0.8 mm, and vert. 7.5 mm).

The Physiological Development of the Fetus and Newborn
ISBN 0 12 389080 2

Copyright © 1985 by Academic Press, London.
All rights of reproduction in any form reserved.

Electrolytic lesions were produced using monopolar electrodes attached to a battery operated DC current lesion generator. An anodal current (5–6 mA) was passed through the electrode for 30 seconds. In the Sham operated animals the electrodes were lowered to the same co-ordinates without passing the current. All fetuses were allowed to recover for 4 days after surgery before being studied.

At the end of the experiments the brains were perfused with saline followed by 10% buffered formalin. They were then blocked in the stereotaxic apparatus and embedded in gelatin. Frozen sections (50 μ thick) were cut and stained with thionin. Lesions were evaluated from photographs of the sections made at $\times 6$ magnification.

Experimental Procedures

The effect of fetal hypotension

Fetal blood pressures were monitored with Statham pressure transducers and recorded on a Grass polygraph. Fetal blood samples (3.25 ml blood each sample) were taken at -15, -5, $+10$, and $+30$ min and monitored for blood gases, pH, haematocrit and hormones. From 0 to $+10$ min nitroprusside in 5% glucose was infused intravenously (starting at 100 μg/min) to reduce mean blood pressure by 50% at $+5$ min. The infusion was stopped at $+10$ min and blood pressure was allowed to recover.

The effect of hypoxaemia

Blood samples were taken at -30, -5, $+40$, and $+60$ min and monitored for blood gases, pH, haematocrit and hormones. From 0–60 min the ewe inhaled a gas mixture (10% O_2, 3% CO_2, 87% N_2) via a face mask. The fetuses were considered hypoxaemic if the arterial PO_2 fell by more than 5 Torr.

The response to synthetic corticotropin releasing factor (CRF)

Blood samples were taken at -15, -5, $+15$, $+30$, and $+60$ min. At time 0, fetuses were given a bolus of 1.0 μg synthetic ovine CRF.

Each experiment was performed on a separate day. Red blood cells were aseptically returned to the fetus at the end of each procedure.

The experiments were done in random order on the fetuses although not all procedures were performed on each fetus. Plasma ACTH was measured as previously described (8) on all samples, as were blood gas, pH and haematocrit.

Results

Surgical outcome

Of the 9 fetuses in which lesions were attempted, 1 died before any experiments were performed, 3 had bilateral lesions of the PVN, 2 had lesions of the basal septal area impinging dorsally on the PVN and 3 had misplaced lesions. The latter were grouped with 4 sham operated fetuses.

The effect of hypotension

The ACTH responses of the fetal sheep to a 50% drop in mean blood pressure induced by nitroprusside infusion are shown in Fig. 1. At − 15 and − 5 min the ACTH levels of all 3 groups of animals were similar and ranged from 15 to 43 pg/ml. At the end of the 10-min nitroprusside infusion, the sham lesioned fetuses had high ACTH levels (285, 305 pg/ml), the fetuses with basal septal lesions had intermediate ACTH levels (111, 123 pg/ml) while the PVN lesioned animals had the lowest ACTH levels (74, 34, 11 pg/ml). Similar differences between the 3 groups were seen 20 min after the end of the nitroprusside infusion.

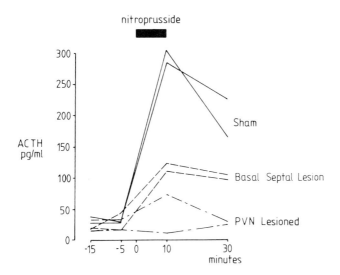

Figure 1. Fetal carotid ACTH concentrations in PVN lesioned, basal septal lesioned and sham lesioned sheep fetuses at 112–114 days gestation, before, during and after fetal hypotension and a 50% reduction in mean blood pressure incuded by nitroprusside infusion (100 μg/min).

The effect of hypoxaemia

The ACTH responses of the fetuses to hypoxemia are shown in Fig. 2. After 40 min of hypoxaemia, the PVN lesioned fetuses had ACTH values of only 71, 30 and 32 pg/ml while the basal septal lesioned and sham operated animals had values ranging from 113 to 232 pg/ml. After 60 min, ACTH concentrations in the basal septal lesioned and sham operated fetuses ranged from 128 to 180 pg/ml while in the PVN lesioned fetuses ACTH values had fallen to 54, 21 and 22 pg/ml.

The response to CRF

The ACTH responses of fetal sheep when given exogenous ovine CRF were similar to the responses observed during the nitroprusside infusion. The levels

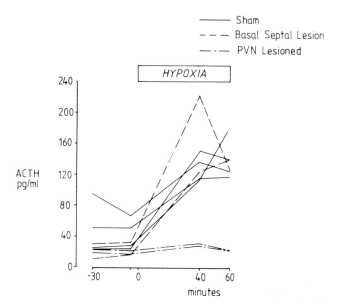

Figure 2. Fetal carotid ACTH concentrations in PVN lesioned, basal septal lesioned and sham lesioned sheep fetuses at 112–114 days gestation, before and during fetal hypotension (5 Torr reduction) enduced by the maternal administration of a 10% O_2, 3% CO_2, 87% N_2 gas mixture for 60 min.

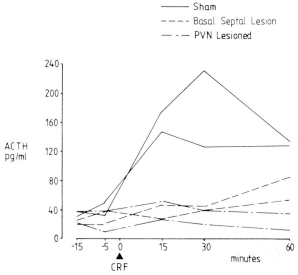

Figure 3. Fetal carotid ACTH concentrations in PVN lesioned, basal septal lesioned and sham lesioned sheep fetuses at 112–114 days gestation, before and after a bolus administration of 1 μg of oCRF to the fetal jugular vein.

of ACTH at + 15 min were highest in the sham operated fetuses (147, 173 pg/ml) but remained low in the basal septal lesioned animals (27, 46 pg/ml) and PVN lesioned animals (27, 36, 52 pg/ml) (Fig. 3).

Discussion

In the fetuses with bilateral ablation of the PVN, basal levels of ACTH secretion were not affected, and no response to both hypotension and hypoxaemia was observed when compared to sham operated animals. Following exogenous ovine CRF, the PVN lesioned fetuses gave no increases in ACTH production. This is in contrast to observations in the adult rat in which lesions of the PVN resulted in hypersecretion of ACTH in response to CRF (9). However these animals were given a dose of CRF that was 8-10 times larger on a weight basis than that administered in the present study. This difference in the CRF challenge may be the basis of this difference in response. Alternatively, it may be that the ability of the fetal pituitary to respond to exogenous CRF has been compromised by lesioning the PVN. Repeated exposure to exogenous CRF may be necessary in the fetus to maintain responsiveness to CRF.

In conclusion, the data from this preliminary study suggest that by 112-115 days of gestation, the fetal PVN mediates ACTH release in response to physiological stimuli via the secretion of a CRF.

References

1. Swanson, L. W., Sawchenko, P. D., Rivier, J. and Vale, W. W. (1982). *Neuroendocrinology* **36**, 165–186.
2. Bloom, F. E., Battenburg, E. L. F., Rivier, J. and Vale, W. W. (1982). *Reg. Peptides* **4**(1), 43–48.
3. Palkovitz, M., Brownstein, M. J. and Vale, W. W. (1983). *Neuroendocrinology* **37**, 302–305.
4. Paul, W. K., Scholer, J., Arimura, C. A., Myers, J. K., Chong, D. and Shimuzu, M. (1982). *Peptides* **3**, 183–191.
5. Bruhn, T. O., Plotsky, P. M. and Vale, W. W. (1984). *Endocrinology* **114**(1), 57–62.
6. Nathanielsz, P. W., Abel, M. H., Bass, F. G., Krane, E. J., Thomas, A. L. and Liggins, G. C. (1978). *Q. J. Exp. Physiol.* **63**, 211–219.
7. Gluckman, P. D. and Parsons, Y. (1983). *J. Develop. Physiol.* **5**, 101–128.
8. Rose, J. C., MacDonald, A. A., Heymann, M. A. and Rudolph, A. M. (1978). *J. Clin. Invest.* **61**, 424–432.
9. Gann, D. S., Ward, D. G. and Carlson, D. E. (1978). *Rec. Prog. Horm. Res.* **34**, 357–400.

Development of Processing of Pro-opiomelanocortin in Pituitary Corticotrophs of Fetal Sheep

Colin T. Jones, J. W. Knox Ritchie and M. Pucklavec

The Nuffield Institute for Medical Research,
University of Oxford, Oxford, UK

Introduction

In most species, with the possible exception of man, the importance of the pituitary and adrenal in the initiation of birth is unquestioned (1–3). For ruminants a sharp rise in fetal cortisol output from the fetal adrenal is the signal to the placenta to initiate a chain of events leading to marked increase in uterine contraction (1–3). The signal prompting this sequence has therefore been sought as the switch to parturition and was thought originally to be simply in increased secretion of ACTH from the fetal pituitary. A number of observations argue against this. ACTH peptides are present at relatively high concentrations for much of gestation and although they increase late in gestation that may come after the cortisol rise (4,5). The demonstration that much of the ACTH in adult and fetal pituitary and plasma is present in high molecular weight precursor forms, and the contribution that these make to total plasma ACTH falls at the time of increased fetal adrenal activity (6–8) implies a complex relationship. Thus the concentration of pro-opiomelanocortion relative (POM) to ACTH falls in the fetal sheep circulation late in gestation (Fig. 1). Physiological significance for this is implied in the fact that POM inhibits steroidogenic effects of ACTH on the fetal adrenal (8–10). Such observations indicate that the factors responsible for the switch from POM to ACTH secretion late in gestation may be one of the important signals initiating a chain of events leading to rapid maturation of the fetal adrenal. This study investigates the possibility that POM processing in the fetal pituitary corticotrophs matures as gestation proceeds.

The Physiological Development of the Fetus and Newborn
ISBN 0 12 389080 2

Copyright © 1985 by Academic Press, London.
All rights of reproduction in any form reserved.

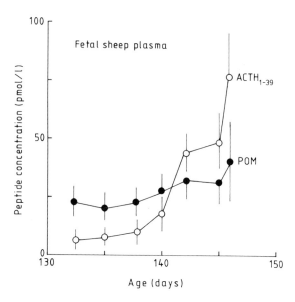

Figure 1. Changes in the concentration of ACTH and of pro-opiomelanocortin (POM) in the plasma of fetal sheep during gestation. ACTH peptides were extracted from fetal plasma and separated by polyacrylamide-gel electrophoresis as described in methods. ACTH was taken as the peptide in the 4.5K region and POM in the 32K region of the gel (Fig. 2). Peptides were measured by RIA.

Methods

Corticotrophs were prepared from the anterior pituitary of fetal sheep by digestion twice at 37°C of minced tissue with 1.25 mg/ml of collagenase (Worthington) in Krebs' bicarbonate buffer for 30 min. Cells (*ca* 10^5/ml) were incubated for 15 min at 37°C in Krebs' bicarbonate buffer then [41]CRF (Peninsular Labs.) or AVP (Ferring) added and the cells incubated for the times indicated below. At the end of the incubation cells were cooled immediately and spun at 1500 g for 5 min. Cells and supernatant were treated with 1 M-HCl containing 1 mM phenylmethylsuphonyl fluoride. ACTH peptides were extracted, separated by polyacrylamide-gel electrophoresis and assayed as described elsewhere (8).

Results

As reported previously much of the ACTH in fetal sheep pituitary is present predominantly in high molecular weight forms (Fig. 2). In the handling of these there are at least two steps in the pathway to secretion—an intracellular breakdown of POM and related peptides to ACTH, and a calcium-sensitive secretion (8,11–14). The calcium sensitivity of secretion by comparison with intracellular processing has been used previously to identify less active breakdown of ACTH precursors in fetal sheep pituitary corticotrophs at about 120 days than near term

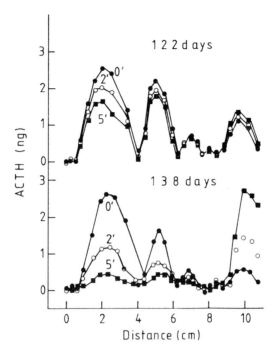

Figure 2. ACTH peptides in the pituitary cells of fetal sheep of 122 days (upper panel) and 138 days (lower panel) at 0, 2 and 5 min after the addition of 1 nmol arginine vasopressin (AVP). Peptides were extracted and separated by gel electrophoresis. Measurement was by RIA.

Table 1. Rates of intracellular formation of ACTH from high molecular weight precursors in pituitary corticotrophs of the fetal sheep

	Rate of ACTH formation (ng/min per 10^5 cells)	
	120–130 days	140–143 days
Control	<0.01	0.05±0.03
[41]CRF (1 nmol)	0.12±0.04	0.73±0.26
AVP (1 nmol)	0.08±0.035	0.50±0.24
CRF+AVP	0.21±0.044	1.46±0.47

Cells (10^5/ml) were incubated in Krebs' bicarbonate buffer at 37°C for 5 min, then immediately cooled and ACTH peptides extracted. Peptides were separated by polyacrylamide-gel electrophoresis and assayed by RIA. The rate of combined intra- and extracellular appearance of the 4.5K peptide running in the same position as ACTH on electrophoresis is taken as the rate of ACTH production.

(14). In the present study intracellular processing was estimated by following the rate of breakdown of precursors and formation of ACTH after the first 5 min of exposure to CRF or to AVP. Thus in cells from fetal sheep around 122 days there was relatively little initial breakdown of precursor, but by 138–140 days it had increased almost 10-fold (Fig. 2 and Table 1). If the rate of breakdown of ACTH *in vivo* is ignored, and this was minimized by adding lima bean trypsin inhibitor, these results indicate that rate of precursor processing to ACTH is in response to CRF or AVP is much greater near term than at 120 days. Over this period there was no significant change in the concentration of corticotrophic peptides per 10^5 cells. Administration of 0.1 mmol butyryl cAMP had an essentially similar effect to CRF (results not shown).

Discussion

Some studies have indicated that between 120–135 days there is a slow rise of plasma "ACTH peptide" concentration (15). This is not a consistent finding. There is a marked increase over this period in the ability of fetal sheep to respond to infusions of CRF (16). This could be explained if CRF receptor density and hence intracellular stimulation of pituitary corticotrophs were low. Thus the relatively low rate of POM processing at 120 days would be explained. Alternatively the poor *in vivo* responses to CRF at this time could be a consequence of the apparently low rates of intracellular processing. This view is confirmed by the effects of cAMP which by-passes the CRF receptor and by the fact that the plasma ACTH peptide concentration is high at this time. The present results thus suggest that in terms of ACTH production the pituitary corticotrophs at 120 days are comparatively unresponsive to stimulation, at least in part, as a consequence of poorly developed intracellular processing. Increased activity of this pathway is likely to contribute to the switch in plasma from relatively inactive to active peptides that have marked effects on adrenal growth and steroid output.

References

1. Liggins, G. C., Fairclough, R. J., Grieves, S. A., Kendall, J. Z. and Knox, B. S. (1973). *Rec. Prog. Horm. Res.* **29**, 111–150.
2. Bassett, J. M. and Thorburn, G. D. (1969). *J. Endocrinol.* **44**, 285–286.
3. Thorburn, G. D. and Challis, J. R. G. (1979). *Physiol. Rev.* **83**.
4. Jones, C. T., Boddy, K. and Robinson, J. S. (1977). *J. Endocrinol.* **72**, 293–300.
5. Rees, L. H., Jack, P. M. B., Thomas, A. L. and Nathanielsz, P. W. (1975). *Nature* **253**, 274–275.
6. Jones, C. T. (1975). *In:* "Radioimmunoassay Techniques in Clinical Biochemistry" (Pasternak, C. A., ed.) pp. 253–260. Heyden and Sons, London.
7. Silman, R. E., Holland, D., Chard, T., Lowry, P., Hope, J., Rees, L. H., Thomas, A. L. and Nathanielsz, P. W. (1979). *J. Endocrinol.* **81**, 19–34.
8. Jones, C. T. and Roebuck, M. M. (1980). *J. Steroid Biochem.* **12**, 77–82.

9. Roebuck, M. M., Jones, C. T., Holland, D. and Silman, R. (1980). *Nature* **284**, 616–618.

10. Roebuck, M. M., Jones, C. T. and Robinson, J. S. (1985). *J. Develop. Physiol.* **7** (in press).

11. Nakanishi, S., Inone, A., Kita, T., Nakamura, M., Chang, A. C. Y., Cohen, S. N. and Numa, S. (1979). *Nature* **278**, 423–427.

12. Eipper, B. A. and Mains, R. E. (1978). *J. Supramol. Struct.* **8**, 247–262.

13. Chang, T.-L. and Loh, Y. P. (1983). *Endocrinology* **112**, 1832–1838.

14. Jones, C. T. (1980). *Biochem. Soc. Trans.* **8**, 585–586.

15. Hennessy, D. P., Coghlan, J. P., Hardy, K. J. and Wintour, E. M. (1982). *J. Develop. Physiol.* **4**, 339–352.

16. Wintour, E. M. (1984). *J. Develop. Physiol.* **6**, 291–299.

The Effects of Food Withdrawal on Uterine Contractile Activity and on Plasma Cortisol Concentrations in Ewes and their Fetuses during Late Gestation

Abigail L. Fowden and Marian Silver

Physiological Laboratory, University of Cambridge,
Cambridge, UK

Introduction

Withdrawal of food for 30–48 h has been shown to increase the production of 13–14 dihydro-15-keto-prostaglandin $F_{2\alpha}$ (PGFM) by the gravid uterus in the mare and ewe (1,2). The PGFM changes during food withdrawal were related to gestational age and were associated with premature delivery when the animals were fasted near to term (1,2). However, little is known about how nutrient restriction may influence the timing of delivery. Enhanced prostaglandin (PG) production might cause myometrial contraction or changes in the fetus may precipitate the natural sequence of events that precede delivery at term. In the present study, the effects of food withdrawal on uterine contractile activity and on fetal hormone and metabolite concentrations have been investigated in chronically catheterized sheep during late gestation.

Material and Methods

Intravascular catheters were inserted under halothane anaesthesia into 14 Welsh Mountain ewes and their fetuses between 120–130 days of gestation as described previously (2). A saline-filled balloon was also placed into the amniotic or allantoic sac to measure intra-uterine pressure (3). Normal feeding patterns were generally

The Physiological Development of the Fetus and Newborn
ISBN 0 12 389080 2
Copyright © 1985 by Academic Press, London.
All rights of reproduction in any form reserved.

restored within 24–48 h of operation but no experiments were carried out until 7–10 days after surgery. Food but not water was withheld for 48 h at gestational ages ranging from 127–141 days. Some animals experienced two 48-h periods of food withdrawal which were separated by at least 7 days. Blood samples were withdrawn from the ewes and their fetuses before, during and after food withdrawal and intra-uterine pressure (IUP) was measured continuously throughout the experimental period. A uterine contraction was defined as a change in IUP greater than 3 mmHg which lasted longer than 5 min (3). Plasma concentrations of cortisol, PGFM and glucose were measured by the methods described previously (2,9).

Results

Outcome of pregnancy

Five of the 9 ewes fasted after 137 days delivered within 12–24 h of ending the fast. In these 5 ewes, delivery occurred at a mean gestational age of 140.3 ± 0.5 days which was significantly less than the age at delivery of the other 4 ewes fasted after 137 days (146 ± 0.8 days, $P < 0.01$) or of similar catheterized ewes not subjected to food withdrawal in late gestation (146.0 ± 0.5 days, $n = 7$). There was no significant difference in the gestational age at the beginning of the fast between the ewes that delivered immediately afterwards and those that did not. All but one of the lambs was alive at birth ($n = 21$).

Plasma hormone and metabolite concentrations

Withdrawal of food for 48 h increased the plasma cortisol concentration in all the fetuses studied (Table 1). The increase in fetal plasma cortisol was significant by 24 h of fasting and was greatest during fasts begun after 137 days of gestation (Table 1, $P < 0.01$); the mean increments in fetal plasma cortisol for 48-h fasts begun at < 134, 134–137 and > 137 days were 20.5 ± 4.1 ng/ml ($n = 5$, $P < 0.05$), 23.8 ± 4.1 ng/ml ($n = 5$, $P < 0.05$) and 60.9 ± 5.4 ng/ml ($n = 10$, $P < 0.01$) respectively. For fast begun after 137 days, the increment in fetal plasma cortisol was similar irrespective of the time of delivery. However, the actual plasma concentrations of cortisol before and at the end of the fast were significantly greater in the fetuses that were delivered within 12–24 h of refeeding than in those that were not (Table 1, $P < 0.05$). In the majority of animals fetal plasma cortisol levels decreased within 24 h of refeeding the fasted ewes but in those animals that delivered immediately after fasting the levels continued to rise after refeeding (Table 1). Maternal plasma concentrations of cortisol did not change from the basal value of 10.6 ± 1.3 ng/ml ($n = 14$) during fasts begun before 137 days of gestation but thereafter there was a small but significant rise in the concentration during the fast ($+ 10.1 \pm 2.6$ ng/ml, $n = 8$, $P < 0.01$).

Fasting increased both the fetal and maternal plasma PGFM concentrations. The rise in fetal PGFM varied widely between animals and showed no obvious gestational trend. The mean increase in fetal plasma PGFM during fasting was 1.24 ± 0.27 ng/ml ($n = 9$, $P < 0.01$). The rise in maternal PGFM during fasting

Table 1. The mean (±SEM) frequency and duration of uterine contractions and the mean plasma concentrations of fetal cortisol before and 36–48 h after beginning a 48-h period of food withdrawal and after refeeding in animals fasted at <133, 134–137 and >137 days of gestation

		<134 days	134–137 days	>137 days	
Uterine contractions				No delivery	Delivery
Frequency (number/h)	Prefasting	1.68±0.26 (5)	1.75 (3)	1.53±0.10 (4)	1.44±0.25 (4)
	Fasted	1.50±0.26 (5)	1.53 (3)	2.19±0.16* (4)	3.02±0.56* (4)
	Postfasting	1.27±0.17 (5)	1.51 (3)	1.50±0.12 (4)	5.09±0.59* (4)
Duration (min)	Prefasting	7.1±0.3 (5)	8.1 (3)	7.7±0.7 (4)	8.2±0.4 (4)
	Fasted	6.8±0.3 (5)	8.3 (3)	7.2±0.3 (4)	7.6±0.7 (4)
	Postfasting	7.3±0.5 (5)	7.9 (3)	7.1±0.7 (4)	8.5±0.6 (4)
Fetal cortisol (ng/ml)					
	Prefasting	10.6±1.4 (5)	20.0±1.6 (5)	21.0±1.6 (6)	44.1±12.2 (4)
	Fasted	31.0±4.9* (5)	44.9±5.2* (5)	85.0±5.7* (6)	111.3±16.6* (4)
	Postfasting	16.9±3.4 (5)	32.9±9.1 (5)	44.1±9.4* (6)	130 (2)

*significant increase from prefasting value. Number of animals in parenthesis.

was similar to that observed previously (2). There was a significant positive correlation between the fetal and maternal plasma PGFM concentrations before, during and after food withdrawal ($r=0.91$, $n=31$, $P<0.01$).

The fetal plasma glucose concentration fell in parallel with the maternal level during fasting; the changes in concentration were not related to gestational age. The mean decreases in fetal plasma glucose for fasts begun at <134, 134–137 and >137 days were 0.11±0.04 mmol/l ($n=5$, $P<0.05$), 0.13±0.04 mmol/l ($n=5$, $P<0.05$) and 0.17±0.03 mmol/l ($n=10$, $P<0.01$) respectively.

Uterine contractile activity

In the fed state, the frequency and duration of the uterine contractions did not vary with gestational age and were similar to the values reported in other studies (Table 1: 3,4). There was no change in uterine activity during fasts begun before 137 days but thereafter food withdrawal increased the frequency of uterine contractions by the end of the fast (Table 1, $P<0.01$). There was no consistent change in the duration of individual contractions during fasting at any of the gestational ages studied (Table 1). The increase in contraction frequency during fasting after 137 days tended to be greater in the ewes that delivered immediately afterwards than in those that did not. However, the difference was not significant (Table 1, $P > 0.05$). In the ewes that did not deliver immediately after fasting, the frequency of uterine contractions returned to the prefasting values within 24 h while in the ewes that delivered the frequency of uterine contractions continued to rise (Table 1), even though the animals ate vigorously.

Discussion

Previous studies of nutrient restriction have demonstrated only a small or insignificant increase in the fetal cortisol concentration which could have been caused by transplacental passage of maternal cortisol (5,6). In the present study, fasting for 48 h produced a significant increase in the fetal cortisol level which was invariably greater than any change in maternal concentration, indicating that, in common with other types of stress (7,8), nutrient restriction can stimulate the release of cortisol in the fetal lamb. The response of the fetal adrenal to fasting increased with gestational age which may explain the relatively small response observed in the younger fetuses used in the previous studies (5,6). The rise in fetal cortisol during fasting after 137 days and the levels attained in some animals were similar to the values observed at term (9). This suggests that activation of the fetal adrenal is responsible, at least in part, for the early parturition in ewes fasted near to term.

Fetal and maternal plasma PGFM levels rose during fasting although fetal arterial concentrations were generally lower than the maternal uterine venous values. This suggests that PGs are metabolized within the uteroplacental tissues and pass into both the fetal and maternal circulations. During most of gestation, the increase in PG metabolism during fasting appeared to be adequate to prevent any change in the uterine contraction pattern. Only after 137 days of gestation was the rise in PGFM associated with increased uterine activity. The increased frequency of uterine contractions followed the rise in PGFM and fetal cortisol and did not always result in active labour. The animals that went into labour after the fast had higher fetal cortisol levels and lower maternal plasma progesterone concentrations (2) at the end of the fast than those that delivered several days after refeeding.

These observations demonstrate that fasting will hasten delivery of viable lambs in animals in which the prepartum increase in fetal cortisol had already begun. Even when ewes are less severely restricted in their diet the length of gestation may be reduced (10). Similar mechanisms may operate in human pregnancy as fasting for 24 h has been shown to increase the number of full-term babies delivered in the subsequent 24 h (11). The rapid rise in fetal cortisol and the increased frequency of uterine contractions observed during fasting near to term emphasize the need for a regular food intake during late gestation and suggests that dietary factors may be important in the precise timing of delivery at term.

References

1. Silver, M. and Fowden, A. L. (1982). *J. Reprod. Fertil. Suppl.* **32**, 511–519.
2. Fowden, A. L. and Silver, M. (1983). *Q. J. Exp. Physiol.* **68**, 337–349.

3. Jansen, C. A. M., Krane, E. J., Thomas, A. L., Beck, N. F. G., Lowe, K. C., Joyce, P., Parr, M. and Nathanielsz, P. W. (1979). *Am. J. Obstet. Gynecol.* **134**, 776-783.
4. Hindson, J. C. and Ward, W. R. (1971). *In:* "The Endocrinology of Pregnancy and Parturition" (Pierrepoint, C. G., ed.), Alpha Omega Alpha, Cardiff.
5. Bassett, J. M. and Madill, D. (1974). *J. Endocrinol.* **61**, 465-477.
6. Mellor, D. J., Matheson, I. C. and Small, J. (1977). *Res. Vet. Sci.* **23**, 119-121.
7. Jones, C. T., Boddy, K., Robinson, J. S. and Ratcliffe, J. G. (1977). *J. Endocrinol.* **72**, 279-292.
8. Rose, J. C., Macdonald, A. A., Heymann, M. A. and Rudolph, A. H. (1978). *J. Clin. Invest.* **61**, 424-432.
9. Barnes, R. J., Comline, R. S. and Silver, M. (1978). *J. Physiol.* **275**, 567-579.
10. Alexander, G. (1956). *Nature* **178**, 1058-1059.
11. Kaplan, M., Eidelman, A. I. and Aboulafia, Y. (1983). *J. Am. Med. Ass.* **250**, 1317-1318.

Maturation of Thermoregulatory and Thermogenic Mechanisms—Studies of the Hypothermic Sheep Fetus

P. D. Gluckman, T. R. Gunn, B. M. Johnston and M. Fraser

Developmental Physiology Laboratory, Department of Paediatrics,
University of Auckland, Auckland, New Zealand

Effective thermoregulatory and thermogenic mechanisms are an essential aspect of the neonatal adaption. Both mature and ACTH induced premature lambs have been demonstrated to exhibit shivering and nonshivering thermogenesis, endocrine, metabolic and cardiovascular responses to cold stress.

We developed a preparation by which the chronically instrumented fetal lamb is exposed to environmental hypothermia *in utero*. A coil of tubing is placed around the fetus between 100 and 130 days of gestation through which cold tap water (14–19°C) can be passed to reduce amniotic and fetal skin temperatures. Passing water at a rate of 300–500 ml/min through the coil for 1 h leads to a fall in fetal core temperature (measured by a thermister within the fetal cranium) of $3.46 \pm 0.50°C$ over 20 min. The fetal temperature is then maintained at this lesser level for the duration of the cooling (1). Recovery takes approximately 50 min at 125 days. Even when the flow rate is reduced to 10–30 ml/min the fetal core temperature still falls by $1.04 \pm 0.04°C$ during the hour of cooling. This suggests that the fetus has little ability to withstand even mild environmental cold stress. Studies between 106 and 139 days of gestation showed no evidence of a maturational change in the ability to withstand cold stress (1) despite evidence that lambs born prematurely following ACTH induction of parturition appear to require a greater degree of cold stress to alter core temperature (2). This suggests that prior to birth there is either relative immaturity of central thermoregulatory mechanisms or of peripheral thermogenic effector systems. Accordingly we have performed a series of observations on the hypothermic fetal lamb to evaluate the maturation of these systems (3).

These studies have demonstrated that by 106 days of gestation, cooling the

The Physiological Development of the Fetus and Newborn
ISBN 0 12 389080 2

Copyright © 1985 by Academic Press, London.
All rights of reproduction in any form reserved.

fetus is associated with the onset of continuous waves of electromyographic activity, typical of shivering, in limb muscles (3). Associated with the cooling there is a significant tachycardia and hypertension. Measurement of umbilical blood flow by means of an electromagnetic flow probe placed on the retroperitoneal segment of the left umbilical artery showed a marked increase in umbilical blood flow during fetal hypothermia. This increase in the blood flow was blocked by α-adrenergic blockage with phentolamine, which abolished the associated hypertension. These observations suggest the fetal response to environmental hypothermia includes a redistribution in blood flow away from the peripheral tissues (Iwamoto *et al.*, and unpublished observations). The fetal arterial PO_2 falls markedly during cooling (1) and in view of the increase in umbilical blood flow this presumably reflects an increase in fetal oxygen consumption although this has not been measured directly.

Plasma adrenaline and particularly noradrenaline concentrations rise markedly during fetal cooling. As would therefore be expected plasma glucose levels rise in association with a fall in fetal insulin concentrations. Plasma thyrotropin (TSH) concentrations also rise rapidly and markedly during cooling. However plasma thyroxine and triiodothyronine (T_3) concentrations do not change significantly (Table 1). Studies in newborn lambs delivered into a waterbath have previously shown that while hypothermia induces the TSH surge at birth, separation from the placenta is necessary for the increase in T_3 to occur (4). The placenta is rich in inner ring deiodinase activity (5) and presumably any thyroxine released by the fetal thyroid in response to the TSH surge is metabolized rapidly to reverse T_3.

In contrast to the above findings, we have failed to demonstrate any rise in free fatty acids (FFA) in 6 fetuses cooled *in utero* between 120 and 137 days of gestation. However, in the neonatal lamb FFA release which is an index of nonshivering thermogenesis, is an essential component of the thermogenic response (Fig. 1).

Table 1. Effects of fetal cooling*

Measurement	Basal	Cooling	P
Heart rate	184 ± 6	231 ± 7	<0.001
Mean blood pressure (mmHg)	44.1 ± 1.2	47.9 ± 1.1	<0.001
Umbilical blood flow (ml/min/kg)	201 ± 24	262 ± 29	<0.001
Triiodothyronine (ng/dl)	16.2 ± 6.5	16.9 ± 7.1	ns
Thyoxine (μg/dl)	9.0 ± 1.4	9.65 ± 1.6	ns
TSH (μU/ml)	1.52 ± 1.56	7.4 ± 1.9	<0.001
Noradrenaline (pg/ml)	336 ± 99	1999 ± 358	<0.001
Adrenaline (pg/ml)	46 ± 12	354 ± 112	<0.001
Glucose (mg/dl)	15.9 ± 1.1	31.3 ± 1.5	<0.001
Insulin (μU/ml)	6.69 ± 1.28	2.16 ± 0.54	<0.01
FFA (μEq/l)	42.7 ± 19.5	46.7 ± 21.2	ns

*Effects of cooling the fetus by a coil in the amniotic cavity.
Mean $\pm$ SEM is shown; ns not significant.

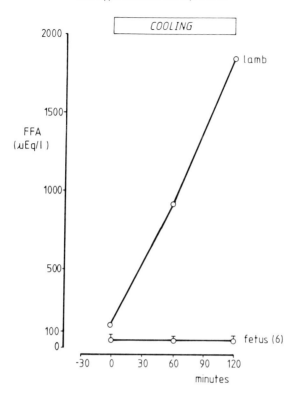

Figure 1. Effect of cooling of plasma FFA levels in 6 fetuses between 120 and 137 days of gestation. Cooling was for 1 h starting at 0 min via a coil surrounding the fetus in the amniotic cavity. The fetal core temperature fell by 2.81 ± 0.14°C. For comparison, the change in FFA following cooling of an infant lamb by ice packs, in which the core temperature fell by 1.5°C is shown.

The studies suggest that the fetus has appropriate central thermoregulatory responses to environmental hypothermia by 106 days of gestation. These regulatory responses include initiation of cardiovascular responses, shivering, catecholamine release and activation of the thyroid axis. However despite these regulatory mechanisms being functional, which presumably reflects differentiation of the hypothalamic thermoregulatory pathways, effective thermogenesis is not observed. As our experimental approach leads to the fetal temperature falling below maternal temperature (1), heat loss is not continuing across the placenta. It therefore seems probable that the inability to mount effective nonshivering thermogenesis, as indicated by the absence of a FFA response is the basis for the inability of the fetus to maintain its fetal temperature against a relatively small thermal gradient across the skin. (The amniotic temperature during cooling is between 33 and 37°C depending on where it is measured in relation to the position of the coil). While immaturity of the skin and wool may contribute to the ease of heat loss in the younger fetuses, it is noteworthy that even in fetuses older than 135 days, thermogenesis appears relatively ineffective.

The explanation for the failure of the fetus to exhibit nonshivering thermogenesis remains to be elucidated. It may simply reflect immaturity of brown fat. Recent *in vitro* studies, however, suggest that there are marked maturational changes in catecholamine stimulated thermogenesis in perirenal brown adipose tissue between 120 and 135 days of gestation with no further increase after birth (6). This may be due to an increase in catecholamine receptors or to the induction of enzymes in the thermogenic metabolic pathways. Despite this *in vitro* evidence for functional thermogenesis in brown fat in late gestation sheep fetuses, we could not demonstrate FFA release *in utero* secondary to hypothermia. In contrast in premature neonates of 130 days postconceptual age delivered following adrenocorticotropin induced labour, nonshivering thermogenesis is observed (7). Although catecholamines induce a FFA response in postnatal lambs (2), our experiments led to a rise in catecholamines without a rise in FFA. The experiments of Sack *et al.* (4) in which lambs were delivered into waterbaths but with intact umbilical cords suggest that a parallel rise in T_3 is necessary for hypothermia to induce FFA release. Thus the primary defect in the fetal response to hypothermia, once the brown adipose tissue has fully differentiated, may be the inability to increase T_3 levels because of the activity of the placental ring deiodinase. A further factor to be considered is that nonshivering thermogenesis is normally reduced under hypoxaemic conditions and the rise in PO_2 at birth may be necessary for effective brown fat thermogenesis. These questions are readily examinable in the fetal lamb.

Acknowledgements

These studies are supported by the Medical Research Council of New Zealand and the Auckland Medical Research Foundation.

References

1. Gunn, T. R. and Gluckman, P. D. 61983). *J. Develop. Physiol.* **5**, 167–179.
2. Alexander, G. and Williams, D. (1968). *J. Physiol.* **198**, 251–262.
3. Gluckman, P. D., Gunn, T. R. and Johnston, B. M. (1983). *J. Physiol.* **343**, 495–506.
4. Sack, J., Beaudy, M., Delameter, P. V., Oh, W. E. and Fisher, D. A. (1976). *Pediat. Res.* **10**, 169–175.
5. Roti, E., Gnudi, A., Braverman, L. E. (1983). *Endocr. Rev.* **4**, 131–149.
6. Klein, A. H., Reviczky, A., Chou, P., Padbury, J. and Fisher, D. A. (1983). *Endocrinology* **112**, 1662–1666.
7. Alexander, G. (1981). *Proc. Aust. Physiol. Pharmacol. Soc.* **12**, 31–36.

Pro-opiomelanocortin Derived Peptides in Fetal Plasma

Raymond I. Stark, Sharon L. Wardlaw, Salha S. Daniel, Connie B. Newman, Mary M. Smeal and L. Stanley James

Columbia University, College of P and S, Division of Perinatology and Department of Medicine, Babies Hospital, New York, USA

We have undertaken studies to characterize the response of the developing hypothalamohypophyseal system to hypoxia. Activation of this system induced by a variety of forms of stress has been extensively examined in the adult of many species and results in the secretion into the circulation of a wide variety of potent hormones from the anterior and posterior lobes of the pituitary (1). During fetal life the intermediate lobe, a third component of pituitary with a distinct hormone content and regulation, must also be considered. This lobe is prominent in the fetuses of mammalian species (2). Of equal importance are the recent demonstrations of independent synthesis of anterior and intermediate lobe peptides in the cell bodies of neurons in the hypothalamus (3). Neuronal projections containing both anterior and intermediate lobe peptides are extensively distributed not only within the hypothalamus but also throughout the central nervous system (4,5). Within the CNS these peptides are believed to act locally as neurotransmitters or neuromodulators. In addition their presence in pituitary portal plexus blood suggests a neurohormonal function (6).

Many of the peptide hormones synthesized within the central nervous system are derived from precursor molecules (4). The pro-opiomelanocortin (POM) protein is synthesized predominantly in the anterior and intermediate lobes of the pituitary and in the hypothalamus (5). Synthesis of POM by the placenta has also been demonstrated (7). The processing of this precursor varies in different tissues resulting in the secretion of peptides with very different biological activities. Thus the anterior pituitary secretes mainly ACTH and β-lipotropin (β-LPH) and some β-endorphin (β-EP) while the intermediate lobe secretes mainly α-melanocyte stimulating hormone (α-MSH), corticotropin like intermediate peptide (CLIP) and N-acetyl β-EP which lacks opiate activity (4,8). The processing of POM in

The Physiological Development of the Fetus and Newborn
ISBN 0 12 389080 2

Copyright © 1985 by Academic Press, London.
All rights of reproduction in any form reserved.

the hypothalamus and placenta resembles that of the intermediate lobe except that in the hypothalamus the peptides are not acetylated. Differences in the secretion of POM peptides in the fetus may be important for adrenal maturation and the prepartum rise in fetal cortisol which has been shown to trigger parturition in the sheep (9). The body of information about the processing of POM in the fetus comes from studies of the pituitary content of these peptides. Measurement of the pituitary content does not necessarily reflect their rate of secretion, and further processing might take place at the time of secretion. Therefore, careful measurements of POM peptides in fetal plasma are required in order to know which peptides are secreted by the fetal pituitary. We present some preliminary results related to the regulation of the release of these peptides.

Methods and Results

Gel filtration and an antibody to β-EP which cross-reacts 30% on a molar basis with β-LPH and 100% with N-acetyl β-EP and specific antibodies to α-MSH ($<0.01\%$ cross-reactivity with ACTH) and N-acetyl-β-EP ($<0.1\%$ cross-reactivity with β-EP) were used for RIA measurement of peptide concentrations. Chronically catheterized fetal lambs were studied under basal and hypoxic conditions. The changes in arterial pH and blood gases with the various experimental protocols is summarized in Table 1.

Table 1. Fetal pHa, $PaCO_2$ (mmHg), and PaO_2 (mmHg) before, during and after exposure of the ewe to various experimental protocols: Control (room air $\times$ 30 min), Hypoxia (10% O_2 in $N_2 \times$ 30 min), and dexamethasone and hypoxia (bolus of 200 μg/h followed by 10% O_2 in $N_2 \times$ 30 min)

		Before	During	After
Control	pHa	7.377 ± 0.016	7.370 ± 0.017	7.379 ± 0.015
	$PaCO_2$	43.9 ± 1.1	41.2 ± 0.6	43.8 ± 1.6
	PaO_2	22.6 ± 1.3	20.6 ± 0.6	22.6 ± 2.1
Hypoxia	pHa	7.386 ± 0.008	$7.305 \pm 0.024^*$	$7.347 \pm 0.011^*$
	$PaCO_2$	43.6 ± 1.0	42.0 ± 1.9	43.1 ± 1.5
	PaO_2	22.1 ± 0.7	$12.4 \pm 0.5^*$	22.9 ± 0.7
Dexamethasone and hypoxia	pHa	7.384 ± 0.016	$7.261 \pm 0.003^*$	$7.327 \pm 0.024^*$
	$PaCO_2$	45.1 ± 1.1	47.2 ± 2.9	41.7 ± 2.8
	PaO_2	18.5 ± 0.7	$11.8 \pm 1.4^*$	18.9 ± 0.9

In other experiments under basal condition molar ratios of total β-EP to β-LP were > 1.0, a ratio higher than that reported for anterior lobe secretion (10). During hypoxia ratios were < 0.4 as we have found in the plasma of human adults who lack an intermediate lobe (11). These data suggested that the POM derived peptide secretion in the undisturbed fetus was of intermediate lobe origin while in the stressed fetus the anterior lobe was activated. By direct measurement under basal conditions total fetal plasma β-EP was almost identical to N-acetyl β-EP

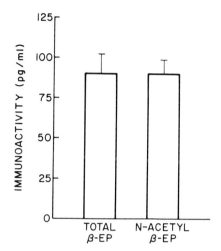

Figure 1. Concentrations (mean±SEM) of total β-endorphin (β-EP) and N-acetyl β-EP under basal conditions defined as mean±SD of pHa 7.388±0.25, $PaCO_2$ 43.6±1.9 mmHg, PaO_2 21.1±2.4 mmHg, BE +0.9±1.6, heart rate 168.4±8.6 beats/min, and mean blood pressure 43.6±3.8 mmHg.

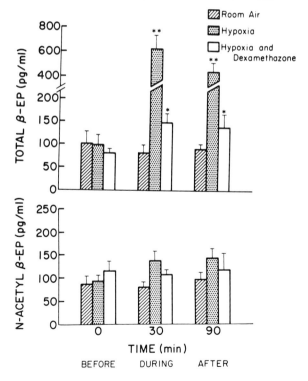

Figure 2. Concentrations (mean±SEM) of total β-endorphin (β-EP) and N-acetyl β-EP in fetal lamb plasma before, during and after various experimental protocols.

R. I. Stark *et al.*

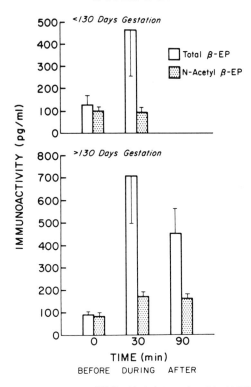

Figure 3. Concentrations (mean ± SEM) of total β-endorphin (β-EP) and *N*-acetyl β-EP before, during and after exposure of the ewe to 10% O_2 in $N_2 \times 30$ min in fetuses < 130 days gestation (upper panel) and > 130 days gestation (lower panel).

(Fig. 1). Thus the majority of fetal plasma β-EP activity under these conditions appeared to be of intermediate lobe origin. When fetal hypoxia was induced by exposure of the ewe to 10% O_2 in N_2 mean total β-EP increased significantly ($P < 0.005$) while mean *N*-acetyl β-EP remained at a value not different from that of the prehypoxia control (Fig. 2). Thus under hypoxic conditions the majority of total β-EP could not be accounted for by *N*-acetyl β-EP. This increase with hypoxia of total β-EP was significantly greater ($P < 0.05$) in fetuses > 130 days gestation than in younger fetuses (Fig. 3). *N*-Acetyl β-EP values were not different. When glucocorticoids were infused to the fetus 30 min prior to hypoxia the increase in mean total β-EP was significantly ($P < 0.05$) less, while mean *N*-acetyl β-EP again remained unchanged (Fig. 3). Under similar basal conditions mean concentration of α-MSH was 33.1 ± 2.4 pg/ml while maternal α-MSH was 8.6 ± 1.2 pg/ml. Intravenous injection of metaclopramide, a dopamine antagonist, to the fetus stimulated α-MSH secretion into fetal plasma (33.9 ± 2.8 to 139 ± 28 pg/ml after 15 min). These data demonstrate a high concentration of α-MSH in fetal plasma which can be further increased by metaclopramide, a known secretagogue of the intermediate lobe.

Conclusions

In prior investigations we described increased levels of total β-EP in the umbilical cord blood of human infants which were inversely correlated with pH and pO_2 (10). We subsequently demonstrated that hypoxia was a potent stimulus to total β-EP and other neuropeptide release in the fetal lamb (12) but the source of the β-EP remained a question. The present studies suggest that in the basal state intermediate lobe peptides predominate in fetal plasma. During fetal hypoxic stress anterior lobe POM related peptides are released and include nonacetylated β-EP and β-LPH. The release of these peptides during hypoxic stress can be inhibited by glucocorticoids. The activation of anterior lobe secretion by hypoxic stress is enhanced by gestational maturation. It is of considerable importance to understand the regulation of POM derived peptides because there is accumulating evidence that these peptides have important physiologic effects. On the other hand excessive release or exogenous administration of neuropeptides or their antagonists at certain stages of fetal development may have long-term detrimental effects (13).

Acknowledgements

This research was supported in part by a grant from the National Institutes of Health HD-13063.

References

1. Axelrod, J. and Reisine, T. D. (1984). *Science* **224**, 452.
2. Silman, R. E. *et al.* (1981). *Peptides Pars Intermedia* **180**.
3. Liotta, A. S. *et al.* (1979). *Proc. Nat. Acad. Sci. USA* **76**, 1448.
4. Kreiger, D. T. (1983). *Clin. Res.* **31**, 342.
5. Roberts, J. L. and Herbert, E. (1977). *Proc. Nat. Acad. Sci. USA* **74**, 5300.
6. Wardlaw, S. L. *et al.* (1982). *J. Clin. Endocrin. Metab.* **55**, 877.
7. Liotta, A., Osathanondh, R. *et al.* (1977). *Endocrinology* **101**, 1552.
8. Mains, R. E. and Eipper, B. A. (1981). *J. Biol. Chem.* **266**, 5683.
9. Silman, R. E., Street, C. *et al.* (1981). *Peptides Pars Intermedia* **180**.
10. Wardlaw, S. L., Stark, R. I. *et al.* (1981). *Endocrinology* **108**, 1710.
11. Wardlaw, S. L. and Frantz, A. G. (1979). *J. Clin. Endocrinol. Metab.* **48**, 176.
12. Stark, R. I., Wardlaw, S. L. *et al.* (1982). *Am. J. Obstet. Gynecol.* **147**, 204.
13. Swaab, D. F. and Boer, G. J. (1982). *J. Develop. Physiol.* **983**, 67.

Inhibition of the Cortisol Response to ACTH$_{1-24}$ by Pro-opiomelanocortin in Lamb and Calf *in vivo*

Deborah J. Tindell*, A. V. Edwards** and C. T. Jones*

*The Nuffield Institute for Medical Research, University of Oxford, Oxford, UK and **Physiological Laboratory, University of Cambridge, Cambridge, UK

It is likely that the fetal pituitary gland is the main determinant of both fetal adrenal growth and steroidogenesis (1). Its importance has been illustrated by the studies of Liggins (2) showing involvement of the pituitary-adrenal axis in the initiation of birth. Thus, a key event preceding parturition in the sheep is a surge of fetal cortisol production.

It has been suggested that until 7–9 days before term the adrenal glands of the fetal sheep *in vivo*, are relatively unresponsive to ACTH stimulation (3,4). In the sheep fetus the increase in glucocorticoid secretion occurs prior to any substantial increase in fetal plasma ACTH, which suggests that either the fetal adrenal sensitivity to ACTH changes late in gestation (5) or that another fetal pituitary trophic factor exists (6).

In the sheep the pituitary hormones ACTH and lipotrophin (LPH) are the principal components of the adult, however, the fetal pituitary gland contains an abundance of large molecular weight material of which there are 3 forms. Two of these contain sequences common to β-LPH, γ-LPH, β-MSH, endorphin and possibly other biologically active peptides, as well as ACTH, α-MSH, and CLIP (7). Investigations on human pituitary glands have revealed a large molecular weight precursor pro-opiomelanocortin (POM) common to ACTH and LPH (8,9). Previous studies have shown with isolated fetal sheep adrenal cells that pro-opiomelanocortin inhibits the steroidogenic response to ACTH and may contribute to the relative inactivity of the adrenal until close to term (10). Thus we have examined the effects of POM, peptide A and ACTH$_{1-24}$ on the output of cortisol by the adrenal gland of the calf, and on the circulation level of cortisol in the lamb.

The Physiological Development of the Fetus and Newborn
ISBN 0 12 389080 2

Copyright © 1985 by Academic Press, London.
All rights of reproduction in any form reserved.

Methods

Pedigree Jersey calves were obtained locally and used at ages ranging from 26–54 days (26–33.8 kg body weight). Food was withheld for at least 6 h prior to surgery, which was carried out under ethylchloride and ether anaesthesia maintained with halothane in oxygen. Preparatory surgery involved hypophysectomizing the calf in order to reduce the basal adrenal output of corticosteroid, before inserting the specially designed adrenal clamp (11). $ACTH_{1-24}$ (Synacthen CIBA) was dissolved in physiological saline calculated to provide a dose of 5 ng/kg/min when infused into the calf via the right jugular vein at a flow rate of 1 ml/min. Similarly, POM (32K prepared from sheep pituitary) was infused to provide a dose of 5 ng/kg/min flowing at 1 ml/min for 15 min. *In vivo* experiments were performed also on newborn lambs at ages ranging from 39–46 days. Vascular catheterization was performed under halothane anaesthesia, with the catheters being implanted into the jugular and carotid arteries, and filled with heparin-saline until experimentation. Studies were performed on the lambs between 9.30–11.00 a.m. Heparinized blood samples (500 μl) were taken at -30, -10, -15, 30 and 60 min for the measurement of plasma cortisol levels. The protocol involved a priming injection of 1 μg of peptide followed by jugular infusion of $ACTH_{1-24}$ at 10 μg/h

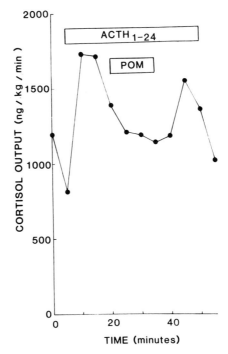

Figure 1. Mean output of cortisol from right adrenal gland in calves infused with 5 ng/kg/min Synacthen and 5 ng/kg/min POM: $n=4$. Period of infusions indicated by horizontal blocks.

with or without POM and Peptide A (12) at 20 μg/h for 30 min. All blood samples were collected into heparinized syringes, centrifuged at 2000 **g** for 15 min at 4°C, and the plasma stored at $-20°$ until analysis. The plasma was left untreated for the cortisol radioimmunoassay used, as described by Abraham (12), in which 5000 μl of redistilled ethanol was used for the extraction of 100 μl of sample.

Results

Calf

Intravenous infusion of $ACTH_{1-24}$ (Synacthen, CIBA) at a dose of 5 ng/kg/min produced a sharp rise in the output of cortisol when given to 4 calves (Fig. 1). The maximum rate of release occurred within 5–10 min reaching a mean value of 1700 ± 360 SEM ng/min/kg. The output of cortisol represents the product of

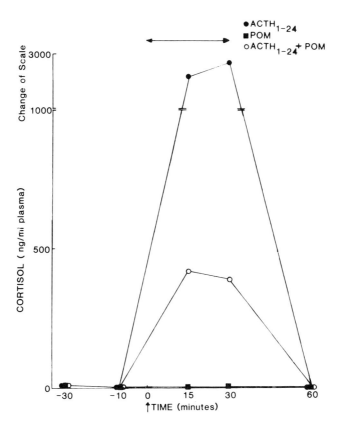

Figure 2. Mean peripheral concentration of cortisol in lambs infused with 10 μg/h $ACTH_{1-24}$, 20 μg/h POM, and $ACTH_{1-24}$+POM: $n=3$. Period of infusion indicated by horizontal bar.

the adrenal vein cortisol concentration and plasma flow through the gland, both
of which were estimated independently (11). The infusion of POM for 15 min
at a dose of 5 ng/kg/min during the ACTH infusion period, caused a dramatic
fall in cortisol output from the gland to a level of approximately two-thirds of
its maximum output. Removal of POM caused the output of cortisol to return
to a near-maximal level again.

Lamb

The peripheral level of cortisol rose abruptly during the intravenous infusion
of $ACTH_{1-24}$ at a dose of $10\,\mu g/h$ (Fig. 2). Infusion of POM ($20\,\mu g/h$) had no
effect on the cortisol level over the initial basal level, and the infusion of POM
($20\,\mu g/h$) simultaneously with $ACTH_{1-24}$ ($10\,\mu g/h$) brought the cortisol
concentration down to a sixth of its $ACTH_{1-24}$-induced maximum level. In
Fig. 3, infusion of $ACTH_{1-24}$ ($10\,\mu g/h$) again led to a rise in the peripheral
cortisol level. Infusion of peptide A ($20\,\mu g/h$) alone had no effect on the initial
cortisol level, and when infused with $ACTH_{1-24}$ ($10\,\mu g/h$) led to the cortisol

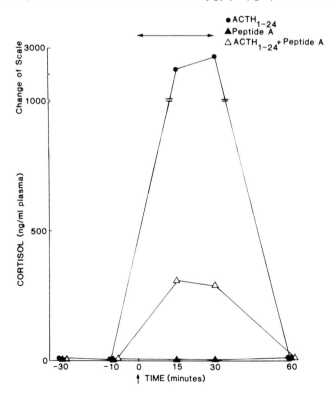

Figure 3. Mean peripheral concentration of cortisol in lambs infused with $10\,\mu g/h$
$ACTH_{1-24}$, $20\,\mu g/h$ Peptide A, and $ACTH_{1-24}$+Peptide A: $n=3$. Period of infusion
indicated by horizontal bar.

concentration coming down to about one-eighth of its maximum $ACTH_{1-24}$-stimulated level.

Discussion

In domestic ruminants and primates control of the growth and steroidogenic activity of the fetal adrenal during the second half of pregnancy depends on trophic agents from the fetal pituitary (13). The nature of these probably change with gestation. For example, as term approaches the concentration ratio of $ACTH_{1-39}$. Pro-opiomelanocortin in the pituitary and in fetal plasma increases at about the same time as the sharp rise in fetal plasma cortisol (10). In the light of the present, and of the previous observations, showing that POM either with isolated adrenal cells (10) or with the intact adrenal *in situ* is relatively nonsteroidogenic, but more important, inhibits ACTH-induced steroidogenesis, a physiological role for circulating POM in the fetus can be proposed. Thus, it is known that the ovine fetal adrenal *in vivo* is relatively unresponsive to ACTH until late in gestation, and some, but not all studies with isolated tissue, are in broad agreement (14,15).

It is important to note, however, that studies with perfused fetal adrenal have shown it to be capable of relatively high rates of steroid production. The present result with the newborn lamb and calf provide a mechanism by which the fetal adrenal may be made acutely and potentially chronically, unresponsive to ACTH stimulation. Also, the natural fall relative to ACTH, in its plasma concentration could provide the signal for the large increase in adrenal activity and growth. No direct studies have been done on the likely mechanism of action of POM but the nature of the ACTH receptor and the structure of POM (16) would be consistent with POM blocking the high affinity nonsteroidogenic site of the ACTH receptor.

Acknowledgements

The work reported in this paper was supported by the Medical Research Council.

References

1. Jost, A. (1966). *In:* "The Pituitary Gland", Harris, G. W. and Donovan, B. T. eds) Vol. 2, pp. 299–323. Butterworth, London.
2. Liggins, G. C., Fairclough, R. J., Grieves, S. A., Kendall, J. Z. and Knox, B. S. (1973). *Rec. Prog. Horm. Res.* **29**, 111–159.
3. Jones, C. T., Boddy, K., Robinson, J. S. and Ratcliffe, J. G. (1977). *J. Endocrinol.* **72**, 279–292.
4. Wintour, E. M., Brown, E. H., Denton, D. A., Hardy, K. J., McDougall, J. G., Oddie, C. J. and Whipp, G. T. (1975). *Acta Endocrinol. Copernh.* **79**, 301–306.
5. Anderson, A. B. M., Pierrepoint, C. G., Griffiths, K. and Turnbull, A. C. (1972). *J. Reprod. Fertil.* suppl. **16**, 25–37.

6. Johnson, P., Jones, C. T., Kendall, J. Z., Ritchie, J. W. K. and Thorburn, G. D. (1975). *J. Physiol.* **282**, 64P.

7. Silman, R. E., Holland, D., Chard, T., Lowry, P. J., Hope, J., Rees, L. H., Thomas, A. and Nathanielsz, P. (1979). *J. Endocrinol.* **81**, 19–34.

8. Mains, R. E. and Eipper, B. A. (1975). *Proc. Nat. Acad. Sci.* **72**, 3565–3569.

9. Kan, K. W., Baird, A., Seidah, N. G., Lis, M., Chrétien, M., Ling, N., Guillemin, R. and Solomon, S. (1977). *Biochem. Biophys. Res. Commun.* **79**, 553–560.

10. Roebuck, M. M., Jones, C. T., Holland, D. and Silman, R. (1980). *Nature* **284**, 616–618.

11. Edwards, A. V., Hardy, R. N. and Malinowska, K. W. (1974). *J. Physiol.* **239**, 477–498.

12. Abraham, G. E., Buster, J. E. and Teller, R. C. (1972). *Analyt. Lett.* **5**, 757–765.

13. Jones, C. T. (1975). *In:* "Radioimmunoassay Techniques in Clinical Biochemistry", (Pasternak, C. A. ed.) p. 253. Van Heyden & Sons, London.

14. Madill, D. and Bassett, J. M. (1973). *J. Endocrinol.* **58**, 75–87.

15. Sayers, G., Swallow, R. L. and Giordano, N. D. (1971). *Endocrinology* **88**, 1063–1068.

16. Nakanishi, S., Inoue, A., Kita, T., Nakamura, M., Chang, A. C. Y., Cohen, S. N. and Numa, S. (1979). *Nature* **278**, 423–427.

Aspects of Fetal Lung Development

G. C. Liggins and J.-C. Schellenberg

Postgraduate School of Obstetrics and Gynaecology,
University of Auckland, Auckland, New Zealand

Investigation of the relative importance of intrinsic and extrinsic factors in promoting growth and maturation of the fetal lung yields conflicting results according to whether the experiments are performed *in vitro* or *in vivo*. The maturation of fetal rat lung maintained in organ culture devoid of hormones (1) follows the same chronological pattern of airsac development and accumulation of lamellar bodies as lungs *in vivo* (2) leading to the conclusion that administered hormones such as corticosteroids may advance development but are unnecessary for normal maturation. In contrast, substantial evidence from *in vivo* experiments points to the need for stimulation by extrinsic physical and hormonal factors if growth and maturation compatible with neonatal survival is to be attained (for recent reviews see (3,4,5)). The complexity of lung structure and function is such that at this early stage in our understanding arbitrary subdivisions of development are needed for descriptive purposes. Development will be regarded as being composed of overall growth, maturation of structure and maturation of function. Obviously, the boundaries between these subdivisions are blurred, each being dependent on the others.

Growth of the Fetal Lung

Fetal rat lung in organ culture containing 1% fetal calf serum grows and shows continued branching of the primitive airway and formation of terminal airsacs (2). The DNA content increases from 1.36 μg/lung at 14 days to 3.65 $\pm$ 0.43 μg/lung after 7 days in culture. This 3-fold increase in DNA content can be compared with the 1000-fold increase over 7 days between day 14 and day 21 in the fetal lung *in vivo* (6). This suggests limited inherent capacity for growth and raises the question of the nature of the stimuli that promote growth *in vivo*. The frequent occurrence of gross pulmonary hypoplasia in human fetuses with a wide variety of malformations having in common a reduction in intrathoracic volume indicates

The Physiological Development of the Fetus and Newborn
ISBN 0 12 389080 2
Copyright © 1985 by Academic Press, London.
All rights of reproduction in any form reserved.

that unrestricted expansion is a necessary component of the stimulus to growth (see 3,4 for reviews). Other fetal organs are able to grow to normal proportions in abnormal locations as illustrated by diaphragmatic hernias when various abdominal viscera may grow at a normal rate within the chest yet the lung is likely to be little more than vestigial. Hormonal influences appear to play little part in lung growth, lung weight:body weight ratio being preserved in various endocrine disorders such as hypopituitarism, hypothyroidism, hypoinsulinaemia or adrenal insufficiency occurring spontaneously in human fetuses or resulting from endocrine organ ablation in experimental animals.

The susceptibility of lung growth to impairment by restricted expansion suggests that distension may normally provide a major stimulus to growth. Alcorn and associates (7) tested this hypothesis experimentally by inducing chronic overdistension. Overdistension was caused by tracheal ligation which led to massive accumulation of secreted lung fluid. The wet weight of the distended lungs corrected by removal of lung fluid was approximately double the expected weight when the fetuses were delivered 3–4 weeks after tracheal ligation and dry weight also was increased (T. M. Adamson, personal communication). Considering the importance of the hypothesis, there is a surprising paucity of experiments designed to test it. Alcorn's work has not been repeated nor have measurements of DNA been made to confirm that alterations in the weight of the lungs reflect increased or decreased cell numbers. A report by Gluck and colleagues (8) describes the surprising findings that the lungs of 6 rhesus monkey fetuses in which tracheal ligation was performed at 108–121 days were not visibly distended when delivered at 148–155 days. The mean wet weight of the lungs of 5.0 g was significantly *less* than the value of 9.5 g in 150-day fetuses reported by other workers (9). Without exception, recent reports have described experiments aimed at retarding rather than accelerating fetal lung growth and the interpretation of results usually is based on the tacit assumption that retarded growth is attributable to loss of a distending force.

Determinants of Lung Volume

Consideration of the determinants of lung volume necessitates a description of the factors regulating lung fluid volume. Detailed reviews will be found elsewhere (3,4,10). The present discussion is limited to a perspective of the conflicting views put forward in the recent literature which may be summed up as the "tonic school" versus the "phasic school".

Tonic Determinants of Lung Volume

The transpulmonary pressure in fetal sheep in late gestation during periods of nonbreathing amounts to 2.5–5.0 torr comprising a positive intratracheal pressure of 1.5–3.0 torr and a negative intrapleural pressure of 1–2 torr (11,12). In a fluid-filled lung in which surface forces are inoperative, a distending pressure of this magnitude is sufficient to account for the volume of lung fluid normally present in the lung. The intratracheal component of the distending force presumably arises from the combined effects of the elastic recoil of the lung and the secretion pressure of lung liquid acting against a tonic resistance to outflow. The relative contributions of the two forces is unknown but it is worthy of note that Alcorn and associates (7) found intratracheal pressures as high as 9 torr after tracheal ligation suggesting that secretion pressure could be a significant factor.

As already pointed out, studies of the influence of tonic forces on lung growth have investigated the effects of reducing rather than increasing those forces. This has been achieved in a variety of ways. Fewell and coworkers (13) drained the lung fluid directly into the amniotic sac through a large, short tube. The dry weight of the lung corrected for body weight was reduced by approximately 25% ($P < 0.02$) in the tracheostomized fetuses. The results were unexpectedly complex in that the reduced growth appeared to involve mainly the apical lobe. Indeed, the DNA concentration of the diaphragmatic lobe was significantly increased (50.3 ± 10.7 mg/g dry wt vs 35.1 ± 10.5; $P < 0.05$). If a ratio of apical:diaphragmatic lobe weights of 1:2.5 is assumed (our unpublished observations) recalculation of the data shows that mean DNA content of the left lung was 129 mg/kg body weight compared to 143 mg/kg in sham operated fetuses suggesting that tracheostomy causes only a small (approx 10%) reduction in overall growth of the lung.

Studies of laryngeal functions in fetal sheep led Harding (14) to propose that tracheal flow is normally retarded by a laryngeal mechanism during apnoea, giving rise to an elevated pressure within the trachea and probably resulting in increased pulmonary distension. They designed a flowmeter capable of measuring the very low flow rates normally present in the trachea and confirmed that the integrated flow rates were similar to the net rate of 4.5 ml/h/kg body weight previously reported by Mescher et al. (15). The flow rate during episodes of fetal breathing was 5–6 times that during apnoea. Denervation of the larynx caused a reduction both in mean overall flow and in the "flow ratio" i.e. the ratio of net flow during breathing to nonbreathing periods. This observation is consistent with the "flow ratio" being determined in the intact animal by accumulation of lung fluid in the lung when outflow resistance is high due to laryngeal adduction during apnoea and by escape of the accumulated fluid when laryngeal abduction occurs during fetal breathing. The alternative explanation that marked changes occur in the secretion rate of lung fluid from a high rate during breathing periods and a low rate during nonbreathing periods to a more constant rate must also be considered since Harding (14) found that preventing breathing movements by paralysing the fetus was associated with a greater than 50% reduction in overall tracheal flow in 4 out of 5 fetuses. However, it cannot be concluded that the change in flow is attributable solely to the absence of breathing movements since the mean overall flow is unaltered by bilateral phrenic nerve sections. Experiments designed to separate the possible effects of breathing movements and of laryngeal resistance on the "flow ratio" are needed to resolve these issues.

Phasic Determinants of Lung Volume

The absence or impairment of fetal breathing movements is associated with pulmonary hypoplasia suggesting that phasic forces contribute to lung growth.

Evidence supporting this hypothesis is both circumstantial and experimental. Congenital disorders of human fetal development that affect diaphragmatic activity are accompanied by gross pulmonary hypoplasia as are also a variety of experimental procedures in rabbit and sheep fetuses that deprive the diaphragm of connections with the central nervous system (see (5) for review). Increasing the compliance of the chest wall by partial removal of ribs to create flexible "windows" has similar effects to diaphragmatic denervation although breathing movements (presumably with less effect on transpulmonary pressure) continue (16).

Attempts to determine the mechanism by which phasic forces may stimulate lung growth have been based on the expectation that fetal breathing movements increase lung volume. Murai *et al.* (17) measured the volume of lung fluid that could be aspirated from the trachea of fetal sheep at 122–138 days of gestation during episodes of fetal breathing and between episodes. In each instance, the tracheal aspiration was performed at least 9 min after the onset of the breathing or nonbreathing episode. When measurements were made during episodes of breathing, the volume aspirated compared to that in nonbreathing episodes increased by 17.5% when the airways were intact and by 38.5% when the trachea was in continuity with an intra-amniotic bag containing lung fluid. The authors propose that lung volume increases during episodes of fetal breathing movements as a consequence of aspiration of fluid; aspiration from the pharynx may be limited by a small available volume or by laryngeal resistance whereas aspiration from a bag is less restricted. The increase in lung volume may be sufficient to stimulate growth of the lung.

Can Opposing Views on Tonic and Phasic Determinants of Lung Growth be Reconciled?

Harding (14) thinks that the lung "deflates" during fetal breathing because he found high flow rates in the trachea at that time and "inflates" during apnoea because flow rates are low and laryngeal resistance is high. In contrast, Murai *et al.* (17) think that the lung "inflates" rather than "deflates" during breathing episodes because the volume of lung fluid that can be aspirated during breathing is higher than when breathing movements are absent. A simultaneous increase in both efflux of lung fluid and lung volume can be explained only by a substantial rise in the rate of secretion of lung liquid. The evidence is against such a rise since Murai *et al.* (17) found that tracheal occlusion for 9 min caused no detectable increase in the volume of fluid that could be aspirated during breathing episodes. Further validation of the techniques used and different approaches to the measurements in question will be needed to gain a clear picture of what happens to lung volume during fetal breathing.

Perhaps the differing views do not matter very much if the wrong question is being asked. If, instead of the question "how is the lung recurrently distended to promote growth?" one asks "how is the lung maintained in the distended state required for the action of some unknown stimulus to growth?", the answers may be at hand. During apnoea, volume could be more or less maintained by laryngeal adductor activity and high outflow resistance; during episodes of breathing movements, volume could be more or less maintained by a fall in mean transpulmonary pressure without the need for sustained outflow resistance. As to the nature of the "unknown" stimulus to growth, it seems most likely to be related in some way to fetal breathing movements. Liggins (5) speculated that since each contraction of the diaphragm causes a change in the shape of the thoracic cavity and thus of the lung (18), fluid shifts of an oscillatory nature must occur in the lung. This suggestion implies that the time course of distending forces related to stimulation of growth should be measured in fractions of seconds rather than fractions of hours. Other physical stresses caused by deformation of the lung during a breathing movement also could have a role. If intrapulmonary fluid redistribution has any importance in promoting lung growth, trachestomy may not be an appropriate experimental preparation for its investigation since the airways could fill during episodes of breathing movements. A better preparation may be laryngeal denervation or laryngeal cannulation in which inflow but not outflow is restricted.

Hormones and Lung Maturation

Detailed descriptions of the morphogenesis of the terminal airway epithelium and the pulmonary vasculature are available (19). Morphological development of the human fetal lung in late gestation was described recently (20). The present discussion is concerned only with the part that hormones may play in the maturation of the fetal lung. The development of a stable, distensible lung depends in part on changes in the structure of walls of the airspaces which become increasingly numerous as septa form and increasingly thin-walled as the epithelium flattens and the mesenchyme thins; in part, maturation depends also on the synthesis, storage and secretion into the air-spaces of surfactant.

Structural Maturation

The role of glucocorticoids in accelerating structual changes in the fetal lung is now well recognized although usually given little emphasis compared to effects on surfactant synthesis. In the rhesus monkey, Beck and associates (21) and Bunton and Plopper (22) showed that maternal corticosteroid treatment caused pronounced changes in distensibility that were independent of surfactant secretion. Fetuses exposed to triamcinolone acetonide (22) during the mid-canicular stage at 110–112 days gestational age (corresponding to about 22 weeks in human fetuses) showed various morphological changes in the lungs when delivered at 150 days (term 168 days). The volume fraction of air space determined by morphometry after fixation by intratracheal infusion of glutaraldehyde at 30 cm H_2O exceeded that of term lungs. Septa were longer, thinner and less cellular, interstitial tissue was reduced and alveolar sacs were more developed than controls of 155 days of gestation.

Kauffman (23) found an increase in volume fraction of air space of dexamethasone-treated mice similar to that in rhesus monkeys. Maximal development of the changes was achieved with doses of corticosteroid that were too low to depress lung weight or fetal weight or to induce the formation of lamellar bodies.

Surfactant Synthesis and Secretion

The extensive experimental studies of the effects of hormones on surfactant synthesis in several species including nonhuman primates, sheep, rabbits, rats and mice have been reviewed by Hitchcock (24), Ballard (3) and Kitterman (4). In contrast, there is a paucity of studies of the temporal relationships between surfactant synthesis and plasma hormone concentrations or of the effects of endocrine ablation. In sheep, the concentration of saturated phosphatidylcholine (SPC), distensibility with air and morphological maturation correlate closely with rising prepartum plasma cortisol concentrations and less closely with gestational age (25). Plasma concentrations of T_3 (26) also rise sharply in the immediate prepartum period in this species when rapid maturation of the lung is occurring. The effects of fetal adrenalectomy on lung maturation have yet to be described. Reports on the effects of thyroidectomy in fetal sheep are conflicting; Erenberg and coworkers (27) found lower L/S ratios in tracheal fluid and retarded Type II cell differentiation whereas Bhakthavathsalan and associates (28) found no decrease in phospholipid/protein ratios in lung homogenates or phospholipid in tracheal fluid.

Studies of the pharmacological effects of hormones *in vivo* and *in vitro* have yielded evidence supporting roles in stimulating lung maturation for corticosteroid, corticotrophin (ACTH), thyroid hormones, thyrotrophin releasing hormone (TRH), oestradiol, prolactin, epidermal growth factor, fibroblast pneumocyte factor, β-adrenergic agonists and prostaglandins. Insulin and testosterone inhibit surfactant synthesis. Experiments *in vivo* in rodents can be difficult to interpret because of stress-related increases in corticosteroid concentrations when the route of administration is fetal (29) and because of possible mediation by unknown factors when the route is maternal. Nevertheless, the usefulness of the maternal route in rabbits is illustrated by the stimulation of alveolar surfactant concentrations by TRH (30), insulin (31), an anti-androgen, flutamide (32) or 3,5 dimethyl-3'-isopropyl-L-thyronine (DIMIT) (33).

Interactions of Hormones

Maturation of the fetal lung in late pregnancy normally occurs in a hormonal environmental in which the concentrations of a number of hormones are rising. In fetal sheep, for example, the prepartum period is characterized by marked increases in the circulating levels of cortisol, triiodothyronine, oestradiol-17β, catecholamines, prostaglandins and prolactin. Each of these hormones singly has been shown to have effects on lung maturation under certain experimental conditions, usually in the rabbit or rat. Thus, prepartum lung maturation normally may represent additive or synergistic effects of several hormones rather than a response limited to one hormone. Most of the work has related to thyroid hormones which are well known to interact with other hormones, especially gluco-corticoids, in a number of systems in maturing and adult tissues (see (24) for review).

Thyroid hormones

The interaction of glucocorticoids with T_4 in the development of the neonatal rat lung was investigated by Hitchcock (34) who determined the effects of T_4 given under conditions of low and high levels of endogenous corticosteroid. Adrenalectomy or inhibition of corticosteroid secretion by metyrapone impaired the response to T_4 and injections of hydrocortisone restored the response. Maximal acceleration of lung development was found when T_4 was given while corticosteroid levels were high as a result of surgical stress. A preliminary communication reports that the combined intra-amniotic injection of T_3 and dexamethasone in fetal rats at Day 17 eliminated the sex difference of choline incorporation into SPC in lung slices at Day 20 (35). The effect of dexamethasone on SPC synthesis in explants of fetal rat lung is enhanced by T_3 (36). The same effect was observed when the hormones were injected into pregnant rats on Days 18 and 19. On Day 20, incorporation of choline into phosphatidylcholine was enhanced by 33% with betamethasone alone, by 34% with T_3 alone and by 69% when the hormones were combined.

The relationship between plasma cortisol and L/S ratio in tracheal fluid of fetal lambs is lost after thyroidectomy suggesting a permissive role for T_3 and T_4 in the action of cortisol on surfactant synthesis (27).

An interaction of thyroid hormones with EGF in the lung is possible since interaction occurs in other tissues. For example, the concentration of EGF in neonatal mouse skin is increased by thyroid hormones (37). In explants of fetal rat lung, the incorporation of choline into PC was increased 35% by EGF, 47% by dexamethasone, 35% by T_3, 75% by EGF plus T_3 and 43% by EGF plus dexamethasone (38).

Prolactin

Incubation of human fetal lung explants in defined medium with cortisol, prolactin or insulin alone and in combination demonstrated that the response to cortisol on the rate of synthesis of phosphatidylcholine was enhanced when prolactin or prolactin plus insulin were present (39).

The possibility of an interaction between thyroid hormones and prolactin in promoting surfactant release was raised by Rooney and coworkers (30) who observed increased phosphatidylcholine in lavage fluid of fetal rabbit lungs after treatment of the does with thyrotrophin releasing hormone (TRH). The hormone crosses the placenta in monkeys (40) and stimulates the secretion of both thyroid hormones and prolactin. The response to TRH differs from that to corticosteroids in that surfactant secretion but not synthesis is affected.

Adrenaline

An interaction between β-adrenergic agonists and glucocorticoids occurs by way of the β-adrenergic receptor. Treatment of rabbits with betamethasone at

25 days of gestation increases the concentration of receptors in fetal lungs (37).

Cortisol treatment of hypophysectomized fetal lambs fails to reverse the retarded lung maturation consequent upon hypophysectomy yet ACTH treatment restores distensibility (41). This paradoxical result raises the possibility that the response to ACTH is mediated by more than one hormone (cortisol). A possible candidate is adrenaline secreted by the adrenal medulla in increased amounts due to enhanced methylation of noradrenaline. Activation of phenylethanolamine-N-methyl transferase by cortisol may depend on high intra-adrenal concentrations of cortisol which are achieved by stimulation with ACTH but not by infusion of cortisol in physiological doses.

Interaction of Cortisol with Other Hormones in Fetal Sheep

We have investigated possible interactions of various hormones with cortisol in 76 fetal sheep at gestational ages of 121–134 days (median 128 days) at delivery. The doses of hormones were similar to those shown by other workers (29,38,42) to have biological effects or to markedly elevate plasma concentrations. The hormones were infused intravenously for 84 hours. Blood samples were taken daily for blood gas determinations and twice daily for hormone analyses. The ewe and fetus were then killed simultaneously by overdoses of phenobarbitone and the fetuses were delivered by hysterotomy. Air pressure-volume curves were performed on the left lung as described previously (41). Preliminary results are shown in Table 1.

Table 1. Effect of cortisol, triiodothyronine (T$_3$), adrenaline, prolactin (PRL) and epidermal growth factor (EGF) singly or in combination on distensibility (V$_{40}$) of the ovine fetal lung. Mean ± SEM.

Experimental group No. Treatment	n	Gestation (days)[†] median (range)	V$_{40}$[‡] (ml/g)
Controls	6	127 (125–129)	0.46±0.11
1. Cortisol (1 mg/h)	7	128 (123–128)	0.97±0.12*
2. Adrenaline (30 μg/h)	6	128 (123–128)	0.44±0.01
3. T$_3$ (0.5 μg/h)	6	128 (127–128)	0.57±0.08
4. T$_3$ (25 μg/h)	6	125.5 (121–128)	0.45±0.07
5. EGF (1 μg/h)	4	127 (128–129)	0.58±0.07
6. Cortisol + adrenaline (30 μg/h)	6	127 (126–129)	1.19±0.03*
7. Cortisol + T$_3$ (0.5 μg/h)	6	128 (128–130)	1.00±0.12*
8. Cortisol + T$_3$ (25 μg/h)	8	128.5 (123–130)	1.20±0.18*
9. Cortisol + PRL (60 μg/h)	6	127 (121–129)	0.66±0.14
10. Cortisol + EGF (1 μg/h)	7	128 (126–129)	0.93±0.15*
11. Cortisol + T$_3$ (25 μg/h) + PRL (60 μg/h)	8	128 (126–129)	1.66±0.11**

[†]age at delivery
[‡]volume of air in left lung at inflation pressure of 40 cm H$_2$O
*$P<0.05$ compared to control
**$P<0.05$ compared to Experiments 1, 7, 8, 9

The gestational age range of 121–134 days was chosen because preliminary studies showed it to be the earliest at which consistent increases in distensibility of the lung could be achieved by infusing cortisol (1 mg/h) for 84 h ($V_{40} = 0.97 \pm 0.12$ ml/g wet weight vs 0.46 ± 0.11 in controls). The distensibility of the lungs of the cortisol-treated fetuses was considerably less than that of untreated fetuses near term (0.97 ± 0.12 ml/g wet weight vs approximately 2.0 ml/g near term) allowing scope for the recognition of synergistic or additive effects by other hormones. Cortisol but not T_3, adrenaline or EGF increased distensibility above control values when infused alone and neither T_3, adrenaline, EGF nor PRL enhanced the response to cortisol when infused together with cortisol (Table 1). But the combination of cortisol with both prolactin and T_3 (25 μg/h) caused a significant increase in distensibility. These results suggest synergism between cortisol, PRL and T_3. Since a combination of PRL and T_3 without cortisol was not tested, the possibility of the two hormones together having effects on the lung cannot be excluded.

The combination of cortisol, PRL and T_3 has not been studied previously to our knowledge. Prolactin enhances the response to cortisol of choline incorporation in explants of human fetal lung (39) and TRH (which stimulates secretion of both T_3 and prolactin) stimulates PC secretion but not synthesis in fetal rabbits (30). The latter study raises the possibility that PRL plus T_3 (or TRH) will stimulate surfactant secretion in sheep, an effect that might be apparent only late in gestation when stores of surfactant are high or when surfactant synthesis and storage is stimulated by cortisol. Assays of SPC in lung washes and tissues from our experimental preparations may help to resolve these issues.

Our results lend some support to Rooney and colleagues' speculation (30) that TRH may have a place in the prevention of respiratory distress syndrome in the human neonate. The very immature human fetus of 26–28 weeks (equivalent to the fetal lamb of 120–125 days) responds relatively poorly to antenatal corticosteroid treatment and it is at this gestational age that the place, if any, of TRH may lie. In term human pregnancies, TRH crosses the placenta and raises T_3 levels but not prolactin levels in cord blood (43). Failure to stimulate prolactin secretion may be a consequence of secretion being already maximal since we have found that maternally administered TRH raises the concentrations of both T_3 and prolactin in the cord blood of neonates of less than 31 weeks gestation (unpublished observations).

Acknowledgements

The work was supported by the Medical Research Council of New Zealand.

References

1. Gross, I. G., Smith, J., Maniscalco, W. M., Czalka, M. R., Wilson, C. M. and Rooney, S. A. (1978). *J. Appl. Physiol.* **45**, 355–362.
2. Gross, J. and Wilson, C. M. (1983). *J. Appl. Physiol.* **55**, 1725–1732.

3. Ballard, P. L. (1982). *In:* "Lung Development. Biological and Clinical Perspectives", Vol. II, (Farrell, P. M. ed.) pp. 205–253, Academic Press, London and Orlando.
4. Kitterman, J. A. (1984). *J. Develop. Physiol.* **6**, 67–82.
5. Liggins, G. C. (1984). *J. Develop. Physiol.* **6**, 237–248.
6. Maniscalco, W. M., Wilson, C. M., Gross, I., Gobran, L., Rooney, S. A. and Warshaw, J. B. (1978). *Biochim. Biophys. Acta* **530**, 333–346.
7. Alcorn, D., Adamson, T. M., Lambert, T. F., Maloney, J. E., Ritchie, B. C. and Robinson, P. M. (1977). *J. Anat.* **123**, 649–660.
8. Gluck, L., Chez, R. A., Kulovich, M. V., Hutchinson, D. L. and Niemann, W. H. (1974). *Am. J. Obstet. Gynecol.* **120**, 524–530.
9. Kerr, G. R., Kennan, A. L., Waisman, H. A. and Allen, J. R. (1969). *Growth* **33**, 201–211.
10. Liggins, G. C. and Kitterman, J. A. (1981). *In:* "The Fetus and Independent Life", (Elliott, K. and Whelan, J., eds) pp. 308–322. Ciba Symp. No. 86. Pitman, London.
11. Vilos, G. A. and Liggins, G. C. (1982). *J. Develop. Physiol.* **4**, 247–256.
12. Fewell, J. E. and Johnson, P. (1983). *J. Physiol.* **339**, 495–504.
13. Fewell, J. E., Hislop, Kitterman, J. A. and Johnson, P. (1983). *J. Appl. Physiol.* **55**, 1103–1108.
14. Harding, R. (1984). *J. Develop. Physiol.* **6**, 249–258.
15. Mescher, E. J., Platzker, A. C. G., Ballard, P. L., Kitterman, J. A., Clements, J. A. and Tooley, W. H. (1975). *J. Appl. Physiol.* **39**, 1017–1021.
16. Liggins, G. C., Vilos, G. A., Campos, G. A., Kitterman, J. A. and Lee, C. H. (1981). *J. Develop. Physiol.* **3**, 275–282.
17. Murai, D. T., Lee, C. T., Wallen, L. D. and Kitterman, J. A. (1984). *Pediat. Res.* **18**, 400A.
18. Poore, E. R. and Walker, D. R. (1980). *J. Physiol.* **301**, 307–315.
19. Meyrick, B. and Reid, L. M. (1977). *In:* "Lung Biology in Health and Disease. Development of the Lung", (Hodson, W. A., ed) pp. 135–214, Marcel Dekker, New York and Basel.
20. Langston, C., Kida, K., Read, M. and Thurlbeck, W. M. (1984). *Am. Rev. Resp. Dis.* **129**, 607–613.
21. Beck, J. C., Mitzner, W., Johnson, J. W. C., Hutchins, G. M., Foidart, J.-M., London, W. T., Palmer, A. E. and Scott, R. (1981). *Pediat. Res.* **15**, 235–240.
22. Bunton, T. E. and Plopper, C. G. (1984). *Am. J. Obstet. Gynecol.* **148**, 203–215.
23. Kauffman, S. (1977). *Lab. Invest.* **36**, 395–401.
24. Hitchcock, K. R. (1980). *Anat. Rec.* **198**, 13–34.
25. Kitterman, J. A., Liggins, G. C., Campos, G. A., Clements, J. A., Forster, C. S., Lee, C. H. and Creasy, R. K. (1981). *J. Appl. Physiol.* **51**, 384–390.
26. Fisher, D. A., Dussault, J. J., Sack, J. and Chopra, I. J. (1977). *Rec. Prog. Horm. Res.* **33**, 59–116.
27. Erenberg, A., Rhodes, M. L., Weinstein, M. M. and Kennedy, R. C. (1979). *Pediat. Res.* **13**, 230–235.
28. Bhakthavathsalan, A., Mann, L. I., Ayromlooi, J., Kunzel, W. and Liu, M. (1977). *Am. J. Obstet. Gynecol.* **127**, 278–284.
29. Ballard, P. L., Gluckman, P. D., Brehier, A., Kitterman, J. A., Kaplan, S. L., Rudolph, A. M. and Grumbach, M. M. (1978). *J. Clin. Invest.* **62**, 879–883.
30. Rooney, S. A., Marino, P. A., Gobran, L. I., Gross, I. and Warshaw, J. B. (1979). *Pediat. Res.* **13**, 623–625.
31. Hallman, M., Wermer, D., Epstein, B. L. and Gluck, L. (1982). *Am. J. Obstet. Gynecol.* **142**, 877–882.

32. Nielsen, H. C., Zinman, H. M. and Torday, J. S. (1982). *J. Clin. Invest.* **69**, 611–616.
33. Ballard, P. L., Benson, B. L., Brehier, A., Carter, J. P., Kriz, B. M. and Jorgensen, E. C. (1980). *J. Clin. Invest.* **65**, 1407–1417.
34. Hitchcock, K. (1979). *Anat. Rec.* **194**, 15–40.
35. Dow, K. and Torday, J. S. (1982). *Pediat. Res.* **16**, 348A.
36. Gross, I. and Wilson, C. M. (1982). *J. Appl. Physiol.* **52**, 1420–1425.
37. Cheng, J. B., Goldfien, A., Ballard, P. L. and Roberts, J. M. (1980). *Endocrinology*, **104**, 1053–1058.
38. Gross, I. and Dynia, D. W. (1984). *Pediat. Res.* **18**, 392A, Abst. 1779.
39. Mendelson, C. R., Johnson, J. M., MacDonald, P. C. and Snyder, J. M. (1981). *J. Clin. Endocrin. Metab.* **53**, 307–317.
40. Azukizawa, M., Murata, Y., Ikenoue, T., Martin, C. B. and Hershman, J. M. (1976). *J. Clin. Endocrin. Metab.* **43**, 1020–1025.
41. Liggins, G. C., Kitterman, J. A., Campos, G. A., Clements, J. A., Forster, C. S., Lee, C. H. and Creasy, R. K. (1981).
42. Lawson, E. F., Brown, E. R., Torday, J. S., Medansky, P. L. and Taeusch, H. W. (1978). *Am. Rev. Resp. Dis.* **118**, 1023–1026.
43. Roti, E., Gnudi, A., Braverman, L. E., Robuschi, G., Emanuele, R., Bandini, P., Benassi, L., Pagliani, A. and Emerson, C. H. (1981). *J. Clin. Endocrin. Metab.* **53**, 813–817.

Synthesis of Surfactant Lipids in the Developing Lung

L. M. G. Van Golde, J. J. Batenburg, M. Post,*
A. C. J. De Vries and B. T. Smith*

Laboratory of Veterinary Biochemistry, State University of Utrecht,
Utrecht, The Netherlands and
*Department of Pediatrics, Harvard Medical School, Boston, USA

Introduction

Pulmonary surfactant prevents alveolar collapse and transudation at low lung volumes by reducing the surface tension at the alveolar surfaces. The production of this lipid-rich material proceeds in the alveolar epithelial Type II cell, one of the approximately 40 different cell types in lung tissue. The bulk of surfactant components are synthesized in the endoplasmic reticulum of the Type II cell and thence transferred, via a still incompletely understood process, to the lamellar bodies. These organelles serve as stores of surfactant before it is secreted onto the alveolar surface, probably via an intermediate form called tubular myelin (1).

The major surface-active component of pulmonary surfactant is undoubtedly dipalmitoylphosphatidylcholine (dipalmitoyl-PC), which comprises almost 50% of total surfactant (2). The exact functions of the remaining components of this complex material such as unsaturated phosphatidylcholines (PC), phosphatidyl-glycerols (PG), phosphatidylethanolamines (PE), phosphatidylinositols (PI), cholesterol and small amounts of specific proteins, are still conjectural. However, physicochemical studies do indicate that the full spectrum of surfactant constituents probably enables surfactant to adsorb and spread rapidly at the alveolar surface (2).

In most mammalian species traces of intracellular (lamellar bodies) or extracellular surfactant are detectable during the immature or early transitional stages of the developing lung. However, there is abundant evidence that the production of surfactant in the fetal lung is set into gear during the transitional period. The surge of surfactant accumulation during this period accompanies

The Physiological Development of the Fetus and Newborn
ISBN 0 12 389080 2

Copyright © 1985 by Academic Press, London.
All rights of reproduction in any form reserved.

the ability of the neonate to establish regular air-breathing. Many observations support the view that surfactant deficiency is indeed a major factor responsible for the occurrence of respiratory distress syndrome in the premature newborn (3). It has been shown for a variety of mammalian species that considerable changes take place in the composition of the surfactant complex as the maturation of the fetal lung progresses (for excellent recent reviews see (4,5)). In the transitional period the percentages of PC and dipalmitoyl-PC increase with a concomitant decrease in the percentage of PE and, particularly, of sphingomyelin. This is reflected by a strong increase in the lecithin to sphingomyelin (L/S) ratio observed in amniotic fluid in this period. The acidic phospholipids of surfactant show a different developmental profile: it has been reported for several mammalian species that the percentage of PI in surfactant declines at term while at the same time the proportion of PG starts to increase (6,7). Interestingly, the appearance of PI in fetal surfactant is preceded by that of yet another acidic phospholipid, phosphatidylserine (7,8).

Intensive research efforts have concentrated on the biosynthesis of surfactant lipids in the developing lung and on the hormonal and metabolic regulation of these processes. Most of these studies have been carried out with preparations of whole fetal lung, such as slices, homogenates and subcellular fractions derived thereof. It is obvious that the results of such studies should be interpreted cautiously because they do not necessarily apply to the alveolar Type II cells, the producers of pulmonary surfactant. In the past few years techniques have become available to isolate Type II cells not only from adult lung (9) but also from fetal lung at different stages of development (10,11). Particularly interesting is the development of methods for isolating immature Type II cells and growing them in culture before inducing the production of lamellar bodies (12). Although studies with models at a higher level of cell and tissue organization will remain necessary, it is clear that isolated fetal Type II cells at various stages of maturation are an attractive model for studies on the biosynthesis of surfactant in the developing lung. After a general survey of the pathways involved in the formation of the major surfactant lipids, this paper will focus on the following questions: (a) which enzyme(s) regulate the *de novo* synthesis of PC in fetal Type II cells (b) which remodeling mechanism could be involved in the conversion of unsaturated PC into dipalmitoyl-PC, a process which is presumably quite active towards the end of gestation and (c) which mechanisms control the switch from PI to PG synthesis around term.

De novo Synthesis of Surfactant Phosphatidylcholines, Phosphatidylinositols and Phosphatidylglycerols in the Developing Lung

The following building stones are required for the synthesis of surfactant phospholipids: glycerol-3-phosphate (glycerol-3-P) or dihydroxyacetone-phosphate (DHAP) as the glycerol backbone, fatty acids, choline and *myo*-inositol. It has been suggested that glycogen may constitute an important source of substrate for surfactant production in the fetal lung. This suggestion is supported by the temporal relationship between the disappearance of glycogen from fetal lung epithelial cells and the onset of surfactant lipid synthesis during the terminal period of fetal lung development (4,5) and by the recent finding (13) that radioactivity from prelabelled endogenous glycogen in explants of fetal lung incorporated into disaturated PC and PG. Glycogen can provide the glycerol backbone for surfactant lipids and, in addition, serve as carbon and NADPH source for the *de novo* synthesis of the fatty acyl constituents of surfactant lipids, a process which is believed to be of vital importance for the rapidly growing and differentiating lung (14,15). Additional fatty acids as well as all of the choline can be provided to the fetal Type II cell by the circulation. The circulation can also supply *myo*-inositol but there is recent evidence that the fetal lung has the capability of synthesizing *myo*-inositol from glucose (16).

The *de novo* synthesis of phospholipids (17) starts with the formation of phosphatidic acid (PA) by step-wise acetylation of glycerol-3-P (Fig. 1). To the best of our knowledge there is no information on the substrate specificity of the enzymes catalysing these two reactions in the fetal Type II cell. However, studies with microsomes isolated from whole adult rat lung indicate that the lung has the potential to synthesize PA with a substantial proportion of dipalmitoyl-PA

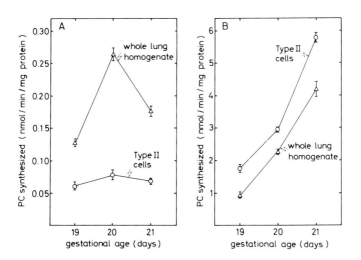

Figure 1. Specific activities of lysophosphatidylcholine: lysophosphatidylcholine acyltransferase (panel A) and lysophosphatidylcholine acyltransferase (panel B) in homogenates of fetal rat lung and in Type II cells isolated from fetal rat lung at different gestational ages. Lysophosphatidylcholine: lysophosphatidylcholine acyltransferase was measured in 50 μl medium containing 160 mmol phosphate buffer (pH 6.0), 0.4 mmol 1-[1-^{14}C]palmitoyl-lysoPC (spec.act. 5.10^3 dpm/nmol) and 30 μg protein. The incubation time was 10 min. Lysophosphatidylcholine acyltransferase was assayed in 50 μl medium of the following composition: 65 mmol Tris/HCl (pH 7.4), 10 mmol MgCl$_2$, 0.2 mmol 1-palmitoyl-lysoPC and 20 μmol [1-^{14}C]palmitoyl-CoA (spec.act. 10^5 dpm/nmol). The reaction was started by the addition of protein (20 μg) and terminated after 5 min.

(18). PA may also be synthesized by acylation of DHAP followed by reduction of the resulting acyl-DHAP to 1-acyl-glycerol-3-P. The relative importance of this acyl-DHAP pathway for the synthesis of PA in the fetal lung remains to be established. However, there is evidence from recent studies on liver that the prime function of the acyl-DHAP pathway lies in the formation of ether lipids (19).

The pathways leading to PC and those producing PG and PI diverge at the PA branchpoint. Phosphatidate cytidylyltransferase commits the utilization of PA to the formation of PG or PI. These acidic phospholipids share CDPdiacylglycerols as a common precursor (see also the section on regulation of PG and PI synthesis in the developing lung). En route to PC, PA is converted into diacylglycerols (DG) by phosphatidic acid phosphatase. Four different forms of this enzyme have been identified in whole fetal and adult lung: two cytosolic forms, one requiring aqueous dispersions of PA as substrate and the other depending on membrane-bound PA, and two membrane-associated forms, one utilizing aqueous dispersions of PA and the other membrane-bound PA as substrate (for reviews see (4,20)). It is likely that the enzyme(s) depending on membrane-bound PA is (are) involved in the formation of PC. The physiological significance of phosphatidic acid phosphatases requiring aqueous dispersions of PA is not clear. This point is important to emphasize because most studies on the activity of this enzyme during development of the fetal lung and on the effects of hormones on this enzyme have employed assays with aqueous dispersions of PA as substrate (for reviews see (4,5)).

The last step in the *de novo* synthesis of PC requires not only DG but also CDPcholine. The latter intermediate is formed by the sequential action of choline kinase, a cytosolic enzyme, and cholinephosphate cytidylyltransferase, an enzyme present both in the cytosol and in the endoplasmic reticulum. The membrane-bound enzyme is probably the active form of cholinephosphate cytidylyltransferase (see also section below). Both in fetal and in adult lung, the conversion of DG into PC proceeds probably entirely in the endoplasmic reticulum. There is evidence from studies on adult lung (21–23) that cholinephosphotransferase does not discriminate between disaturated and unsaturated DG as substrates. If this is also true for cholinephosphotransferase of fetal Type II cells, surfactant dipalmitoyl-PC could be synthesized in the fetal lung by direct synthesis *de novo*, provided that sufficient amounts of dipalmitoylglycerol are generated in the Type II cells.

Regulation of *de novo* Synthesis of PC in Fetal Type-II Cells

Studies with various labelled precursors have shown that the increase in PC content of surfactant at the end of gestation is correlated with enhanced rates of pulmonary PC synthesis (24,25). For example, in a number of mammalian species a strong increase in the rate of choline incorporation occurs at about 90% of term, which corresponds to the time of increased surfactant production (5). The biochemical basis of this enhanced PC synthesis remains to be determined. Numerous studies, conducted with a variety of mammalian species, have shown that pulmonary development is accompanied by a number of changes in the specific activities of the enzymes involved in the synthesis of PC (for reviews see (4,5,20)). Although some general conclusions can be drawn, these studies have not led to a clear unifying hypothesis explaining an overall mechanism by which the synthesis of surfactant PC (or that of other surfactant lipids) could be regulated. A major problem is that such studies have so far been carried out with preparations of whole fetal and neonatal lung. Hence, the results cannot be directly extrapolated to events occurring specifically in the fetal Type II cells during development. In addition, the enzyme activities are generally measured under conditions which are optimal *in vitro*. In the cells *in vivo*, the actual conditions may be different. Moreover, different conditions may exist in the various subcellular compartments.

Post *et al.* (26) carried out pulse-label experiments with Type II cells isolated from fetal rat lung using [*Me*-³H]choline as radioactive precursor. The choline taken up by the cells was rapidly converted to cholinephosphate. At all times investigated, most of the water-soluble radioactivity was associated with cholinephosphate whereas less than 5% was in the form of CDPcholine. After 3 h of incubation, the labelling of choline, cholinephosphate and CDPcholine appeared to be constant whereas the entry of label into PC increased for at least 5 h. These observations suggested, in agreement with earlier studies with adult Type II cells (27) that the cholinephosphate pool in the Type II cell is much larger than the choline and CDPcholine pools, supporting the concept that cholinephosphate cytidyltransferase catalyses a rate-limiting reaction in the CDPcholine pathway. Chemical measurement of the pool sizes of choline and its intermediates shows (Table 1) that the cholinephosphate pool in whole fetal lung and in fetal Type II cells is indeed much larger than the choline and CDPcholine pools. The levels of the intermediates in the whole fetal lung are comparable to those reported earlier (28). Interestingly, the Type II cells are highly enriched in intracellular choline and its intermediates, most notably in cholinephosphate. That the rate-limiting step in the formation of PC from choline in the fetal Type II cell is indeed catalysed by cholinephosphate cytidylyl-transferase is also supported by pulse-chase experiments with labelled choline. The radioactivity remaining as free choline decreased rapidly during the chase period

Table 1. Pool sizes of choline and its metabolites in fetal rat lung and in Type II cells isolated from fetal rat lung

Type II cells were isolated from fetal rat lung at 19 days gestation as described earlier (11,26). Values of the pool sizes represent means ± SEM for the number of experiments indicated in parentheses. For further details see (26).

	Fetal lung	Type II cells
	(pmol/µg DNA)	
Choline	14.1 ± 2.5 (4)	130.3 ± 9.2 (3)
Cholinephosphate	110.5 ± 18.4 (4)	1989.8 ± 298.5 (3)
CDPcholine	5.5 ± 1.2 (4)	57.3 ± 12.0 (3)
Phosphatidylcholine	735 ± 70 (4)	937 ± 124 (3)

whereas the radioactivity lost from choline-phosphate during the chase appeared in PC without any significant change in the radioactivity of CDPcholine (26).

Several other approaches support the concept that cholinephosphate cytidylyltransferase plays an important role in the regulation of PC synthesis in the fetal Type II cell. A number of studies have indicated this enzyme to be an important target in the hormonal regulation of surfactant PC synthesis in the fetal lung (for reviews see (4,5)). Furthermore, it has been shown that acidic phospholipids, such as PS, PI and PG (29) and fatty acids (30) activate cytosolic cholinephosphate cytidylyltransferase in the fetal lung. It was suggested that this activation was accomplished by conversion of the enzyme from a low molecular into a high molecular weight form. However, recent studies (31) provided strong evidence that the microsomal, rather than the cytosolic, cytidylyltransferase regulates the rate of PC synthesis. The intriguing hypothesis was proposed that reversible translocation between cytosol and endoplasmic reticulum may be the major determinant of the activity of cholinephosphate cytidylyltransferase (31). In this respect, it may be important to point out that most studies on the effects of hormones on the activity of this enzyme in the fetal lung have been focussed on only the cytosolic form of the enzyme (4,5).

Synthesis of Dipalmitoyl-PC in the Fetal Lung by Remodeling of Unsaturated PC

Studies with whole lung and with isolated Type II cells have provided evidence that dipalmitoyl-PC is produced not only by direct synthesis *de novo* but also by remodeling of PC species containing palmitate at position 1 and an unsaturated fatty acid at position 2. At least two mechanisms have been proposed for this remodeling (for review see (32)): (a) a deacylation-reacylation cycle involving cleavage of the unsaturated fatty acid by phospholipase A_2 followed by reacylation of the resultant 1-palmitoyl-lysoPC with palmitoyl-CoA by lysoPC acyltransferase and (b) a deacylation-transacylation process in which one 1-palmitoyl-lysoPC produced by phospholipase A_2 donates its palmitate moiety to a second 1-palmitoyl-lysoPC to yield dipalmitoyl-PC and glycero-3-phosphocholine. This transacylation reaction is catalysed by lysoPC: lysoPC acyltransferase.

Convincing evidence has been provided that the conversion of 1-palmitoyl-lysoPC into dipalmitoyl-PC proceeds in the mature Type II cell by reacylation (mechanism (a)) rather than by transacylation (mechanism (b)) (32,33). However, it has been reported that the activity of lysoPC: lysoPC acyltransferase increases strongly just before term in the developing mouse (34) and rat (35) lung. These observations suggested that the transacylation process might be an important remodeling mechanism in the prenatal lung. However, these studies (34,35) had been carried out with whole fetal lung preparations. Therefore, it was deemed of interest to compare the activities of lysoPC acyltransferase and lysoPC: lysoPC acyltransferase in Type II cells isolated from fetal rat lung at different gestational ages. The results are shown in Fig. 1. The specific activity of lysoPC acyltransferase in fetal Type II cells and in whole fetal lung homogenate increases with gestational age. At all ages examined the activity of this enzyme appears to be enriched in Type II cells when compared to whole lung. The activity of lysoPC acyltransferase in Type II cells is at least an order of magnitude higher than that of lysoPC: lysoPC acyltransferase. Furthermore, the activity of the latter enzyme is much lower in Type II cells than in whole lung homogenates and the activity of the Type II cell enzyme does not increase with gestational age. These observations, which are similar to those reported earlier for adult Type II cells (33), strongly suggest that a deacylation-transacylation process does not play an important role in the synthesis of dipalmitoyl-PC in the fetal Type II cell. The deacylation-reacylation cycle appears to be a more likely candidate as remodeling mechanism, although its relative importance in the formation of dipalmitoyl-PC in the fetal lung remains unknown.

Regulation of Phosphatidylglycerol and Phosphatidylinositol Synthesis

As described above, PG starts to appear in surfactant around term with a concomitant decrease in the proportion of PI. Studies with whole fetal lung (36) and with Type II cells from adult lung (37,38) have shown that the availability of myo-inositol is an important factor which modulates the distribution of the common precursor CDPdiacylglycerols between PI and PG synthesis. The decrease in serum inositol at the end of gestation is probably at least partially responsible for the switch-over from PI to PG formation. In addition, it has been shown (7) that the activity of microsomal glycerol-phosphate phosphatidyl-transferase increases during perinatal development of the rabbit lung. This may also contribute to the increased PG content of surfactant around term. Recently, we could demonstrate that a competition between PG and PI synthesis for the common substrate CDPdiacylglycerol also takes place in isolated fetal Type II cells. Histotypic cultures of fetal Type II cells were incubated with radioactive glycerol in the presence and absence of myo-inositol. Figure 2 shows the incorporation of glycerol into PI and PG of the surfactant fraction isolated from the cultures as described by Engle et al. (39). Whereas the incorporation of glycerol into PC is not significantly affected by the addition of inositol, a significant reduction of PG formation can be observed with a concomitant increase in the formation of PI. Evidence was obtained (J. J. Batenburg et al. in prep.) that the competition between PG and PI formation proceeds in the endoplasmic reticulum of the fetal Type II cells.

An alternative or additional explanation for the reciprocal relationship between PG and PI in surfactant was proposed by Bleasdale and colleagues (40,41). According to their hypothesis the increased PC synthesis in late gestation leads to an enhanced level of CMP. This CMP may slow down the PI synthesis and thus increase the availability of CDPdiacylglycerol for PG synthesis. In an attempt to provide evidence for this hypothesis (37), Type II cells isolated from adult rat lung were incubated in the presence of choline which led to increased synthesis of PC from labelled glucose. This was, indeed, accompanied by an increased formation of PG. However, there was also an increased rather than decreased

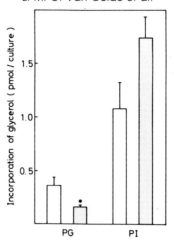

Figure 2. The incorporation of glycerol into surfactant PG and PI by fetal rat lung Type II cells. Ten histotypic cultures (DNA content 54 μg/culture) on Gelfoam pads (10) were incubated for 3 h in 15 ml medium of the following composition: 125 mmol NaCl, 5 mmol KCl, 2.5 mmol Na$_2$HPO$_4$, 2.5 mmol CaCl$_2$, 1.2 mmol MgCl$_2$, 17 mmol Hepes and 50 μg/ml gentamycin supplemented with 0.2 mmol palmitate (complexed to bovine serum albumin), 0.2 mmol choline, 0.25 mmol [1(3)-^{3}H]glycerol (spec. act. 2.10^5 dpm/nmol) and, if added, 5 mmol *myo*-inositol. After the incubations, the cultures were homogenized and the surfactant fraction isolated from the Type II cells as described in (39). Open bars: without inositol; dotted bars: with inositol; ✳: significantly different from control (0.025 < P < 0.05).

synthesis of PI. These observations do not support a CMP-mediated decrease of PI synthesis as a mechanism to explain the reciprocal relationship between PI and PG synthesis, although it should be emphasized that these experiments have been carried out with Type II cells isolated from adult lung (37).

The importance of the sequential appearance of the acid phospholipids PS, PI and PG in surfactant is unknown. It has been speculated (8) that this sequence may be critical for normal lung development, possibly because these three lipids may sequentially activate cholinephosphate cytidylyltransferase and in that way regulate the synthesis of the major surfactant lipid, dipalmitoyl-PC.

Acknowledgements

These investigations were supported by the Nederlands Foundation for Chemical Research (SON) with financial aid from the Netherlands Organization for the Advancement of Pure Research (ZWO) and by the United States National Institutes of Health (HL-27372, Specialized Center of Research in Pediatric Lung Disease).

References

1. Goerke, J. (1974). *Biochim. Biophys. Acta* **344**, 241–261.
2. King, R. J. (1982). *J. Appl. Physiol.* **53**, 1–8.

3. Farrell, P. M. and Avery, M. E. (1975). *Am. Rev. Resp. Dis.* **111**, 657–688.
4. Possmayer, F. (1984). *In:* "Pulmonary Surfactant", (Robertson, B., Van Golde, L. M. G. and Batenburg, J. J., eds) Elsevier Biomedical Press, Amsterdam, (in press).
5. Rooney, S. A. (1983). *In:* "The Biological Basis of Reproductive and Developmental Medicine" (Warshaw, J. B., ed.) pp. 239–287, Elsevier Biomedical, New York, Amsterdam and Oxford.
6. Hallman, M., Feldman, B. H., Kirkpatrick, E. and Gluck, L. (1977). *Pediat. Res.* **11**, 714–720.
7. Hallman, M. and Gluck, L. (1980). *Pediat. Res.* **14**, 1250–1259.
8. Benson, B. J., Kitterman, J. A., Clements, J. A., Mescher, E. J. and Tooley, W. H. (1983). *Biochim. Biophys. Acta* **753**, 83–88.
9. Mason, R. J. (1982). *In:* "Lung Development: Biological and Clinical Perspectives", (Farrell, P. M., ed.) Vol. 1, pp. 135–150, Academic Press, New York and London.
10. Douglas, W. H. J. and Teel, R. W. (1976). *Am. Rev. Resp. Dis.* **113**, 17–23.
11. Post, M., Torday, J. S. and Smith, B. T. (1984). *Exp. Lung Res.* (in press).
12. Scott, J. E., Possmayer, F. and Harding, P. G. R. (1983). *Biochim. Biophys. Acta* **753**, 195–204.
13. Bourbon, J. R., Rieutort, M., Engle, M. J. and Farrell, P. M. (1982). *Biochim. Biophys. Acta* **712**, 382–389.
14. Maniscalco, W. M., Finkelstein, J. N. and Parkhurst, A. B. (1982). *Biochim. Biophys. Acta* **711**, 49–58.
15. Freese, W. B. and Hallman, M. (1983). *Biochim. Biophys. Acta* **750**, 47–59.
16. Bleasdale, J. E., Maberry, M. C. and Quirk, J. G. (1982). *Biochem. J.* **206**, 43–52.
17. Kennedy, E. P. (1961). *Fed. Proc.* **20**, 934–940.
18. Yamada, K. and Okuyama, H. (1979). *Arch. Biochem. Biophys.* **196**, 209–219.
19. Declercq, P. E., Haagsman, H. P., Van Veldhoven, P., Debeer, L. J., Van Golde, L. M. G. and Mannaerts, G. P. (1984). *J. Biol. Chem.* (in press).
20. Possmayer, F. (1982). *In:* "Biomedical Development of the Fetus and Neonate", (Jones, C. T., ed.) pp. 337–391, Elsevier Biomedical Press, Amsterdam.
21. Ide, H. and Weinhold, P. A. (1982). *J. Biol. Chem.* **257**, 14926–14931.
22. Van Heusden, G. P. H. and Van den Bosch, H. (1982). *Biochim. Biophys. Acta* **711**, 361–368.
23. Post, M., Schuurmans, E. A. J. M., Batenburg, J. J. and Van Golde, L. M. G. (1983). *Biochim. Biophys. Acta* **750**, 68–77.
24. Epstein, M. F. and Farrell, P. M. (1975). *Pediat. Res.* **9**, 658–665.
25. Maniscalco, W. M., Wilson, C. M., Gross, I., Gobran, L., Rooney, S. A. and Warshaw, J. B. (1978). *Biochim. Biophys. Acta* **530**, 333–346.
26. Post, M., Batenburg, J. J., Van Golde, L. M. G. and Smith, B. T. (submitted).
27. Post, M., Batenburg, J. J., Schuurmans, E. A. J. M. and Van Golde, L. M. G. (1982). *Biochim. Biophys. Acta* **712**, 390–394.
28. Tokmakjian, S. and Possmayer, F. (1981). *Biochim. Biophys. Acta* **666**, 176–180.
29. Feldman, D. A., Dietrich, J. W. and Weinhold, P. A. (1980). *Biochim. Biophys. Acta* **620**, 603–611.
30. Feldman, D. A., Brubaker, P. G. and Weinhold, P. A. (1981). *Biochim. Biophys. Acta* **665**, 53–59.
31. Vance, D. E. and Pelech, S. L. (1984). *Trends Biochem. Sci.* **9**, 17–20.
32. Batenburg, J. J. and Van Golde, L. M. G. (1979). *In:* "Reviews in Perinatal Medicine" (Scarpelli, E. M. and Cosmi, E. V., eds) Vol. 3, pp. 73–114, Raven Press, New York.
33. Batenburg, J. J., Longmore, W. J., Klazinga, W. and Van Golde, L. M. G. (1979). *Biochim. Biophys. Acta* **573**, 136–144.

34. Oldenborg, V. and Van Golde, L. M. G. (1976). *Biochim. Biophys. Acta* **441**, 433–442.
35. Okano, G. and Akino, T. (1978). *Biochim. Biophys. Acta* **528**, 373–384.
36. Hallman, M. and Epstein, B. L. (1980). *Biochem. Biophys. Res. Commun.* **92**, 1151–1159.
37. Batenburg, J. J., Klazinga, W. and Van Golde, L. M. G. (1982). *FEBS Lett.* **147**, 71–74.
38. Bleasdale, J. E., Tyler, N. E., Busch, F. N. and Quirk, J. G. (1983). *Biochem. J.* **212**, 811–818.
39. Engle, M. J., Sanders, R. L. and Douglas, W. H. J. (1980). *Biochim. Biophys. Acta* **617**, 225–336.
40. Bleasdale, J. E. and Johnston, J. M. (1982). *In:* "Lung Development: Biological and Clinical Perspectives", (Farrell, P. M., ed.) Vol. 1, pp. 259–294, Academic Press, New York and London.
41. Bleasdale, J. E., Wallis, P., MacDonald, P. C. and Johnston, J. M. (1979). *Biochim. Biophys. Acta* **575**, 135–147.

The Development of Breathing

P. Johnson

Nuffield Department of Obstetrics,
University of Oxford, Oxford, UK

Introduction

The notion that the respiratory system is primarily chemically controlled with other factors such as metabolism, thermoregulation and airway mechanosensory reflexes acting as modulators seems well established. This account questions the validity of that assumption, during development at least, and considers new evidence from fetal and postnatal animal and human studies. Considered in conjunction with earlier well-documented experimental and clinical evidence against a chemical primacy the implications have both fundamental and clinical importance. Convincing clinical studies have clearly described the immense importance of mechanosensory reflexes in the establishment of effective lung volume (1) and breathing in the immediate postnatal period. The active expiratory component was well-described, both in the healthy term baby and particularly in the preterm infant grunting with the respiratory distress syndrome (2), although its significance in normal respiratory control mechanisms was not fully appreciated. Nonetheless it was clearly shown that effective gas exchange depended on the expiratory grunt which was enhanced by hypoxaemia. Glottic constriction in response to hypoxia, as opposed to the dilation observed in deeply anaesthetized animals (3) has only recently been recognized (4).

Despite the clear recognition a few years ago that breathing activity, albeit intermittent, was a normal feature of fetal life (5), the activation of chemoreceptors at, or shortly after, birth has still been presumed in the onset of independent respiration after birth. Fetal breathing in the healthy fetus was only partially stimulated by carbon dioxide and was promptly inhibited by hypoxaemia. The time spent in high voltage electrocortical slow wave sleep (SWS) increased by hypoxia. In the fetal lamb, which is relatively precocial, it is now evident from a number of studies that breathing activity becomes inhibited as SWS develops (6). Further support for the notion of an active inhibition of breathing in SWS

The Physiological Development of the Fetus and Newborn
ISBN 0 12 389080 2

Copyright © 1985 by Academic Press, London.
All rights of reproduction in any form reserved.

has come from experiments in which prostaglandin synthetase inhibitors infused into the fetus caused rhythmic breathing to occur during the high voltage state (7), thus effectively causing fetal breathing to be continuous. This occurred despite the denervation of peripheral chemoreceptors. Selective midbrain sections and lesions have shown that breathing activity can, firstly be divorced from its association with high and low voltage electrocortical state, and secondly, with a low midbrain section, be stimulated by hypoxia rather than inhibited (8). In tracheostomized lambs it was found that carotid body denervation or dopamine infusion caused a fall in breathing frequency by lengthening of expiratory time in the second week of life but not in the immediate newborn period (9). This suggestion that carotid body function is of greater importance in the older lamb is supported by the observation that 4 of 7 carotid body denervated lambs died "unexpectedly" at 4–6 weeks of postnatal age (10). Recently it has been shown that the arterial chemoreceptors in the newborn lamb at birth were silenced when the arterial oxygen tension rose abruptly with the onset of air breathing and remained so for a day or so before "resetting" to adult oxygen values had occurred (11). So what is the stimulus that sustains breathing in the newborn period?

It had been known for some time that the fetus breathed vigorously when exposed to a cold environment (12) and that brisk airway reflexes were readily elicited in the neonatal period. A very convincing demonstration of this association was seen in studies in which the exterior of the fetus was cooled *in utero* when it was observed that fetal breathing became vigorous and occurred in the high voltage electrocortical state (13), thus again apparently "releasing" the inhibition of breathing associated with this behavioural state. Nonetheless this breathing activity was still inhibited by hypoxaemia. Thus sleep state, or factors associated with it, and temperature control appeared the most powerful factors influencing normal fetal breathing.

Fetal breathing is obstructed breathing with inspiratory abductor activity of the larynx failing to prevent adduction of the cords in inspiration (14). It has been suggested that the alar nasae and genioglossus muscles lack a respiratory rhythmicity during fetal breathing. However the newborn must have effective dilation of the upper airway muscles and this has to occur in advance of diaphragmatic inspiration for breathing to be effective ie for upper airway obstruction not to occur. The fact that this co-ordination depends on sensory stimuli from air flow through the upper airway was clearly shown when obstructive apnea leading to asphyxial death occurred in newborn rabbits in which the upper airways had been anaesthetized (15).

In earlier studies in which chronically monitored telemetred lambs reared with their ewes had been observed for sleep state, breathing frequency and heart rate, from 1 until 32 days of age it had been noted that both breathing frequency and heart rate rose after birth before declining between the second and third week of postnatal life (6). It has been tacitly assumed that the higher respiratory rates of the newborn are due to the high metabolic demands of the neonatal period. However, the rise in the heart rate, not commented on in earlier studies, has now been well described in a number of species. In 1959 Dawes and Mott described the remarkable 3-fold increase in oxygen consumption that occurred in the first 24 hours of life in anaesthetized newborn lambs (16). It was clearly shown that the rise in minimal oxygen consumption had a time course of many hours and equally the decline in oxygen consumption to fetal and adult values took place over many weeks. Examination of the time course of the rise and fall in the heart rate and respiratory frequencies in our chronically monitored lambs and recently in a group of unanaesthetized lambs in which heart rate, cardiac output, oxygen consumption, amongst other variables were measured serially (17) during postnatal life indicated that these changes approximated very closely with the changes in minimal oxygen consumption already described. In a large study of free-ranging lambs over the first 36 h of life the progressive rise in minimal oxygen consumption was also clearly confirmed, however these studies included observations on breathing frequencies as well (18). They showed the marked increase in breathing frequency that occurred during the first 36 h of postnatal life as minimal oxygen consumption rose while thermal efficiency, as judged by a marked fall in the lower critical temperature, was increasing. Notably, breathing frequencies were lower when the lambs were below the lower critical temperature suggesting that increased metabolic demands were probably met by an increase in tidal volume and a reduction in frequency. Joining these sets of observations with our own, in which oxygen consumption was not measured, and those in which oxygen consumption, cardiac output and heart rate were (17), but minute ventilation and breathing frequency were not, it is not difficult to speculate at the close relationship between metabolic demands and breathing frequency.

In our earlier studies, we had noted that as the breathing frequency fell during SWS in the second, third and fourth weeks of postnatal life, so the appearance of prominent laryngeal expiratory constrictor activity appeared. The fall in frequency was almost entirely accounted for by an increased expiratory time and in many instances anything from 60–100% of breaths in SWS were associated with marked expiratory glottic constriction (19). Breathing frequency in rapid eye movement (REM) sleep at this stage was significantly higher than that observed in SWS whereas, remarkably perhaps, in the first 10 days of life breathing frequencies were higher in SWS than in REM sleep. At a month of age a tracheal window was implanted under halothane anaesthesia. When this "window" was subsequently opened during SWS there was a marked drop in breathing frequency, often an arrhythmia, with prolonged and enhanced laryngeal constrictor activity. This only occurred during SWS and was entirely consistent with the absence of this phasic laryngeal expiratory activity, as with the loss of intercostal muscle activity, that occurs during REM sleep. A specific study conducted into the significance of the role of the larynx during SWS in lambs of this age showed that the ventilatory response to hypoxia, after the acute arousal response was not sustained if the tracheal window was open (4). It was evident that laryngeal constrictor activity was enhanced by hypoxaemia. Applying positive expiratory pressure, reconnecting the upper airway, stimulating to arousal, adding carbon dioxide, and sometimes pulsing air through the redundant upper airway would restore effective breathing. Although we had defined an age between 2 and 6 weeks in which respiratory failure could be readily induced by hypoxaemia, the variability both within an animal and between animals was considerable suggesting

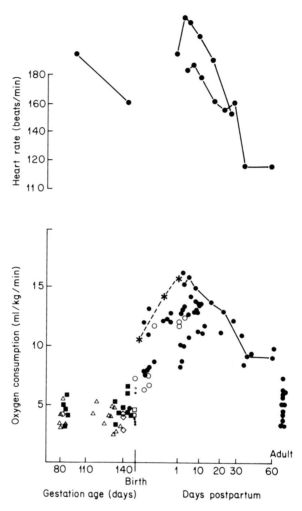

Figure 1. This is a composite illustration with data from several studies replotted on the same axes. *Oxygen consumption.* The isolated points are those of Dawes (16). The broken line those of Mercer (18). The solid line those of Lister (17). *Heart rate.* Fetal data from Johnson (6). Postnatal upper solid line — Johnson (6). Lower solid line — Lister (17): Note the postnatal rise and fall in heart rate related to oxygen consumption.

that other factors modulated the response. It was evident that the vagally mediated "braking" mechanism, elegantly demonstrated in unanaesthetized cats (20) as a response to opening a tracheal window, was in fact an essential component of spontaneous breathing in the intact postneonatal lamb, especially during SWS when breathing frequencies were lowest. It was evident that rhythmogenesis and sometimes effective breathing was apparently entirely dependent on the presence of this mechanism. Older lambs demonstrated the same mechanism and a qualitatively similar response, although the marked arrhythmia, lung collapse and asphyxia did not occur. We reasoned then that either chemical control was still developing during this period or that lung volume was not so readily compromised in the older lambs with a more rigid thoracic cage.

It was decided to study in closer detail the developmental changes in these mechanisms after birth. Thus a group of lambs (chronically instrumented under fluothane anaesthesia after separation from their ewes and establishment on an ad-lib artificial milk regime) were then studied serially. The intention of these studies, dealt with in detail in a separate paper in this volume (Andrews *et al.* p. 258) was to determine the influence of ambient temperature, first on the high breathing frequencies after birth, and secondly on the lower breathing rate observed in later postnatal life. Two findings stand out. The first was that the initial breathing frequencies in the first 12 days of life in the artificially reared lambs were markedly lower than those observed in the ewe-reared lambs. Although studied in the same ambient temperature (Ta) range we were able to see from closed circuit video that the younger lamb, raised with its ewe, slept against the maternal flank which is known to be a potent heat source. We are unable to say whether the marked difference in breathing frequencies were due to this factor or some other factor related to natural feeding. Breathing frequencies fell significantly with age and were then influenced by an ambient temperature range considered to be within the thermoneutral range for this species. Thus we were able to influence breathing frequency in the very age group in which we had demonstrated a specific vulnerability to breathing irregularity and respiratory failure when the regulation of the upper airway had been removed. Since we had observed shivering in lambs at 3 and 6 days of age at 10°C Ta, it seemed reasonable to conclude that these animals were subject to a cold stimulus to breathing and that any Ta between this and 30°C when breathing frequencies were noted to abruptly increase, represented a cold stimulus to thermogenic metabolism and with it breathing. Only at 12 days of age was it observed that breathing frequency was influenced by Ta such that comparatively low breathing frequencies were observed at Ta's within the thermoneutral range.

Thus we had an explanation for the possible variability in the degree of dysrhythmia that followed the bypassing of the upper airway in lambs aged between 2 and 6 weeks. In a number of these animals it had been noted that the fall in breathing frequency and irregularity was sufficient to lead to hypoxaemia and hypercapnia, clearly demonstrating that the chemical drive to breathing was insufficient to restore effective breathing. Either a cold stimulus or a hot stimulus were adequate breathing and restore effective gas exchange. Our previous results had suggested that lambs older than about 50 days of age were relatively immune from this form of failure although the dysrhythmia was still apparent. This finding accords with the report that carotid denervated fetal lambs will establish effective breathing after birth (21) and that they, as well as lambs carotid denervated in the neonatal period, while having a measurably lower oxygen tension and higher CO_2 tension than normals, gradually improve these variables over the first weeks of life. However, 4 of 7 chemodenervated animals were found unexpectedly dead at about 40 days of age (10). This finding if substantiated might be interpreted

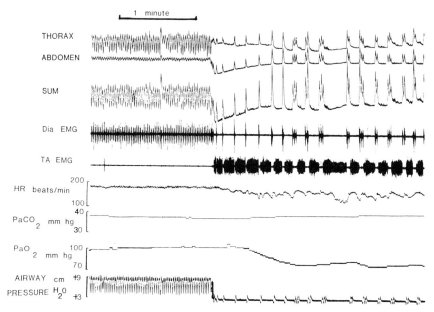

Figure 2. This record shows the effect of abruptly reducing expiratory pressure applied to a tracheostomy tube in a 41-day-old lamb in SWS. Instant "primary" respiratory and "secondary" cardiac arrhythmia occurred. Marked expiratory laryngeal (thyroarytenoid) constrictor activity, a fall in PaO_2 and a rise in $PaCO_2$ occurred which did not stimulate the return of effective breathing.

as indicating that chemoregulation of breathing becomes particularly important at this age when the metabolic and thermal stimuli to respiration decrease.

It is concluded that, in the development of control of breathing after birth, there are at least three phases during which different factors are prominent in sustaining rhythmic and effective breathing. First a major metabolic demand, largely to achieve effective thermoregulation, with feeding and ingestion playing a part, followed by a period when mechanosensory pathways are prominent as thermal efficiency improves and ambient thermal factors assume an importance before the chemical regulation of breathing achieves primacy. It should be appreciated that even in this final phase there are other factors which play a role in the maintenance of effective lung volume such as the increasing elastic recoil as the chest walls develops rigidity. It follows from this proposal that deficiencies in any of these three (or four) factors will only become apparent as the relevant developmental periods are reached. For example a depression of metabolism such as with starvation (18) or hypothyroidism, will decrease the metabolic demands and increase dependence on mechanosensory reflexes for sustaining breathing before the chemical drive is adequately developed. Thus although the regulation of breathing is clearly multifactorial, there is a changing hierarchy of these factors with increasing postnatal age. The fact that these effects were prominent during SWS suggest that, as in fetal life, SWS, or an associated factor, can operate as

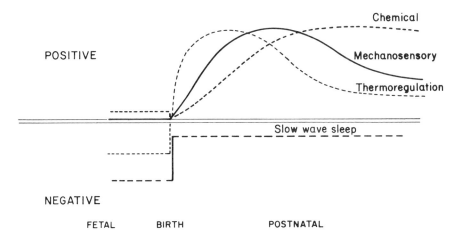

Figure 3. Schematic of the major factors in the perinatal regulation of breathing. *In utero* vagal mechanosensory information has little effect on breathing; chemoreceptor activity has at best an intermittent functional effect; temperature and SWS have substantial inhibitory effects. After birth thermal effects rapidly provide a stimulus which is a major factor for several weeks; chemoreceptor activity is normally silenced initially and probably takes many weeks to mature; in the meantime vagal mechanosensory reflexes are important for maintenance of lung volume and rhythmic breathing as the metabolic demands decline with increased thermal efficiency.

a potential inhibition to breathing if an adequate afferent sensory input is not sustained.

Another demonstration of the well organized powerful mechanisms that conserve metabolic demands in the perinatal period was seen in studies where newborn rabbits were allowed to select their optimal ambient temperature (Ta). These rabbits quickly found the Ta which equated with minimal oxygen consumption and this "self-selected" Ta fell with increasing postnatal age in direct relation to their increasing thermal efficiency (D. Hull, unpublished work).

Recent evidence in the human infant suggests that similar factors may operate. Firstly it has been observed that infants studied in SWS at 27°C Ta have breathing frequencies of 33 ± 5 1SD and 32 ± 7 1SD SWS at 1 and 4 weeks of age (22) when lying in an open cot, but 41 ± 4 1SD and 38 ± 5 1SD at 1 and 4 weeks when heavily swaddled (23) at the same Ta. Frequencies in excess of 60/min occurred at 33°C Ta (24). Breathing frequencies were still noted to fall with increasing postnatal age. It was noteworthy in the last study that frequencies, as in our naturally reared lambs in the laboratory, were higher in SWS than in REM sleep, which is the converse to that found in infants at an ambient temperature of 27°C. Again the influence of SWS on temperature regulation is suggested whereas in REM sleep poikilothermic regulation occurs. In this context it is noteworthy that REM sleep defined a much narrower thermoneutral range than did minimal metabolic rate in rats where the incidence of REM sleep at 29°C was twice that observed at 23°C (25). On the other hand the incidence of periodic breathing has been found to be highest at 1–2 months postterm by a number of investigators (22,23) studying infants serially between 1 week and 6 months of age. This pattern of breathing, once considered to be a feature of the premature infant, would suggest that there is a marked change in the regulation of rhythmic breathing at that age. It has been shown that this periodic breathing usually follows a sigh at this age and has been taken to suggest an instability due to poorly developed chemical control of breathing (26). It has also been noted that the Dejour hyperoxic test, as well as the single CO_2 breath test, are submaximal until 2–3 months of postterm age (27). These observations suggest that the same factors, albeit operating to different degrees and on different time scales, occur in another species, namely the human.

A central feature of rhythmogenesis in the newborn is the recognition of an active expiratory contribution to breathing, very similar to the original Hering Breuer reflex when they showed not only an inflationary inhibition of breathing, but an active expiratory response proportional to the magnitude of the inflation. This component of the reflex had been considered by others to be an artefact of the opiates used for anaesthesia in their experiments and recognition of the importance of this phase of the respiratory cycle has continued to escape recognition despite the clear demonstration that 10 cm H_2O of expiratory pressure was sufficient to stimulate expiratory activity of the abdominal oblique muscle (28) which was abolished by lung vagal afferent denervation. Our own studies confirm this and suggest that the mechanism operates normally in quiet breathing during SWS when some 5–7 cm H_2O of endogenous expiratory pressure are generated mainly by the elastic recoil of the lungs against the closed glottis, but this rapidly becomes an active expiratory phenomenon if lung collapse, hypoxaemia, increased expiratory resistance or obstruction occurs. Such a mechanism is thought to lead to pneumothorax when preterm infants with RDS actively expire against positive pressure ventilation (Greenough et al. this volume, p. 259). This reflex is therefore the "forgotten" active expiratory component originally described by Hering Breuer in response to lung inflation. There is convincing evidence that the newborn, who cannot assume maintenance of lung volume by passive mechanisms, normally recruits the use of increased intercostal muscle, postinspiratory diaphragmatic activity and, if necessary, abdominal oblique muscle activity as well as laryngeal adduction for this purpose. The experimental evidence is convincing that the afferent message for this response comes from vagal pathways from the upper and lower airways. The use of these mechanisms are greatly modulated by sleep state, metabolism, temperature regulation, as well as the peripheral chemoreceptors which would appear to modulate this activity. What is also quite clear from these studies is that rhythmogenesis is also sustained by lung afferents, presumptively pressure, particularly in the expiratory phase of breathing in older lambs breathing at lower frequencies. Prior to that high breathing frequencies stimulated by a high metabolic rate achieve an adequate lung volume by virtue of a short expiratory time. Since the metabolic requirements of temperature regulation are a major stimulus to breathing in the newborn the much discussed biphasic ventilatory response to hypoxia is very likely to simply reflect a reduction in metabolic rate and is certainly not a depression of breathing even in the unanaesthetized newborn (29).

We believe therefore that these observations have considerable implications for a range of neonatal respiratory problems, particularly that of persistent oxygen dependence or chronic lung disease and later on possibly sudden infant death syndrome. Certainly a postneonatal vulnerability for abnormal chemical control would be examined by the progressive changes in factors that determine effective breathing that have been described here. It also follows from these observations that simple tests of respiratory control, such as occlusion responses claimed to test the Hering Breuer reflex responses, hyperoxic or CO_2 tests of chemical control are going to vary depending on the age of the infant and the presence of other factors such as changes in the ambient temperature. Specifically it is evident that lambs, even in an apparently comfortable laboratory temperature live with a cold stress during the first 4–5 days of life before their improved thermal efficiency "transfers" them as it were, into a thermoneutral zone at the same Ta, whereas in the older age group it is possible that despite minimal oxygen consumption, the respiratory system is then engaged in the cooling function of thermoregulation at the warm end of the range.

Finally, the information gained from these types of observations clearly endorse the need for descriptive physiological studies particularly in the perinatal period where developmental changes are rapid. Classical respiratory physiology has been found wanting in this area in much the same way as in the understanding of respiratory control in the adult during sleep. These observations are probably more in accord with clinical observations than many of the conventional views of respiratory control.

References

1. Karlberg, P., Cherry, R. B., Escardo, F. E. and Koch, G. (1962). *Acta Paediatrica* **51**, 121–136.
2. Harrison, V. C., de Heese, H. and Klein, M. (1968). *Pediat.* **41**, 549.
3. Dixon, M., Szereda-Przestazewska, M., Widdicombe, J. G. and Wise, J. C. M. (1974). *J. Physiol.* **239**, 347–363.
4. Fewell, J. E. and Johnson, P. (1981). *J. Physiol.* **320**, 57.
5. Boddy, K., Dawes, G. S., Fisher, R., Pinter, S. and Robinson, J. S. (1974). *J. Physiol.* **243**, 599.
6. Johnson, P. (1978). *In:* "Central Nervous Control Mechanisms in Breathing", (von Euler, C. and Lagercrantz, H., eds) pp. 337–351, Pergamon Press, Oxford.
7. Kitterman, J. A., Liggins, G. C., Clements, J. A. and Tooley, W. H. (1975). *J. Develop. Physiol.* **1**, 453–466.
8. Dawes, G. S., Gardner, W. N., Johnston, N. M. and Walker, D. W. (1983). *J. Physiol.* **335**, 535–553.
9. Maycock, D. E., Standaert, T. A., Guthrie, R. D. and Woodrun, D. E. (1983). *J. Appl. Physiol.* **54**(3), 814–820.
10. Bureau, M. A. (1983). *Am. Rev. Resp. Dis.* **127**, 215.
11. Blanco, C. E., Dawes, G. S., Hanson, M. A. and McCooke, H. B. (1984). *J. Physiol.* **351**, 25–38.
12. Dawes, G. S. (1968). "Fetal and Neonatal Physiology". p. 35 Year Book Medical Publishers, Chicago.

13. Gluckman, P. D., Gunn, T. R. and Johnston, B. M. (1983). *J. Physiol.* **343**, 495–506.
14. Fewell, J. E. and Johnson, P. (1983). *J. Physiol.* **339**, 495–504.
15. Yousef, K. A. O., Oommen, P. M. and Thach, B. T. (1981). *Pediat.* **68**, 67–96.
16. Dawes, G. S. and Mott, J. C. (1959). *J. Physiol.* **146**, 294–315.
17. Lister, G., Walker, T. K., Versmold, H. T., Dallman, P. R. and Rudolph, A. M. (1979). *Am. J. Physiol.* **237**, H668–H675.
18. Mercer, J. B. (1974). Ph.D. Dublin University.
19. Harding, R., Johnson, P. and McClelland, M. E. (1980). *Resp. Physiol.* **40**, 165–180.
20. Remmers, J. E. and Bartlett, Jr. D. (1977). *J. Appl. Physiol.* **42**, 80–87.
21. Jansen, A. H., Ioffe, S., Russell, B. J. and Chernick, V. (1981). *J. Appl. Physiol.* **51**(3), 630–633.
22. Carse, E. A., Wilkinson, A. R., Whyte, P. L., Henderson-Smart, D. J. and Johnson, P. (1981). *J. Develop. Physiol.* **3**, 85–100.
23. Hoppenbrouwers, T., Harper, R. M., Hodgman, I. E., Sterman, M. B. and McGinty, D. J. (1978). *Pediat. Res.* **12**, 120–125.
24. Steinschneider, A. and Weinstein, S. (1983). *Pediat. Res.* **17**, 35–41.
25. Szymusiak, R. and Satinoff, E. (1981). *Physiol. Behaviour.* **26**, 887–890.
26. Bryan, A. C. and Bryan, H. (1984). "Sudden Infant Death Syndrome" Harper, R. M., ed. Interscience Foundation" (in press).
27. Fleming, P. J., Goncalves, A. L., Levine, M. R. and Woolhard, S. (1984). *J. Physiol.* **347**, 1–16.
28. Bishop, B. and Bachofen, H. (1972). *J. Appl. Physiol.* **32**, 798–805.
29. Blanco, C., Hanson, M., Johnson, P. and Rigatto, H. (1984). *J. Appl. Physiol.* **56**(1), 12–17.

Ventilatory Response to CO_2 in Preterm Infants with Idiopathic Apnoea

Manuel Durand, Sami Georgie, Carl Barberis,
Luis A. Cabel, Felipe Gonzalez,
Toke Hoppenbrouwers and Joan E. Hodgman

Newborn Division of the Los Angeles County-University of Southern California
Medical Center; Department of Pediatrics, University of Southern California
School of Medicine, Los Angeles, USA

Introduction

With increasing gestational age the incidence of apnoea in preterm infants decreases (1). Further, severe idiopathic apnoea in larger preterm infants, > 30 weeks of gestation, after the first week of life is uncommon and poorly understood. In spite of the current interest in apnoea, surprisingly little information is available for this group of infants.

We designed this study to assess the ventilatory response to hypercapnia in these infants. Changes in resting ventilation and oxygenation were also analysed.

Patients and Methods

Nine healthy pre-term infants and 8 infants with 3 or more episodes of central apnoea (≥ 20 s) in 24 h after the first week of life were studied during active sleep, while the infants were on a radiant heat warmer. The mean birth weight of the control group was 1771 ± 67 g (SEM); gestational age 33 ± 0.4 weeks; and postnatal age 14 ± 2.2 days. The mean birth weight of the study group with apnoea was 1899 ± 151 g; gestational age 33 ± 0.5 weeks; and postnatal age 17 ± 2.9 days. None were receiving methylxanthines. Small for gestational age infants were excluded. In the study group only infants with evidence of apnoea the day of the study were included. Specific causes of apnoea, e.g., infection, biochemical abnormalities, cardiopulmonary disease and other diagnosed medical conditions, were excluded from the study group.

The Physiological Development of the Fetus and Newborn
ISBN 0 12 389080 2

Copyright © 1985 by Academic Press, London.
All rights of reproduction in any form reserved.

Using a nosepiece and a pneumotachograph attached to the outflow part of the system, tidal volume, flow, and end-tidal CO_2 and O_2 concentrations, were recorded continuously on a Gould Brush recorder (2,3,4,5). Transcutaneous PO_2 was monitored continuously (TCO_2M 818, Novametrix Medical Systems, Inc.). Heart rate and impedance changes with respirations were recorded continuously on a Corometrics 512 neonatal monitor. Skin temperature was servocontrolled to 36.5°C and sleep state in our patients was documented by behavioural observation as suggested by Prechtl (6). Active sleep was defined by the presence of somatic and eye movements.

We measured minute ventilation (V_E), tidal volume (V_T), respiratory frequency (f), alveolar PCO_2 ($PACO_2$), alveolar PO_2 (PAO_2), the slope and intercept of the CO_2 response curve, and transcutaneous PO_2 ($PtcO_2$). The ventilatory response to CO_2 was analysed by measuring and summing each tidal volume during one minute periods, before and during the fifth minute following administration of 4% CO_2 in air. End-tidal PCO_2 was estimated during the same time interval and assumed to be equivalent to alveolar PCO_2. Transcutaneous PO_2 was analysed from the appropriate tracings, during the same time that minute ventilation was estimated (5,7).

Ventilation and oxygenation were compared for both groups of infants, while they were breathing air. The slope and intercept of the CO_2 response curves were also compared. Statistical significance of the differences between the groups was assessed with the unpaired t-test.

Results

Changes in ventilation

Infants with apnoea had a lower resting minute ventilation (213.6 *vs* 274.5 ml/min/kg, $P < 0.01$), lower respiratory frequency (31 *vs* 40 breaths/min, $P < 0.005$), and higher alveolar PCO_2 (38 *vs* 33 mmHg, $P < 0.01$) than healthy preterm infants. Tidal volumes was slightly higher in infants with apnoea, but the difference was not significant (Table 1).

Ventilatory response to CO_2

Preterm infants with apnoea as compared with healthy preterm infants had a significantly reduced slope of the ventilatory response to CO_2 19.0 ± 2.0 (Mean $\pm$ SEM) *vs* 40.4 ± 3.2 ml/min/kg/mmHg $PACO_2$ ($P < 0.001$). In addition, in the study group the intercept at 300 ml/min/kg was shifted to the right ($P < 0.001$) (Table 1, Fig. 1).

Changes in oxygenation

Infants with apnoea had a lower resting alveolar PO_2 and a slightly lower transcutaneous PO_2 than healthy preterm infants, although the differences were not significant. Alveolar-transcutaneous oxygen gradients were essentially the same (Table 1).

Table 1. Ventilation, CO₂ response and oxygenation in 9 healthy preterm infants and 8 preterm infants with apnoea*

	$\dot{V}_E$ ml/min/ kg Air	f breaths/ min Air	V_T ml/kg Air	PACO₂ mmHg Air	Slope ml/min/ kg/ mmHg	Inter- cept† mmHg	PAO₂ mmHg Air	PtcO₂ mmHg Air
Control	274.5 ±10.4	40 ±2	6.8 ±0.2	33 ±1	40.4 ±3.2	34.0 ±1.1	114 ±2	83 ±4
Apnoea	213.6ᶜ ±16.3	31ᵇ ±2	7.0 ±0.3	38ᶜ ±1	19.0ᵃ ±2.0	43.3ᵃ ±1.8	108 ±2	76 ±3

*Values are means ± SEM. Abbreviations used are: $\dot{V}_E$, minute ventilation; f, respiratory frequency; V_T, tidal volume; PACO₂, alveolar PCO₂; PAO₂, alveolar PO₂; PtcO₂, transcutaneous PO₂. Significant difference from control value as follows: (a) $P < 0.001$, (b) $P < 0.005$, (c) $P < 0.01$. †Alveolar PCO₂ at 300 ml/min/kg.

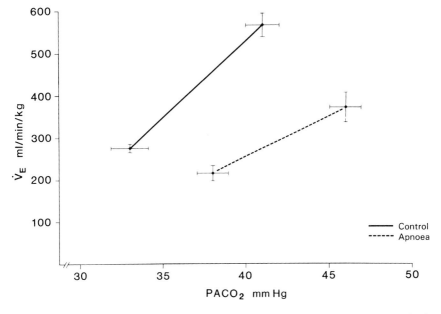

Figure 1. Ventilatory response to CO₂ in healthy preterm infants and preterm infants with apnoea (Mean ± SEM). The slope was significantly reduced in infants with apnoea. In addition, the intercept was shifted to the right in this group.

Discussion

During a year's surveillance of our large service with aproximately 14 000 deliveries only a dozen cases were found which met the criteria for this study. We found that infants with apnoea had a lower resting minute ventilation than healthy preterm infants. This was primarily due to a decreased respiratory frequency, tidal volume being essentially unchanged. These results are in agreement with the report of Rigatto and Brady (2) of 6 preterm infants with periodic breathing. Our results extend these earlier observations to large preterm infants in whom significant episodes of apnoea (≥ 20 s) were documented within 24 h of the ventilatory study. Associated with this decreased minute ventilation, alveolar PCO_2 increased and alveolar PO_2 decreased. Our patients with apnoea had a significantly decreased slope of the ventilatory response to CO_2 as compared to slope values in control infants, suggesting a decreased CO_2 sensitivity. In addition, the intercept was shifted to the right, probably related to an increase in the respiratory centre threshold to CO_2. Measurements of the ventilatory response to hypercapnia in large preterm infants with severe idiopathic apnoea are not available for comparison. Rigatto and Brady (2) documented in their infants with periodic breathing a significant shift of the CO_2 response curve to the right with a slight decrease in slope (22%). In our patients the decrease in slope was 53%.

The infants with apnoea did not have cardiopulmonary disease; thus mechanical factors leading to increased airway resistance and increased work of breathing could not account for our findings. Further, although obstructive apnoea has been documented recently in preterm infants (8,9) with increased frequency, we only studied infants with central apnoea as identified by absence of chest movements by thoracic impedance.

Changes in alveolar PO_2 are seldom reported in studies of ventilatory control in newborn infants. We found a lower alveolar PO_2 in our patients with apnoea; this is probably related to the decreased minute ventilation. In addition, transcutaneous PO_2 values were slightly lower than in control infants. These findings account for essentially unchanged alveolar-transcutaneous O_2 gradients suggesting that the major deficit in these infants is not in the lungs.

Our findings suggest that the deficit in infants with apnoea is in the respiratory centre. Interestingly, these changes appear to be transient. We restudied the ventilatory response to CO_2 in 3 of our infants with apnoea prior to discharge, once their apnoea had resolved, and found that their slopes were comparable to those in healthy preterm infants. Hazinski et al. (10) recently reported preliminary data using transcutaneous PCO_2 changes as a measure of ventilation. They documented that apnoeic infants had a reduced response to CO_2 and that the resolution of apnoea was associated with a normal CO_2 response. Several reports suggest that the ventilatory response to CO_2 in newborn infants is not different during active versus quiet sleep (11,12). We evaluated our data during active sleep because preterm infants spend more time in this stage of sleep than in quiet sleep.

Our study has documented that large preterm infants, > 30 weeks of gestation, with serious apnoea after the first week of life have: (1) significantly decreased resting minute ventilation, primarily as a result of decreased respiratory frequency; (2) a significantly reduced ventilatory response to CO_2, e.g., decreased CO_2 responsivity; (3) normal alveolar-transcutaneous oxygen gradients. These findings suggest that the major deficit in these infants is a central disturbance in the regulation of breathing.

Acknowledgements

Supported in part by National Institutes of Health, Child Health and Human Development, Program Project Grant RO1 HD 13689-03.

References

1. Henderson-Smart, D. J. (1981). *Aust. Pediat. J.* **17**, 273–276.
2. Rigatto, H., Brady, J. P. (1972). *Pediat.* **50**, 202–218.
3. Durand, M., Leahy, F. N., MacCallum, M., Cates, D. B., Rigatto, H., Chernick, V. (1981). *Pediat. Res.* **15**, 1509–1512.
4. Gerhardt, T. and Bancalari, E. (1981). *J. Appl. Physiol.* **50**, 1282–1285.
5. Durand, M., McCann, E. and Brady, J. P. (1983). *Pediat.* **71**, 634–638.
6. Prechtl, H. F. R. (1974). *Brain Res.* **76**, 185–212.
7. Brady, J. P., Durand, M. and McCann, E. (1983). *Am. Rev. Resp. Dis.* **127**, 422–424.
8. Mathew, O. P., Roberts, J. L. and Thach, B. T. (1982). *J. Pediat.* **100**, 964–968.
9. Milner, A. D., Boon, A. W., Saunders, R. A. and Hopkin, I. E. (1980). *Arch. Dis. Child.* **55**, 22–25.
10. Hazinski, T. A., Severinghaus, J. W., Marin, M. S. and Tooley, W. H. (1982). *Pediat. Res.* **16**, 290A.
11. Davi, M., Sankaran, K., MacCallum, M., Cates, D. and Rigatto, H. (1979). *Pediat. Res.* **13**, 982–986.
12. Haddad, G. G., Leistner, H. L., Epstein, R. A., Epstein, M. A. F., Grodin, W. K. and Mellins, R. B. (1980). *J. Appl. Physiol.* **48**, 684–688.

Arousal and Cardiorespiratory Responses to Upper Airway Obstruction during Sleep in Lambs

James E. Fewell

Department of Pediatrics and Physiology, University of Arkansas
for Medical Sciences, Little Rock, Arkansas, USA

Introduction

Upper airway obstruction has recently been recognized to cause apnoea in new-borns as well as in adults (1,2). It has been suggested that newborns are particularly vulnerable from the standpoint of developing hypoxaemia during cessation of airflow because of their high rate of oxygen consumption in relation to their lung oxygen stores (3). Since little information is available concerning the physiological response to upper airway obstruction in newborns, experiments were done to investigate the arousal and cardiorespiratory responses to upper airway obstruction during sleep in lambs.

Methods

Seven lambs ranging in age from 13 days to 20 days were studied. Each lamb was anaesthetized and instrumented for recordings of electrocorticogram, electro-oculogram, nuchal electromyogram, diaphragm electromyogram and for measurements of pulmonary blood flow (electromagnetic flow transducer) and systemic arterial blood pressure. A fiberoptic catheter oximeter (Oximetrix, Inc.) was placed in the thoracic aorta, a tracheotomy done, and a fenestrated tracheostomy tube (Shiley, Inc.) placed in the trachea. Following surgery, the tracheostomy tube was situated so that airflow during tidal respiration would be through the upper airway. The lambs were not studied before the third postoperative day.

During a study, a 5F balloon-tipped catheter was inserted through the

The Physiological Development of the Fetus and Newborn
ISBN 0 12 389080 2

Copyright © 1985 by Academic Press, London.
All rights of reproduction in any form reserved.

decannulation cannula into the tracheostomy tube so that airflow could be obstructed by inflating the balloon. Measurements were made during a 1-min control period and during an experimental period of airway obstruction during 24 epochs of quiet sleep and during 18 epochs of active sleep; airway obstruction was terminated by deflating the balloon once the animal aroused from sleep. Control measurements were begun approximately 2 min after the lamb entered quiet sleep and approximately 30 s after the animal entered active sleep. In an additional 15 epochs of quiet sleep and 14 epochs of active sleep, the balloon was not inflated following the control measurements so that the time to spontaneous arousal from sleep could be determined.

Results

Arousal occurred from both sleep states during airway obstruction (Figs 1, 2) but was significantly delayed ($P < 0.05$ by Student's paired t-test) during active sleep (19.6 ± 6.0 s, mean ± 1 SD) compared to quiet sleep (6.6 ± 1.5 s). Arousal occurred after 13 ± 3 obstructed breaths in active sleep and after 4 ± 1 obstructed breaths in quiet sleep. The arterial haemoglobin oxygen saturation at the point of arousal was $74 \pm 13\%$ in active sleep and $90 \pm 3\%$ in quiet sleep; control values were similar in both sleep states (active sleep $92 \pm 3\%$, quiet sleep $92 \pm 2\%$).

Small increases in systemic arterial blood pressure occurred during airway obstruction before arousal in both sleep states (active sleep 70.9 ± 5.5 to 75.5 ± 9.7 mmHg, quiet sleep 78.9 ± 4.5 to 82.7 ± 4.6 mmHg). Cardiac output decreased more following upper airway obstruction during active sleep (1204 ± 243 to 919 ± 190 ml/min) than during quiet sleep (1328 ± 211 to 1356 ± 196 ml/min).

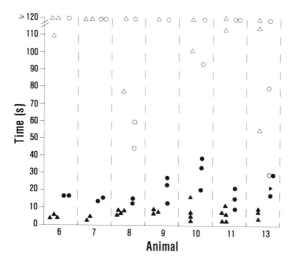

Figure 1. Time to arousal following upper airway obstruction (solid symbols) and to spontaneous arousal (open symbols) in quiet sleep (▲, △) and active sleep (●, ○) in 7 lambs.

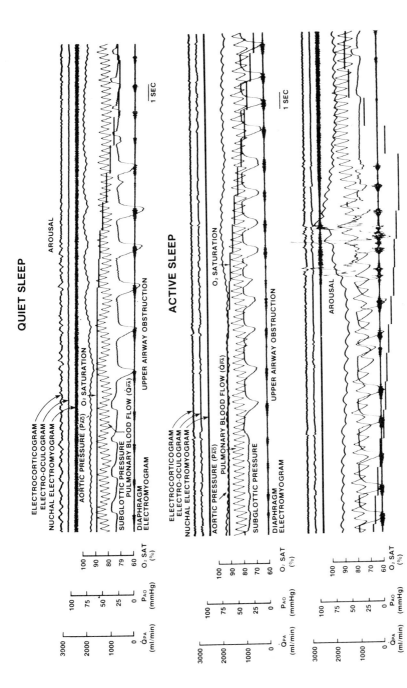

Figure 2. Arousal and cardiorespiratory response to upper airway obstruction during quiet sleep (upper) and active sleep (lower) in lamb No. 10.

Heart rate decreased as the arterial oxygen saturation decreased during upper airway obstruction.

The diaphragm electromyogram was successfully recorded in 6 lambs (i.e. 21 epochs of quiet sleep and 14 epochs of active sleep). The respiratory response to upper airway obstruction depended upon sleep state. During quiet sleep, there was increased activity on the diaphragm electromyogram from the first occluded breath in 20 of 21 epochs; this activity was maintained but did not increase progressively. Respiratory frequency decreased on the first occluded breath in 15 of 21 epochs because of an increase in inspiratory time but then returned toward control levels because of a gradual decrease in expiratory time. During active sleep, there was increased activity on the diaphragm electromyogram from the first occluded breath in 12 of 14 epochs but this activity was not maintained. The respiratory frequency response to upper airway obstruction was variable.

Discussion

These results provide evidence that sleep state influences the arousal and cardiopulmonary responses to airway obstruction in young lambs. The rapid arousal response to upper airway obstruction in quiet sleep suggests that afferent stimuli from receptors other than the peripheral chemoreceptors (e.g. lung and airway receptors and/or respiratory muscle and chest wall receptors) initiate the arousal response. Arousal occurred during some epochs of quiet sleep before any changes in arterial oxygen saturation had occurred. In contrast, the arterial oxygen saturation decreased significantly before arousal occurred from active sleep. More experiments are needed to investigate the mechanism of arousal following upper airway obstruction in lambs.

Cardiac output, measured continuously using an electromagnetic flow transducer, decreased more in active sleep than in quiet sleep during upper airway obstruction. These differences most likely relate to the length of occlusion before arousal and the resultant blood gas changes rather than to specific effects of sleep state on the cardiovascular response to chemoreceptor stimulation. The changes in cardiac output were similar in quiet sleep and active sleep when measured approximately 6 s (i.e. the average time to arousal in quiet sleep) following upper airway obstruction. Furthermore, we have previously found that sleep state does not affect the cardiovascular response to chemoreceptor stimulation (i.e. isocapnaeic hypoxaemia) in lambs (4). Since our measurements of cardiovascular variables were made at end-expiration, the early changes in aortic pressure and pulmonary blood flow most likely resulted from an increased fluctuation of these variables in phase with respiration caused by the mechanical effects of loaded breathing (5). The later changes (i.e. decreased pulmonary blood flow and bradycardia particularly during active sleep) were most likely the result of arterial chemoreceptor stimulation at a fixed lung volume (6,7).

During quiet sleep there was evidence of an active lung inflation reflex as inspiratory time increased following upper airway obstruction. In contrast, there was no consistent change in inspiratory time following upper airway obstruction in active sleep. This finding may be related to the absence of volume related phasic vagal input to the central nervous system or may be caused by an indirect reflex effect of ribcage distortion on inspiratory time during loaded breathing (8). During quiet sleep, there was an immediate increase in diaphragm electrical activity; this activity was maintained but did not increase progressively. Thus, the animals exhibited immediate load compensation but not progressive load compensation. This most likely results from an intact α-motorneuron drive and fusimotor system which have been suggested to mediate immediate load compensation and the lack of a hypoxic stimulus which has been suggested to mediate progressive load compensation (9–11). During active sleep, there was an immediate increase in diaphragm electrical activity which was not maintained. The reason for this is not clear.

Acknowledgements

The technical assistance of Mrs Cheryl Orintas and Mr Thomas Sziszak is greatly appreciated.

References

1. Milner, A. D., Boon, A. W., Saunders, R. A. and Hopkin, I. E. (1980). *Arch. Dis. Child.* **55**, 22–25.
2. Thach, B. T. (1983). *In:* "Sudden Infant Death Syndrome" (Tildon, J. T., Roeder, L. H., Steinschneider, A., ed.) pp. 279–292, Academic Press, New York and London.
3. Henderson-Smart, D. T. (1980). *Sleep* **3**, 331–342.
4. Fewell, J. E., Williams, B. J. and Hill, D. E. (1985). *J. Develop. Physiol.* (in press).
5. Bromberger-Barnea, B. (1981). *Fed. Proc.* **40**, 2172–2177.
6. Daly, M. D. and Scott, M. J. (1958). *J. Physiol.* **144**, 148–166.
7. Zwillich, C., Devlin, T., White, D., Douglas, W., Weil, J. and Martin, R. (1982). *J. Clin. Invest.* **69**, 1286–1292.
8. Knill, R. and Bryan, A. C. (1976). *J. Appl. Physiol.* **40**, 352–356.
9. Campbell, E. J. M., Dinnick, O. P. and Howell, J. B. L. (1961). *J. Physiol.* **156**, 260–273.
10. Callanan, D. and Read, D. J. C. (1974). *J. Physiol.* **241**, 33–44.
11. Biscoe, T. J. and Purves, M. J. (1967). *J. Appl. Physiol.* **190**, 413–424.

Postnatal Maturation of the Respiratory Rhythm Generator*

Phyllis M. Gootman, Andrew M. Steele,*
Howard L. Cohen and Lawrence P. Eberle

Department of Physiology, Downstate Medical Center, State University of New York, New York and *Division of Neonatology, Schneider Children's Hospital, Long Island Jewish-Hillside Medical Center, New York, USA

Introduction

Knowledge of neonatal respiration and its postnatal maturation is still quite limited (1–3). Central respiratory activity is usually defined by reference to efferent phrenic (PHR) activity (4,5); the high frequency oscillations (HFO) (5) observed in PRH discharge are considered to be indices for identification of neurons (4–7) making up the respiratory rhythm generator (RRG) (5). In this paper we will report some of our preliminary findings concerning the age-related changes in the HFO of piglet PHR activity.

Methods

PHR activity was recorded in piglets, < 1–46 days old, lightly anaesthetized with Althesin® (4 mg/kg/h) (8), immobilized with C-10 and artificially ventilated. Blood gases were sampled and pH and $PaCO_2$ maintained within normal limits. Recordings were made on magnetic tape of left and/or right PHR activity (bandpass 10–10 000 Hz), integrated PHR (TC 0.1 s), intratracheal pressure, aortic pressure, EKG, and pulses marking the phases of the central respiratory cycle: inspiratory (I: abrupt onset of PHR activity) or expiratory (E: abrupt offset of PHR activity) phase and the ventilatory cycle. Computer analyses (PDP 11/45) included correlation and averaging techniques as well as power spectral analysis. Power spectral densities of PHR activity were investigated at sampling intervals of 0.244 ms; 1024 or 2048 point Fast Fourier Transforms (FFT) (9), depending upon epoch (sampling interval of PHR activity during I or E), were computed.

The Physiological Development of the Fetus and Newborn
ISBN 0 12 389080 2

Copyright © 1985 by Academic Press, London.
All rights of reproduction in any form reserved.

Aliasing was avoided by determining the Nyquist foldover rate and using the appropriate low pass filter setting. Hanning windows (9) were applied to reduce sidelobe leakage. Averages of 50–200 epochs were plotted as peak power/frequency interval; by calibration, the ordinate was converted from a linear power function (uV²) to a nonlinear voltage function (uV/unit frequency). The experimental protocols included ventilating the animals with appropriate gas mixtures to produce either hypoxia or hypercapnia and, under control conditions, carrying out No Lung Inflation Tests (5,10–12).

Results

Examples of PHR power spectra from piglets of four different ages are presented in Fig. 1. It can be seen that peak power increased with increasing postnatal age. At the younger ages, peak power was *ca* 100–110 Hz. As the piglets matured, the peak frequency increased to *ca* 140–150 Hz.

During hypoxia PHR activity increased; the increase was not sustained in younger piglets. In addition, neither hypoxia or hypercapnia altered the peak frequency although magnitude could be affected, as shown in the example from a 16-day-old piglet (Fig. 2). Note that, in this animal, the power of the peak frequency was increased during hypercapnia but not during hypoxia.

The effect of depth of anaesthesia on the PHR responses to the No Lung Inflation Test is shown in Fig. 3. Under deep anaesthesia (40 mg/kg/h Althesin; right panel) PHR discharge, in this 13-day-old, was increased in both amplitude and duration. However, under light anaesthesia (4 mg/kg/h; left panel), PHR discharge was not altered, although onset of I occurred earlier.

Discussion

The peak frequency observed in PHR activity of neonatal swine increased with increasing postnatal age, 100–150 Hz from < 1 day to 4 weeks (Fig. 1). Age-related changes in the HFO have been reported in kittens (0–80 days: 20–60 Hz; adult: 100 Hz) and puppies (0–25 days: 20–60 Hz) (5,6,13). Unpublished observations (K. Koizumi, M. Kollai, L. P. Eberle) indicated a peak frequency in adult canine PHR discharge of *ca* 100–120 Hz. These results suggest both species differences and age-related maturation of HFO.

The inability of preterm infants (1–3) and neonates of other species (14–18), to maintain increased ventilation in the presence of hypoxia is still not explained. We have shown (Fig. 2) that the amplitude of peak power in PHR bursts also can reflect this immaturity. On the other hand, neonates are capable of a maintained response (augmented respiration) to hypercapnia. This result is now supported by the increased power in PHR activity observed during hypercapnia (Fig. 2). The lack of an increase in PHR activity during hypoxia suggests a central site (RRG) of inhibition (1–3, 14–18).

Traditionally, pulmonary stretch receptor activity has been considered to be inhibitory to the RRG (5). However, facilitation has recently been reported in adult cats under light pentobarbitone anaesthesia (19). We have now demonstrated

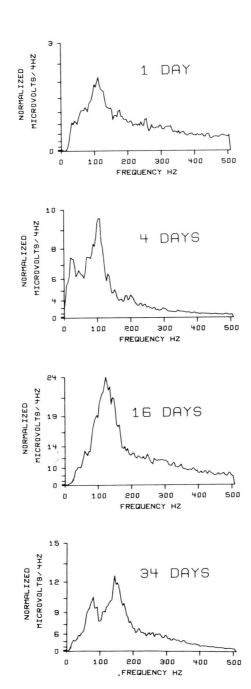

Figure 1. Power spectra (uV/4 Hz) of PHR activity (computed during I) from piglets of 4 different ages. Note differences in gains.

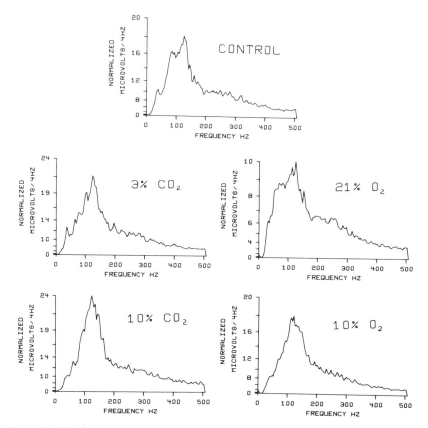

Figure 2. Effects of changes in inspired CO_2 or O_2 on PHR activity (power spectra) from a 16-day-old piglet. CONTROL — 100% inspired O_2. Note differences in gains.

that the latter phenomenon can also be observed in piglets under Althesin (Fig. 3) and halothane anaesthesia (P. M. Gootman, S. M. DiRusso, unpublished observations).

Our results, to date, indicate that neonatal swine is an appropriate model for investigations of postnatal maturation of the RRG. Furthermore, integration, correlation and power spectral analysis are appropriate analytical tools for delineating age-related responses of the RRG to alterations in afferent inputs.

Acknowledgements

This work was supported by a USHS grant from the HLBI of NIH awarded to PMG. Althesin was supplied by Glaxo Group Research Ltd.

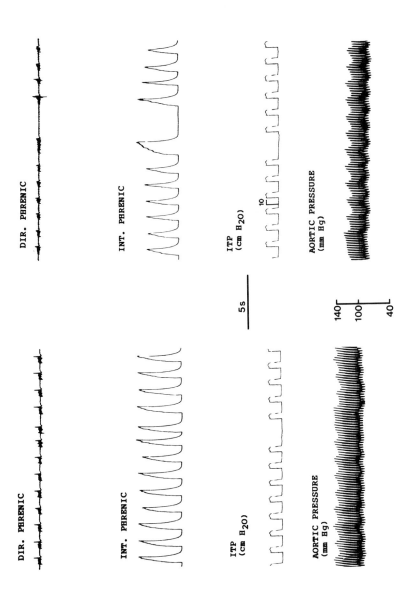

Figure 3. Effect of anaesthesia (left panels: low Althesin: 4 mg/kg/h; right panels: high Althesin: 40 mg/kg/h) on the No Lung Inflation Test from a 13-day-old piglet. Polygraph records of PHR (Top traces: DIR. – direct, Second traces; INT. – integrated (TC 100 ms), intratracheal pressure (Third traces: ITP), aortic blood pressure (Bottom traces).

References

1. Rigatto, H. (1984). *Ann. Rev. Physiol.* **46**, 661-674.
2. Rigatto, H. and Brady, J. P. (1972). *Pediat.* **50**, 219-228.
3. Jansen, A. H. and Chernick, V. (1983). *Physiol. Rev.* **63**, 437-483.
4. Richter, D. W. (1982). *J. Exp. Biol.* **100**, 93-107.
5. Cohen, M. I. (1979). *Physiol. Rev.* **59**, 1105-1173.
6. Richardson, C. A. and Mitchell, R. A. (1982). *Brain Res.* **223**, 317-336.
7. Euler, C. von (1983). *J. Appl. Physiol.* **55**, 1647-1659.
8. Hilton, S. M. and Marshall, J. M. (1982). *J. Physiol.* **326**, 425-513.
9. Brigham, E. O. (1974). "The Fast Fourier Transform", Prentice-Hall, New York.
10. Gootman, P. M. and Cohen, M. I. (1983). *Brain Res.* **270**, 134-136.
11. Cohen, M. I., Gootman, P. M. and Feldman, J. L. (1980). *In:* "Arterial Baroreceptors and Hypertension" (Sleight, P., ed.) pp. 161-167, Oxford University Press, Oxford.
12. Feldman, J. L. and Gautier, H. (1976). *J. Neurophysiol.* **39**, 31-44.
13. Suthers, G. K., Henderson-Smart, D. J. and Read, D. J. C. (1977). *Brain Res.* **132**, 537-540.
14. Schwieler, G. H. (1968). *Acta Physiol. Scand.* (suppl.) **304**, 1-123.
15. Lawson, E. E. and Long, W. A. (1983). *J. Appl. Physiol.* **55**, 483-488.
16. Steele, A. M., Gootman, P. M., Cohen, H. L., Eberle, L. P. and Rudell, A. P. (1984). *Pediatric. Res.* **18**, 406A.
17. Gootman, P. M., Steele, A. M., Cohen, H. L., Rudell, A. P. and Eberle, L. P. (1983). *Neurosci. Abst.* **9**, 1162.
18. Blanco, C. E., Hanson, M. A., Johnson, P. and Rigatto, H. (1984). *J. Appl. Physiol.* **56**, 12-17.
19. DiMarco, A. F., Euler, C. von, Romaniuk, J. R. and Yamamoto, Y. (1981). *Acta Physiol. Scand.* **113**, 375-386.

Effects of Thyroid Hormones and Glucocorticoids on Phosphatidylcholine Synthesis in Cultured Fetal Lung

Philip L. Ballard and Linda K. Gonzales

Cardiovascular Research Institute and the Department of Pediatrics,
University of California, San Francisco, California, USA

Surfactant is a complex mixture of lipids and protein which lines the alveolar air-spaces and maintains lung expansion after birth. Production of this material during late gestation is critical to normal function of the pulmonary system; insufficient surfactant is a major cause of neonatal Respiratory Distress Syndrome (RDS). The principal phospholipid and surface active component of surfactant is saturated phosphatidylcholine (PC). Accordingly, regulation of the synthesis and secretion of PC has been extensively studied both *in vivo* and *in vitro*.

Production of surfactant, and specifically PC, is influenced by the hormonal milieu. The stimulatory effect of glucocorticoids on PC synthesis and release has been described in many studies with experimental animals (1), and glucocorticoids have been used clinically to prevent RDS in premature human infants (2-4). A positive effect of thyroid hormones on lung maturation, including PC synthesis and accumulation in air spaces, has been demonstrated both *in vivo* (5-8) and *in vitro* (9-14), and intra-amniotic administration of T_4 to human fetuses was associated with a low incidence of RDS (15). The precise mechanism of action has not been described for either glucocorticoids or thyroid hormones. However, we recently demonstrated that the glucocorticoid effects on PC synthesis in fetal lung are receptor-mediated and require *de novo* protein synthesis (16). The presence of T_3 receptors in fetal lung nuclei (17-19) led us to postulate that thyroid hormone effects on PC synthesis are also receptor-mediated. This study further characterizes the glucocorticoid and thyroid hormone effects on PC synthesis with regard to receptor-mediation and synergistic interaction.

The Physiological Development of the Fetus and Newborn
ISBN 0 12 389080 2
Copyright © 1985 by Academic Press, London.
All rights of reproduction in any form reserved.

Materials and Methods

The methodology has been described in detail in recent reports (14,16). Lungs from New Zealand White rabbit fetuses (23 days gestation) and human abortuses (15-22 weeks gestation) were chopped into $1\,mm^3$ pieces and placed in organ culture with Waymouth's MB-752/1 medium without serum for 3 or 7 days, respectively. PC was isolated by TLC and phospholipid was quantified by phosphorus assay. Statistical significance was assessed by paired or unpaired t-test and by least squares linear regression.

Results and Discussion

Stimulation of phosphatidylcholine synthesis

Choline incorporation in explant cultures of both rabbit and human fetal lung is stimulated by T_3 and dexamethasone (Dex) (Table 1). The amount of stimulation was similar for the two tissues at the time of optimal exposure to the hormones (3 days and ~ 6 days in the rabbit and human, respectively). The effect of T_3 in the presence of Dex was more than additive in most experiments for both the rabbit (21/22), and human (12/15) lung. These results provide further evidence that T_3 and Dex stimulate PC synthesis via independent biochemical sites, as suggested by previous studies with lung (10,11,14,20).

Table 1. Stimulation of choline incorporation into PC by T_3 and dexamethasone

Tissue (n)	Exposure (days)	Choline Incorporation		
		T_3	Dex	$T_3 + Dex$
		(% stimulation vs control)		
Rabbit (22)	3	50.0 ± 5.8	62.1 ± 6.5 $P < 0.0001$	161.4 ± 11.4
Human (7)	2	11.8 ± 4.8	36.6 ± 11.7 $P < 0.05$	107.4 ± 36.5
Human (12)	6	51.6 ± 12.6	103.4 ± 14.2 $P < 0.01$	165.2 ± 16.8

Lung explants (rabbit, 23 days gestation; human 16-22 weeks gestation) were cultured in the presence of T_3 (2-5 nmol) and/or Dex (10-100 nmol). Choline incorporation (nmol/4 h/mg DNA) was determined as in Methods, and values are the mean $\pm$ SEM of the number of experiments (n) shown.

The time course of response to addition of T_3 plus Dex was more rapid for rabbit than human lung. With rabbit tissue, choline incorporation was stimulated as early as 14 h and stimulation was optimal at 46 h. The response to T_3 plus Dex, compared to either T_3 or Dex alone, was greater than additive at all times (28, 46, 68 h) after 14 h. Stimulation of incorporation was observed in human tissue after 1 day of exposure and plateaued between 4 and 7 days. Choline incorporation into PC reflects an accumulation of PC in explant cultures of both rabbit ($r=0.94$, $n=22$) and human lung ($r=0.97$, $n=14$) as determined by linear regression analysis, similar to previous reports (16,21).

The saturated fraction of total PC in rabbit explants remains at 20–24% of the newly synthesized PC in the presence or absence of T_3 and/or Dex, in agreement with previous studies in this species (14,16,22). In contrast, both T_3 and Dex have a stimulatory effect on the percent saturation of newly synthesized PC in human lung. After 6 days exposure to hormone ($n=8$), T_3 increased the percent saturation of newly synthesized PC to $19.2\pm1.5\%$, vs the control value of $17.6\pm1.0\%$ ($P<0.01$), and Dex and T_3 plus Dex increased the saturation to $25.2\pm1.0\%$ and $23.9\pm1.3\%$, respectively. Therefore, both T_3 and Dex had a significantly greater stimulatory effect on synthesis of saturated PC than on unsaturated PC, but this effect was not additive when both hormones were present.

Incorporation of other radioactive precursors ($[^3H]$glucose, $[^3H]$glycerol, $[^3H]$acetate) into PC by rabbit lung was also stimulated by T_3 (25.5%, 8.1%, and 28.9%, respectively), by Dex (8.3%, 28.9%, and 33.4%, respectively), and by T_3 plus Dex (51.1%, 78.0%, and 51.4%, respectively). The incorporation of glucose and glycerol was more than additive in the presence of both hormones compared to each hormone alone ($P<0.03$), similar to the results with $[^3H]$choline, and incorporation of acetate was additive. The hormones affect not only the total incorporation of precursor, but also its distribution among phospholipids. In rabbit lung, Dex in either the absence or presence of T_3 increased the percentage incorporation of $[^3H]$acetate into PC to $77.2\pm0.5\%$ and $80.3\pm0.2\%$, respectively, compared to a control value of $74.1\pm0.5\%$ ($P<0.05$); in human lung, Dex and T_3 plus Dex increased the percentage incorporation of $[^3H]$glycerol into PC to 13.6 and 11.9%, respectively, compared to a control value of $4.9\pm0.4\%$. These results indicate that Dex, but not T_3 alone, selectively stimulates synthesis of those phospholipids which increase in relative abundance during normal lung maturation (23,24).

Mediation of T_3 action by nuclear receptors

The response to T_3 in rabbit explants is dose-dependent, with half-maximal stimulation of choline incorporation at a mean T_3 concentration of 0.12 ± 0.02 nmol ($n=6$). A somewhat lower concentration of 0.03 ± 0.01 nmol ($n=4$) produces a half-maximal response by human lung. These doses compare closely to the equilibrium dissociation constants (K_D) for receptor binding of 0.11 ± 0.04 nmol (18) and 0.04 ± 0.003 nmol (19) for rabbit and human fetal lung nuclei, respectively. Dose-response studies with several thyroid hormone analogues were performed with both rabbit and human explants; concentrations required for half-maximal response are plotted versus the K_Ds for receptor binding in Fig. 1. The values are grouped around the line of identity indicating a close correlation between potency and the affinity for receptor binding in both species. The relative potency of these analogues was triiodothyroacetic acid (TRIAC)> T_3-proprionic acid>L-T_3~D-T_3>L-T_4≫3,5-diethyl-3′-isopropyl-DL-thyronine (DIET)~3,5-dimethyl-3′-isopropyl-L-thyronine (DIMIT)~rT_3. Of particular note, the naturally occurring analogues L-T_4 and rT_3, which are present in

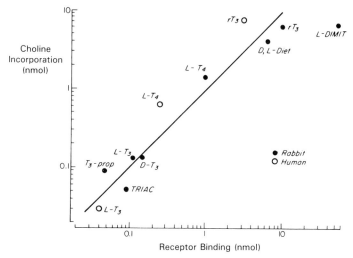

Figure 1. Comparison of potency and binding affinity for thyroid hormone analogues in rabbit (●) and human (○) lungs. Dose-response experiments were done for each analogue and mean values (2–4 experiments) for half-maximal stimulation of choline incorporation were plotted *vs* the K_D for binding to receptors in isolated fetal rabbit (18) and fetal human (19) lung nuclei. The line of identity is shown.

relatively high concentrations in the fetal circulation, have about 10% and 1% the potency of L-T_3 both in stimulating PC synthesis and binding to the receptor. The synthetic analogues DIMIT and DIET have low biological potency as predicted by their low receptor affinities. This positive correlation between receptor binding and potency in stimulating PC synthesis strongly suggests that nuclear receptors mediate the thyroid hormone effect.

RNA and protein synthesis

The requirement for macromolecular synthesis in the T_3 effect was investigated in rabbit lung using the inhibitors of RNA and protein synthesis, Actinomycin D and cycloheximide, respectively. In dose-response studies in Actinomycin D concentration of 0.2 μg/ml (14) completely inhibited the T_3 stimulation of choline incorporation when the inhibitor was continuously present during hormone treatment (46 h), and greatly reduced the stimulation of choline incorporation by T_3 plus Dex (Table 2). If Actinomycin D was present during only the last 24 h of hormone treatment, the T_3 effect was inhibited ~ 50% (data not shown).

Cycloheximide (0.04 μg/ml) reduced incorporation only slightly in control cultures (Table 2), but eliminated the T_3-induced stimulation of incorporation. The responses to Dex and to T_3 plus Dex were reduced but not eliminated. Cycloheximide was equally effective when added during the last 24 h or the entire 46 h of hormone exposure (data not shown). These results are consistent with a requirement for *de novo* synthesis of both mRNA and protein in the hormonal

Table 2. Inhibition of choline incorporation by Actinomycin D and cycloheximide

Hormones Added	Culture Condition			
	Actinomycin D		Cycloheximide	
	−	+	−	+
	(nmol choline incorporation/4 h/mg DNA)			
None	12.09 ± 0.62	7.91 ± 0.48	9.84	8.46
	(% stimulation *vs* control)			
T_3	19.5 ± 1.0	0	36.7	3.8
Dex	27.9 ± 1.9	21.4 ± 8.8	73.7	32.3
T_3 + Dex	98.5 ± 1.9	42.0 ± 16.4	143.6	104.2

Rabbit fetal lung was cultured for 72 h. For the Actinomycin D study, hormones (1 nmol T_3, 100 nmol Dex) were present for the last 46 h of culture, in the presence or absence of Actinomycin D (0.2 µg/ml). Values are the mean ± SEM of 3 experiments. For the cycloheximide study, hormones were present during the entire 72 h and cycloheximide (0.04 µg/ml) for the last 24 h. Values are the mean of duplicate determinations which varied < 10%.

stimulation of PC synthesis. The greater effectiveness of cycloheximide than Actinomycin D when added during the last day of culture is consistent with sequential stimulation of RNA and protein synthesis, and/or a relatively longer half-life of induced RNA *vs* protein.

Conclusions

T_3 and Dex appear to act at different and complementary biochemical sites to stimulate PC synthesis in explant cultures of both rabbit and human fetal lungs, producing a synergistic effect on the biosynthesis of PC. Dose-response studies with several T_3 analogues suggest that nuclear T_3-receptors mediate the T_3 effect in lung, and studies with inhibitors of RNA and protein synthesis provide evidence that T_3-receptor interaction promotes sequential synthesis of new mRNA and protein. Combined hormonal treatment may be more effective than glucocorticoid alone in stimulating surfactant production and preventing RDS in premature infants.

Acknowledgements

This work was supported in part by grants from the NIH (HL-24075 and HL-29564).

References

1. Ballard, P. L. (1982). *In:* "Development of the Lung and the Pathobiology of Hyaline Membrane Disease" (Farrell, P. M., ed.) pp. 205–253, Academic Press, New York and London.

2. Papageorgiou, A. N., Colle, E., Farri-Kostopoulos, E. and Gelfand, M. M. (1981). *Pediat.* **67**, 614–617.
3. Collaborative Group on Antenatal Steroid Therapy (1981). *Am. J. Obstet. Gynecol.* **141**, 276–286.
4. Liggins, G. C. and Howie, R. N. (1972). *Pediat.* **50**, 515–525.
5. Hitchcock, K. R. (1979). *Anat. Rec.* **194**, 15–40.
6. Wu, B., Kikkawa, Y., Orzalesi, M. M., Motoyama, E. K., Kaibara, M., Zigas, C. J. and Cook, C. D. (1973). *Biol. Neonate* **22**, 161–168.
7. Ballard, P. L., Benson, B. J., Brehier, A. and Carter, J. P. (1980). *J. Clin. Invest.* **65**, 1407–1417.
8. Erenberg, A., Rhodes, M. L., Weinstein, M. M. and Kennedy, R. L. (1979). *Pediat. Res.* **13**, 230–235.
9. Gross, I., Wilson, C. M., Ingleson, L. D., Brehier, A. and Rooney, S. A. (1980). *J. Appl. Physiol.* **48**, 872–877.
10. Gross, I. and Wilson, C. M. (1982). *J. Appl. Physiol.* **54**, 1420–1425.
11. Smith, B. T. and Sabry, K. (1983). *Proc. Nat. Acad. Sci. USA* **80**, 1951–1954.
12. Smith, B. T. and Torday, J. S. (1974). *Pediat. Res.* **8**, 848–851.
13. Longmuir, K. J., Bleasdale, J. E., Quirk, J. G. and Johnston, J. M. (1982). *Biochim. Biophys. Acta* **712**, 356–364.
14. Ballard, P. L., Hovey, M. L. and Gonzales, L. K. (1984). *J. Clin. Invest.* (in press).
15. Mashiach, S., Barkai, G., Sack, J., Stern, E., Brish, M., Goldman, B. and Serr, D. M. (1979). *J. Perinat. Med.* **7**, 161–170.
16. Gross, I., Ballard, P. L., Ballard, R. A., Jones, C. T. and Wilson, C. M. (1983). *Endocrinology* **112**, 829–837.
17. Lindenberg, J. A., Brehier, A. and Ballard, P. L. (1978). *Endocrinology* **103**, 1725–1731.
18. Gonzales, L. W. and Ballard, P. L. (1982). *Endocrinology* **111**, 542–552.
19. Gonzales, L. W. and Ballard, P. L. (1981). *J. Clin. Endocrin. Metab.* **53**, 21–28.
20. Gross, I., Dynia, D. W., Wilson, C. M., Ingleson, L. D., Gewolb, I. H. and Rooney, S. A. (1983). *Pediat. Res.* **18**, 191–196.
21. Mendelson, C. R., Johnston, J. M., MacDonald, P. C. and Synder, J. M. (1981). *J. Clin. Endocrin. Metab.* **53**, 307–317.
22. Rooney, S. A., Gobran, L. I., Marino, P. A., Maniscalco, W. M. and Gross, I. (1979). *Biochim. Biophys. Acta* **572**, 64–76.
23. Hallman, M., Kulovich, M., Kirkpatrick, E., Sugarman, R. G. and Gluck, L. (1976). *Am. J. Obstet. Gynecol.* **125**, 613–617.
24. Hallman, M. and Gluck, L. (1980). *Pediat. Res.* **14**, 1250–1259.

The Relationship between the Mg-dependent and Mg-independent Phosphatidic Acid Phosphohydrolases and Glycerolipid Biosynthesis in Rat Lung Microsomes

Fred Possmayer, Paul Walton and Paul G. R. Harding

Departments of Obstetrics/Gynaecology and Biochemistry,
University of Western Ontario, London, Ontario, Canada

Introduction

Phosphatidic acid phosphohydrolase occupies a central role in glycerolipid metabolism. The product of this enzyme, diacylglycerol (DG), acts as the immediate precursor of neutral triacylglycerol (TG) and of the nitrogen-containing phospholipids, phosphatidylethanolamine (PE) and phosphatidylcholine (PC) (Fig. 1). The disaturated PC, dipalmitoyl-phosphatidylcholine is the major constituent of pulmonary surfactant.

A potential role for phosphatidate phosphohydrolase in the control of surfactant biosynthesis has been inferred from the observation that the specific activity of this enzyme increases during fetal development and after treatment with glycocorticoids (see (1) for review). In the studies cited above, phosphatidate phosphohydrolase activity was assayed using liposomes of phosphatidic acid (PA) and Mg was not added. Studies from the authors' laboratory have reported that the properties of this Mg-independent enzyme assayed with aqueous dispersions of PA differs considerably from the properties of the enzyme assayed with biosynthetically formed membrane-bound PA. It can be shown that this latter enzyme activity is equivalent to the Mg-dependent phosphatidate phospho-hydrolase activity assayed with mixed liposomes of PA and PC (data not shown). The observation that the Mg-independent activity possesses K_m and

The Physiological Development of the Fetus and Newborn
ISBN 0 12 389080 2
Copyright © 1985 by Academic Press, London.
All rights of reproduction in any form reserved.

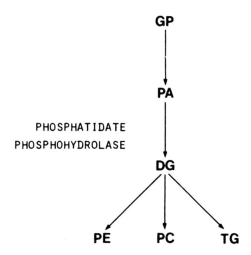

Figure 1. *De novo* pathway for glycerolipid biosynthesis. Abbreviations: GP, glycerol-3-P; PA, phosphatidic acid; DG, diacylglycerol; PE, phosphatidylethanolamine; PC, phosphatidylcholine; TG, triacylglycerol.

V_{max} values which are 10 and 35-fold, respectively greater than the Mg-dependent activity explains the relative lack of investigation with this latter enzyme.

In view of previous suggestions for a role of the Mg-independent phosphatidate phosphohydrolase in the control of surfactant synthesis, it is important to determine whether the Mg-dependent, or independent phosphohydrolase activities are responsible for the formation of DG for the synthesis of surfactant PC *in vivo*. The present studies provide strong evidence of the view that the Mg-dependent phosphatidate phosphohydrolase activity is specifically involved in glycerolipid synthesis.

Methods

Mg-Independent phosphatidate phosphohydrolase activity was assayed using 1.0 mmol (^{32}P)-labelled PA liposomes at pH 6.5 (2). The Mg-dependent activity was assayed using 0.2 mmol mixed PA-PC (1:1) liposomes, at pH 7.4, 1.25 mmol EDTA, in the presence and absence of 6 mmol $MgCl_2$. The Mg-dependent activity was calculated from this difference. Formation of PC from (^{14}C) glycerol-3-P was estimated by a modification of the incubation system of Fox and Zilversmit (3) followed by thin-layer chromatography as described by Ide and Weinhold (4).

Results

The effect of washing rat lung microsomes through centrifugation with different concentrations of NaCl on the Mg-dependent phosphatidate phosphohydrolase activities is illustrated in Fig. 2. The total phosphohydrolase activity exhibited a marked decline between microsomes pelleted in 0.1 and 0.3 M NaCl. This decline was accounted for by a decrease in the Mg-dependent activity. Neither the Mg-independent component assayed with mixed PA-PC liposomes or the Mg-independent activity assayed with higher concentrations of aqueously dispersed PA (data not shown), were affected by salt washing.

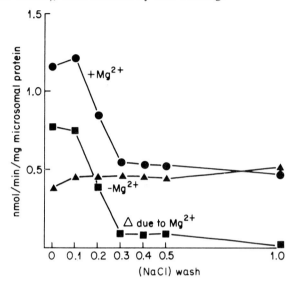

Figure 2. Effect of salt washing on Mg-dependent phosphatidic acid phospho-hydrolase activity of rat lung microsomes.

The effect of salt washing on the incorporation of (^{14}C) glycerol-3-P into lipids as illustrated in Fig. 3. It can be observed that washing lung microsomes with increasing levels of NaCl resulted in a decrease of the incorporation into PG and TG and a corresponding increase in the labelling of PA. These observations indicate that removing the Mg-dependent phosphohydrolase from rat lung microsomes results in the accumulation of radioactivity from (^{14}C) glycerol-3-P in PA (Fig. 1).

The results presented in the first two sections of this paper are consistent with the view that the selective removal of the Mg-dependent phosphohydrolase activity from microsomes results in a diminution of the formation of DG and TG. However, other possibilities exist. For example, salt washing could remove a factor which confers Mg-dependency on the phosphohydrolase activity remaining on the microsomes (5). Consequently, it was important to show that the Mg-dependent activity lost from the microsomes could be recovered in the washes. Figure 4A demonstrates that washing microsomes with 500 but not 50 mmol NaCl results in the recovery of the major proportion of the Mg-dependent activity in the wash supernatants. In contrast, washing microsomes in 50 and 500 mmol NaCl had little effect on the localization of the Mg-independent phosphohydrolase

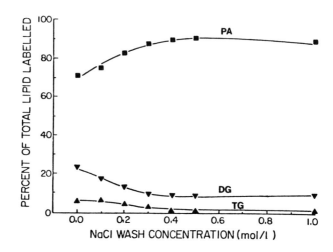

Figure 3. Effect of salt-washing on the incorporation of (^{14}C) glycerol-3-P into PA and neutral lipids.

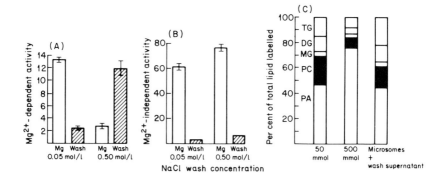

Figure 4. Effect of salt-washing on (A) the Mg-dependent phosphohydrolase activity, (B) the Mg-independent phosphohydrolase activity, and (C) the incorporation of (^{14}C) glycerol-3-P, of rat lung microsomes.

(Fig. 4B). These results clearly demonstrate that the Mg-dependent and Mg-independent phosphohydrolase activities are catalysed by separate enzymes.

The effect of washing rat lung microsomes with NaCl on PC biosynthesis is illustrated in Fig. 4C. Although salt washing did not produce a significant effect on choline-phosphotransferase activity microsomes (data not shown), the incorporation of (^{14}C) glycerol-3-P into PC was markedly depressed. Salt washing also resulted in a diminution of the incorporation into neutral lipids. Addition of the wash supernatants to the microsomes resulted in a restoration of the labelling patterns.

Discussion

The presence of both Mg-dependent and Mg-independent phosphatidate phosphohydrolase activities in microsomal preparations has been known for a number of years (1,2). Circumstantial evidence has indicated that only the Mg-dependent activity was involved in glycerolipid metabolism. However, direct evidence of a role for either activity in the production of PC in lung, or other tissues, was still lacking. The present results indicate that Mg-dependent phosphatidate phosphohydrolase is a peripheral protein which can be removed from microsomal membranes by washing with high salt. The activity removed from the microsomes can be quantitatively recovered in the washed supernatants. Washing microsomes results in a marked decrease in the ability to process membrane-bound PA for the formation of neutral lipids, or PC. The ability of the washed microsomes to incorporate radioactive glycerol-3-P into neutral lipids and PC is restored by the addition of the wash supernatants.

Washing of lung microsomes does not decrease the activity of the Mg-independent phosphatidate phosphohydrolase. Actually, this activity increased slightly, possibly due to the removal of peripheral proteins from the microsomal membrane surface. It appears that the Mg-independent phosphatidate phosphohydrolase is an integral protein. This may partially explain its resistance to inactivation by heat or trypsin (2). Since salt-washed microsomes, possessing the original complement of this enzyme, exhibit an impairment in the ability to process membrane-bound PA, it appears unlikely that this enzyme is involved in glycerolipid metabolism. The function of this Mg-independent phosphohydrolase activity remains unknown.

Acknowledgements

These studies were supported by grants from the Medical Research Council of Canada.

References

1. Possmayer, F. (1982). *In:* "The Biochemical Development of the Fetus and Neonate", (Jones, C. T., ed.) pp. 336–391, Elsevier Biomedical Press, Amsterdam.
2. Casola, P. G. and Possmayer, F. (1981). *Biochim. Biophys. Acta* **664**, 298–315.
3. Fox, P. L. and Zilversmit, D. B. (1982). *Biochim. Biophys. Acta* **712**, 605–615.
4. Ide, H. and Weinhold, P. A. (1983). *J. Biol. Chem.* **251**, 14926–14931.
5. Possmayer, F., Harding, P. G. R. and Walton, P. (1982). *Soc. Gynecol. Invest.* **30**, 202.

Metopirone Inhibits the Maturational Effect of ACTH in the Ovine Fetal Lung even in the Presence of Exogenous Glucocorticoids

George A. Vilos, John R. G. Challis, Stephen J. Lye, Fred Possmayer and Paul G. R. Harding

MRC Group in Reproductive Biology, Department of Obstetrics and Gynaecology, Research Institute, St Joseph's Hospital, The University of Western Ontario, London, Canada

Introduction

The relationship of ACTH to lung maturation was first recognized by Liggins in 1969 (1). He observed that infusion of ACTH accelerated lung maturation in lambs as early as 120 days of gestation. The mechanism was thought to be mediated through cortisol, produced by the fetal adrenal.

We have recently reported that physiological doses of ACTH (12 μg/day) infused for 72 h markedly accelerated maturation of the fetal sheep lung at 127–130 days of gestation (2). None of these lungs however had reached maturity comparable to term lungs.

In the present study we asked the following questions:

1. Does the lung attain full maturity when the fetus is pulsed with ACTH until labour is established?
2. If so, is the advanced maturation due to ACTH or due to the mechanics of labour?
3. Does metopirone, which blocks cortisol production in the fetal adrenal inhibit the maturational effect of ACTH?
4. If so, would exogenous glucocorticoids restore lung maturation when pulsed together with ACTH in the presence of metopirone?

The Physiological Development of the Fetus and Newborn
ISBN 0 12 389080 2
Copyright © 1985 by Academic Press, London.
All rights of reproduction in any form reserved.

Methodology

Forty-six accurately dated pregnancies were used for these experiments. Surgery was performed at 115–120 days of gestation as previously described (3). Blood sampling was started on day 125. The fetuses were infused from day 127 according to the following protocol.

Group 1. (ACTH-pulse, Singletons)
ACTH was infused as a pulse in sterile isotonic saline (66.7 ng/min for 15 min, at 2 ml/h) once every 2 h until labour was well established as judged by uterine activity, opening of the cervix and descent of the presenting part.

Group 2. (ACTH-pulse, Twins)
ACTH was infused as in group 1 to one fetus in twin pregnancies.

Group 3. (ACTH-pulse + metopirone)
Metopirone was infused via the fetal artery continuously at 32 mg/h for 100 h.

Group 4. (ACTH-pulse + metopirone + Low cortisol-pulse)
Cortisol was infused together with the ACTH-pulse at 200 μg/pulse for 100 h.

Group 5. (ACTH-pulse + metopirone + High cortisol-pulse)
Cortisol infusion was increased to 2 mg/pulse for 100 h.

Group 6. (ACTH-pulse + metopirone + dexamethasone-pulse)
Dexamethasone was infused together with ACTH at 8.3 μg/pulse for the first 48 h and increased to 83.3 μg/pulse from 48–100 h.

Group 7. (Saline-pulse)
Saline was pulsed at 2 ml/h for 15 min and subsequently at 0.35 ml/h for 105 min every 2 h for 100 h.

Group 8. (Term)
Seven fetuses were allowed to go to term spontaneous labour.

The protocol for fetal and maternal sampling, plasma cortisol and ACTH measurements as well as assessment of the various pulmonary maturation indices have been previously described (2,4).

Results

The mean period of infusion before labour was established was found to be 102.6 ± 6.6 h and 181.0 ± 18.0 h in the singleton and twin pregnancies respectively.

In Table 1 we list the number of animals (n), the adrenal to body weight ratio, the fetal basal plasma cortisol, the lung distensibility and the concentration of phosphatidylcholine measured in lung lavage.

Adrenal weight

We found that the adrenal to body weight ratio was 2.90 ± 0.16 in the ACTH singleton and 2.84 ± 0.52 in the ACTH infused twin fetuses. This represents a 2-fold increase in adrenal weight when compared to 1.43 ± 0.12 in the saline and 1.22 ± 0.13 in the twin intact fetuses.

There was no significant increase in the fetuses that received metopirone alone or in combination with glucocorticoids.

Table 1. Adrenal to body weight ratio, basal fetal plasma cortisol concentration and various indices of pulmonary maturation in all the groups studied

Group	n	Adrenal: body weight $\times 10^{-4}$	Plasma cortisol (ng/ml)	Lung distensibility[†] (ml air/g lung)	Phosphatidyl-choline (mg/g)
Term	7	1.63±0.16	(50–70	2.06±0.07***	0.63±0.13
Saline-pulse	8	1.43±0.12	3.69±0.96	1.10±0.14	0.07±0.02
ACTH-pulse (singletons)	5	2.90±0.16**	31.80±12.25*	1.90±0.20***	0.23±0.11****
ACTH-pulse (twins)	5	2.84±0.52**	23.01±8.59*	2.11±0.28***	0.20±0.06****
—intact	5	1.22±0.13	—	0.93±0.12	0.11±0.03
ACTH+metopirone	5	1.47±0.14	15.52±3.94*	0.99±0.17	0.25±0.08****
ACTH+metopirone +low cortisol	3	1.77±0.35	20.05±5.80*	1.29±0.34	0.11±0.02
ACTH+metopirone +high cortisol	4	1.48±0.15	29.95±5.97*	1.21±0.31	0.16±0.11
ACTH+metopirone +dexamethasone	4	1.27±0.08	8.79±1.79	1.42±0.34	0.32±0.10****

Results are mean±SEM
[†]Lung distensibility: V 40-ml of air/g of lung at 40 cm H_2O pressure
*$P<0.005$ vs saline, **$P<0.005$, ***$P<0.01$, ****$P<0.1$ vs all groups
Students' t-test

Fetal plasma cortisol

Basal levels of cortisol were less than 5 ng/ml prior to ACTH or saline infusion. Saline pulse had no demonstrable effect on fetal plasma cortisol while ACTH pulses resulted in a significant increase in fetal cortisol by 24 h. The increase in basal cortisol reached 31.80±12.25 ng/ml and 23.01±8.59 ng/ml just prior to the delivery of the singleton and twin ACTH infused fetuses respectively. In both Groups 1 and 2 there was an acute increase in cortisol temporally related to each ACTH pulse reaching levels of up to 100 ng/ml.

The fetal basal plasma cortisol increased to 15.52±3.94 ng/ml ($P<0.005$) in the ACTH+metopirone group and there was a small rise in cortisol associated with each ACTH pulse.

With the infusion of exogenous glucocorticoids there was a significant increase ($P<0.005$) in basal plasma cortisol up to 20.05±5.80 ng/ml and 25.95± 5.97 ng/ml for the low and high cortisol groups respectively. Following each ACTH+cortisol pulse there was also an acute rise in cortisol comparable to the rise in groups 1 and 2.

There was no significant rise in basal cortisol following the dexamethasone infusion. The cortisol level in this group reached up to 8.79±1.79 ng/ml just prior to caesarean delivery.

Pulmonary maturation

The distensibility, defined as the amount of air in the lung/g of wet lung at 40 cm H_2O pressure determined by pressure–volume curves, was 1.90±0.20 ml/g and

2.11±0.28 ml/g in the ACTH pulsed singleton and the infused twin respectively. In the intact twin it was 0.93±0.12 ml/g. This was not different from the distensibility of 1.10±0.14 of the saline infused fetuses. There was no significant increase in distensibility in the groups that received metopirone and glucocorticoids.

The saturated phosphatidylcholine measured in lavage fluid was increased in several of the groups studied but the levels were far below the level measured in term fetal lungs.

Histologically only the lungs of the fetuses treated with ACTH alone were indistinguishable from term lungs while in the other groups the lungs were partially expanded with thick-walled future airsacs.

Discussion

In the present study we have demonstrated that ACTH plays a major role in maturation of the fetal lung. Infusion of ACTH in physiological doses advances the lung to the same degree of maturity as that of the term fetuses. Since the animals were in active labour it was not clear whether the maturation was due to ACTH or due to the mechanics of labour. However when the experiment was repeated with twin pregnancies we found that only the twin that received ACTH had mature lungs while the lungs of its counterpart were similar to saline-infused fetuses. In two preparation EMG electrodes and intra-uterine pressure catheters were placed in both uterine horns and the activity recorded during labour was similar in both horns. This demonstrated that the maturation was due to ACTH and not due to the mechanics of labour.

In the first two experimental groups we found that the ACTH treated fetuses had increased their adrenal weight by 2-fold. The fetal plasma cortisol had risen in a stepwise manner to levels similar to those reported in term fetal lambs prior to spontaneous labour (5).

These two observations implied that the effect of ACTH on the lung was mediated through the fetal adrenal and the production of cortisol. This hypothesis was strengthened even further when metopirone which blocks the production of cortisol in the fetal adrenal inhibited the maturational effect of ACTH.

However, when the metopirone block was bypassed by infusion of exogenous cortisol in doses sufficient to raise the plasma cortisol to levels similar to those measured at term the lungs failed to advance in maturity.

Similarly, dexamethasone, a potent glucocorticoid infused together with ACTH failed to advance pulmonary maturation in the presence of metopirone.

These observations allow us to make the following conclusions:
1. Pulsed ACTH in physiological doses until labour was established advanced the fetal lung to full maturation. This was achieved in a period of 100 h.
2. Since only the lungs of the ACTH infused twin were found to be mature although both twins were subjected to the same forces of labour we conclude that labour plays no role in lung maturation.
3. Metopirone inhibited the effect of ACTH on the lung by preventing an increase in adrenal weight and rise in fetal plasma cortisol.

4. Exogenous glucocorticoids failed to restore lung maturation when pulsed together with ACTH in the presence of metopirone.
5. The effect of ACTH is exerted through activation of the fetal adrenal and it may be mediated through endogenous cortisol or some other unknown factor.

Acknowledgements

This work was supported by the Medical Research Council of Canada (Group Grant in Reproductive Biology to J.R.G.C., Post-doctoral Fellowship to S.J.L. and MRC Grant MT-4952).

References

1. Liggins, G. C. (1969). *J. Endocrinol.* **42**, 323–329.
2. Vilos, G. A., Challis, J. R. G., Lye, S. J., Possmayer, F. and Harding, P. G. R. (1983). *J. Develop. Physiol.* **5**, 341–350.
3. Challis, J. R. G., Patrick, J. E., Cross, J., Workweych, J., Manchester, E. and Power, S. (1981). *Can. J. Physiol. Pharmacol.* **59**, 261–267.
4. Lye, S. J., Sprague, C. L., Mitchell, B. F. F. and Challis, J. R. G. (1983). *Endocrinology* **113**, 770–776.
5. Strott, C. A., Sundel, H. and Stahlman, M. T. (1974). *Endocrinology* **95**, 1327–1339.

Laryngeal Resistance and Lung Liquid Flow in Relation to Breathing Activity in Fetal Sheep

R. Harding, A. D. Bocking,
J. N. Sigger and P. J. D. Wickham

Department of Physiology, Monash University,
Clayton, Victoria, Australia

Introduction

The purpose of this study was to identify factors which regulate the movement of fluid, via the trachea, into and from the mammalian fetal lungs. Such information is necessary for an understanding of the control of fetal pulmonary volume which has been shown to be a major determinant of lung growth (1,2,3,4). There is a growing body of evidence that fetal breathing movements (FBM), which take place throughout a large proportion of late fetal life, also play a role in development of the lungs (5,6,7). Since it has been shown that FBM move fluid within the trachea (8,9) we have made a study of the flow of liquid in the fetal trachea and of the influence of respiratory activity.

Using a newly developed flowmeter sensitive to very low flow rates (10) we have found that the mean rate of fluid flow from the lungs of fetal sheep is 3.0–8.4 times greater during episodes of FBM than during apnoea (11). This difference was not present in fetuses in which the recurrent laryngeal nerves were sectioned, indicating that the muscles of the larynx play a regulatory role in the passage of fluid along the trachea. In preliminary experiments to investigate the role of the fetal larynx measurements of upper-airway resistance were made during episodes of FBM and apnoea and were partitioned into laryngeal and supralaryngeal components (12). These experiments showed that upper airway resistance to the efflux of fluid was higher during episodes of apnoea than during FBM and that the larynx was the major source of resistance.

Subsequently, we have extended these observations in fetuses with laryngeal

The Physiological Development of the Fetus and Newborn
ISBN 0 12 389080 2
Copyright © 1985 by Academic Press, London.
All rights of reproduction in any form reserved.

nerve sections and have measured upper airway resistance to the passage of fluid into the trachea from the pharynx. The function of the upper respiratory tract in influencing the flow of fluid to and from the trachea has been evaluated by measuring the flow of tracheal fluid when it was allowed to enter the amniotic sac directly, thus bypassing the entire upper airway.

Methods

The experiments were carried out in 15 fetal sheep between 119 and 140 days of gestation. Under halothane anaesthesia a 3 m re-entrant cannula was inserted into the cervical trachea of each fetus (12). Catheters were also implanted into the fetal trachea for the detection of FBM, into the pharynx and amniotic sac, and into the carotid artery and/or the jugular vein. The flow of liquid within the trachea was measured with a pressure-sensitive flowmeter incorporating a servo-controlled peristaltic pump (10). In 5 fetuses a large-diameter cannula with a "basket" tip to prevent blocking, was placed in the amniotic sac; this was used in the upper airway bypass experiments. Tracheal flow rates were calculated from polygraph recordings of integrated flow made over at least 8 h. Mean flow rates were derived by summing the flow during episodes of FBM or apnoea, or over the total period and dividing by the appropriate summed time intervals. The values expressed below are mean values for the 5 fetuses±SEM.

Results

Resistance to liquid entering the trachea from the pharynx

These experiments were performed by attaching a syringe to the ascending tracheal cannula and withdrawing fluid at a constant rate (0.2 or 0.5 ml/min) while measuring pressures within the cannula, pharynx, amniotic sac and lower trachea. When the fetuses were apneic an immediate fall in pressure occurred within the tracheal cannula indicating a very high resistance to the passage of fluid through the larynx towards the lungs. In the presence of FBM fluid could sometimes be withdrawn without a substantial fall in pressure, but only for short periods. When saline was simultaneously infused into the pharynx via a pharyngeal catheter (0.5 ml/min) fluid could be withdrawn for as long as continuous FBM were present. When they ceased, pressure within the tracheal cannula dropped sharply indicating laryngeal closure.

Resistance to the flow of liquid leaving the trachea via the larynx

Isotonic saline was infused into the ascending tracheal cannula at 0.2 to 0.5 ml/min while pressures were measured as described above. By subtracting amniotic from upper tracheal cannula pressure an estimate of total upper airway resistance could be obtained. In other experiments this resistance was partitioned into a laryngeal component (upper tracheal minus pharyngeal pressure) and a subtralaryngeal component (pharyngeal minus amniotic pressure). The mean resistance of the entire upper airway ($n=6$) was significantly greater ($P<0.025$) during periods of apnoea (24.7 ± 6.9 mmHg/ml/min) than when FBM were present ($4.6\pm2/4$ mmHg/ml/min). When upper airway resistance during apnoea was partitioned in 4 fetuses the larynx was found to present a greater resistance than the nasal or oral cavities. In 4 fetuses in which the recurrent laryngeal nerves had been sectioned the resistance of the upper airway during apnoea was significantly lower ($P<0.05$) than in intact fetuses.

Tracheal flow when the upper airway was bypassed

Flow measurements were made in 5 fetuses for at least 8 h before and after connecting the lower tracheal cannula to the amniotic sac cannula via the flowmeter. With the airway "intact" the mean flow rate from the lungs was 7.8 ± 0.9 ml/h. During episodes of FBM it was 12.9 ± 2.7 ml/h, representing a mean loss of 2.7 ± 0.5 ml from the lungs per episode. During periods of apnoea the mean efflux rate was 2.5 ± 1.0 ml/h, equivalent to 0.4 ± 0.1 ml per episode.

When the upper airway was bypassed, the mean rate of efflux from the lungs was 5.7 ± 1.1 ml/h. (In 2 fetuses, it was more than halved while it was altered little in the others). During episodes of FBM there was a net shift of fluid *into* the lungs from the amniotic sac in each fetus; the mean flow rate was 19.4 ± 6.9 ml/h representing a movement of 4.2 ± 1.2 ml into the lungs during each episode of FBM. When the fetuses became apnoeic there was a rapid flow of fluid out of the lungs; the mean flow rate was 37.0 ± 11.6 ml/h, equivalent to a loss of 6.7 ± 1.0 ml from the lungs during each period of apnoea. The flow of fluid from the lungs was often augmented during nonlabour uterine contractions. During 53 contractions which occurred in the 5 fetuses in the absence of FBM episodes, there was a mean flow rate of 81.3 ± 17.0 ml/h equivalent to a loss of 11.6 ± 2.7 ml from the lungs.

Discussion

The importance of the upper airway to fetal lung development has recently been demonstrated by the studies of Fewell et al. (4) in which fetal tracheostomy led to impaired lung growth. This manoeuvre abolishes the slight distending pressure present in the lungs when fetal breathing movements are absent (13). Our data demonstrate that the major component of upper airway resistance is the larynx; it is largely dependent upon the integrity of the recurrent laryngeal nerves and is abolished by fetal paralysis (12). This conclusion contrasts with that of Fewell and Johnson (14) who considered that the major site of resistance to outward movement of fluid lay above the larynx; insertion of nasopharyngeal tubes in 2 fetuses caused the apparent equalization of tracheal and amniotic pressures. It is possible that in some fetuses the pharyngeal muscles contribute to upper airway resistance, but the major contribution is likely to be the laryngeal adductor muscles (15).

The resistance of the larynx to fluid movement towards the lungs is also dependent upon fetal breathing movements. Fluid could only be drawn through the larynx when FBM were present, presumably due to rhythmical abductor muscle activity (15). However, the ability to do this depends on the presence of fluid in the pharynx. It seems probable that the fetal pharynx does not normally contain fluid because (a) it was rarely possible to sample fluid from the pharyngeal catheters and (b) it was usually necessary to introduce fluid into the pharynx to permit a flow of fluid through the larynx towards the lungs. In the absence of FBM, the larynx behaves as a valve (16) allowing flow towards the pharynx but not towards the lungs.

That the upper airway plays a major role in regulating the flow of fluid from the lungs, and hence in the maintenance of lung volume is amply demonstrated by the altered pattern of flow during its bypass. Allowing the lower trachea to connect directly with the amniotic sac led to a reversal of the normal pattern of flow of pulmonary fluid during episodes of FBM; instead of a net efflux there was a substantial influx. Furthermore the flow of fluid out of the lungs during periods of apnoea was greatly increased in the absence of the upper airway, particularly when the uterus contracted. Thus the upper airway, during episodes of FBM, has the effect of promoting efflux of fluid against a normal tendency for influx generated by FBM. This effect may be achieved by fluid entering the pharynx, due to rhythmical abduction of the larynx, to be either swallowed or lost to the amniotic sac. It is unlikely that this fluid normally pools in the pharynx, but appears to be expelled leaving the pharynx devoid of contents. Rhythmical abduction of the larynx is capable of generating negative pressures in the upper trachea which may contribute to the expulsion of fluid into the pharynx.

Bypass of the upper respiratory tract allowed amniotic fluid to enter the lungs when FBM were present. In 2 fetuses there was a striking irreversible reduction in overall production of lung liquid but the cause of this is not clear. The greater viscosity of amniotic fluid may have led to an increase in resistance to flow in the tracheal loop, retarding efflux of fluid, but this was not evident in the other fetuses.

In conclusion, the upper airway seems to be essential for the net loss of fluid from the lungs in the presence of FBM, protecting the pulmonary epithelium from the entry of amniotic fluid which may contain potentially harmful substances such as meconium (17). During periods of apnoea egress of lung liquid is retarded, principally by the action of the laryngeal adductor muscles. In the absence of the retarding effect of the upper airway, substantial volumes of fluid may be lost from the lungs, particularly during uterine contractions, adversely affecting their growth.

References

1. Alcorn, D., Adamson, T. M., Lambert, T. F., Maloney, J. E., Ritchie, B. C. and Robinson, P. M. (1977). *J. Anat.* **123**, 649-660.
2. Harrison, M. R., Bressack, M. A., Chung, A. M. and De Lorimier, A. B. (1980). *Surgery* **88**, 260-268.
3. Liggins, G. C. and Kitterman, J. A. (1981). *In:* "The Fetus and Independent Life", Ciba Foundation Symposium no. 86, pp. 308-330. Pitman, London.

4. Fewell, J. E., Hislop, A. A., Kitterman, J. A. and Johnson, P. (1983). *J. Appl. Physiol.* **55**, 1103-1108.
5. Wigglesworth, J. S. and Desai, R. (1979). *Early Human Dev.* **3**, 51-65.
6. Liggins, G. C., Vilos, G. A., Campos, G. A., Kitterman, J. A. and Lee, C. H. (1981). *J. Develop. Physiol.* **3**, 267-274.
7. Liggins, G. C., Vilos, G. A., Campos, G. A., Kitterman, J. A. and Lee, C. H. (1981). *J. Develop. Physiol.* **3**, 275-282.
8. Dawes, G. S. (1973). *In:* "Fetal and Neonatal Physiology" (R. S. Comline, K. W. Cross, G. S. Dawes and P. W. Nathanielsz, eds) pp. 49-62, Cambridge University Press.
9. Maloney, J. E., Adamson, T. M., Brodecky, V., Cranage, S., Lambert, T. F. and Richie, B. C. (1975). *J. Appl. Physiol.* **39**, 423-428.
10. Wickham, P. J. D. and Harding, R. (1984). *Med. Biol. Eng. Comput.* (in press).
11. Harding, R., Sigger, J. N., Wickham, P. J. D. and Bocking, A. D. (1984). *Resp. Physiol.* (in press).
12. Harding, R. (1984). *J. Develop. Physiol.* **6** (in press).
13. Vilos, G. A. and Liggins, G. C. (1982). *J. Develop. Physiol.* **4**, 247-256.
14. Fewell, J. E. and Johnson, P. (1983). *J. Physiol.* **339**, 495-504.
15. Harding, R., Johnson, P. and McClelland, M. E. (1980). *Resp. Physiol.* **40**, 165-180.
16. Brown, M. J., Olver, R. E., Ramsden, C. A., Strang, L. B. and Walters, D. (1983). *J. Physiol.* **344**, 137-152.
17. Jose, J. H., Schreiner, R. L., Lemons, J. A., Gresham, E. L., Mirkin, L. D., Siddiqui, A. and Cohen,M. (1983). *Pediat. Res.* **17**, 976-981.

The Effects of Arginine Vasopressin on Lung Liquid Secretion in Chronic Fetal Sheep

A. M. Perks and S. Cassin

Department of Physiology, College of Medicine, J. Hillis Miller Health Center, University of Florida, Gainesville, Florida, USA and Department of Zoology, University of British Columbia, Vancouver, BC, Canada

The fetal lungs produce large quantities of fluid, which pass to the fetal gut and amniotic cavity (1). The production is probably important for correct lung development (1), and for fetal salt and water regulation (2). However, it is vital to stop production, and clear the lungs at birth. One possible factor in these changes is arginine vasopressin (AVP). AVP is known to direct water movement towards the fetus through many fetal membranes (3), and it is liberated in large quantities at birth (4,5). Our initial studies, in late fetal goats under anaesthesia, showed that intravenous AVP could slow lung liquid secretion, and promote reabsorption (6). However, it was important to extend investigations to other species, and to chronic preparations free of the immediate effects of surgery and anaesthesia. Accordingly, the results given here follow lung liquid production through development and birth in chronic fetal sheep, and investigate the effects of AVP.

Methods

Thirty pregnant sheep of 122–134 days of gestation were used for developmental studies, 12 for investigations of AVP. Mothers were anaesthesized with halothane. Under sterile conditions, a loop of silicone tubing was inserted into the lower trachea of the fetus (length of loop, 230 cm; internal diameter, 0.264 cm; volume, 15.0 ml). In normal conditions, the loop allowed lung liquid to continue to the buccal cavity; during experiments, the closing of a T-piece halfway along the loop allowed withdrawal of fluid from the lungs. Polyvinyl catheters were placed

The Physiological Development of the Fetus and Newborn
ISBN 0 12 389080 2

Copyright © 1985 by Academic Press, London.
All rights of reproduction in any form reserved.

in the fetal carotid artery and jugular vein, the amniotic space, and the maternal femoral artery and vein. Cannulae were tunneled under the maternal skin to a pouch on the flank. After 5 days, the tracheal loop was clamped, and impermeant tracers were added to the lungs (450 mg Blue Dextran 2000, Pharmacia, and 500 000 dpm albumen $-I^{125}$). Rates of secretion of fluid and ions were determined from rates of dilution of tracers, and concentrations of ions, as described elsewhere (2). Fetal weights were determined according to Robillard and Weitzman (7).

Results

Lung liquid production through gestation and delivery

Fifty-four estimates of lung liquid production from 30 chronic fetal sheep between 128–145 days gestation averaged 3.1 ± 0.3 ml/kg/h (9.2 ± 1.0 ml/h). However, production rates changed through gestation (Fig. 1). Both the 2.2-fold rise to

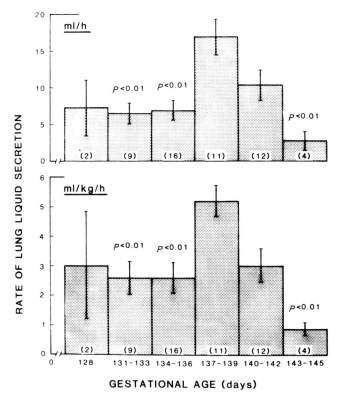

Figure 1. Lung liquid secretion rates in chronic fetal sheep through late gestation. Vertical bars represent standard errors of the mean. Numbers of fetuses are shown on each column. Significances are relative to fetuses at 137–139 days gestation.

5.2 ± 0.6 ml/kg/h at 137–139 days gestation, and the subsequent 83% fall by 143–145 days gestation, were significant at $P < 0.01$ (ANOVA/Newman-Keuls). The levels at 143–145 days gestation were the lowest recorded (0.87 ± 0.42 ml/kg/h). However, a more dramatic fall was seen during a spontaneous delivery at 142 days gestation. Over the 3 h before delivery, production averaged 3.1 ml/kg/h (ion production: Cl^-, 0.41; Na^+, 0.48; K^+, 0.018 mEquiv./h). There was no change at rupture of the membranes. During the 10 min taken for delivery, the lungs remained closed, and no air entered. However, 3 samples of fluid were obtained, and there was a 30.2% fall in the fluid, Cl^-, Na^+ and K^+ ions present in the lungs, mainly within the last 5 min. The average rate of reabsorption during the delivery was 4.4 ml/min, or 73.0 ml/kg/h.

The effects of AVP on lung liquid secretion

Twelve fetuses of 128–142 days gestation, with an average secretion rate of 3.7 ± 0.6 ml/kg/h (12.3 ± 2.3 ml/h), were used in studies of AVP (8 tests), or as controls (8 tests), as follows:

Older fetuses (134–142 days gestation). Four fetuses with an average secretion rate of 4.9 ± 1.1 ml/kg/h were infused with synthetic AVP (Sigma) for 2 h (7.4–20.5 mU/kg/min), in intravenous saline (0.0764 ml/min). All fetuses showed prolonged decreases in secretion. Reductions were significant in 3 fetuses in the first hour ($P < 0.05$–0.001), and in all fetuses by the second hour ($P < 0.01$–0.001). In all cases, the effects continued and increased during the 2 h after termination of infusion. One fetus showed reabsorption by the final hour (0.3 ml/kg/h). Average values for these fetuses are shown in Fig. 2a; reductions in successive hours were 1.1, 0.9, 2.6 and 3.0 ml/kg/h, or 23, 19, 53 and 62% (all significant, $P < 0.01$–0.0005). It is probable that this prolonged response eventually reversed, since one fetus, tested 18 hours after infusion, had returned to 8% above its original rate. Changes in electrolyte secretion followed those for volume. Chloride secretion fell 44, 43, 76 and 87% in successive hours (all significant, $P < 0.05$–0.005; initial rate, 0.66 ± 0.21 mEquiv./h). Na^+ ion secretion fell similarly: K^+ ion secretion also fell, but the reductions were less consistent and the average changes were not significant.

Younger fetuses (128–134 days gestation). In contrast, younger fetuses, with an average secretion rate of 3.8 ± 0.8 ml/kg/h, did not respond to AVP in similar doses (6.6–11.3 mU/kg/min; Fig. 2b). In fact, electrolytes showed small increases in secretion. The possibility that the responses to AVP developed at 134 days gestation was confirmed in 1 fetus, which gave no response on day 133, but responded strongly to a lower dose on day 134. However, one additional fetus at 131 days showed a transitory reabsorption during the second hour of AVP.

Control fetuses showed no responses similar to those treated with AVP. Four older fetuses (136–141 days gestation; average secretion rate 4.6 ± 0.9 ml/kg/h)

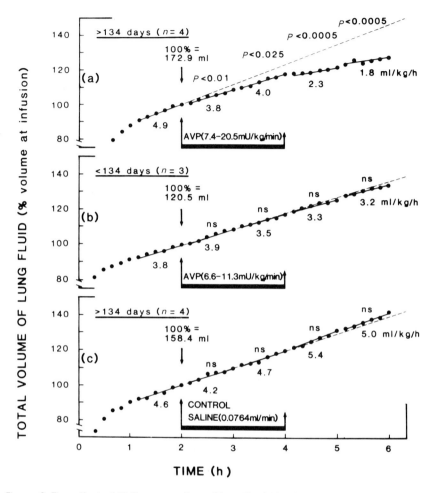

Figure 2. The effect of AVP on secretion of lung liquid in chronic fetal sheep. (a) i.v. to fetuses above 134 days gestation (average of 4 fetuses). (b) i.v. to fetuses below 134 days gestation (average of 3 fetuses). (c) i.v. to fetuses above 134 days gestation (average of 4 fetuses). *Ordinates:* Total volume of lung secretion, expressed as a percentage of the volume at infusion (100% volume = (a) 172.9 ± 59.3 ml; (b) 120.5 ± 5.0 ml; (c) 158.4 ± 18.8 ml). Regressions are lines of best fit (least squares), over 1 h intervals. Rates (ml/kg/h) are given below the regressions; significance of changes from the rate before infusion are given above the regressions.

given saline infusions at the usual rate, showed slight increases in secretion later in the experiments, but on average these were not significant (Fig. 2c). One younger fetus (131 days gestation) increased production significantly with saline. Three fetuses (140–142 days gestation) left without infusion, showed no significant change over 4 h.

Discussion

These results suggest that lung liquid production in chronic fetal sheep falls in the last week before delivery, but reabsorption over birth is more dramatic. This confirms other workers (8,9,10), but differs from our previous results in acute fetal goats, where there was an exponential increase until term. However, the ability of AVP to cause prolonged reduction in secretion, or reabsorption, is similar in both species. The emergence of the response close to term is also similar, although 3 days later in the sheep. The mechanism of the effect of AVP is unknown, although it differs from that of lung expansion, since there was no movement of K^+ ions into the lungs (6).

The effect of AVP may well be physiological. All except the single highest dose would raise plasma AVP to plateau levels of 300–470 μU/ml (Rurak (11) private communication). Despite large variations in published fetal plasma levels, these values lie below limits reported for vaginal deliveries in sheep (4,12) and humans (5,13). In addition, they do not represent threshold values. Finally, AVP is unlikely to act alone; epinephrine (6,10) and lung expansion (6) have similar effects. However, all these factors produce slow, prolonged responses, more adapted to long-term drainage of the lungs than to the rapid reabsorption which we saw at birth. Therefore, there may be further stimuli which act at birth, or other changes, such as a rapid surge of blood through newborn lungs, which augment and maximize their effects.

References

1. Strang, L. B. (1977). "Neonatal Respiration; Physiological and Clinical Studies." p. 316, Blackwell Scientific Publications, Oxford.
2. Cassin, S. and Perks, A. M. (1982). *J. Develop. Physiol.* **4**, 311–325.
3. Perks, A. M., Vizsolyi, E., Holt, W. F. and Cassin, S. (1978). *In:* "Comparative Endocrinology" (Gaillard, P. J. and Boer, H. H., eds) pp. 231–234, Elsevier/North-Holland Biomedical Press, Amsterdam.
4. Stark, R. I., Daniel, S. S., Husain, K. M., James, L. S. and Vande Wiele, R. L. (1979). *Biol. Neonate* **35**, 235–241.
5. Pohjavuori, M. and Fyhrquist, F. (1980). *J. Pediat.* **97**, 462–465.
6. Perks, A. M. and Cassin, S. (1982). *Chest* **81** (suppl.) 63S–65S.
7. Robillard, J. E. and Weitzman, R. E. (1980). *Am. J. Physiol.* **238**, F407–F414.
8. Kitterman, J. A., Ballard, P. L., Clements, J. A., Mescher, E. J. and Tooley, W. H. (1979). *J. Appl. Physiol.* **47**, 985–989.
9. Dickson, K. A., Wilkinson, M. H., Berger, P. J. and Maloney, J. E. (1983). *Proc. Int. Union Physiol. Sci.* **15**, 82.
10. Brown, M. J., Olver, R. E., Ramsden, C. A., Strang, L. B. and Walters, D. V. (1983). *J. Physiol.* **344**, 137–152.
11. Rurak, D. W. (1978). *J. Physiol.* **277**, 341–357.
12. Stark, R., Hussain, K., Daniel, S., Milliez, J., Morishima, H. and James, S. L. (1977). *Pediat. Res.* **11**, 412.
13. Chard, T., Hudson, C. N., Edwards, C. R. W. and Boyd, N. R. H. (1971). *Nature* **234**, 352–354.

An Active Expiratory Reflex in Preterm Ventilated Infants

Anne Greenough, C. J. Morley and P. Johnson[*]

Department of Paediatrics, University of Cambridge, UK
[*]Department of Obstetrics and Gynaecology, University of Oxford, Oxford, UK

Introduction

We have previously demonstrated that preterm infants suffering from the respiratory distress syndrome (RDS) were not simply the passive recipients of artificial ventilation (1). Their spontaneous respiration interacted with artificial ventilation in 5 distinct patterns, which were in part due to stimulation of mechanical respiratory reflexes by the positive pressure inflation (2). One of these interactions, an active expiratory response was shown to proceed the development of pneumothoraces (1). Although paralysis of infants demonstrating this particular response successfully prevented the development of air leaks in the majority of infants, this was not without side-effects (3). The present study tried to elucidate why some infants "fight the ventilator" in this manner and in particular whether the exact timing of ventilator inflation during the infant's spontaneous respiratory cycle was important.

Patients

Seventy infants, of gestational ages from 24–33 weeks, were included in the study. All the babies were less than 1 week old and were ventilated to treat the respiratory distress syndrome (RDS) by Bourne ventilators (no. 202) through 3.0 or 3.5 nasotracheal tubes. The infants were included in the study if they were able to breathe spontaneously during a temporary disconnection from the ventilator.

Methods

The 70 infants had respiratory recordings on 88 separate occasions. A pneumo-tachograph (Mercury F10L) placed between the endotracheal tube and the

The Physiological Development of the Fetus and Newborn
ISBN 0 12 389080 2

Copyright © 1985 by Academic Press, London.
All rights of reproduction in any form reserved.

ventilator circuit recorded flow changes, both due to the infant and the ventilator. This was connected to a Mercury differential pressure transducer and the signal was then integrated electronically to volume. The infant's spontaneous respiratory activity was recorded by a hand-made latex oesophageal balloon (2.0×0.6 cm, wall thickness 0.05 mm) connected to a Mercury pressure transducer. The balloon was placed in the lower third of the oesophagus. Ventilator pressure was recorded from the infant's side of the pneumotanchograph using a third Mercury pressure transducer. All the pressure transducers used had identical speeds of response confirmed by a balloon burst technique.

The signals were recorded on a Gould 6 channel recorder, which had a maximum full scale response frequency of 60 Hz. Respiratory recordings were made at a paper speed of 10 mm/second.

From these recordings dynamic compliance was calculated during a temporary disconnection from the ventilator, using the oesophageal pressure changes due to a spontaneous breath between periods of zero flow and the tidal volume. Static compliance was also calculated, using peak ventilator pressures maintained for a plateau of at least 0.5 s and the resultant tidal volume. In the babies who were actively expiring against the ventilator only dynamic compliance could be measured, because their active expiratory efforts interfered with the measurement of static compliance (4).

From the respiratory recordings the average inspiratory time (Ti) and expiratory time (Te) of 10 regular spontaneous breaths during intermittent ventilation were calculated, this was found to be Ti of 0.39 ± 0.02 s ($\bar{x}\pm$SEM) and Te of 0.38 ± 0.02 s. The relationship of the timing of spontaneous respiration and positive pressure inflation was determined by measuring the time from the onset of ventilator inflation to the end of spontaneous inspiration.

The type of respiratory response the infant was making inflation was determined from 100 ventilator breaths. Infants were actively expiring against positive pressure inflation if on more than 80% of ventilator inflations the oesophageal pressure recording showed the infant was expiring and this corresponded to a reduction in tidal volume compared to that which occurred as a result of unimpeded inflation. Infants who were making this response on less than 20% of ventilator inflations were considered to be not actively expiring.

This study had the approval of the Cambridge Ethical Committee.

Statistical Analysis

Students *t* test.

Results

Thirty four infants on 46 occasions were actively expiring against the ventilator. Those infants were more mature (29.5 ± 1.7 $\bar{x}\pm$SD) than the nonactive expiratory group (28.2 ± 2.3 weeks, gestational age) $P<0.05$. The active expiratory group also had stiffer lungs (0.4 ± 0.2 ml/cm H_2O, $\bar{x}\pm$SD) when compared to the infants passively expiring (0.6 ± 0.2 ml/cm H_2O) ($P<0.01$).

The 2 groups of infants were of similar postnatal ages, 17.2 h (median, range 1 h to 6 days) for the nonactive expiration group (NS).

On 44 of the occasions infants were studied active expiration was stimulated only when ventilator inflation commenced within a "window" approximately 0.2 s before or after the end of spontaneous inspiration 0.08 ± 0.01 ($\bar{x}$ SEM) before and 0.05 ± 0.01 s after. On the other 2 occasions an active expiratory response was stimulated in one when the start of ventilator inflation occurred at 0.25 s before the end of inspiration and in the second at the start of inspiration.

Analysis of the data from the infants not actively expiring showed that during their recordings the start of ventilator inflation rarely occurred within this "window", that is ± 0.2 s from end inspiration. Instead if ventilator inflation occurred at the start of a spontaneous breath, inspiration continued or at slow ventilator rates an augmented inspiration was provoked (2). Inflation late in expiration prolonged the expiratory period. On only 5 ventilator inflations, during all the study occasions involving the nonactive expiratory infants, did positive pressure inflation occur within the previously defined window. Once at 0.2 s before the end of inspiration provoking an augmented inspiration and on the other 4 occasions ventilator inflation occurred after the end of inspiration (0.2, 0.15, 0.2, 0.2 s) and stimulated a lengthened expiration.

Following reconnection to the ventilator, following the measurement of dynamic compliance, infants in the active expiration group altered their respiratory pattern in such a manner that within 6 ventilator breaths, the start of positive pressure inflation again occurred at the end of inspiration and the infants were stimulated to actively expire. No such trend was seen in the passive expiration group, whose spontaneous respiratory pattern tended to be more irregular than the actively expiring infants. Both active expiration and other respiratory responses were seen at all frequencies of ventilation studied, (10, 20, 30, 40, 60/min).

Discussion

We have attempted to define a respiratory window at end inspiration, in which positive pressure inflation provoked an active expiratory response. Although infants passively expiring tended to have more compliant lungs, both groups of infants were ventilated in a similar manner. Infants actively expiring even altered their respiratory pattern following disconnection from the ventilator so that the start of positive pressure inflation again coincided with the "respiratory window". Further investigation is necessary to determine why certain infants become entrained in this manner, which is so disadvantageous to them (3). However the present results may have practical potential, if servo assisted ventilation could be simply directed away from this "window" it might be possible to reduce the amount of active expiration and its sequalae without having to resort the two-edged sword of paralysis (3).

Acknowledgements

This work was supported by a grant from the Medical Research Council.

References

1. Greenough, A., Morley, C. J. and Davis, J. A. (1983). *J. Pediat.* **103**, 769–773.
2. Greenough, A., Morley, C. J. and Davis, J. A. (1983). *Early Hum. Dev.* **8**, 65–75.
3. Greenough, A., Wood, S., Morley, C. J. and Davis, J. A. (1984). *Lancet* **1**, 1–3.
4. Greenough, A., Morley, C. J. and Wood, S. (1983). *Biol. Neonate* **44**, 322–323.

Provoked Augmented Inspirations in Ventilated Premature Infants

Anne Greenough and C. J. Morley

Department of Paediatrics, University of Cambridge,
Cambridge, UK

Introduction

Augmented inspirations, likened to Head's paradoxical reflex (1), can be provoked
by lung inflation in human neonates (2). Mead and Collier (3) demonstrated this
reflex to be important in increasing and maintaining lung compliance and
suggested that it may have a role in reopening collapsed airways. Positive pressure
inflation by artificial ventilation in preterm infants can, under certain
circumstances, stimulate augmented inspirations (4,5). This paper describes
the possible stimulating and moderating effects of this reflex in ventilated
neonates and a subsequent study which investigated the effectiveness of
theophylline to increase the occurrence of this reflex and so possibly increase
compliance.

Methods

Forty neonates were studied on 112 different 30-min occasions. Their postnatal
ages were 1 h to 8 weeks and gestational ages 24–33 weeks. The infants were
suffering from respiratory distress syndrome (RDS) or bronchopulmonary
dysplasia. All the infants were ventilated through 3.0 mm endotracheal tubes by
time-cycled, pressure limited Bourne ventilators. The ventilator rates, pressures,
inspiratory-expiratory ratio and oxygen concentrations were adjusted only by the
clinical team caring for the infant. During the study period the infants remained
in their incubators receiving full supportive care.

The infant's response to positive pressure inflation was recorded using a hand-
made latex oesophageal balloon on a 6 french gauge nasogastric feeding tube which
was attached to a Mercury pressure transducer. Tidal flow was measured by a

The Physiological Development of the Fetus and Newborn
ISBN 0 12 389080 2

Copyright © 1985 by Academic Press, London.
All rights of reproduction in any form reserved.

pneumotachograph (Mercury F2L), placed between the endotracheal tube and the ventilator circuit. This was attached to a Mercury differential pressure transducer and its signal was then integrated electronically to volume. Ventilator pressure changes were measured from the endotracheal tube, by another pressure transducer, on the infant's side of the pneumotachograph. These signals were recorded simultaneously on a Gould polygraph. All the transducers were matched and had identical response frequencies.

Static compliance was measured using peak pressure inflation maintained at a plateau for 0.5 s and the resultant volume change. Dynamic compliance was measured, during a temporary disconnection from the ventilator, using the oesophageal pressure changes between periods of zero airflow and tidal volumes. To minimize errors due to possible leaks around the endotracheal tube expiratory volumes were used. Both static and dynamic compliance were calculated from of 10 breaths on at least 3 separate occasions during the study period. If there was not good agreement between the 2 measurements then the results from that study occasion were not used.

Each recording was analysed for ventilator provoked augmented inspirations. These were present, if during ventilator inflation, there was a sharp negative deflection in the oesophageal pressure trace, at least twice that caused by spontaneous inspiration (see Fig. 1). The inspiratory reflex started at the beginning of the augmented negative deflection in the oesophageal pressure recording (A).

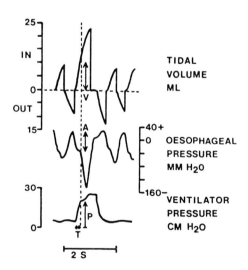

Figure 1. This demonstrates a provoked augmented inspiration. The upper trace is the volume recording, the integrator resets to zero at zero airflow. An upward deflection represents inspiration and a downward deflection expiration. The middle trace is the oesophageal pressure recording, downward deflection are caused by spontaneous inspiratory activity. The lower trace is the ventilator pressure. Reproduced with permission from *Early Human Development* (5).

At that point the inflating volume (V) and pressure (P) were noted. The time from the start of inflation to the beginning of the augmented inspiration was calculated (T). The frequency of elicitation of the reflex was expressed as the percentage of ventilator inflations which provoked the infant to make an augmented inspiration.

In another study 6 infants (gestational ages 27–30 weeks) were given theophylline orally, 5 mg/kg/24 h in 4 divided doses. Theophylline was given when the infant's RDS had improved sufficiently to reduce the ventilator settings to a rate of 20/min and a peak inflating pressure to 20 cm H_2O. The effect of theophylline was assessed by comparing closely for gestational and postnatal age, sex, type of delivery and place of birth. Lecithin to sphingomyelin ratios were measured from gastric aspirates obtained at birth. Compliance was measured before treatment with theophylline, at a similar postnatal age in the controls and again 6 h later in both groups.

This study was approved by the Cambridge ethical committee.

Statistical Analysis

Wilcoxon rank sum test.

Results

Augmented inspirations were seen in 18% of the studies. The frequency of elicitation on each occasion was independent of the infant's gestational age and blood gas status. However, regardless of the infant's maturity, augmented inspirations could only be provoked during the first five postnatal days.

The frequency of elicitation of the augmented inspirations and the ventilator pressure (P) which provoked the reflex were inversely proportional to lung compliance. The volume (V) at which the reflex occurred was similar in all infants especially when related to body weight, $(5.7 \pm 1.1$ ml/kg body weight, $\bar{x} \pm$ SD).

Augmented inspirations always occurred within 0.22 ± 0.05 s ($\bar{x} \pm$ SD) after the onset of ventilator inflation.

The highest incidence of provoked augmented inspirations was 50% of ventilator inflations. The reflex only occurred if the ventilator rate was less than or equal to 15 breaths/min. If the ventilator rate was increased above this, augmented inspirations were no longer provoked. This suggested that the refractory period of the reflex was at least 8 s.

The 6 infants given theophylline in the recovery phase of RDS had significantly better compliances 6 h after commencing treatment than the matched controls

Table 1			
L/S Ratio compliance		1.45 ± 0.43	1.58 ± 0.42
Pre-treatment	(ml/cmH$_2$O)	0.4 ± 0.1	0.5 ± 0.2
compliance			
6 h later		1.0 ± 0.2	0.5 ± 0.2
($\bar{x} \pm$ SD)			

of a similar postnatal age ($P<0.01$), see Table 1. During treatment with theophylline the frequency of provoked augmented inspirations had increased with respect to the infant's compliance.

Discussion

These results suggest that a rapidly adapting stretch receptor is involved in mediating this reflex, as augmented inspirations were always provoked at the start of positive pressure inflation by a similar volume in all infants, when related to body weight. The inverse relationship both between the frequency of elicitation of this reflex and the provoking pressure (P) and the compliance also supports this hypothesis.

Preliminary evidence suggests that theophylline may have a role in weaning preterm infants from ventilation (6). The results presented here suggest a possible mechanism for theophylline's action. Infants treated with theophylline in this study had more compliant lungs than matched controls, who had similar L/S ratios. This improvement in compliance could have been due to the increase in the frequency of elicitation of provoked augmented inspirations seen in the "theophylline" infants.

Acknowledgements

This work was supported by a grant from the Medical Research Council. Dr C. M. Hill and Mrs B. Brown performed the analysis of the gastric aspirates.

References

1. Head, H. (1889). *J. Physiol.* **10**, 1-70.
2. Cross, K. W., Klaus, K., Tooley, W. H. and Weisser, K. (1960). *J. Physiol.* **151**, 551-556.
3. Mead, J. and Collier, C. (1959). *J. Appl. Physiol.* **14**, 669-678.
4. Greenough, A., Morley, C. J. and Davis, J. A. (1983). *Early Hum. Dev.* **8**, 65-75.
5. Greenough, A., Morley, C. J. and Davis, J. A. (1984). *Early Hum. Dev.* **9**, 111-117.
6. Barr, P. A. (1978). *Arch Dis Child.* **53**, 598-600.

Stability of the Control of Breathing in Newborn Infants: A Non-linear Mathematical Analysis

J. P. Cleave, P. J. Fleming, M. R. Levine and A. M. Long

Departments of Mathematics, Child Health and Physiology,
University of Bristol, Bristol, UK

The respiratory responses to spontaneous disturbances of respiration (e.g. sighs), in QS, change with age in normal infants (1). When expressed as sequential values of the fractional deviation of $\dot{V}_E$ (the breath-by-breath minute ventilation), from the mean, these responses can be fitted with linear second order equations representing a critically damped or underdamped response

$$y = A\,(1 + \beta t)e^{-\beta t} \text{ or } y = Ae^{-\beta t}\cos\,(\omega t + \phi) \tag{1}$$

The early responses are of long period and highly damped. With increasing age both period and damping decrease, until at a time between 1 and 3 months marked oscillations are seen. Thereafter the damping increases but the period remains short. The response is therefore rapid and the oscillations die away rapidly. These responses are stable, i.e. the disturbance dies away and the ventilation returns to the pre-sigh level. Mathematically the condition for stability is that $-\beta$ (eq. 1) is negative. The question arises as to the meaning to be attached to instability. We have investigated this mathematically using a simple nonlinear physiological model (2).

As a first step we define a simple model (2) in terms of the CO_2 feedback alone. The model is intended to describe the response of the respiratory system, initially in a state of equilibrium, to a sudden change in the concentration of CO_2 in the lungs brought about by a deep breath or sigh.

The Physiological Development of the Fetus and Newborn
ISBN 0 12 389080 2
Copyright © 1985 by Academic Press, London.
All rights of reproduction in any form reserved.

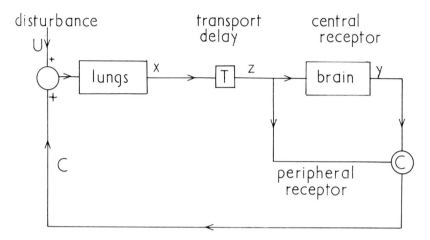

Figure 1. Control system diagram. $x = C_{aCO_2}$ at the lungs; $y = C_{BCO_2}$ the concentration of CO_2 within the brain compartment; $z = C_{aCO_2}$ at the brain. C is the controller function; T is the transport delay between the lungs and brain compartment and also between lungs and peripheral receptors. U is the disturbance.

We regard the lungs as a box of constant volume and homogeneous content ventilated by a continuous stream of gas. The rate of flow of gas through the lung compartment is a continuous variable $\dot{V}_E$.

A block diagram of the model is given in Fig. 1. The output of the lung compartment, $PaCO_2$ (mmHg), is conveyed via the blood stream to the central chemoreceptor, which senses PCO_2 in the brain compartment, and to the peripheral chemoreceptor, which senses PCO_2 in the carotid artery. $\dot{V}_E$ is in turn a function C of the receptor outputs. Changes in PaO_2 are not dealt with explicitly here but would exert their effect by altering the function C. The venous concentration of CO_2, C_VCO_2, is assumed to be at a constant steady value as in the cardiac output Q and the cerebral blood flow Q_B.

The behaviour of the model is defined in terms of three variables, x, y, z, which are concentrations of CO_2 at the points shown on the figure. We express the relations between these variables in eqs 2–4. Note that the eq. 2 for x is non-linear.

From Millhorn (3) we get equations for x and y.

$$\frac{dx}{dt} = \frac{\dot{Q}}{V_A k} (C_{VCO2} - x) - \frac{\dot{V}_E}{V_A} \cdot x \qquad (2)$$

$$\frac{dy}{dt} = \frac{MR_{BCO2}}{V_B} + \frac{\dot{Q}_B}{V_B} (z - y) \qquad (3)$$

In order to represent z in terms of x and the circulatory delay T, we may approximate a finite delay (T) in a feedback loop by a distributed delay.

Thus $z(t) = \int_{\sigma}^{\infty} De^{-D\tau} x(t-\tau)d\tau$, where $D = 1/T$,

then $\quad \dfrac{dz}{dt} = D(x-z)$ \hfill (4)

also $\quad \dot{V}_E = C(z, y)$.

The concepts of dynamical systems can be used to investigate this model (4,5). First we find where the equilibrium points lie in the three-dimensional phase space (x, y, z). Secondly we classify the equilibrium points in terms of the response to small displacements of x from equilibrium. Trajectories will move towards a stable equilibrium point away from an unstable one. They may move in an oscillatory pattern or follow a monotonic path.

There is a unique equilibrium point x_0 y_0 z_0 defined by $\dot{x} = \dot{y} = \dot{z} = 0$. Near this point the solutions of 2, 3, 4 are approximately those of the linearized form of 2, 3, 4 and so of the form

$$y = k_1 e^{\lambda_1 t} + k_2 e^{\lambda_2 t} + k_3 e^{\lambda_3 t}, \hfill (5)$$

where $\lambda_1, \lambda_2, \lambda_3,$ —are the eigenvalues of the linearized form of 2,3,4. If $\lambda_2, \lambda_3,$ are complex conjugates with $\lambda_2 = -\beta + i\omega$

$$y = k_1 e^{\lambda_1 t} + k_4 e^{-\beta t} \cos(\omega t + \phi). \hfill (6)$$

When the first term (third-order component) in this equation is small, this equation is similar to the empirically derived second-order model described above (eq. 1).

Stability of the system is defined in terms of the values of λ_1 and β. If λ_1 or $-\beta$ are positive the equilibrium point is unstable.

We have derived a condition for instability in terms of the model parameters, namely that there exist values of the parameters for which the equilibrium point is unstable with two conjugate eigenvalues having positive real parts if:

$$\frac{k\, x_0\, C_y}{\dot{Q} + kC} > 4\left\{1 + \sqrt{1 + \frac{k\, x_0\, C_z}{\dot{Q} + kC}}\right\},$$

where C, C_y and C_z are respectively the controller function and its derivatives with respect to y and z at the equilibrium point. We have shown mathematically that when the two complex conjugate eigenvalues have small but positive real parts then the equilibrium point is unstable and the system will respond to a disturbance by going into a limit cycle, i.e. the trajectory of the solution in the three-dimensional space defined by x, y, z, will approach a closed path around the equilibrium point. In dynamical systems theory this transition is called a Hopf bifurcation.

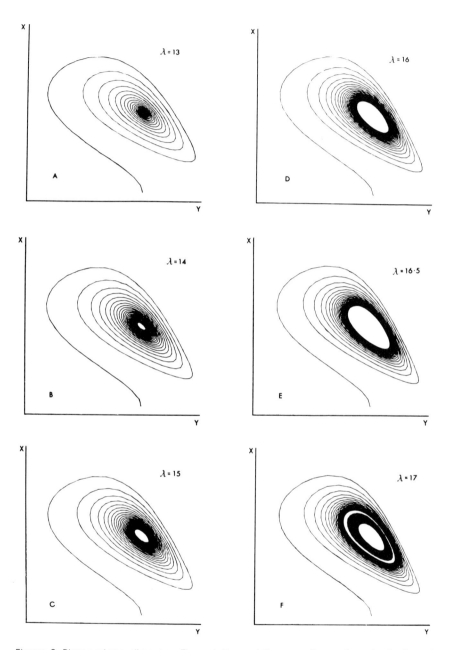

Figure 2. Phase plane diagram. The solutions of the equations after x is displaced to 0.1 of its equilibrium value. The response of the system is illustrated by plotting x versus y. In addition the result of displacing x to 0.9 of its equilibrium value is superimposed on F.

Using the Runge Kutta algorithm we have solved some differential equations of the type 2, 3, 4, numerically to demonstrate the transition from stability to instability.

$$\dot{x} = 1 - x. \exp\left(\lambda\left(\frac{5}{6}y + \frac{1}{6}z - 2\right)\right)$$

$$\dot{y} = \frac{6}{5} - y + z$$

$$\dot{z} = x - z$$

For $0 < \lambda < 16$ the equilibrium point is asymptotically stable (Figs 2A,B,C). As λ increases through 16, two eigenvalues cross into the right-hand half of the complex plane. A Hopf bifurcation ensues — the equilibrium point becomes unstable and a stable limit cycle in created (Figs 2D,E,F).

If we examine the form of the function C, (6) we can see a simple way in which instability could occur. There are thresholds for each receptor below which there is no response to CO_2, and these thresholds are different for central and peripheral chemoreceptors. Thus, if the equilibrium point is near one of these thresholds then a small change in equilibrium point can result in a large change in either C_y or C_z. Thus a change in regime, from stable to unstable, can result from a small change in equilibrium point. The slope of the peripheral response curve C_z is also dependent upon the oxygen tension (PaO_2) so that a change in regime could also be caused by a small change in arterial oxygen tension.

This analysis shows that with small changes in equilibrium point the system may switch from one regime to another — e.g. from damped oscillations to continuous undamped oscillation or vice versa. Such changes might occur with alterations in C_z (e.g. from hypoxic potentiation of the peripheral chemoreceptor response to CO_2).

Respiration pattern in QS in healthy preterm infants commonly shows sudden transitions from regular respiration with occasional sighs followed by damped oscillations to continuous oscillations (periodic breathing) and vice versa. The mathematical model described accounts qualitatively for these observations, and may thus provide a conceptual framework for their further investigation.

Acknowledgements

These studies were generously supported by a grant from the Foundation for the Study & Infant Deaths.

References

1. Fleming, P. J., Goncalves, A. L., Levine, M. R. and Wollard, S. (1984). *J. Physiol.* **347**, 1-16.

2. Cleave, J. P., Levine, M. R. and Fleming, P. J. (1984). *J. Theoret. Biol.* **108**, 261–283.
3. Milhorn, H. T. (1966). "The Application of Control Theory to Physiological Systems". W. B. Saunders, Philadelphia.
4. Arrowsmith, D. K. and Place, C. M. (1982). "Ordinary Differential Equations". Chapman and Hall, London.
5. Pontryagin (1962). "Ordinary Differential Equations". Addison-Wesley, London.
6. Duffin, J. (1972). *Resp. Physiol.* **15**, 277–301.

Respiratory Pauses and REMs in Sleeping Premature and Full-term Infants

Lilia Curzi-Dascalova and Genevieve Korn

Hôpital de Port Royal, Paris, France

Mechanisms involved in respiratory pauses (RP) continue to be uncertain (7,10). Correlations between RP and some phasic events of REM sleep have been reported. In 1965, Aserinski (1) found, in humans, an association between hypopnoea and apnoea and bursts of rapid eye movements (REMs). Netick *et al.* (6) described, in cats, an association between intense firing of REM-specific medular neurons and irregular respiration with rapid swings of small amplitude around zero airflow. Orem (8) found, in cats, variable relationships between diaphragmatic activity and PGO wave incidence: "the correlationships between these phenomena were in some cases negative and in other cases positive". On the contrary, Watanabe *et al.* (11) reported that in newborns, at all conceptional ages, >3 s duration apnoeic episodes were observed mostly (in $>85\%$ of cases) when REM bursts were absent. These authors concluded that "REM sleep prevents sudden infant death syndrome". The aim of the present work, begun 3 years ago, was to study whether some relationship exists between RP and REM. It was performed in normal, 31–41 week conceptional age infants. Our method was not identical to, and our results and conclusions showed some differences from previous studies.

Subjects

The study was carried out on 46 normal, 31–41 week conceptional age infants: 35 of them were recorded during the neonatal period (up to 10 days of legal age); 11 prematurely born infants were recorded when they reached the term of 37–40 weeks.

Age and normality of the infants were determined according to criteria previously described (2,3).

The Physiological Development of the Fetus and Newborn
ISBN 0 12 389080 2

Copyright © 1985 by Academic Press, London.
All rights of reproduction in any form reserved.

Methods

Polygraphic recordings were performed during the morning, between two meals. They included:

1. EEG;
2. ECG;
3. Eye movements recorded with a piezo-electrical quartz accelerometer attached to one eyelid (9);
4. Thoracic and abdominal respiratory movements recorded with mercury strain gauges fixed 1 cm above the nipples and 2 cm above the umbilicus;
5. Airflow recorded with a nasal thermistor;
6. Diaphragmatic inspiratory EMG recorded with surface EMG electrodes, attached bilaterally at the subcostal level on the mamillary line.

Sleep states were coded according to EEG (5) and REMs criteria. All RP of >2 s duration were noted (method in (2)).

We counted REMs recorded during RP and during an equal number of control periods (CP) of similar duration; CP were established 20 s after the end of a given RP.

Results were statistically tested by analysis of variance and by computing correlation coefficients.

Results

No RP longer than 15 s was seen. Only 2 RP (lasting 3 and 4 s) were obstructive. We counted 3705 central RP: 2447 in active sleep, 689 in indeterminate sleep and 565 in quiet sleep.

First we studied REMs occurring during RP of different duration (2–4.9 s, 5–9.9 s, 10–15 s) and during corresponding CP. We did not find any differences related to RP duration. Results obtained for all 2–15 s RP and CP were as follows:

1. During *active sleep* (Table I), at 35–36 weeks and 37–38 weeks conceptional age, mean number of REMs recorded during CP was significantly higher, compared to REMs during RP. But only less than half of RP (1057 out of 2447) and of CP (1345 out of 2447) were accompanied by REMs. REMs densities during RP and during CP were usually correlated ($P<0.01$ except for 35–36 week group). However, sometimes we noted numerous REMs during a given RP but no REMs during the CP and vice versa.

2. No significant differences or correlations were found when REMs during RP and CP of *indeterminate sleep* were studied.

3. 565 RP occurred during *quiet sleep*. Their duration was similar to that observed in active and in indeterminate sleep. None of these RP or CP were related to REMs.

Discussion

RP of short duration are usually observed in normal premature and full-term infants (4). At this age they are more numerous than in older infants. As early

Table 1. Correlations between rapid eye movements (REM) and respiratory pauses (RP) during active sleep in prematures recorded during the neonatal period (the first 4 groups) or when they reached 37–40 weeks conceptional age (CA, the 5th group)

CA in weeks	Total No. of RP	No. with REM RP	CP	m REM in RP	m REM in CP	F	r
30–34				1.9	2.2		
	241	144	127	$\pm$	$\pm$	2.4	0.34**
$n=5$				2.6	3.2		
35–36				1.5	2.0		
	771	327	408	$\pm$	$\pm$	13.6***	0.13
$n=11$				2.8	3.0		
37–38				1.6	2.1		
	390	183	333	$\pm$	$\pm$	7.0**	0.34**
$n=10$				2.8	3.1		
39–41				.59	0.7		
	105	31	37	$\pm$	$\pm$	0.9	0.34**
$n=9$				1.1	1.2		
Prem. reaching 37–40				1.4	1.6		
	940	372	410	$\pm$	$\pm$	6.6	0.31**
$n=11$				2.5	2.8		
Total $n=46$	2447	1057	1315				

No. with REM = number of RP or control periods (CP) accompanied by REM. m REM in = F = coefficient of analysis of variance for comparison of mean number of REM occurring in RP and CP. r = correlation coefficient. **$P<0.01$. ***$P<0.001$.

as 31–34 weeks conceptional age, they predominate in active, REM sleep, compared to quiet NREM sleep (2). So normal premature and full-term infants can be a good "model" for the study of correlations between RP and the other phasic phenomena characterizing REM sleep.

The present study does not give any data suggesting a significant correlation between RP and REMs. A coincidence between both phenomena occurred only for 43.2% of RP in active sleep and for 10.3% in indeterminate sleep; no RP recorded in quiet sleep was accompanied by REMs. Our percentages of coincidence are higher than those of Watanabe et al. (11), but we studied all REMs, including single REMs, while Watanabe et al. studied only coincidence between RP and bursts of REMs. The mean number of REMs we recorded during RP was between 1.4 and 1.9, i.e. many REMs did not occur in bursts. However, both studies confirm the absence of a positive correlation between REMs and RP in young infants.

Do REMs prevent the occurrence of RP as suggested by Watanabe et al. (11)? Our study shows, in active sleep, a higher density of REMs during CP than during RP. However, the density of REMs in both RP and CP was frequently correlated: if REMs were numerous during RP, they were numerous during CP and vice versa. We did not find any differences between duration of RP occurring with or without REMs. In spite of the presence of REMs, RP were more numerous in active sleep, compared to quiet NREM sleep. We consider that all these facts do not permit the conclusion that REMs protect infants from the occurrence of RP.

Conclusion

The present study does not show any significant positive or negative correlations between respiratory pauses and REMs occurring in normal premature and full-term infants. Respiratory pauses and REMs, numerous in active, REM sleep, do not seem to be causally related.

References

1. Aserinski, E. (1965). *Science* **150**, 763–766.
2. Curzi-Dascalova, L. and Christova-Gueorguieva, E. (1983). *Biol. Neonate* **44**, 325–332.
3. Curzi-Dascalova, L., Christova-Gueorguieva, E., Lebrun, F. and Firtion, G. (1984). *Neuropediatrics* **15**, 13–17.
4. Curzi-Dascalova, L., Radvanyi, M. F., Couchard, M., Monod, N. and Dreyfus-Brisac, C. (1976). *In*: "Respiratory Centers and Afferent Systems" (B. Duron, ed.) pp. 287–297, INSERM Paris.
5. Dreyfus-Brisac (1979). *In*: "Human Growth, a Comprehensive Treatise" (Folkner, F. and Tanner, J. M. eds) pp. 157–182, Plenum Corporation, New York.
6. Netick, A., Orem, J. and Dement, W. (1977). *Brain Res.* **20**, 197–207.
7. Orem, J. (1980). *In*: "Physiology in Sleep" pp. 273–313, Academic Press Inc., New York and London.
8. Orem, J. (1980). *J. Appl. Physiol.* **48**, 54–65.
9. Pajot, N., Vicente, G. and Dreyfus-Brisac, C. (1976). *J. Electrophysiol. Technol.* **2**, 29–38.
10. Philipson, E. A. (1978). *Am. Rev. Resp. Dis.* **118**, 909–939.
11. Watanabe, K., Inokuma, K. and Negoro, T. (1983). *Eur. J. Pediat.* **140**, 289–292.

Studies of the Biphasic Respiratory Response of Conscious Kittens to Acute Hypoxia

H. B. McCooke and M. A. Hanson

Department of Physiology and Biochemistry, University of Reading,
Reading, UK

Introduction

In previous work (1) the "biphasic" respiratory response of anaesthetized, tracheotomized kittens aged 5–34 days was studied when inspired oxygen fraction (F_I,O_2) was reduced from 0.21 to between 0.06 and 0.12. The fall in $\dot{V}_E$ in the second phase was predominantly due to a fall in respiratory frequency (f), with a smaller and more variable fall in inspired tidal volume (V_T). We have now developed a noninvasive method which permits rapid reduction in $F_I O_2$ to be made whilst respiration is measured in conscious kittens. We have made repeated observations of the biphasic response of kittens from the day of birth to 1 month old.

Methods

Kittens were studied on the day of birth, then on day 4, 7, 14 and 28. For each trial a kitten was placed in a perspex chamber, a loose-fitting seal around the neck holding the animal in position without discomfort. Respiration was measured as airflow in or out of the chamber by a pneumotachometer head (Fleisch No. 0). This provided a low resistance to gas movement. Hence there was no need for the chamber to be airtight and changes in ambient pressure or temperature do not produce baseline drift. The airflow signal was integrated electronically to derive tidal volume. At the start of each experiment the temperature of the chamber was allowed to stabilize (range 28–32°C), then kept at this temperature ±0.5°C with an infra-red lamp. The system was calibrated by passing known

The Physiological Development of the Fetus and Newborn
ISBN 0 12 389080 2

Copyright © 1985 by Academic Press, London.
All rights of reproduction in any form reserved.

volumes of air in or out of the chamber using a syringe. The chamber was placed in a nylon hood through which gas was passed at *ca* 61/min. Parallel gas lines delivered air or a hypoxic mixture to a T-piece connected to the hood. Each line incorporated a low resistance side leak. Rapid changes of FO_2 in the hood were produced by opening one side leak and simultaneously closing the other, FO_2 in the hood was measured continuously by a fast gas analyser (Beckman OM11).

After being placed in the chamber, a kitten was allowed a period of about 5 min to become accustomed to the apparatus. Respiration was recorded for a control period of 1 min and then F_IO_2 was reduced abruptly to 0.12 for 5 min. During the control the test periods general behaviour observations were made on whether the kitten was awake or asleep; we did not attempt to define sleep state more precisely. The procedure was repeated at F_IO_2 0.10 and 0.08, 5–10 min being left for recovery between each trial.

Table 1. Degree of the bisphasic response (mean ± SEM) (0 = no biphasic response; 1 = complete return to control)

Age, days	1	4	7	14	28
F_IO_2					
0.12	0.46 ±0.03	0.39 ±0.07	0.34 ±0.08	0.33 ±0.04	0.40 ±0.07
0.10	0.32 ±0.05	0.28 ±0.08	0.33 ±0.05	0.31 ±0.06	0.14 ±0.07
0.08	0.30 ±0.05	0.45 ±0.08	0.21 ±0.05	0.34 ±0.05	0.44 ±0.09

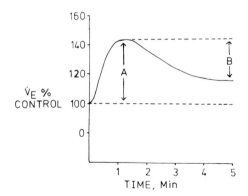

$$\text{Size of Biphasic Response} = \frac{B}{A}$$

Figure 1. Diagram of biphasic ventilatory response to an abrupt reduction in F_IO_2, showing the method used for quantifying the degree of the response.

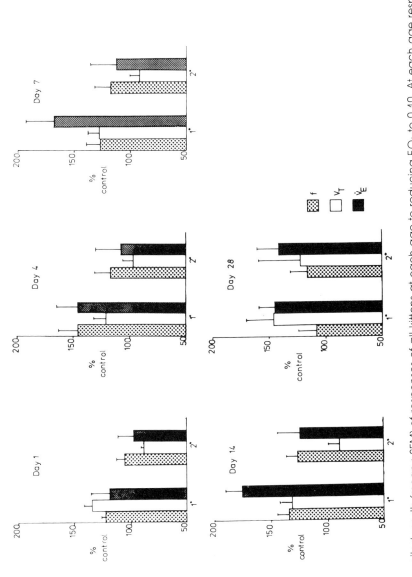

Figure 2. Compiled results (mean ± SEM) of responses of all kittens at each age to reducing FO_2 to 0.10. At each age response is shown as frequency (f, stippled bars), tidal volume (V_T, open bars) and minute ventilation ($\dot{V}_E$, cross-hatched bars) in the first phase, 1°, of the response about 1 min after reducing F_IO_2 and in the second phase, 2°, 3 min later.

Results

A biphasic respiratory response to hypoxia was observed in the majority of trials at each F_IO_2 level and at each age. Its incidence did not decrease with age up to 28 days, and there was no significant correlation between the occurrence of the response and the level of F_IO_2. Table 1 shows the degree of the bisphasic response (where present), quantified as in Fig. 1. The response was not greater at 0.08 than at 0.12 F_IO_2, nor was there any consistent reduction in the response with age up to 28 days. The percentage time spent in arousal was significantly greater in the 2nd phase compared with that in the 1st phase at each age. This was true at each F_IO_2. There were no significant differences in the percentage times spent in arousal in the 1st phase or the 2nd phase between the three F_IO_2 levels, however.

Figure 2 shows the components of the ventilatory response to reducing F_IO_2 to 0.10. In the 1st phase the increase in $\dot{V}_E$ was due to an increase in both f and V_T. The size of this increase in $\dot{V}_E$ became in general greater as the kittens became older. In the 2nd phase $\dot{V}_E$ was reduced, predominantly by a fall in V_T. The changes in f were more variable; usually it fell during the 2nd phase but sometimes it remained at its phase 1 value or even increased above this value. This pattern was observed in all trials at F_IO_2 0.08 and 0.12.

Discussion

In this study we have used a noninvasive method to measure the breathing of conscious kittens continuously, and have studied their responses to abrupt reductions in F_IO_2. We observed a biphasic response in the majority of trials, as reported for anaesthetized kittens (8,1) and rabbits (4). A biphasic response has been reported in conscious monkeys (9) and in full-term or premature infants (3,2,7).

Our results differ from those of Blanco et al. (1) in two important respects. First, they showed that in anaesthetized kittens $\dot{V}_E$ fell during the 2nd phase of the response due predominantly to a fall in f, but we found in conscious kittens that the fall in $\dot{V}_E$ was due to a consistent fall in V_T. It is likely that the difference is due to the fact that our animals were conscious, as Blanco et al. noted that a fall in f during the 2nd phase correlated with a concurrent fall in arterial blood pressure, and suggested that anaesthesia might play a role in producing this effect. Secondly, in our experiments $\dot{V}_E$ fell in the 2nd phase to ca 66% of its value in the 1st phase whereas in the experiments of Blanco et al. the fall was much greater, to ca 11% of its 1st phase value. This difference may again be due to anaesthesia but a difference in ambient temperature must also be considered, for their experiments were conducted at room temperature whereas ours were conducted at 28–32°C, close to the thermoneutral temperature for the kitten (5). VO_2 is known to fall during hypoxia in the kitten (6), the fall being greater below the thermoneutral temperature. More work is needed to establish whether there is a causal link between VO_2, or the concurrent V_{CO_2}, and $\dot{V}_E$ during hypoxia in the newborn.

We did not observe differences in the degree of the biphasic response which correlated with the level to which F_IO_2 was reduced; thus in kittens up to 28 days the 2nd phase of the response is not more pronounced at F_IO_2 0.08 than it is at 0.12. We have not been able to make detailed observations of the state of sleep or wakefulness of the kittens during the periods of hypoxia, because we wanted to study the biphasic response from the day of birth without causing any disturbance to feeding and development. Nonetheless, at each age the percentage time spent in arousal was greater during the 2nd phase than in the 1st phase, irrespective of the level of F_IO_2. This is further evidence against the notion that "depression" of respiration by hypoxia plays a role in the production of the 2nd phase, since if such depression occurred it should be greater the more intense the hypoxia.

References

1. Blanco, C. E., Hanson, M. A., Johnson, P. and Rigatto, H. (1984). *J. Appl. Physiol.* **56**, 12–17.
2. Cross, K. W. and Oppé, T. E. (1953). *J. Physiol.* **117**, 38–55.
3. Cross, K. W. and Warner, P. (1951). *J. Physiol.* **114**, 282–295.
4. Grunstein, M. M., Hazinski, T. A. and Schlueter, M. A. (1981). *J. Appl. Physiol.* **51**, 122–130.
5. Hill, J. R. (1959). *J. Physiol.* **149**, 346–373.
6. Moore, R. E. (1956). *J. Physiol.* **133**, 69–70P.
7. Sankaran, K., Wiebe, H., Seshia, M. M. K., Boychuk, R. B., Cates, D. and Rigatto, H. (1979). *Pediat. Res.* **13**, 875–878.
8. Schweiler, G. H. (1968). *Acta Physiol. Scand.* (Suppl.) **304**, 1–123.
9. Woodrum, D. E., Standaert, T. A., Maycock, D. E. and Guthrie, R. D. (1981). *Pediat. Res.* **15**, 367–370.

Carotid Bodies Mediate the Attenuating Effect of β-Adrenergic Agonists on Apnoea Reflex Response to Laryngeal Water Stimulation in Newborn Lambs

Jens Grögaard and Håkan Sundell

Department of Pediatrics, Vanderbilt University Medical School,
Nashville, Tennessee, USA

Reflex apnoea from water stimulation of the laryngeal chemoreceptorreflex (LCR) has previously been described in several animal species (1,2,3) and in human infants (4). The reflex is thought to be a protective mechanism through which animals and humans prevent aspiration to the lungs and preserve vital function while they are not breathing. Besides inducing apnoea, the laryngeal chemoreflex response consists of bradycardia, hypertension and blood flow redistribution (2). Frequent swallowing also occurs during laryngeal stimulation in order to remove the stimulus from the sensory receptors.

During stimulation there is a decrease in arterial oxygen tension which should stimulate arterial chemoreceptors. In a previous study (2), we proposed that part of the cardiovascular response to laryngeal water administration in newborn lambs might be due to stimulation of arterial chemoreceptors.

Administration of terbutaline, a β-adrenergic agonist, to newborn lambs attenuated the apnoea response (5), and we postulated that the terbutaline effect might be mediated by the carotid bodies.

Material and Methods

Seven healthy, normal full-term lambs were studied. The lambs were studied awake and unanaesthetized after 2 weeks of age when the immediate postnatal

The Physiological Development of the Fetus and Newborn
ISBN 0 12 389080 2

Copyright © 1985 by Academic Press, London.
All rights of reproduction in any form reserved.

carotid body maturation is said to have occurred (6). The lambs were chronically instrumented on the 10–12th day after birth according to a previously described method (2) with placement of a low tracheostomy and arterial and venous catheters. Six preterm lambs (gestational age 135 days) were instrumented in the same way and studied between age 4–10 days.

Experimental Protocol

The LCR response to laryngeal water administration was tested in a standardized manner with distilled water at body temperature. Each water stimulation consisted of a baseline period of 30 s followed by the retrograde injection of 1 ml of water into the larynx through the balloon catheter during a 5 s period. Reflex responses were tested before and after terbutaline administration. Terbutaline was given as an infusion of 2–4 μg/kg/min mixed in 5% dextrose water over 1–2 h period. Carotid body denervation (CBD) was performed in 5 lambs in each group: 2 lambs in the term group and in the preterm group were sham operated. The sinus nerves were cut on both sides and the junctions of the carotid artery and the occipital and lingual arteries were stripped clean down to the adventitia. After CBD, the lambs were allowed a 48 h recovery period before studies were repeated. Airway occlusions were performed for measurements of airway pressure 0.1 s after onset of inspiration (P0.1) in all the lambs (7) in order to evaluate neuromuscular inspiratory drive.

The reflex response was expressed as percent change from baseline values for respiration, heart rate and blood pressure. The effect of LCR stimulation on respiration was assessed as apnoea response (% change in ventilation volume) measured with a pneumotachograph as the volume of gas inspired during the 30 s baseline or stimulation periods.

Results

Figure 1 shows that the apnoea response to LCR stimulation remained unchanged after CBD in the 4 to 10-days-old preterm lambs. The 14 to 28-day-old term lambs are included in the figure for comparison. The older lambs had a significantly smaller response before CBD compared to the preterm lambs. A significantly increased apnoea response was seen after CBD in the older, but not in the younger lambs.

Terbutaline infusion given before CBD to the preterm lambs resulted in an insignificant decreased response was seen in the older lambs. To apnoea response to LCR stimulation was not significantly altered in either group of lambs by terbutaline given after CBD.

Figure 2 shows that P 0.1 did not change significantly when terbutaline was given to the 4 to 10-day-old preterm lambs either before or after CBD. The sham operated preterm and term lambs, however, had an increased P 0.1 after surgery. P 0.1 increased significantly after the terbutaline infusion in all the 14 to 28-day-old term lambs before CBD but not afterwards.

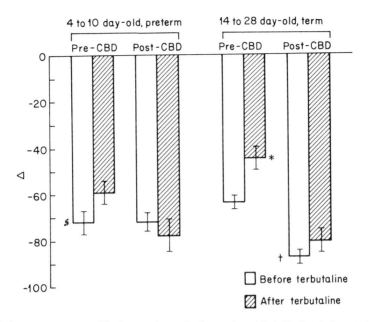

Figure 1. Apnoea response (% change in ventilation volume) to LCR stimulation during wakefulness in five 4 to 10-day-old preterm lambs and five 14 to 28-day-old term lambs performed before and after an i.v. terbutaline (T) infusion given both pre- and post-CBD. Mean ± SEM N = 18–23 stimulations. * indicates significant difference between responses obtained before and after terbutaline. † indicates significant difference between responses obtained before and after CBD. § indicates significant difference between responses obtained in preterm and term lambs.

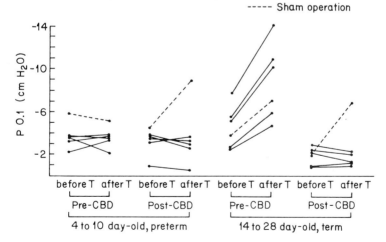

Figure 2. Airway occlusion pressure (P 0.1) in five 4 to 10-day-old preterm lambs and five 14 to 28-day-old term lambs performed before and after iv terbutaline infusion given both pre- and post-CBD. One sham operated lamb was also studied in each group.

Before terbutaline, P 0.1 was significantly lower after CBD in the term lambs but not in the preterm lambs.

Cardiovascular Response to LCR Stimulation

Blood pressure (hypertension) and heart rate (bradycardia) response to LCR stimulation were significantly reduced following CBD in the 4 to 10-day-old preterm lambs. Terbutaline did not significantly alter blood pressure and heart rate response to LCR whether given before or after CBD. The older lambs showed similar changes in the cardiovascular response.

During hypoxia the older lambs had a greater and more sustained hyperventilation response than the younger lambs before CBD. Ater CBD the ventilatory response to hypoxia was significantly decreased in both groups of lambs.

Conclusion

This study demonstrates the modifying role of the carotid bodies on the respiratory and cardiovascular responses of the laryngeal chemoreflex. After CBD, the apnoea response was enhanced, while the hypertension and bradycardia responses were diminished. The study also shows that the attenuating effect of terbutaline is partially mediated by the carotid bodies. The prerequisite for the attenuating effect of terbutaline, however, is a mature carotid body function.

References

1. Downing, S. E. and Lee, J. C. (1975). *Pediat.* **55**, 640–649.
2. Grögaard, J., Lindström, D. P., Marchal, F., Stahlman, M. T. and Sundell, H. (1982). *J. Develop. Physiol.* **4**, 353–370.
3. Harding, R., Johnson, P. and McClelland, M. E. (1978). *J. Physiol.* **277**, 409–422.
4. Perkett, E. and Vaughan, R. (1982). *Acta Paediatr. Scand.* **71**, 969–972.
5. Grögaard, J. and Sundell, H. (1983). *Pediat. Res.* **17**, 213–219.
6. Belenky, D. A., Standaert, T. A. and Woodrum, D. E. (1979). *J. Appl. Physiol.* **47**, 927–930.
7. Whitelaw, W. A., Derenne, J. and Milic-Emili, J. (1975). *Resp. Physiol.* **23**, 181–199.

Perinatal Respiratory Activity in the Lamb

Philip J. Berger, Adrian M. Walker, Rosemary Horne,
Vojta Brodecky, Malcolm H. Wilkinson, Fiona Wilson,
and John E. Maloney

Monash University Centre for Early Human Development,
Queen Victoria Medical Centre,
Melbourne, Australia

Introduction

Within the last 12 years there have been a number of studies of the development of the respiratory system before birth in experimental animals (1,2) and man (3). Likewise the onset of rhythmical respiration at birth in the newborn (4) has received some attention. There is however a paucity of continuous information which describes respiratory activity in the same fetus during labour, birth and the newborn period at the onset of air breathing.

This paper briefly reports a study of respiratory activity in the perinatal period during the spontaneous and unassisted birth of the fetal lamb.

Methods

The operating and instrumentation procedures used in this study have been described elsewhere (5) and will be briefly reviewed. Seven fetal lambs of gestational ages between 129 and 136 days were exposed under sterile operating conditions via a midline laparotomy for the attachment of recording electrodes and the implantation of catheters. Parameters to be measured from the fetus in this series of experiments included diaphragmatic electrical activity, electrocortical activity (ECoG) in 4 animals, and electrocardiographic activity. Catheters were also implanted into the jugular vein and carotid artery of each fetus which enabled measurements of blood pressure and the analysis of arterial blood gases. A catheter

The Physiological Development of the Fetus and Newborn
ISBN 0 12 389080 2

Copyright © 1985 by Academic Press, London.
All rights of reproduction in any form reserved.

was sewn onto the chest wall of the fetus in the mid clavicular line at the level of the xiphisternum for the measurement of amniotic fluid pressure. Following the operation all leads were exteriorized to enable monitoring from late gestation onwards; all incisions were closed and the ewe and the fetus were allowed to recover. All the ewes commenced successful labour and delivery between 7-17 days after the operation when the gestational ages of the fetal lambs were between 141 and 147 days. The parameters reported in this paper were recorded continuously on a Hewlett-Packard (7858B) multichannel pen recorder and simultaneously on a Hewlett Packard (3968A) eight channel electromagnetic tape recorder, for subsequent computer analysis. The computer software developed for the identification of diaphragmatic electrical activity has been detailed previously (5).

Results

All animals in this series of experiments proceeded through labour, birth, and the newborn period without complication. The average oxygen and carbon dioxide partial pressures, pH, heart rate and arterial blood pressure (corrected for amniotic fluid pressure) between 1 and 3 days prior to birth were 24.6 ± 1.2 mmHg, 46.2 ± 1.0 mmHg, 7.36 ± 0.1 units, 154 ± 5 b/m, and 72.0 ± 1.3 cm H_2O in 6 fetal lambs. The measurements of these parameters were not made in this interval on one fetal lamb due to catheter blockage; this animal also proceeded to a successful delivery. Within 1-5 min prior to birth oxygen and carbon dioxide partial pressures and pH varied from 11.0-16.0 mmHg, 46.9-58.6 mmHg; and 7.25-7.32 units in 4 animals on which measurements were available. Following the establishment of air breathing arterial oxygen tensions rapidly rose to >50 mmHg within the first 5 min with an arterial oxygen saturation of approximately 80%.

The frequency with which electrocortical activity changed between high voltage (HV) and low voltage (LV) in the period of approximately 1 h prior to delivery was 22, 7, 8 and 10 cycles/h with epochs of low voltage activity varying between 2.1 ± 0.3 and 4.7 ± 1.4 min in the 4 animals studied. This represents a significant alteration in the partitioning and electrocortical activity from that seen in late gestation. All the 4 animals in which ECoG was studied were in low voltage electrocortical activity by the time the fetus was exposed to the level of the xiphisternum, though a HV-LV change occurred following the delivery of the fetal head in 1 animal.

Two patterns of respiratory activity exemplifying different features of birth are shown in Fig. 1. In the upper panel prior to the presentation of the head there is tonic electrical activity in the diaphragm for periods of up to 43 s and the head presents during such an epoch. The diaphragm then enters a series of rhythmic bursts of activity until the exposure of the xiphisternum when following several longer breaths phasic respiratory activity continues with respiratory pauses being $\leqslant 3$ s. The lower panel of Fig. 1 illustrates the establishment of air breathing in a fetus which had not made any respiratory effort for the 30 min prior to the delivery of the thorax which was preceded 30 s earlier by the appearance of the

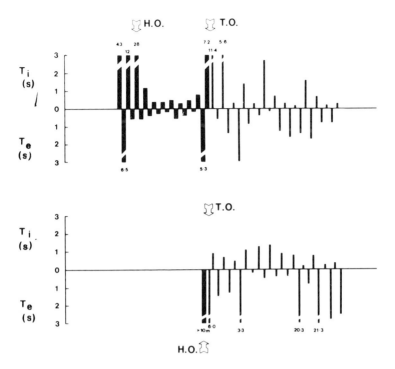

Figure 1. This figure depicts consecutive breaths at birth for 2 fetal lambs both born at 142 days gestation. T_i and T_e represent inspiratory and expiratory times measured directly from the recording of diaphragmatic electrical activity during birth. In the upper panel the head of the fetus was delivered (H.O) approximately midway (13 s) from the end of a 28 s tonic burst of diaphragmatic electrical activity and the thorax was completely born (T.O) 7.2 s into a further 18.6 s interval of diaphragmatic activity. In the lower panel the diaphragm is electrically silent during an interval of > 10 min up to and including the presentation of the head (H.O) and following presentation of the thorax there is a further 6 s before phasic breathing commences. The thin bars represent the time intervals following the delivery of the xiphisternum.

fetal head. In the establishment of phasic breathing the inspiratory time did not exceed 1.5 s. The complete absence of tonic as well as phasic diaphragmatic electrical activity in the 30 min preceding birth was also observed on this one occasion. In the 6 other fetuses there was a significant reduction in respiratory rate during labour prior to delivery. In the 60 min preceding the first air breath average minutely respiratory rate did not exceed 11 "breaths"/min while in the 30 min after delivery the average rate rose to between 37–76 breaths/min.

Discussion

These studies are among the first continuous descriptions of the electrical activity of the diaphragm and cortex during the immediate perinatal period and indicate that there is a significant alteration in both the pattern of diaphragmatic and electrocortical activity in this period.

The 7 fetal births discussed in this pilot series proceeded to healthy newborn status. Within 5 min of air breathing arterial oxygen saturations were ~ 80% despite significant pulmonary oedema. Bland et al. (6,7) have indicated that although there is a significant reduction of extravascular water content of the lungs during labour it does not decrease further for at least 30 min postnatally. At this time approximately 75% of the extravascular water is found in perivascular cuffs. Thus in the immediate newborn period extensive perivascular oedema has only a minor effect on gas exchange in the immediate newborn period.

The noted change in electrocortical activity during parturition has been previously recognized (8). In late fetal life the ECoG LV-HV change has a period of approximately 40 min (~ 1.7c/h) compared with the rapid alterations during labour of 7–22 c/h in the ~ 60 min prior to labour. During LV cortical activity it was not possible in our study to distinguish between rapid eye movement sleep and the awake state. Ruckebusch (8) has indicated however that in the majority of low voltage activity during parturition the fetus is awake. In all of our experiments where electrocortical activity was measured LV electrocortical activity was present by the time the thorax was delivered, though on one occasion the fetus was in HV activity (non rapid eye movement sleep) during delivery of the head.

Finally, the variable and irregular manner with which phasic breathing is established in the fetal lamb (Fig. 1) has been noted also for the human infant (9,10). While inspiratory efforts which exceed 1.5 s in duration are commonly observed within seconds of the exposure of the thorax, they are not a necessary condition for the establishment of air breathing (lower panel Fig. 1). Such an observation supports an earlier suggestion (11) that upon air breathing the respiratory muscles may not always be required to develop a significant opening pressure in the lung.

Acknowledgements

We wish to acknowledge the skilled technical assistance of Mr J. Cannata and Mr A. Pearson in these experiments and thank our secretary Mrs A. Carruthers for the help in the production of this manuscript.

References

1. Maloney, J. E. and Bowes, G. (1983). In: "Hypoxia, Exercise and Altitude" Proceeding of the Third Banff International Hypoxia Symposium. pp. 17–37, A.R. Liss Publishers.
2. Dawes, G. S. and Henderson-Smart, D. J. (1981). In: "International Review of Physiology: Respiratory Physiology" III: 23. (Widdicombe, J. G., ed.) pp. 75–110, University Park Press, Baltimore.
3. Patrick, J., Campell, K., Carmichael, L., Natale, R. and Richardson, B. (1980). Obstet. Gynecol. 56, 24–30.

4. Mortola, J. P., Fisher, J. T., Smith, J. B., Fox, G. S., Weeks, S. and Willis, D. (1982). *J. Appl. Physiol. Respirat. Environ. Exercise Physiol.* **52**, 716–724.
5. Bowes, G., Adamson, T. M., Ritchie, B. C., Wilkinson, M. H. and Maloney, J. E. (1981). *J. Appl. Physiol. Respirat. Environ. Exercise Physiol.* **50**, 693–700.
6. Bland, R. D., McMillan, D. D., Bressack, M. A. and Dong, L. (1980). *J. Appl. Physiol. Respirat, Environ. Exercise Physiol.* **49**, 171–177.
7. Bland, R. D., Hansen, T. N., Haberkern, C. M., Bressack, M. A., Hazinski, T. A., Usha Raj, J. and Goldberg, R. B. (1982). *J. Appl. Physiol. Respirat. Environ. Exercise Physiol.* **53**, 992–1004.
8. Ruckebusch, Y., (1972). *Electroenceph. Clin. Neurophysiol.* **32**, 119–128.
9. Karlberg. P., Cherry, R. B., Escardo, F. E. and Koch, G. (1962). *Acta Paediatrica* **51**, 121–136.
10. Milner, A. D. and Saunders, R. A. (1977). *Arch. Dis. Child.* **52**, 918–924.
11. Saunders, R. A. and Milner, A. D. (1978). *J. Pediat.* **93**, 667–673.

Lung Hypoplasia and Breathing Movements Following Oligohydramnios in Fetal Lambs

A. C. Moessinger, J. E. Fewell, R. I. Stark,
M. H. Collins, S. S. Daniel, M. Singh,
W. A. Blanc, J. Kleinerman, and L. S. James

The Departments of Pediatrics, Physiology and Pathology, College of
Physicians and Surgeons of Columbia University, New York; University of
Arkansas for Medical Sciences, Little Rock, Arkansas; Mt Sinai School of
Medicine, New York, USA

Introduction

Congenital lung hypoplasia has now become a common pathological finding in perinatal deaths (1). The emergence of lung hypoplasia in recent autopsy series results mainly from a decrease in the incidence of the once more common pulmonary pathologies such as severe meconium aspiration, congenital pneumoni and hyaline membrane disease (2). The majority of infants with lung hypoplasia have multiple associated malformations such as diaphragmatic hernia, renal anomalies, rightsided cardiac lesions or musculoskeletal disorders (3). Lung hypoplasia is however also found as an isolated anomaly (4), or in association with minor deformities compatible with intact survival, i.e. oligohydramnios deformation sequence following premature rupture of the fetal membranes and continued leakage of amniotic fluid (5).

Little is known about the pathogenesis of lung hypoplasia, particularly when associated with oligohydramnios (6). In this short communication, we present work done to answer three questions: 1) Does a short period of amniotic fluid drainage lead to lung hypoplasia in fetal lambs? 2) Does oligohydramnios decrease the incidence of breathing movements (7,8) which have been demonstrated to be important determinants of fetal lung growth (9,10)? 3) Does oligohydramnios decrease the small airway distending pressure produced by lung fluid secretion

The Physiological Development of the Fetus and Newborn
ISBN 0 12 389080 2

Copyright © 1985 by Academic Press, London.
All rights of reproduction in any form reserved.

against the resistance of the upper airway (11,12) which has also been demonstrated to be an important determinant of lung growth in the fetal lamb (13)?

In order to investigate these possible mechanisms we used the fetal lamb in which physiologic measurements can be recorded in a stable chronic preparation. We performed our studies during the canalicular stage of lung development for two reasons: 1) fetal instrumentation is easily feasible then, 2) interference with lung growth by oligohydramnios is more marked during this stage than later on (14).

Methods and Results

Documentation of lung hypoplasia

To determine the impact of oligohydramnios on fetal lung growth, 6 pregnant mixed-breed ewes (4 with singletons and 2 with twins), were instrumented with only amniotic catheters exteriorized to the ewe's flank. Two days following surgery (mean: 100 days), amniotic fluid volume was determined by dye-dilution technique using Congo red. The amniotic fluid surrounding 4 fetuses (2 singletons and 1 fetus in each pair of twins) was chronically drained for a mean period of 18 days. Four fetuses with intact amniotic fluid volume served as controls (2 singletons and the second of twins mentioned above). At caesarean section (mean 118 days, range 117–120 days) the amniotic fluid volume was measured, the fetal trachea was ligated, and the fetuses were killed, weighed and dissected. Fetal lung fluid volume was determined by tracheal suction and the fetal lungs as well as other organs were weighed. After trying the left mainstem bronchus, the right lung was fixed-inflated at a constant pressure of 20 cm H_2O with Ito-Karnovsky's solution for 24 h. Two experimental and two control lungs did not leak and were processed for morphometry, including the measurement of elastic fibre length (15,16). Portions of both the upper and lower lobes of the left lung

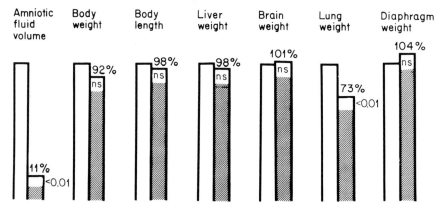

Figure 1. Amniotic fluid volume, fetal body and organ weights following 18 days of oligohydramnios in the sheep. Measurements obtained at a mean gestational age of 118 days and expressed in percent of controls. Data derived from 4 experimental and 4 sham-control fetuses.

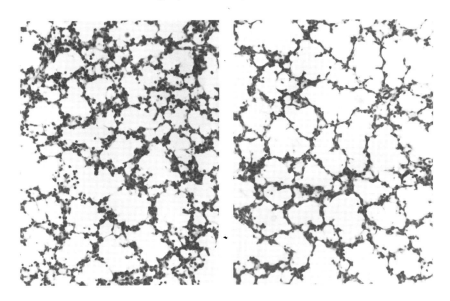

Figure 2. The impact of oligohydramnios on lung growth is illustrated by these two microphotographs (right upper lobes) of a set of twins (120 days gestation). A = control lung, B = experimental lung, (HαE, ×98). Both lungs were fixed — inflated at the same pressure and neither leaked. There are more smaller (newer) saccules in the control lung, A.

Table 1. Fetal lung growth following oligohydramnios

(Days 100–119 of gestation, sheep)
Values on day 118, expressed in percent of controls

General data*	%	P
Lung wet wt.	73	0.01
Lung dry wt.	80	0.02
% dry wt.	110	0.06
Lung fluid vol.	35	0.01
Total lung DNA	73	0.04
Lung SPC/DNA	96	0.39
Morphometry**	%	
Lung volume	62	N.T.
Total no. saccules	46	N.T.
Internal surface area	58	N.T.
Elastic tissue length	42	N.T.

* Data derived from 4 experimental and 4 sham-control fetuses.
** Data derived from 2 experimental and 2 sham-control fetuses (see text).
N.T. = not tested.

were used for determinations of dry weight, DNA and saturated phosphatidyl-choline (SPC) contents using standard techniques.

The results are presented in Figs 1 and 2 and Table 1. The lung DNA and SPC/DNA results were derived combining upper and lower lobe measurements for each fetus.

Physiologic measurements

To investigate possible mechanisms by which amniotic fluid drainage leads to lung hypoplasia we prepared an additional 4 pregnant ewes for measurements of tracheal and amniotic fluid pressure. The amniotic catheter used for pressure measurement was sutured to the anterior aspect of the fetal neck with its tip located at the same level as that of the tracheal catheter, i.e. 3 cm below the thyroid isthmus. Two additional amniotic catheters were inserted for amniotic fluid drainage. The ewes were operated between days 107 and 110 of gestation and were not studied until the 7th postoperative day. For each experiment, pressure measurements were made during a 24 h control period and a 24 h experimental period in which oligohydramnios was produced by draining amniotic fluid. Typically most of the amniotic fluid volume (500–700 ml) was drained within 30–90 min but the catheters were left open throughout the experimental period yielding only small volumes of fluid (150–250 ml) after the initial gush. We have so far limited our analysis to incidence of fetal breathing activity, excluding fetal gasps, and have not looked for changes in amplitude. Airway distending pressure was derived by substracting amniotic pressure from tracheal pressure during periods of apnea. These pressure measurements were made within 5 min after the strain gauges had been zeroed to atmospheric pressure and balanced. The results are presented in Table 2.

Table 2. Fetal breathing and airway distending pressure following acute drainage of amniotic fluid (mean 117 days)*

	Before drainage	P	After drainage
Incidence of fetal breathing, %	25 ± 10	n.s.	24 ± 7
Airway distending pressure, mmHg	1.2 ± 0.6	n.s.	1.4 ± 0.7

*Data derived from 4 animals over 24 h periods.

Discussion

Chronic drainage of amniotic fluid in the sheep leads to a selective pattern of fetal growth retardation with a predominant impact on lung growth and sparing other organs. We have already described a similar pattern in three other species, suggesting that amniotic fluid volume is a determinant of lung growth in the mammalian fetus (6,14,17). In the sheep, during the canalicular stage of lung development, chronic oligohydramnios does not affect lung maturation as judged by tissue SPC content per mg of lung DNA. The lungs show a striking reduction in the total number of saccules (future alveoli) which tend to be larger. Parenchymal elastic tissue and internal surface area are markedly reduced. These morphological changes were also noted in the guinea-pig in a previous study of the impact of oligohydramnios on lung growth (14). It is not known whether the hypoplastic lungs of human fetuses seen in association with prolonged leakage of amniotic fluid have the same characteristics since no complete morphometric study of such lungs has been published to date. So far we have not looked at pulmonary vasculature nor airway size in the animal model.

The incidence of fetal breathing movements is unchanged by amniotic fluid drainage on day 117 of gestation in the sheep. The impact of long term (weeks) drainage on the incidence of fetal breathing movements is not presented here, however, preliminary results (2 fetal preparations) indicate that the incidence of fetal breathing is again not affected. Using longitudinal axis linear array B mode sonography we recently demonstrated that the percent of time spent breathing by human fetuses was also not markedly altered by oligohydramnios (18). Whether other characteristics of fetal breathing, such as the transient increase in lung volume (19), are modified under this condition is unknown at this point.

As noted previously by others and ourselves, fetal tracheal pressure is greater than amniotic fluid pressure during periods of apnoea (11,12). This gradient of pressure is not changed during the first 24 h following the onset of amniotic fluid drainage. This suggests that oligohydramnios does not alter lung fluid secretion nor the upper airway resistance to lung fluid secretion. We need to measure this pressure gradient over a more prolonged period following the onset of oligohydramnios.

Acknowledgements

This work was supported by grants #HL-14218 and #HL-20585 from the National Institutes of Health.

References

1. Wigglesworth, J. S. and Desai, R. (1982). *Lancet* **1**, 264–267.
2. Moessinger, A. C., Abbey-Mensah, M., Driscoll, J. M., Jr. and Blanc, W. A. (1983). *Pediat. Res.* **17**, 327A.
3. Page, D. V. and Stocker, J. T. (1982). *Am. Rev. Resp. Dis.* **125**, 216–221.
4. Swischuk, L. E., Richardson, C. J., Nichols, M. M. and Ingman, M. J. (1979). *J. Pediat.* **95**, 573–577.
5. Blanc, W. A., Apperson, J. W. and McNally, J. (1962). *Bull. Sloane Hosp. Women* **8**, 51–64.
6. Moessinger, A. C., Bassi, J. A., Ballantyne, G., Collins, M. H., James, L. S. and Blanc, W. A. (1983). *Early Hum. Devel.* **8**, 343–350.
7. Gruenwald, P. (1957). *J. Mount Sinai Hosp.* **24**, 913–919.
8. Wigglesworth, J. S. (1976). *J. Clin. Path.* **29**, (suppl.) *(Roy. Coll. Path.)*, **10**, 27–30.
9. Alcorn, D., Adamson, T. M., Maloney, J. E. and Robinson, P. M. (1980). *J. Anat.* **130**, 683–695.

10. Fewell, J. E., Lee, C. C. and Kitterman, J. A. (1981). *J. Appl. Physiol.* **51**. 293–297.
11. Vilos, G. A. and Liggins, G. C. (1982). *J. Develop Physiol.* **4**, 247–256.
12. Fewell, J. E. and Johnson, P. (1983). *J. Physiol.* (London) 339, 495–504.
13. Fewell, J. E., Hislop, A. A., Kitterman, J. A. and Johnson, P. (1983). *J. Appl. Physiol.* **55**, 1103–1108.
14. Moessinger, A. C., Collins, M. H., Blanc, W. A., Kleinerman, J. and James, L. S. (1984). *Pediat. Res.* **18**, 336A.
15. Dunnill, M. S. (1962). *Thorax* **17**, 320–328.
16. Niewoehner, D. E. and Kleinerman, J. (1977). *Am. Rev. Resp. Dis.* **115**, 15–21.
17. Naeye, R. L. and Blanc, W. A. (1972). *Am. J. Pathol.* **67**, 95–105.
18. Fox, H. E. and Moessinger, A. C. (1984). *Am. J. Obstet. Gynecol.* (in press).
19. Murai, D. T., Lee, C. C., Wallen, L. D. and Kitterman, J. A. (1984). *Pediat. Res.* **18**, 400A.

Arachidonic Acid and the Pressor Response to Hypoxia in Perinatal and Adult Sheep

S. Cassin and M. L. Tod

Department of Physiology, College of Medicine,
University of Florida, Gainesville, Florida, USA

Many conflicting reports appear in the literature describing effects of arachidonic acid on the pulmonary circulation. Some studies suggest only vasoconstriction of the pulmonary circulation in response to arachidonic acid (1–4), while others report dose dependent vasodilation (5). Hyman et al. (6) proposed that pre-existing pulmonary vascular tone in adult cats determines the response to arachidonic acid. In adult dogs, Gerber et al. (7) report that infusion of arachidonic acid diminishes the pressor response to hypoxia. In previous studies on fetal and neonatal goats, we found dose dependent pulmonary pressor responses to arachidonic acid associated with systemic hypotension. Based on the above observations we performed the present experiments to clarify effects of age, species, and hypoxia on the pulmonary pressor response to arachidonic acid infusions.

Methods

Thirteen newborn lambs (2–9 days of age), 18 fetal lambs (0.91–0.97 gestation), and 10 nonpregnant ewes anaesthetized with chloralose (50 mg/kg), were used in these studies. The methodology employed in these experiments is described in detail elsewhere (8).

The following treatment were applied in random order to each animal group after establishing baseline values for pressure and flow and obtaining normal arterial blood gases and pH:

    1. Arachidonic acid was infused directly into the left pulmonary arterial perfusion circuit for 2 min at varying rates. Doses of arachidonic acid were expressed as amount/kg body wt/min.

The Physiological Development of the Fetus and Newborn
ISBN 0 12 389080 2
Copyright © 1985 by Academic Press, London.
All rights of reproduction in any form reserved.

2. Hypoxia was produced by lowering the inspired O_2 to 6% for 3 min in fetal and newborn animals (10% for 15 min in adults).

3. A combination of the two treatments was given, with hypoxia started for 1 min, and arachidonic acid infused during the second and third min of hypoxia in fetal and newborn animals (fifth to tenth min of 15 min of hypoxia in adults). A recovery period of at least 10 min was allowed between each experimental period in order to return to control values.

4. Following the above treatments perinatal animals received 50 mg OKY 1581 (ONO Pharmaceutical Co), a thromboxane synthetase inhibitor, slowly into the pulmonary artery. Hypoxia and arachidonic acid treatments were then repeated.

5. Perinatal lambs were treated with authentic PGH_2, prepared according to Egan et al. (9) and modified by She et al. (10). Injections of 0.1 ml of 1.0, 10.0, 20.0 and 40.0 μg/ml directly into the pulmonary artery were performed within 15 s of PGH_2 dilution with saline.

6. In preliminary studies in which 4 fetal lambs were treated only with arachidonic acid, pulmonary venous blood was sampled and assayed (RIA) for 6-keto-$PGF_{1\alpha}$ and TXB_2.

Results

Intrapulmonary arterial infusion of arachidonic acid (134 and 164 μg/kg min) in ventilated ($FIO_2 = 0.30$) fetal and newborn lambs resulted in a marked pressor response (Fig. 1). Hypoxia ($FIO_2 = 0.06$) also induced a marked pressor response (peak fetal, 160% increase in PVR; peak newborn, 140% increase in PVR). When fetal sheep were subjected to 3 min of hypoxia during which arachidonic acid ($+1.0$ min) was infused into the pulmonary artery for 2 min, the pulmonary pressor response was greater than that seen with arachidonic acid or hypoxia alone (Fig. 2). In contrast, the pulmonary pressor response to hypoxia and arachidonic acid in newborn lambs was not altered from that seen with arachidonic acid alone. Adult sheep subjected to infusions of arachidonic acid (12.3–17.6 μg/kg/min) gave similar pulmonary pressor responses. The adult pulmonary pressor response to arachidonic acid was not altered by hypoxia (10%) or another pressor agent ($PGF_{2\alpha}$, 4.4 μg/kg/min). In addition, the pulmonary pressor response to hypoxia was not affected by concomitant arachidonic infusions. In all 3 age groups arachidonic acid produced a systemic hypotension. Similarly, in all 3 age groups hypoxia seemed to enhance formation of dilators from the lung as evidence by a greater fall in systemic pressure.

Following thromboxane synthetase inhibition with OKY 1581 in newborn lambs, 2 doses of arachidonic acid (53 and 164 μg/kg/min) produced peak increases in pulmonary vascular resistance (PVR) which were 80 and 50% less than the peak responses to arachidonic acid prior to OKY 1581. In fetal lambs treated with OKY 1581, arachidonic acid (296 μg/kg/min) produced peak increases in PVR which were 54% less than the PVR prior to the blocker.

Bolus injections of PGH_2 (0.24–0.61 μg/kg) produced significant ($P < 0.05$) increases in PVR of unventilated fetal lambs.

Analyses of pulmonary venous concentrations of 6-keto-$PGF_{1\alpha}$ and TXB_2

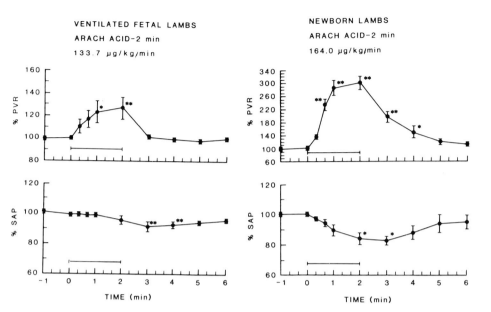

Figure 1. Average pulmonary and systemic responses to 2-min infusions of arachidonic acid (8 fetuses, ave. dose = 133.7 ± 11.7 μg/kg/min) (Newborn, ave. dose = 164.0 ± 15.9 μg/kg/min) Vertical bars = SEM; horizontal bars = duration of treatment. Points marked with asterisks are slightly different from value at 0 min; $*P = <0.05$, $**P = <0.01$.

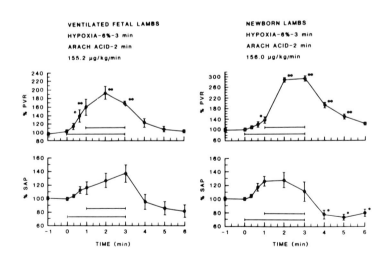

Figure 2. Average pulmonary and systemic responses to a combination of 3-min periods of hypoxia (FIO$_2$ = 0.06) and 2-min infusion of arachidonic acid. (n=4 ventilated fetuses, 5 newborn). Symbols as in Fig. 1.

were made before and after infusions of arachidonic acid directly into the pulmonary artery (200 μg/kg/min). Results showed a significant increase in TXB_2 (64%) (above control levels) after the injection. Although there was a small increase in pulmonary venous plasma concentration of 6-keto-$PGF_{1\alpha}$, following arachidonic acid infusion, the increment was not statistically significant.

Discussion

In ventilated fetal lambs, newborn lambs, and adult sheep, arachidonic acid always produced pulmonary vasoconstriction and generally systemic hypotension. This was not due to pre-existing pulmonary tone in adult sheep, since elevation of PVR with hypoxia or $PGF_{2\alpha}$ does not modify response to arachidonic acid. In ventilated fetuses, the effect of arachidonic acid infusion was additive to the hypoxic pulmonary pressor response, while the pulmonary vascular response to arachidonic acid in newborn lambs was unaltered by hypoxia. Thus, differences observed between the present studies and reports by others (5-7, 10) on the pulmonary response to arachidonic acid, do not appear to be age related, but may be due to species variation. A portion of the response to arachidonic acid was due to formation of thromboxanes as shown by significant reduction of the pulmonary pressor response following OKY 1581, as well as by the pulmonary venous plasma concentration elevation of TXB_2. The elevation of PVR is not due to platelet aggregation since similar responses were observed in isolated saline perfused lungs (12). Additionally, injections of authentic PGH_2, caused pulmonary vasoconstriction in ventilated fetal lambs. These studies suggest that: (a) the perinatal pulmonary vasculature does not produce primarily dilator substances from exogenous arachidonic acid; and (b) the pressor response to arachidonic acid in (fetal, newborn, and adult) sheep is due in part to thromboxanes, perhaps PGF_2 and/or intermediate cycle endoperoxides.

References

1. Kadowitz, P. J., Spannhake, E. W., Greenberg, S., Feigen, L. P. and Hyman, A. L. (1977). *Can. J. Physiol. Pharmacol.* **55**, 1369-1377.
2. Tyler, T. L., Leffler, C. W. and Cassin, S. (1978). *Prostaglan. Med.* **1**, 213-229.
3. Wicks, T. C., Rose, J. C., Johnson, M., Ramwell, P. W. and Kot, P. A. (1976).
4. Hyman, A. L., Mathe, A. A., Leslie, C. A., Matthews, C. C., Bennett, J. T., Spannhake, E. W. and Kadowitz, P. J. (1978). *J. Pharmacol. Exp. Ther.* **207**, 388-401.
5. Mullane, K. M., Dusting, G. J., Salmon, J. A., Moncada, S. and Vane, J. R. (1979). *Eur. J. Pharmacol.* **54**, 217-228.
6. Hyman, A. L., Spannhake, E. W. and Kadowitz, P. J. (1980). *Am. J. Physiol.* **239**, H40-H46.
7. Gerber, J. G., Voelkel, N., Nies, A. S., McMurtry, I. F. and Reeves, J. T. (1980). *J. Appl. Physiol.* **49**, 107-112.
8. Cassin, S., Tyler, T., Leffler, C. and Wallis, R. (1979). *Am. J. Physiol.* **236**, H828-H832.
9. Egan, R. W., J. Paxton and F. A. Kuehl, Jr. (1976). *J. Biol. Chem.* **251**, 7329-7335.

10. She, H. S., McNamara, D. B., Spannhake, E. W., Hyman, A. L. and Kadowitz, P. J. (1981). *Prostaglandins* **25**, 531–541.
11. Moon, M., Lemen, R. J., Quan, S. and Whitten, M. (1982). *Physiologist* **25**, 275.
12. Leffler, C. W., Greene, R. S., Jenning, S. R. V. and Cassin, S. (1984). *Prostaglan. Leuk. Med.* (in press).

The Regulation of CTP: Cholinephosphate Cytidylyltransferase in Human Fetal Lung

A. D. Postle, A. N. Hunt and I. C. S. Normand

Child Health, Faculty of Medicine,
Southampton General Hospital, Southampton, UK

Introduction

CTP: cholinephosphate cytidylyltransferase catalyses the rate-limiting, and hence regulatory, reaction of phosphatidylcholine (PC) biosynthesis in liver (1) and lung (2) of the rat. The enzyme from both sources has many similar properties. It exists as a relatively inactive protomer of mol. wt 200 000 and as a more active aggregate of mol. wt in excess of 10^6. The stimulation of PC synthesis in neonatal rat liver (3) and of surfactant PC synthesis in late fetal and neonatal rat lung (4) are associated with an increased aggregation state and stimulated activity of cytidylyltransferase. This was interpreted for neonatal rat liver as a translocation of enzyme from the cytoplasmic to the microsomal fraction of the hepatocyte. The protomeric L-form of cytidylyltransferase from 16 to 18-day fetal rat lung, before the initiation of surfactant synthesis, can be stimulated extensively and aggregated to the H-form of the enzyme by incubation with an emulsion of phosphatidylglycerol (PG). (5) It has been proposed that the increased concentrations of fetal lung PG in late gestation could regulate surfactant PC synthesis by activation of cytidylyltransferase. However, information about the enzyme activity in rat lung might not be directly applicable to the study of human fetal lung development. Little is known about the enzyme activity, subcellular distribution or PG-activation properties of cytidylyltransferase from either fetal or adult human lung. We report here preliminary observations on these parameters.

The Physiological Development of the Fetus and Newborn
ISBN 0 12 389080 2
Copyright © 1985 by Academic Press, London.
All rights of reproduction in any form reserved.

Materials and Methods

Fetal human lung was obtained at 14–17 weeks of gestation after therapeutic abortion. Samples of adult human lung were obtained at postmortem. Tissue was stored at $-70°C$ until use. Lung samples were homogenized in 4 volumes of buffer (150 mmol NaCl, 50 mmol TrisHCl, pH7-4, 1 mmol DTT, 1 mmol EDTA-Na$_2$, 1 mmol sodium azide and 0.2 mmol PMSF). Mitochondrial fractions obtained by centrifugation at 10 000**g** for 15 min were not analysed due to the extensive tar contamination of all adult samples. Microsomal and cytosolic fractions were prepared from the pellet and supernatant of a subsequent centrifugation at 100 000**g** for 1 h. Cytidylyltransferase activity was measured at 37°C by the incorporation over 20 min of [^{14}C-methyl] choline phosphate into CDP: choline both before and after pre-incubation with 0.25 mmol PG. (4) Gel filtration through Sepharose 6B was performed using a 2.6 × 90 cm column. SDS-polyacrylamide gel electrophoresis was performed in 10% gels according to Laemmli. (6) Protein was measured using the Phenol: Ciocalteau reagent. (7)

Results and Discussion

Distribution of enzyme

Table 1. Cytidylyltransferase activity in adult and fetal human lung (nmol/min/g dry wt in the presence of 0.25 mmol PG, mean ± SEM)

	Microsomes		Cytosol	
Fetal human lung ($n = 10$)	80 ± 19	(16.6%)	401 ± 67	(83.4%)
Adult human lung ($n = 5$)	159 ± 27	(21.8%)	569 ± 145	(78.2%)

The fraction of enzyme activity measurable in the microsomal fraction of fetal lung (16.6%) was not significantly different from that of adult lung (21.8%). Neither enzyme activity was stimulated by PG. Results are expressed per g dry weight of lung to account for the differing percentage dry weight of fetal (9.2%) and adult human (15.9%) lung. These results argue against a progressive translocation during development of cytidylyltransferase from the cytosolic to the microsomal compartments. However, no information is available about the subcellular distribution of the enzyme in perinatal lung.

Activation of cytosolic cytidylyltransferase activity by phosphatidylglycerol

There was no significant difference between the maximal (PG-stimulated) cytosolic cytidylyltransferase activities of adult and fetal human lung (Table 2). In the absence of PG, fetal enzyme activity was half that of the adult and the extent of PG stimulation was greater (134 *vs* 71%). However, it is hard to interpret these figures as representing a predominantly inactive enzyme in fetal human lung compared with adult lung, especially as the enzyme activity of immature fetal rat lung at a comparable stage of gestational development (16–18 days) was

Table 2. Cytosolic cytidylyltransferase activity (nmol/min/mg protein, mean ± SEM)

	No PG	+0.25 mmol PG	PG stimulation
Fetal human lung (14–17 weeks, $n = 10$)	0.30 ± 0.04	0.72 ± 0.12	134%
Adult human lung ($n = 5$)	0.59 ± 0.16	0.98 ± 0.25	71%
Fetal rat lung (16–18 days, $n = 8$)	0.23 ± 0.04	1.24 ± 0.18	440%

stimulated 440% by PG. These results were further complicated by modulation of enzyme activities *in vitro* independently of PG. For instance, adult lung cytosolic activity in the absence of PG was stimulated by 50% after incubation either overnight at 4°C or for 2 h at 37°C. Consequently, we investigated the molecular weight distribution of cytidylyltransferase for both adult and fetal human lung.

Molecular weight distribution of cytidylyltransferase

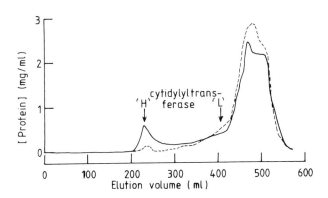

Figure 1. Eution profile of human adult lung cytosol on Sepharose 6B (2.6 × 90 cm). – – – No pre-incubation; ———— +0.25 mmol phosphatidyl glycerol.

Samples (15 ml) of cytosol from adult of fetal human lung were incubated at 37°C for 2 h either with or without 0.25 mmol PG and were then applied to a column of Sepharose 6B at 4°C. A typical elution profile of protein from adult lung cytosol is shown in Fig. 1. The fractions containing the high mol. wt form (H) and the low mol. wt form (L) of cytidylyltransferase are indicated. The results obtained were unexpected and showed little difference between adult and fetal enzymes. Cytidylyltransferase present as H-form was respectively 49% and 41%

for fetal and adult lung cytosol. For both tissue sources the total enzyme activity recovered from the column was about three times that applied. In neither case was the relative distribution of enzyme forms affected by pre-incubation of cytosol with PG. Also, no enzyme activity recovered from the Sepharose 6B column was significantly stimulated by PG. Ammonium sulphate at 40% fractional saturation precipitated over 60% of both H and L-cytidylyltransferase, the activity being recoverable in the centrifuge pellet after dialysis. One problem encountered here was that ammonium sulphate inhibited enzyme activity at concentrations much lower than required for precipitation.

H-cytidylyltransferase was very unstable, 90% of activity being lost on storage at 4°C for 1 week. By contrast, L-cytidylyltransferase remained stable under identical conditions. The instability of H-enzyme might be related to the major quantitative effect of PG on lung cytosol. This is shown in Fig. 1, and was confirmed by SDS-PAGE of column fractions, to be polymerization of G-actin (mol. wt 42 500) into F-actin, which eluted in the void volume. This aggregation occurred spontaneously but was greater accelerated by incubation with PG. It was easily shown to occur after preparation of the cytosolic fraction by centrifugation at 100 000g for 1 h. Virtually all protein in the void fractions from the Sepharose 6B column, including F-actin and H-cytidylyltransferase, were pelleted by a repeat centrifugation at 100 000g for 1 h. Similar centrifugation of L-cytidylyltransferase fractions did not affect enzyme activity. It is possible that the loss of H-cytidylyltransferase activity on storage was due to the formation of increasingly insoluble aggregates with F-actin.

Summary

The discrepancy between the PG-stimulation, albeit slight, of fetal human lung cytosolic cytidylyltransferase and the properties of the enzyme after gel filtration is hard to reconcile. Presumably some regulatory factor was separated by the Sepharose 6B column. It is not known whether this is related to enzyme interaction with actin polymerization or to the putative enzyme phosphorylation. (8) No precautions were taken in these experiments against the actions of phosphoprotein phosphatases. On reflection, the similarity between the fetal and adult cytidylyltransferase need not be surprising as alveolar Type II cells account for only about 16% of the lung parenchyma. (9) A developmental change in the surfactant-specific cytidylyltransferase of Type II cells could easily be masked by the lack of response of the overall tissue enzyme. This observation emphasized the problem encountered when using measurements on whole lung to investigate the regulation of the enzymes of surfactant biosynthesis. Such studies ideally require the isolation of fetal pre-alveolar and adult alveolar Type II cells.

Acknowledgements

This work was supported by a grant from the National Medical Research Fund.

References

1. Infante, J. P. and Kinsella, J. E. (1978). *Biochim. Biophys. Acta* **526**, 440–449.
2. Rooney, S. A. (1979). *Trends Biochem. Sci.* **4**, 189–191.
3. Pelech, S. L., Power, E. and Vance, D. E. (1983). *Can. J. Biochem. Cell Biol.* **61**, 1147–1152.
4. Stern, W., Kovac, C. and Weinhold, P. A. (1976). *Biochim. Biophys. Acta* **441**, 280–293.
5. Feldman, D. A., Kovac, C. R., Dranginis, P. L. and Weinhold, P. A. (1978). *J. Biol. Chem.* **253**, 4980–4986.
6. Laemmli, U. K. (1970). *Nature*, **227**, 680–685.
7. Lowry, O. H., Rosebrough, N. J., Farr, A. L. and Randall, R. J. (1951). *J. Biol. Chem.* **193**, 265–275.
8. Pelech, S. L. and Vance, D. E. (1982). *J. Biol. Chem.* **257**, 14198–14202.
9. Crapo, J. D., Barry, B. E., Gehr, P., Bachofen, M. and Weibel, E. R. (1982). *Am. Rev. Resp. Dis.* **125**, 332–337.

Surfactant Replacement Therapy for Respiratory Distress Syndrome

Z. Weintraub[1], Y. Sorokin[2], E. Flohr[3], T. C. Lancu[1],
H. Abramovici[2], G. D. Eitan[4] and N. Gruener[3]

Departments of Pediatrics and Neonatal Intensive Care[1], Obstetrics and
Gynecology[2], and Clinical Chemistry[3], Carmel Hospital;
Faculty of Medicine[1] and Department of Biology[4], Technion-Israel Institute
of Technology, Haifa, Israel

Surfactant (SF) deficiency is crucial in the pathogenesis of neonatal respiratory distress syndrome (RDS). There are recent reports concerning surfactant replacement therapy (SRT) in premature animals (1,2) and man (3) using synthetic dipalmitoylphosphatidyl choline (DPPC) and phosphatidylglycerol (PG) (4,5), natural surfactant (N-SF) (6,7), or mixture of both (3). Some of the reports are encouraging; however, very recent reports are somewhat disappointing (8,9). This report describes preliminary results with SRT in premature babies with severe RDS.

Materials and Methods

Synthetic DPPC and PG were purchased and DPPC in powder form was mixed with PG dispersed in chloroform in weight ratio of 7:3. The chloroform was evaporated under a nitrogen stream and the remaining mixture was resuspended in ether which was re-evaporated under nitrogen stream. This last step was repeated several times until a dry precipitate was obtained. The precipitate was diluted with sterile phosphate buffer and sonicated in a bath sonicator until the suspension cleared. The material was kept at $-20\,^{\circ}\mathrm{C}$ and bacterial cultures were obtained periodically. Just before use, the artificial surfactant (A-SF) was heated to $40\,^{\circ}\mathrm{C}$ and sonicated for 10 min. Each 1 ml of the material contained 25 mg of A-SF. One ml of A-SF was instilled endotracheally as a rapid bolus injection and the ventilator peak inspiratory pressure (PIP), positive end expiratory pressure (PEEP), and inspiratory time were increased by 10–20% for 20 s in order to facilitate A-SF delivery to atelectatic areas.

The Physiological Development of the Fetus and Newborn
ISBN 0 12 389080 2

Copyright © 1985 by Academic Press, London.
All rights of reproduction in any form reserved.

Twenty-two newborns at 26–34 weeks of gestation ($x \pm$ SD: 29.2 ± 2.7) were included in the study. Inclusion criteria were: Severe RDS necessitating endotracheal intubation; use of the ventilator with at least 20 cm of PIP; inspired oxygen concentration (FiO_2) of 0.6 or more; clinical deterioration prior to treatment. Similar criteria were used for retreatment.

There were 32 A-SF instillations. The initial dose was given at 0.5–140 hours of age ($x \pm$ SD: 7.42 ± 12.5). Seven infants received a second dose at 2–80 h ($x \pm$ SD: 4.38 ± 2.13) after the initial dose. A third dose was given to 3 infants, 15–24 h ($x \pm$ SD: 19.66 ± 3.68) after the second dose.

Effects of therapy were assessed by comparing alveolar-arterial oxygen gradient ($AaDO_2$), partial arterial carbon dioxide pressure ($PaCO_2$) and PIP shortly before and 10–180 min ($x \pm$ SD: 70.8 ± 44.4) after SRT. Intermittent frequent sampling of arterial blood were performed during the 3 h posttherapy and the samples showing the greatest improvement were used for analysis. Paired t test was used for statistical analysis of significance. Chest X-rays were compared as well.

Results

In most individual treatments, SRT produced improvements in pulmonary functions, with significant reductions in $AaDO_2$, $PaCO_2$ and PIP (Table 1). A marked improvement in the roentgenographic findings was also noticed: There was clearing of the air-bronchogram and of the reticulogranular pattern and increased lung volumes. When changes in $AaDO_2$ and PIP were displayed against postnatal age, there seemed to be an inverse relationship between the 2 parameters: The earlier A-SF administration, the better the response. The response of all 3 parameters to repeated doses seemed to be less pronounced than the initial response.

Table 1. Mean and standard deviation of 32 surfactant administration

Parameter	Units	Mean	Standard Deviation	t	P
$AaDO_2$ I	Torr	385.0	181.8	4.31	<0.01
$AaDO_2$ II	Torr	262.0	140.6		
$PaCO_2$ I	Torr	35.6	12.9	4.98	<0.01
$PaCO_2$ II	Torr	27.0	9.5		
PIP I	CmH_2	27.5	5.2	4.26	<0.01
PIP II	CmH_2	22.6	5.2		

I: Before therapy. II: After therapy.

Eight infants died, most of them with birthweights of less than 1000 g. Their weight was significantly ($P < 0.01$) smaller than that of surviving infants. The patients had the following diagnoses: sepsis (2 infants); asphyxia and intraventricular haemorrhage (birthweight 720 g); renal malformation; intestinal obstruction and liver failure; symptomatic patent ductus arteriosus and bronchopulmonary dysplasia; and severe pulmonary interstitial emphysema

(2 infants). Among the 14 survivors, the following complications were observed: Patent ductus arteriosus, bronchopulmonary dysplasia, first degree retinopathy of prematurity and pneumothorax.

Discussion

Most artificial surfactants are composed of mixtures of synthetic DPPC and PG which provide the rapid spreading characteristics. In surfactant-depleted adult rats, such a mixture was the most effective in restoring the lung pressure-volume characteristics (2). The presently available preparations present some problems. The aqueous dispersions may trap the phospholipids (PL) in liposomes (*in vitro*) thus inhibiting their spreading as a monolayer (10). In addition, dry powder SF may adhere to the endotracheal tube and may be degraded by the wet environment, could swell and obstruct small airways. A desirable preparation would be a synthetic, nonantigenic SF, which performs *in vivo* effectively as a surface-tension reducing material.

The results of this limited study suggest that aqueous dispersion of synthetic DPPC-PG may be temporarily effective in improving neonatal respiratory performance in most patients. This was a very selected group of infants, with severe RDS and continuous clinical deterioration despite mechanical ventilation and with high inflative pressures and high inspired oxygen concentrations, prior to SRT. The clinical improvement of the patients was paralleled by improvement of blood gas values and of chest roentgenograms, as well as a significant decrease in mechanical inflation pressures and FiO_2. The effect of SRT lasted for a variable time but the impression was that the maximum effect was of 3–6 h duration. Several instillations are probably required for optimal results. The dosage needed seemed to be much larger than the one theoretically calculated. Exogenous SF may undergo inhibition, metabolism and could form large aggregates in the airways.

The risks of using A-SF are difficult to estimate from this study: 6 out of the 8 deaths in our groups were not related to SRT. Nevertheless, the possible connection between rapid improvement in lung compliance after SRT and the appearance of severe pulmonary interstitial emphysema in 2 patients needs further consideration. Artificial SRT appears to be effective in some newborns and its benefits seem to outweigh the potential risks. At present, in addition to A-SF, we are using natural surfactant in the treatment of severe RDS of very small premature babies. The natural SF is obtained from amniotic fluid. While no conclusive data is yet available, our preliminary impression is that natural surfactant is probably more effective than the artificial compounds.

References

1. Enhorning, G., Hill, D., Sherwood, G. *et al.* (1978). *Am. J. Obstet. Gynecol.* **132**, 529–536.
2. Ikegami, M., Silverman, J. and Adams, F. H. (1979). *Pediat. Res.* **13**, 777–780.

3. Fujiwara, T., Maeta, H. and Chida, S. T. (1980). *Lancet* **1**, 55-57.
4. Ivey, H. H., Kattwinkel, J. and Roth, S. (1980). *In: "Liposomes and Immunology"* (Tom, H. B. and Six, H. R., eds) pp. 301-314, Elsevier-North Holland, New York.
5. Morley, C. J., Bangham, A. D. and Miller, N. *et al.* (1981). *Lancet* **1**, 64-67.
6. Smythe, J. A., Metcalfe, I. L. and Duffy, P. (1983). *Pediat.* **71**, 913-917.
7. Hallman, M., Merritt, T. A. and Schneider, H. (1983). *Pediat.* **71**, 473-482.
8. Halliday, L. H., Reid, M. N. and Meban, C. *et al.* (1984). *Lancet* **1**, 476-478.
9. Milner, A. D., Vyas, H. and Hopkin, I. E. (1984). *Arch. Dis. Child.* **59**(4), 369-371.
10. Morley, C. J., Bangham, A. D., Miller, N. *et al.* (1978). *Nature* **271**, 162-163.

Fetal Surfactant Maturation in Diabetic Pregnancy

D. K. James

Consultant Senior Lecturer in Obstetrics, Southmead Hospital,
Westbury on Trym, Bristol, UK

The association between maternal diabetes and neonatal respiratory distress has been recognized for a long time (1,2). Yet the relationship between the two conditions is controversial (3) and a number of unresolved questions remain:

1. Does maternal diabetes produce a delay in fetal surfactant production and directly *cause* a higher incidence of respiratory distress syndrome (RDS)?

2. Why is the lecithin:sphingomyelin (L/S) ratio generally recognized to be of diminished value in diabetic pregnancies (4,5,6).

To answer these questions fetal surfactant phospholipid maturation was compared during normal and diabetic pregnancies. Surfactant phospholipids were studied using a technique employing two-dimensional thin layer chromatography (TLC) and assay of inorganic phosphorus. The details of this method have been published elsewhere (7,8,9).

Figure 1 illustrates the changes in amniotic fluid phospholipids over the last 10 weeks of normal pregnancy. The concentration of sphingomyelin (SM) remained relatively low and constant over this time, but the concentration of PC rose progressively after the 33rd week. The concentration of PI also rose after 33 weeks but fell off towards term. PG did not appear in significant amounts until 36 or 37 weeks but thereafter became the second most common phospholipid after PC. It is now accepted that during normal pregnancy two kinds of surfactant are made by the fetus: an "early" one (PC and PI only) from 34 to 36 or 37 weeks and a "late" one (PC, PI and PG) from 36 or 37 weeks onwards.

The influence of maternal diabetes on fetal surfactant maturation was studied by examination of the phospholipids in amniotic fluid (obtained by amniocentesis) over the last 10 weeks of pregnancy in 3 groups of patients (Table 1).

Comparisons were made using 3 gestational subgroups: 33 weeks and less, 34–36 weeks and 37 weeks or more (verified by ultrasonic scan in the first half of pregnancy).

The Physiological Development of the Fetus and Newborn
ISBN 0 12 389080 2

Copyright © 1985 by Academic Press, London.
All rights of reproduction in any form reserved.

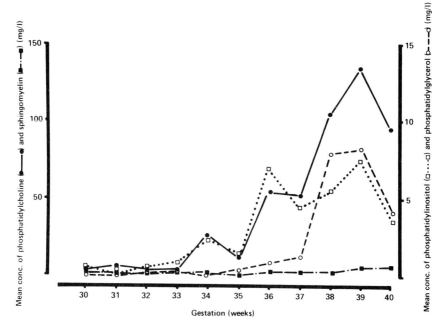

Figure 1. Mean concentration of phospholipids in amniotic fluid over the last 10 weeks of normal pregnancy.

Table 1. Sources of amniotic fluid

Group	Characteristics	Number of patients
Normals	Totally normal pregnancies; free of all factors claimed to influence fetal lung maturation (10)	33
Diabetics — excellent control	Mean peak value of sequential 24 h blood glucose series over the second and third trimesters < 8.5 mmol/l	17
Diabetics — suboptimal control	Mean peak value of sequential 24 h blood glucose series over the second and third trimesters of > 8.5 mmol/l	27

The median PC levels (Table 2) in all gestational periods of the well controlled diabetics patients were higher than the median PC concentrations in the nondiabetic and poorly controlled diabetic patients. The differences for 34–36 weeks were statistically significant ($P < 0.05$). The median PC concentrations in the poorly controlled diabetics were similar to the levels found in the nondiabetic patients.

Table 2. Concentration of phosphatidylcholine in amniotic fluid

Gestational age (weeks)	Concentration of PC (mg/l)		
	Nondiabetics	Poorly controlled diabetics	Well controlled diabetics
≤ 33	5.53 (2.96–9.97) (n = 7)	7.48 (4.73–13.3) (n = 3)	20.73 (5.45–36.01)* (n = 2)
34–36	24.74 (8.81–79.41) (n = 8)	25.87 (2.29–137.02) (n = 21)	60.06 (17.18–208.83)** (n = 12)
≥ 37	55.45 (41.47–287.56) (n = 18)	85.71 (18.65–380.31) (n = 6)	110.04 (54.08–202.13)* (n = 4)

Results are median (range).
*Not significant.
**Well controlled vs nondiabetics P = 0.04; well controlled vs poorly controlled P = 0.02.

Table 3. Concentration of sphingomyelin (SM) in amniotic fluid

Gestational age (weeks)	Concentration of SM (mg/l)		
	Nondiabetics	Poorly controlled diabetics	Well controlled diabetics
≤ 33	3.26 (2.88–4.12) (n = 7)	0.79 (0.70–1.10)* (n = 3)	3.57 (2.78–4.36) (n = 2)
34–36	2.37 (0.96–5.25) (n = 8)	2.99 (0.75–14.99) (n = 21)	2.43 (1.61–6.70) (n = 12)
≥ 37	3.20 (1.40–17.04) (n = 18)	3.08 (1.35–7.18) (n = 6)	4.02 (3.54–5.64) (n = 4)

Results are median (range).
*Poorly controlled vs nondiabetic P = 0.04; poorly controlled vs well controlled P = 0.04.

The median concentrations of SM (Table 3) in the well controlled diabetics were constant (at 2–4 mg/l) and similar to these in the nondiabetic samples for all 3 gestational periods. In the poorly controlled diabetics the median SM concentrations for 34–36 weeks and > 37 weeks were also similar to those values in normal pregnancy. However, in those of < 33 weeks the median SM concentration was significantly lower than in normal pregnancy ($P < 0.05$) and the well controlled pregnancy ($P < 0.05$).

In both the poorly and well controlled preterm diabetic patients the median PC/SM ratios, as well as the majority of the individual values were > 4.21 (that ratio corresponding to a conventional L/S ratio of 2.0 measured planimetrically using single dimension TLC). This observation is especially relevant in those diabetics who were < 33 weeks. In those well controlled diabetics (< 33 weeks) the elevation of the PC/SM ratio was due to a real elevation of PC levels; whilst in the poorly controlled diabetics of comparable gestational age, the elevation of the PC/SM ratio was mainly the result of a lowering of SM concentration.

In all 3 gestational periods the median PI concentrations in the well controlled diabetics were greater than in both the nondiabetic and the poorly controlled diabetic patients. This was statistically significant at 34–36 weeks ($P < 0.05$). The concentrations of PI were similar in the poorly controlled diabetic and normal patients for each gestational period.

There were very low median concentrations of PG at < 33 weeks in all 3 groups of patients, but at 34–36 weeks, whilst the median concentration of PG remained low in the normal and poorly controlled diabetic patients, there was a significant rise in median PG concentration in the well controlled diabetics ($P < 0.05$). At term (> 37 weeks) there were similar levels of PG in all 3 groups of patients.

Infants born to diabetic mothers have a higher morbidity which includes hypoglycaemia, polycythaemia, jaundice and being large for dates. It have been unable to demonstrate that the association with respiratory distress syndrome was due to a delayed appearance of fetal lung surfactant in such babies. Indeed, in the well controlled diabetic pregnancy there was evidence of enhanced surfactant maturation. The PC/SM ratio in diabetic pregnancies was generally greater for any gestational age than in normal pregnancies. Whilst in most cases this was due to a higher PC concentration, in a few poorly controlled preterm diabetics it was the result of a lower concentration of SM. This undoubtedly explains why the L/S ratio is of questionable value in diabetic pregnancy. It is speculated that elective preterm delivery together with a falsely reassuring L/S ratio are major contributory factors to the documented association between maternal diabetes and neonatal respiratory distress.

References

1. Gellis, S. S. and Hsia, D. Y. Y. (1959). *Am. J. Dis. Child.* **97**, 1–41.
2. Lemons, J. A., Vargas, P. and Delaney, J. J. (1981). *Obstet. Gynecol.* **57**, 187–192.
3. Robert, M. F., Neff, R. K., Hubbell, J. P., Taensch, H. W. and Avery, M. E. (1976). *N. Engl. J. Med.* **294**, 357–360.
4. Dahlenburg, G. W., Martin, F. I. R., Jeffrey, P. E. and Horacek, I. (1977). *Br. J. Obstet. Gynecol.* **84**, 294–299.
5. Donald, I. R., Freeman, R. K., Goebelsmann, U., Chan, W. H. and Nakamura, R. M. (1973). *Am. J. Obstet. Gynecol.* **115**, 547–552.
6. Mueller-Heubach, E., Caritas, S. N., Edelstone, D. I. and Turner, J. H. (1978). *Am. J. Obstet. Gynecol.* **130**, 28–34.
7. James, D. K., Harkes, A., Williams, M., Chiswick, M. L., Tindall, V. R., Richardson, T. and Gowenlock, A. (1984). *J. Obstet. Gynaecol.* **4**, 166–169.
8. James, D. K., Chiswick, M. L., Harkes, A., Williams, M. and Tindall, V. R. (1984). *Br. J. Obstet. Gynaecol.* **91**, 316–324.
9. James, D. K., Chiswick, M. L., Harkes, A., Williams, M. and Tindall, V. R. (1984). *Br. J. Obstet. Gynaecol.* **91**, 325–329.
10. Gluck, L. (1980). *Mead Johnson Symp. Perinat. Dev. Med.* **14**, 40–49.

Accelerated Fetal Lung Maturation and Fetal Catecholamines

Norimasa Sagawa, Takeshi Okazaki,
Akira Muneshige and Takahide Mori

Department of Gynecology and Obstetrics, Kyoto University,
Faculty of Medicine, Kyoto, Japan

Phosphatidylglycerol (PG), a second major component of the surfactant, appears and increases in amniotic fluid at approximately 36 weeks gestation and thereafter. In certain pregnancies complicated with maternal diabetes mellitus, amniotic fluid PG has been shown to be most predictive for fetal lung maturity. Recently, it was reported that amniotic fluid levels of catecholamines increased as pregnancy progressed, a sharp increase in late pregnancy (1,2). The recent identification of β-adrenergic receptor in fetal lung (3), a significant increase of both PG and catecholamines in pregnancies of growth-retarded fetus (4), and a decrease in the incidence of respiratory distress syndrome (RDS) after treatment of premature labour with β_2-adrenergic agonist in low-birth weight infant (5), all indicated a close relationship between fetal lung maturation and fetal adrenergic activity.

In this paper, amniotic fluid PG, measured enzymatically, was correlated with amniotic fluid content of catecholamines and their monoamine oxidase (MAO) metabolites, 3,4-dihydroxyphenylglycol (DOPEG) and 3,4-dihydroxyphenylacetic acid (DOPAC) from norepinephrine and dopamine, respectively, determined by radioenzymatic assay. A physiological role of catecholamines in the development of fetal lung maturation will be discussed.

Material and Methods

Amniotic fluid samples were obtained from women undergoing amniocentesis for medical indications or elective caesarian section, or vaginally collected from women complicated with premature rupture of the membrane or at normal vaginal delivery. The first urine from newborns was obtained immediately after delivery: 1 ml amniotic fluid was placed into a tube containing 1.2 mg glutathione, and

The Physiological Development of the Fetus and Newborn
ISBN 0 12 389080 2

Copyright © 1985 by Academic Press, London.
All rights of reproduction in any form reserved.

1.8 mg ethylene glycol-bis(β-aminoethylether) N,N'-tetracetic acid, mixed thoroughly and centrifuged at 800**g** for 10 min at 4°C. The resulting supernatant was stored at -80°C until use.

Catecholamines and the deaminated metabolites were determined using radioenzymatic assay kit (Cat REA Kit, Upjohn Diagnostic) with some modifications.

Phosphatidylglycerol (PG) and phosphatidylcholine (PC) were determined enzymatically as described previously (6).

Results

Amniotic fluid concentrations of catecholamines and its MAO metabolites were determined from 21–41 weeks gestation. Figure 1 shows that dopamine (DA) content increased progressively with the advance of gestational age. Although data are not shown, epinephrine (E) was found detectable in significant amounts in the second half of pregnancy, but did not show any significant increase in late third trimester; in contrast, norepinephrine (NE) remained to be low up to 35 weeks' gestation, after which it rose sharply until term. Concentrations of DOPEG and DOPAC were found to be 5–6 times higher than those of their

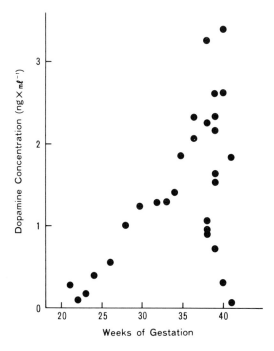

Figure 1. Concentrations of dopamine in amniotic fluid as a function of gestational age.

parent catecholamines, and elevated significantly late in pregnancy (data not shown).

Highly significant elevations of DA and PG values were noted with the samples obtained before 37 weeks gestation ($r = 0.712$, $P < 0.001$) as shown in Fig. 2, but not with those obtained after 37 weeks gestation. Similar results for NE ($P < 0.05$), E ($P < 0.02$), and DOPEG ($P < 0.001$) were also observed *vs* PG levels with the amniotic fluid samples only before 37 weeks gestation. However, DOPAC, which thought to reflect intraneuronal dopaminergic activity, did not show any significant correlation with PG throughout pregnancy.

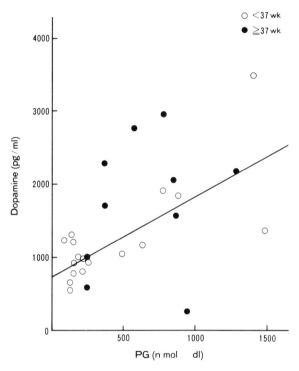

Figure 2. The correlation between concentrations of dopamine and phosphatidyl-glycerol in amniotic fluid. $y = 744 + 1.08x$; $r = 0.712$; $P < 0.001$.

Concentrations of catecholamines in the first urine of newborns were compared with those in the amniotic fluid obtained from the same patient at the time of delivery (Table 1). Catecholamines were 6–12 times higher in the first urine than in the amniotic fluid. The MAO metabolites were 2–3 times higher in the urine than in the amniotic fluid. As demonstrated in Table 1, DA constituted a considerable portion of both fetal urine (69%) and amniotic fluid (65%). The ratios of DA/DOPAC and NE/DOPEG in the amniotic fluid were 0.26 and 0.25, respectively, while these same ratios in the urine were 1.57 and 0.66, respectively.

Table 1. Concentrations of catecholamines and MAO metabolites in the amniotic fluid and fetal urine obtained at the time of delivery (37–40 weeks gestation)

	Amniotic fluid (pg/ml)	Fetal urine (pg/ml)	Fetal urine/ amniotic fluid
Dopamine (DA)	1 720	19 197	11.2
DOPAC	6 445	12 520	1.9
DA + DOPAC	8 165	31 717	3.9
Epinephrine (E)	571	6 854	12.0
Norepinephrine (NE)	345	1 956	5.7
DOPEG	1 548	4 297	2.8
NE + DOPEG	1 893	6 253	3.3
DA/DOPAC	0.26	1.57	
NE/DOPEG	0.25	0.66	

All figures are expressed as means of 7 cases.

Discussion

For intra-uterine fetal development, catecholamines are known to play an important role as first demonstrated by Zuckerkandl in 1901. Using experimental animals, an acute increase in fetal plasma catecholamines in response to hypoxia (7), and to hypoglycaemia (8) were recently reported. Significant correlation of umbilical plasma norepinephrine and epinephrine versus fetal blood pH and/or PO_2 was also demonstrated (9). Divers *et al.* found that in the smoking pregnant mother, who is known to associate with intra-uterine growth retardation (IUGR) and premature delivery, norepinephrine and DOPEG increased significantly in the amniotic fluid (10). This, together with the fact that both PG and catecholamines elevated in IUGR pregnancies (4), indicated that fetal adrenergic activity increased in response to chronic fetal distress and the increased catecholamines facilitated the process of fetal pulmonary maturation.

It is also suggested that under chronic distress, the fetus redistributes the fuel nutrients and oxygen systematically, possibly by activating intra-neuronal adrenergic tissue, as was reflected by increased content of MAO metabolites in the amniotic fluid. This hypothesis, although speculative, is consistent with the view that limiting supply of the fuel and oxygen that is found at term of normal pregnancy, might produce a trigger for extra-uterine life of the fetus; for the maturational changes of fetal organs including lung, followed by initiation of parturition. Limiting supply of glucose and/or oxygen present in IUGR pregnancies or other chronic fetal distress, may induce fetal maturation by mobilizing catecholamines systematically, as was reported a case of accelerated maturation of fetal lung in IUGR pregnancies (11). It still remains to be clarified that accelerated maturation found before 37 weeks gestation is the same as seen at term.

Concentrations of (DA + DOPAC) and (NE + DOPEG) were 3–4 times higher in the fetal urine than those in the amniotic fluid (Table 1), and dopamine is by far the predominant catecholamine in both fetal urine and amniotic fluid. These results clearly indicated that most, if not all, of catecholamines and its MAO metabolites in amniotic fluid are of fetal urine origin. It is also noted that DA/DOPAC and NE/DOPEG ratios were much higher in the urine than in amniotic fluid. Since dopamine occupied most of the catecholamines in the amniotic fluid (69%), and DA/DOPAC ratio was 6-fold higher in the urine than in the amniotic fluid, dopamine could have the potential to initiate parturition through direct myometrial dopaminergic stimulation, after it voided into amniotic compartment.

References

1. Phillippe, M. and Ryan, R. J. (1981). *Am. J. Obstet. Gynecol.* **139**, 204-208.
2. Divers, W. A., Wikes, M. M., Babaknia, A. and Yen, S. S. C. (1981). *Am. J. Obstet. Gynecol.* **139**, 483-486.
3. Jacobs, M. M., O'Brien, A. T., Goldfien, A. and Roberts, J. M. (1982). *In:* "Proceedings of the 29th Annual Meeting of the Society for Gynecologic Investigation", abstr. 318.
4. Divers, W. A., Babaknia, A., Hopper, B. R., Wilkes, M. M. and Yen, S. S. C. (1982). *Am. J. Obstet. Gynecol.* **142**, 440-444.
5. Boog, G., Brahim, M. B. and Gandar, R. (1975). *Br. J. Obstet. Gynaecol.* **82**, 285-288.
6. Muneshige, A., Okazaki, T., Quirk, J. G., MacDonald, P. C., Nozaki, M. and Johnston, J. M. (1983). *Am. J. Obstet. Gynecol.* **145**, 474-480.
7. Cohen, W. R., Piasecki, G. J., Cohn, H. E., Young, J. B. and Jackson, D. T. (1984). *Endocrinology* **114**, 383-390.
8. Phillippe, M. and Kitzmiller, J. L. (1981). *Am. J. Obstet. Gynecol.* **139**, 407-415.
9. Padbury, J. F., Roberman, B., Oddie, T. H., Hobel, C. J. and Fisher, D. A. (1982). *Obstet. Gynecol.* **60**, 607-611.
10. Divers, W. A., Wikes, M. M., Babaknia, A. and Yen, S. S. C. (1981). *Am. J. Obstet. Gynecol.* **141**, 625-628.
11. Divers, W. A., Wilkes, M. M., Babaknia, A., Hill, L. M., Quilligan, E. J. and Yen, S. S. C. (1981). *Am. J. Obstet. Gynecol.* **141**, 608-610.

Properties of Artificial Pulmonary Surfactant Containing Hexagonal H$_{II}$ Phase Promoters

Paul G. R. Harding, Shou-Hwa Yu and Fred Possmayer

Departments of Obstetrics and Gynaecology and Biochemistry, University of Western Ontario, London, Ontario, Canada

Introduction

The mammalian lung is stabilized by an extraordinary material, the pulmonary surfactant, which reduces the surface tension at the air–liquid interface of the alveoli. Presence of surfactant is particularly critical at birth when the newborn infant must clear its lungs and establish regular breathing. Absence of sufficient surfactant stores to maintain appropriate surface tensions appears to be a major factor contributing to the development of the Neonatal Respiratory Distress Syndrome, the major cause of perinatal morbidity and mortality in developed countries.

The ability of pulmonary surfactant to reduce the surface tension of an air-liquid interface to near zero is dependent upon the formation of a relatively pure monolayer of dipalmitoyl-phosphatidylcholine (DPPC) during exhalation (1). At 37°C hydrated bilayers of DPPC exist in the gel state. The other lipids and the apoproteins present in surfactant apparently facilitate the adsorption of DPPC. The realization that only DPPC and possibly phosphatidylglycerol (PG) are required in the monolayer has prompted workers to attempt to develop artificial mixtures which could transfer DPPC to the surface at a sufficient rate to maintain normal lung function (1). The present paper describes studies in which DPPC is dispersed under conditions designed to produce hexagonal H$_{II}$ phase. The latter state (Fig. 1B) consists of elongated cylinders of lipids in the inverted micellar form with fatty acids extending outwards and polar groups binding an inner core, or pore of water, which extends along the elongated cylinder (2). These studies demonstrate that artificial surfactant systems, containing DPPC

The Physiological Development of the Fetus and Newborn
ISBN 0 12 389080 2

Copyright © 1985 by Academic Press, London.
All rights of reproduction in any form reserved.

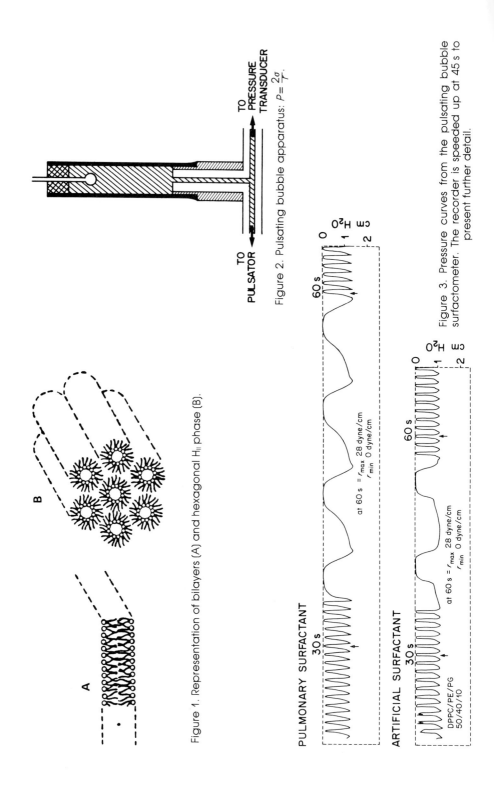

Figure 1. Representation of bilayers (A) and hexagonal H_{II} phase (B).

Figure 2. Pulsating bubble apparatus: $P = \frac{2\sigma}{r}$.

PULMONARY SURFACTANT

at 60 s = r_{max} 28 dyne/cm
r_{min} 0 dyne/cm

ARTIFICIAL SURFACTANT

DPPC/PE/PG
50/40/10

at 60 s = r_{max} 28 dyne/cm
r_{min} 0 dyne/cm

Figure 3. Pressure curves from the pulsating bubble surfactometer. The recorder is speeded up at 45 s to present further detail.

and phosphatidylethanolamine (PE), or DPPC plus PE and PG can mimic the essential properties of natural surfactant on the pulsating bubble apparatus. The effects of lipid composition, calcium ion concentration, temperature of mixing and mechanical agitation were investigated. Formation of active preparation correlated with the appearance of particles of aggregated lipids indicative of H_{II} phase.

Methods

Natural surfactant and its lipid extracts were prepared from freshly slaughtered cows as previously described (3). The ability of natural surfactant, or artificial dispersions, to reduce surface tension was assayed with a pulsating bubble surfactometer, as described by Enhorning (4). The samples are loaded into a small chamber which has a small capillary open to the atmosphere (Fig. 2). Sufficient fluid is withdrawn to produce a bubble with a radius of 0.55 mm. The bubble is pulsated at 20 cpm between 0.55 mm (r_{max}) and 0.40 mm (r_{min}) at 37°C. The pressure difference across the bubble is continuously monitored by a pressure transducer. The surface tension at any point is calculated from the Laplace equation which states that the pressure difference equals twice the surface tension divided by the radius. Artificial surfactants were prepared by hydrating the N_2-dried lipids with vigorous agitation with a wrist-action shaker for 1 h at room temperature. The dispersions were incubated 1 h at 37°C before testing on the pulsating bubble surfactometer as indicated above.

Results

Figure 3 depicts representative pressure tracing obtained with dispersions (1% w/v) of natural surfactant and for an artificial surfactant composed of DPPC/PE/PG (5:4:1). Within a few pulsations, the surface tension at r_{max} fell rapidly to 25–30 dynes/cm. This surface tension corresponds to the equilibrium surface tension for monolayers of DPPC. It can be seen that by 1 min after the initial formation of the bubble, the surface tension at minimum bubble size (r_{min}) was close to 0 dynes/cm. The recorder speeds were accelerated for a few pulsations at 45 s in order to display more detail. In contrast, artificial mixtures containing DPPC and PG alone fail to achieve surface tensions below 40 dynes/cm at r_{max} and 15 dynes/cm at r_{min} even after pulsation for several minutes (3).

Figure 4 illustrates the effect of phospholipid composition and calcium concentrations on surfactant activity. The surface tensions at r_{max} are depicted by open bars, while the surface tensions at r_{min} are depicted by closed bars. Somewhat lower surface tensions were observed with pure PE than with DPPC alone. Artificial surfactant composed of DPPC/PE (5:5) produced surface tension characteristics similar to those observed with natural surfactant. While the presence of Ca^{++} had little effect on the surfactant activity of the mixture containing PC and PE, this divalent cation was required to obtain low surface tensions with mixtures containing the acidic phospholipid PG.

During the course of these experiments, it became evident that the production

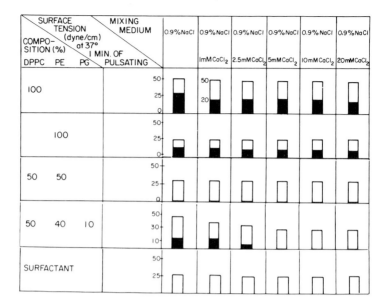

Figure 4. Effects of composition and Ca^{2+} on surface tension of mixed phospholipids.

of dispersions of artificial surfactant which were capable of reducing the surface tension of the pulsating bubble to between 25–30 dynes/cm at r_{max} and near 0 dynes/cm at r_{min} required mixing the samples at room temperature and subsequent incubation of the samples at 37°C for approximately 1 h (data not shown). It was observed that as the smooth lipid dispersions were incubated at 37°C, large flocculated lipid aggregates became visible. The appearance of these lipid aggregates correlated with the formation of active dispersions. When the lipids were mixed at 37°C which is above the phase transition of the mixture, lipid aggregates were not observed and the dispersions were not active. The appearance of lipid aggregates constitutes circumstantial evidence for the presence of H_{II} phase. Further support for the view that the formation of a surface active

Table 1. Effects of sonication on surface tension

Composition (%)				Surface tension (dyne/cm)	
DPPC	PE	PG		Before sonication	After sonication
50	50		r_{max}	29	46
(1 mmol $CaCl_2$)			r_{min}	0	20
50	40	10	r_{max}	28	40
(5 mmol $CaCl_2$)			r_{min}	0	18

Surface tension was estimated after pulsation of a 1% solution for 1 min at 37°C.

monolayer is dependent upon the presence of H_{II} phase was obtained in experiments in which active samples prepared as described above were vigorously agitated by immersion in a bath sonicator for 10 min at room temperature. Sonication resulted in the loss of surfactant activity (Table 1). The presence of lipid aggregates was also lost. Incubation at 37°C for several hours did not restore the surfactant activity, or the aggregated appearance of the sample.

Discussion

The ability to pack very closely in a monolayer at 37°C allows DPPC to bind surface water very effectively, and thereby reduces surface tension from 70 dynes/cm to near 0 dynes/cm (1). However, below 41°C hydrated bilayers of DPPC are in the solid gel state which adsorb only slowly to the air-liquid interface. The other lipids in pulmonary surfactant, divalent cations and surfactant apoproteins are all thought to promote the adsorption of DPPC to the monolayer. The present studies demonstrate that the surface adsorbability of DPPC can also be enhanced by mixing with the H_{II} phase promoter PE. Whether the artificial surfactants described in this paper contain H_{II} has not yet been proven. The following observations are consistent with this view.

First, the surfactant activity of the artificial dispersions correlated with the appearance of aggregated lipid particles. It should be clear from Fig. 1 that cylinders of H_{II} phase could be stabilized through the formation of lipid aggregates which minimize methyl-group-water interactions. Second, the bilayer to H_{II} phase transition of unsaturated PE occurs within 15°C above the high temperature end of the hydrocarbon phase transition (5). Fluorescence polarization studies demonstrated that the transition temperature of the active mixtures was near 34°C. These observations are consistent with previous observations suggesting that below the hydrocarbon chain transition, mixed lipid systems prefer the bilayer structure. Above the transition temperature, the cone-shape of PE is enhanced and the formation of inverted micellar structures is favoured (5).

Third, when mixtures are dispersed in a fluid form above the phase transition, the formation of stable closed liposomes can be promoted (5). This could explain the inability to produce active surfacts at 37°C.

Fourth, mechanical agitation can facilitate phospholipid hydration and thereby favour the formation of stable, closed liposomes (5). In contrast to the mixed lipid systems, the flaking appearance of dispersions of PE and their surface tension reducing properties were not affected by mixing temperature, temperature of incubation, or the presence of calcium.

Acknowledgements

This paper was supported by grants from the Medical Research Council of Canada.

References

1. Possmayer, F., Yu, S.-H., Weber, J. M. and Harding, P. G. R. (1984). *Can. J. Biochem. Cell. Biol.* (in press).
2. Cullis, P. R. and deKruiff, B. (1979). *Biochim. Biophys. Acta* **559**, 399–420.
3. Yu, S.-H., Harding, P. G. R., Smith, N. and Possmayer, F. (1983). *Lipids* **18**, 522–529.
4. Enhorning, G. (1977). *J. Appl. Physiol.* **42**, 976–979.
5. Tyrrell, D. A., Heath, T. D., Colley, C. M. and Ryman, B. E. (1976). *Biochim. Biophys. Acta* **457**, 259–302.

Lung Lymph Studies in Newborn Lambs with Hyaline Membrane Disease

H. W. Sundell, J. Rojas, J. Grogaard,
P. Mohan, B. Engelhardt, A. Van den Abbeele,
T. R. Harris and K. L. Brigham

Vanderbilt University School of Medicine, Department of Pediatrics and
Medicine, Nashville, Tennessee, USA

Proteinaceous pulmonary oedema is characteristically found in lungs of humans and animals with hyaline membrane disease (HMD). Increased alveolar epithelial permeability has been demonstrated in this disease (1). There is, however, reason to suspect that increased vascular endothelial permeability also exists. Other abnormalities of the pulmonary vascular bed include increased vascular resistance and decreased pulmonary blood flow (2) indicating a decrease in perfused surface area of the pulmonary vasculature.

In order to elucidate these pathophysiologic mechanisms, two sets of studies were undertaken in preterm lambs with and without hyaline membrane disease. Studies with indicator dilution technique for determination of ^{14}C-urea permeability-surface area products (PS) (3,4) and studies of lung lymph clearance for proteins were performed in two separate groups of lambs. The results should be interpreted together, since neither study alone can independently separate effects of changing vascular permeability from changing surface area of the pulmonary exchange vessels.

Methods

Indicator dilution studies

Twelve lambs were delivered by caesarian section. The umbilical cord was cut and the lambs were intubated and ventilated with a Babybird® (Bird Corporation,

The Physiological Development of the Fetus and Newborn
ISBN 0 12 389080 2

Copyright © 1985 by Academic Press, London.
All rights of reproduction in any form reserved.

Palm Springs, CA). Inspired oxygen and pressures were adjusted to maintain a PaO_2 between 60 and 90 torr and $PaCO_2$ between 35 and 45 torr. Repeated measurements were performed of cardiac output and ^{14}C-urea permeability-surface area products using an earlier described multiple indicator method (3,4) which employed injections of multiple indicators in the right ventricle and sampling from the carotid artery. ^{125}I human albumin and ^{51}Cr-labelled erythrocytes were used to establish a composite intravascular reference curve. Separate determination of right and left cardiac output, shunts through the ductus arteriosus and pulmonary blood flow was performed with a microsphere method (5). The effect of ductal shunts on PS calculations was accounted for by methods described by Harris (6). Thirteen studies were performed in HMD lambs and 12 in nonHMD lambs. Mean values for each group were calculated for the average results of 1–4 studies in each lamb. Histological examination of the lungs showed that 7 of the lambs had HMD with evidence of cell slough and hyaline membrane formation, and that 5 of the lambs lacked such pathology. The gestational age was 131 ± 1 days (mean $\pm$ SEM) for the lambs with HMD and 140 ± 1 days for the lambs without HMD.

Lung lymph studies

The efferent duct from the caudal mediastinal lymph duct was catheterized in 7 lambs with histologically verified HMD and in 7 lambs without HMD. The gestational age for the HMD lambs was 130 ± 1 and for the nonHMD lambs 135 ± 1. Vascular catheters were placed and the tail of the node was resected. Lung lymph was collected for 2 h before and for 4 h after delivery. Total protein concentration was measured in plasma and lymph using a modified Biuret method (7). Polyacrylamide gradient gel electrophoresis was used to separate proteins in lymph and plasma samples (8).

Results

Indicator dilution studies

Table 1 summarizes the results. The lambs with HMD had significantly higher mean pulmonary arterial pressure and significantly lower PS.

In 4 HMD lambs with repeated measurements PS decreased significantly from 0.47 ± 0.21 ml/s/kg at 2 h after birth to 0.22 ± 0.18 ml/s/kg at 4 h after birth, while

Table 1. Summary of measurements with indicator dilution method

| | No. of Animals | Pulmonary blood flow | | PA Pressure (Torr) | Permeability surface area | |
		(ml/s)	(ml/s/kg)		(ml/s)	(ml/s/kg)
HMD	7	10.9 ± 1.8	3.1 ± 0.6	$54 \pm 3^{\star}$	$1.06 \pm 0.33^{\star}$	$0.29 \pm 0.08^{\star}$
NonHMD	5	12.3 ± 2.0	3.2 ± 0.6	45 ± 2	3.06 ± 0.38	0.80 ± 0.12

Results are means $\pm$ SEM
*Significantly different at $P < 0.05$ (unpaired t test)

PS remained essentially unchanged in 2 lambs without HMD (0.71 ± 0.16 and 0.88 ± 0.04, respectively).

A significant inverse correlation according to an exponential function PS$=(5.8)e^{-04(PVR)}$, ($r = -0.79$, $P = 0.035$) between mean ^{14}C-urea PS products was found for each lamb and mean pulmonary vascular resistances.

Lymph studies

Table 2 summarizes the results of the lymph study. Normalized to fetal values mean lymph flow increased 3.3 times at 1 hour after birth in lambs without HMD and decreased thereafter to 1.7 times the fetal value. Lymph flow in HMD lambs increased progressively to 2.7 times the fetal value. Mean lymph/plasma protein ratios decreased with time in both groups of lambs and were always higher in HMD lambs but significantly so only at 2 h. Lymph protein clearance for total protein and all 7 protein fractions increased progressively in lambs with HMD but decreased between 1 and 4 h in lambs without HMD. At 4 h after birth protein clearance was 50% higher and the pulmonary arterial pressure was 8% higher in the HMD lambs compared to the nonHMD lambs. At 4 hours after birth, clearance in HMD lambs was 260% higher than fetal values for the three smallest fractions and 290% higher for the largest fraction. Postmortem extravascular lung water was 13.1 ± 1.1 ml/kg in nonHMD lambs and 17.8 ± 0.2 ml/kg in HMD lambs ($P < 0.025$).

Table 2. Summary of lung lymph study

	PA pressure (torr)	Lymph plasma protein conc.	Lymph flow (ml/kg)	Lymph flow (% of fetal)	Protein clearance (ml/kg)	Protein clearance (% of fetal)
HMD						
In uteru	50 ± 3	0.79 ± 0.04	0.28 ± 0.05	—	0.22 ± 0.05	—
After birth						
1 h	45 ± 3	0.69 ± 0.04	$0.36 \pm 0.09\star$	$164 \pm 28\star$	$0.30 \pm 0.06\star$	$142 \pm 25\star$
2 h	43 ± 2	$0.68 \pm 0.03\star$	0.49 ± 0.08	190 ± 30	0.34 ± 0.07	162 ± 30
3 h	42 ± 3	0.67 ± 0.03	0.55 ± 0.08	239 ± 63	0.37 ± 0.05	189 ± 41
4 h	47 ± 2	0.65 ± 0.04	0.64 ± 0.11	274 ± 83	0.42 ± 0.09	224 ± 65
NonHMD						
In uteru	55 ± 3	0.77 ± 0.03	0.38 ± 0.11	—	0.30 ± 0.08	—
After birth						
1 h	43 ± 2	0.66 ± 0.03	0.82 ± 0.16	329 ± 115	0.54 ± 0.10	289 ± 111
2 h	34 ± 2	0.58 ± 0.05	0.51 ± 0.13	258 ± 92	0.36 ± 0.07	178 ± 62
3 h	39 ± 2	0.62 ± 0.04	0.54 ± 0.11	216 ± 78	0.33 ± 0.06	159 ± 51
4 h	44 ± 3	0.63 ± 0.04	0.45 ± 0.08	175 ± 60	0.28 ± 0.05	135 ± 86

Results are mean $\pm$ SEM
$\star$Significantly different compared to nonHMD lambs at $P < 0.05$ (unpaired t test).

Discussion

These studies have shown that preterm lambs with HMD have significantly wetter lungs than lambs without HMD. There is also a progressive decrease of permeability surface area for ^{14}C-urea and an increase of pulmonary vascular resistance in HMD lambs but not in nonHMD lambs, indicating a decreasing surface area or derecruitment of the pulmonary exchange vessels, with advancing severity of the disease as the lambs became older. A decreased permeability would be extremely unlikely. Lymph flow and protein clearance showed a progressive increase in the HMD lambs in spite of vascular derecruitment, which one would assume was present in both groups of lambs with HMD. Although statistical significance was not obtained at 4 h after birth, the trend of increasing protein clearance for all protein fraction in HMD lambs compared to the decreasing trend in nonHMD lambs would suggest that increased vascular permeability was present in lungs of lambs with HMD. Mean lymph/plasma protein ratios were consistently higher in the HMD lambs, so that an effect of increased microvascular pressures is not likely.

The rapidly increasing lymph flow which peaks at 1 h after birth in nonHMD lambs represents clearing of fetal lung liquid, the fluid which in fetal life fills the potential airways. This finding is consistent with earlier described results by Bland *et al.* (9) and Normand *et al.* (10). Delayed resorption of fetal lung liquid in the HMD lambs has also been described by Normand *et al.* who suggested that the high surface tension in the alveoli could account for retention of this fluid (10). Their studies were, however, not extended beyond 2 h after birth. An accumulation and delayed elimination of the almost protein free fetal lung liquid from the interstitial space is not likely to be the sole explanation for the increased extravascular water, increased lymph flow and protein clearance at 2–4 h after birth in HMD lambs, since protein concentration in lymph fell proportionally less in the HMD lambs compared to the nonHMD lambs.

Summary

These studies have shown that lambs with HMD have increased extravascular lung water and low ^{14}C-urea permeability-surface area products indicating a decreased surface area for exchange due to derecruitment of pulmonary exchange vessels. In spite of this, there was increased lymph clearance of all plasma protein fractions suggesting increased microvascular permeability. Delayed elimination of fetal lung liquid was also found.

References

1. Egan, E. A., Nelson, R. M. and Beale, E. F. (1980). *Pediat. Res.* **14**, 314.
2. Chu, J., Clements, J. A., Cotton, E. K., Klaus, M. H., Sweet, A. Y. and Tooley, W. H. (1967). *Pediat.* **40**, 709.

3. Brigham, K. L., Sundell, H., Harris, T. R., Catterton, Z., Kovar, I. and Stahlman, M. T. (1978). *Circulat. Res.* **42**, 851.
4. Sundell, H. W., Brigham, K. L., Harris, T. R., Lindstrom, D. P., Catterton, W. Z., Green, R., Rojas, J. and Stahlman, M. T. (1980). *J. Develop. Physiol.* **2**, 191.
5. Cotton, R. B., Lindstrom, D. P., Kanarek, K. S., Sundell, H. and Stahlman, M. T. (1977). *J. Appl. Physiol.* **43**, 352.
6. Harris, T. R. (1978). *Proc. 31st Annual Conf. on Eng. in Med. Biol.* **20**, 17.
7. Failing, J., Buckley, M. and Zak, D. (1960). *Am. J. Clin. Pathol.* **33**, 83.
8. Brigham, K. L. and Owen, P. J. (1975). *Circulat. Res.* **36**, 761.
9. Bland, R. D., Hansen, T. N., Haberkern, C. M., Bressack, M. A., Hazenski, T. A., Raj, J. V. and Goldberg, R. B. (1982). *J. Appl. Physiol. Resp. Environ. Exercise Physiol.* **53**, 992.
10. Normand, I. C. S., Reynolds, E. O. R., Strang, L. B. and Wigglesworth, J. S. (1968). *Arch. Dis. Child.* **43**, 334.

Studies on Developmental Physiology in the Preterm Using Liquid Ventilation

Thomas H. Shaffer, Vinod K. Bhutani and Marla R. Wolfson

Department of Physiology, Temple University School of Medicine
and Section of Newborn Pediatrics, Pennsylvania Hospital,
University of Pennsylvania, Philadelphia, Pennsylvania, USA

Introduction

The *in vivo* study of physiological development has been limited by the relative inaccessibility of the fetus and nonviability of the preterm extra-uterine animal. The majority of studies are those in lamb fetuses at various stages of development (1), exteriorized lambs (2,3), or in older lambs delivered by caesarean section after 125 days of gestation (4,5,6). These studies have offered significant basic biological information. However, the many physiological, anatomical and biochemical changes associated with birth limit the applicability of these preparations for understanding development of the immature lamb after delivery.

In recent studies, we have demonstrated that it was possible to establish effective pulmonary gas exchange in 106-days-old preterm lambs independent of umbilical-placental circulation by utilizing liquid ventilation (LV) techniques (7). This procedure eliminates the air liquid interface in the immature lung and permits uniform expansion at lower alveolar pressures.

The objective of the present study was to employ this experimental preparation to investigate age related changes in cardiopulmonary function of the preterm extra-uterine lamb.

Methods

Preterm lambs Group I: ($n=8$), 105-111 days of gestation, 1.75 ± 0.5 SEM kg and Group II: ($n=8$), 132–138 days of gestation, 3.14 ± 0.2 SEM kg were

The Physiological Development of the Fetus and Newborn
ISBN 0 12 389080 2

Copyright © 1985 by Academic Press, London.
All rights of reproduction in any form reserved.

delivered by caesarean section and instrumented. The umbilical cord was then clamped, tied, and cut while 2.5 mg/kg of 50% sodium bicarbonate solution were administered intravenously. The animal's rectal temperature was monitored continuously with a digital centigrade thermometer. Pancuronium bromide (Pavulon® 0.1 mg/kg) was administered. Arterial blood gas tensions and pH were determined on 1 ml samples and corrected to body temperature of the animal (8).

In Group I the tracheal tube was connected to the liquid ventilation system at birth. Group II animals were initially ventilated with a volume controlled gas ventilator ($FIO_2 = 1.0$, for 30–60 min). LV was maintained in the lambs for 1–3 h at a functional residual capacity (FRC) of 30 ml/kg, a tidal volume of 15 ml/kg and a frequency of 4–9 breaths/min. Liquid ventilation with fluorocarbon was achieved using a previously described and modified liquid-breathing system (7,9). Fluorocarbon liquid was warmed to 39°C and oxygenated (P_IO_2 gauged from 600–620 mm HG).

Pulmonary mechanics were measured during LV (after arterial blood gases and pH of the lambs were stabilized) by simultaneously monitoring transpulmonary pressure, inspiratory and expiratory flow rates, and tidal volume on a Polygraph recorder and X-Y recorder. Values of respiratory rate were ascertained directly from the polygraph record and dynamic lung compliance was determined graphically by the method of Neergard and Wirz (10).

Oxygen consumption was determined by a closed-circuit spirometry method (11). Central venous pressure (CVP) and mean arterial pressure (MAP) were monitored and recorded on a polygraph recorder. Heart rate was obtained from blood pressure recordings.

Results

The summarized blood chemistry profile for both groups is presented in Table 1. As shown, it was possible to maintain effective gas exchange and acid-base status for a duration of 3 h.

Table 1. Summarized blood chemistry profile (mean ± SEM)

	105–111 days gestation	130–138 days gestation
Pa O_2 (mmHg)	214 ± 32	203 ± 19
Pa CO_2 (mmHg)	40 ± 6	37 ± 2
pH	7.28 ± 0.02	7.35 ± 0.03
A-a DO_2 (mmHg)	338 ± 29	317 ± 22

Figure 1 illustrates a typical dynamic pressure-volume (P-V) relationship of the lungs during LV. The P-V loop displays characteristic hysteresis during inflation and deflation. As compared to Group II animals, the lung compliance in Group I animals during LV appeared reduced. The mean data for lung compliance are shown in Table 2. The cardiopulmonary status of this experimental preparation remained relatively stable and is presented in Table 2.

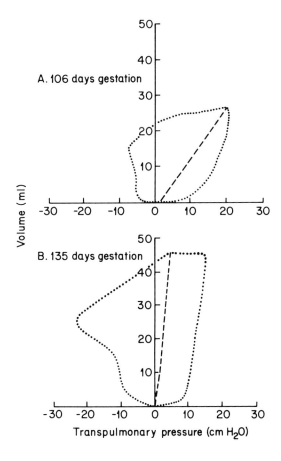

Figure 1. Dynamic Pressure-volume curves during LV in lamb from each age group (A) Group I, and (B) Group II.

Table 2. Summarized cardiopulmonary profile (mean ± SEM)

	105–111 days gestation	130–138 days gestation
Heart rate (beats/min)	209 ± 9	146 ± 8
Mean arteriol pressure (mmHg)	40 ± 2	63 ± 7
Functional residual capacity (ml)	50 ± 4	102 ± 6
Pulmonary compliance (ml/cmH$_2$O/kg)	0.58 ± 0.12	2.1 ± 0.2
Oxygen consumption (ml/min/kg)	7.67 ± 0.23	2.9 ± 0.6

Discussion

Effective gas exchange, acid-base status, and cardiopulmonary function was demonstrated in preterm lambs (105–138 days of gestation) ventilated with oxygenated fluorocarbon. These findings indicate that we have extended the viability of the preterm lamb to the limit of pulmonary capillary development rather than that of the pulmonary surfactant system. Thus, this approach provides the flexibility and unique opportunity to sequentially study biological development under conditions heretofore restrained by *in utero* and exteriorized preparations.

In comparing Group I and Group II animals, there were no apparent differences in gas exchange or acid-base status. Furthermore, the similarity in A-a DO_2 for both age groups indicates the same degree of intrapulmonary and intracardiac shunting. These data also suggest that the responsiveness of the pulmonary vasculature is not significantly dependent on developmental age over the range studied.

Since the air-liquid alveolar interface is eliminated during LV the observed increase in compliance with developmental age reflects structural and morphological alterations of the alveoli. A point of further significance was the finding that lung compliance in the very preterm lambs (Group I) during LV was very similar to that in more mature lambs during conventional gas ventilation (5). The onset of neonatal circulation has been associated with an increase in oxygen consumption (VO_2) (12). The VO_2 for Group I was slightly higher than *in utero* fetal levels (12). Surprisingly VO_2 for Group II was less than that for Group I and more in line with fetal data. Furthermore, the observed decrease in heart rate and increase in arterial blood pressure with maturity parallels that seen in the developing fetal lamb (13). Previous studies have demonstrated that pulmonary blood flow in the liquid-filled lung is more evenly distributed than in the gas-filled lung (14). Therefore, the ventilation/perfusion distribution in the LV lung may be ultimately responsible for the effective gas exchange, even at the very early stages of lung development. In conclusion, this experimental approach provides an opportunity to study physiological development in an animal preparation resembling the perinatal status of the extremely preterm neonate.

Acknowledgements

The authors are indebted to Drs C. A. Lowe, S. D. Rubenstein, E. M. Sivieri, and N. Tran for their collaboration.

The research leading to this paper was supported in part by Public Health Service grant HL-22843. Fluorocarbon liquid was supplied by RIMAR CHIMICA, S.P.A., represented in the United States by Mercantile Development, Inc.

References

1. Rudolph, A. M. and Heyman, M. A. (1970). *Circulat. Res.* **26**, 289–294.
2. Born, G. V. R., Dawes, G. S. and Mott, J. C. (1955). *J. Physiol.* **130**, 191–198.

3. Heyman, M. A. and Rudolph, A. M. (1968). *Circulat. Res.* **21**, 741–747.
4. Reynolds, E. O. R., Jacobson, H. N., Motoyoma, E. K. *et al.* (1965). *Pediat.* **35**, 382–391.
5. Shaffer, T. H., Delivoria-Papadopoulos, M., Arcinue, E., Paez, P. and Dubois, A. B. (1976). *Resp. Physiol.* **28**, 179–188.
6. Stahlman, M., Lequire, V. S., Young, W. C. *et al.* (1964). *Am. J. Dis. Child.* **108**, 375–381.
7. Shaffer, T. H., Tran, N., Bhutani, V. K. and Sivieri, E. M. (1983). *Pediat. Res.* **17**, 680–684.
8. Nunn, J. F., Bergman, N. A., Sunatyan, A. and Coleman, A. J. (1965). *J. Appl. Physiol.* **20**, 23–26.
9. Shaffer, T. H., Rubenstein, S. D., Moskowitz, G. D. and Delivoria-Papadopoulos, M. (1976). *Pediat. Res.* **16**, 227–231.
10. Neergard, K. and Wirz, K. (1927). *Klin, Med.* **105**, 35–39.
11. Sivieri, E. M., Moskowitz, G. D. and Shaffer, T. H. (1981). *Undersea Biomed. Res.* **8**, 75–83.
12. Dawes, G. S. and Mott, J. C. (1959). *J. Physiol.* **146**, 295–302.
13. Dawes, G. S. (1968). "Foetal and Neonatal Physiology" pp. 110–120, Yearbook Medical Publishers, Inc., Chicago.
14. West, J. B., Dollery, C. T. and Naimaito, A. (1964). *J. Appl. Physiol.* **19**, 713–719.

Organization and Control
of the Fetal Circulation

Abraham M. Rudolph

Departments of Pediatrics, Physiology, and Obstetrics, Gynecology, and Reproductive Sciences, and the Cardiovascular Research Institute, University of California, San Francisco, California, USA

In the adult mammal, blood circulates sequentially through the systemic and pulmonary vasculature and there is essentially no mixing of blood oxygenated in the lungs and systemic venous blood. During fetal life, blood is oxygenated in the placenta and returns to the fetal body via the umbilical vein, which joins the portal vein in the hepatic sinus; the oxygenated blood subsequently enters the inferior vena cava, which also receives blood from the lower portion of the fetal body. The fetal circulation is characterized by the presence of several shunts, which facilitate venous return from the placenta (ductus venosus) and reduce blood flow through the lungs (foramen ovale and ductus arteriosus). These shunts account for considerable mixing of well oxygenated (umbilical venous) and poorly oxygenated systemic venous blood. These features of the fetal circulation raise interesting and important questions concerning mechanisms utilized to provide oxygen and energy substrates to different organs. In addition, the ductus arteriosus provides such a large communication between the pulmonary trunk and the aorta that pulmonary arterial and aortic pressures are almost equal, whilst the foramen ovale similarly tends to equalize atrial pressures. Under these circumstances of similar filling and ejection pressures, the performance of the left and right ventricles and their ability to provide cardiac output and oxygen blood flows are of great interest.

Venous Return to the Heart

Using radionuclide-labelled microspheres, we have shown that, in fetal sheep, about 70% of venous return to the heart is derived from the lower body, about 20% from the superior vena cava, 3% from the heart muscle, and the remaining

The Physiological Development of the Fetus and Newborn
ISBN 0 12 389080 2

Copyright © 1985 by Academic Press, London.
All rights of reproduction in any form reserved.

7% from the lungs (1). About half of the total venous return to the heart is derived from blood that passes through the hepatic circulation and the ductus venosus. This comprises about 5% of the combined ventricular output which is distributed to the gastrointestinal tract and spleen, and the 40–45% distributed to the umbilical-placental circulation. Because of this large proportion of the combined ventricular output, which enters the portal sinus, the functional behaviour of the ductus venosus and the hepatic microcirculation could have an important influence on venous return to the heart.

Hepatic and ductus venosus blood flows

Brinkman *et al.* (2) suggested that the ductus venosus is important in regulating blood flow to the liver, but Edelstone (3) concluded that the ductus venosus responds passively to intraluminal pressures. We have studied the distribution of umbilical venous and portal blood flows in fetal lambs *in utero* by injecting radionuclide-labelled microspheres into tributaries of these vessels (4). About 55% of umbilical venous return passes through the ductus venosus, the remainder being distributed to the liver. The right and left lobes of the liver both receive large contributions of umbilical venous blood, but portal venous blood is distributed almost completely to the right lobe; a small proportion (5–10%) may pass through the ductus venosus, but none enters the left lobe. Blood flow to the liver from the hepatic artery is quite low during fetal life.

Because of its large blood flow and highly vascular nature, the liver may be an important organ in regulating fetal blood volume and venous return to the heart. Greenway and Stark (5) estimate that blood occupies about 25% of the liver volume of adult animals, which represents about 10% of total blood volume. The fetal liver probably also has a large volume and, as shown by Gilbert *et al.* (6), is a highly compliant organ. Recent studies suggest that the liver plays a major role in regulating the distribution of umbilical blood flow during fetal stress. When fetal hypoxaemia is induced by maternal hypoxia, umbilical blood flow does not change significantly from its normal value of about 200 ml/min/kg fetal weight (7). However, the proportion of umbilical venous blood entering the hepatic microcirculation is reduced from 45 to about 35%, whereas the proportion distributed through the ductus venosus increases from 55 to 65%, representing an 18% increase in actual ductus venous flow (8). Reduction of total umbilical venous blood flow by about 30%, induced by lowering blood volume by haemorrhage, also increases the proportion of umbilical venous return that is distributed through the ductus venosus (9). Because total umbilical venous blood flow is reduced, flow through the hepatic microcirculation is markedly decreased. When umbilical venous return is reduced either by inflating a balloon in the fetal descending aorta (10) or by umbilical venous compression (11), the proportion of umbilical venous blood passing through the ductus venosus increases markedly, and actual hepatic blood flow is greatly reduced. Whereas the blood flow to each liver lobe from the umbilical vein is usually similar in relation to tissue weight (4), umbilical venous supply to the right lobe is preferentially decreased to a considerably greater extent than that to the left lobe when umbilical blood flow is reduced (10). Total blood flow to the right lobe, although reduced, is similar to that of the left lobe, but a much greater proportion of its flow is derived from portal venous blood than under normal circumstances.

The mechanisms responsible for the reduction in hepatic blood flow, and relative or actual increase in ductus venosus flow have not been elucidated. The changes might be related to simple haemodynamic alterations. Thus, when umbilical blood flow is reduced and assuming umbilical venous pressure falls, hepatic vascular resistance could be increased by reduction of distending pressure in the vascular bed, with a resulting fall in blood flow relatively greater than flow through the ductus venosus. This would assume that the ductus venosus is more compliant than the hepatic vascular bed. However, during hypoxaemia induced by maternal hypoxaemia, unbilical blood flow is maintained (7). Yet hepatic blood flow decreases and actual ductus venosus flow increases. This can be explained only by dilation of the ductus venosus or an increase in hepatic vascular resistance.

Sphincters have been demonstrated in the adult liver both at the entrance of the portal venules into the central sinusoids (12) and at the junction of the hepatic veins with the central sinusoid (13). Vascular reactivity in the fetal liver may be controlled by autonomic neural and/or hormonal mechanisms, which regulate blood flow during fetal hypoxia, or in association with reduced umbilical venous return.

Distribution of hepatic venous and inferior vena caval blood

Chronic catheterization of the left and right hepatic veins in fetal sheep liver shows that the O_2 saturation is higher in the left (approx. 70%) than in the right (approx. 55%) vein (14). This difference can be accounted for by the fact that the left lobe of the liver receives predominantly umbilical venous blood, which is well oxygenated, whereas the right lobe receives almost all the portal venous blood, with a low O_2 saturation, as well as umbilical venous blood.

The concept has generally been held that the blood of the few vessels entering the thoracic inferior vena cava via the distal inferior vena cava, the ductus venosus, and the left and right hepatic veins mixes adequately, and the mixed venous blood passes through the foramen ovale and the tricuspid valve. Behrman et al. (1970) demonstrated preferential streaming of ductus venosus blood across the foramen ovale rather than through the tricuspid valve by means of radionuclide-labelled microspheres in acute studies in primate features. We have confirmed that in the sheep fetus, distal inferior vena caval blood is preferentially directed to the tricuspid valve, whilst ductus venosus blood preferentially passes through the foramen ovale. This streamlining of blood flow in the inferior vena cava is present during both normoxia and hypoxia (16,17) and is at least partly responsible for the higher oxygen saturation in ascending aortic as compared with descending aortic blood (vide infra).

Recently we have shown that the left and right hepatic venous blood is also preferentially distributed. The left hepatic venous blood, which has a relatively high O_2 saturation, preferentially streams through the foramen ovale in a similar manner to ductus venosus blood. However, right hepatic venous blood, with a lower O_2 saturation, joins the distal inferior vena caval blood stream to pass preferentially through the tricuspid valve (Bristow and Rudolph—unpublished observations). Figure 1 illustrates the various venous flow patterns in the fetal portal sinus.

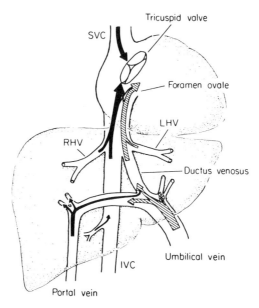

Figure 1. The course and distribution of venous blood entering the heart in the fetus. Umbilical venous blood enters the hepatic hilum and gives off branches to the left lobe. The ductus venosus carries predominantly umbilical venous blood directly to the inferior vena cava. The umbilical vein then arches to the right to join the portal vein. Almost all portal venous blood enters the right lobe of the liver. The right hepatic venous blood joins the abdominal inferior vena caval stream to be preferentially distributed through the triscuspid valve. Left hepatic venous blood joins the ductus venosus stream and these two well oxygenated bloods are preferentially directed through the foreamen ovale. The superior vena caval blood is almost completely directed through the tricuspid valve. From (32).

Superior vena caval return

Superior vena caval blood entering the right atrium is almost completely directed through the tricuspid valve to the right ventricle. Less than 5% of superior vena caval blood passes across the foramen ovale into the left atrium and left ventricle in the normoxemic fetus (1). Initially it was suggested that during fetal hypoxaemia the proportion of superior vena caval blood crossing the foramen ovale increased; we have now shown that fetal hypoxaemia induced by maternal hypoxia does not significantly alter superior vena caval blood flow across the foramen ovale. Increased shunting of superior vena caval blood into the left atrium probably occurs as a result of increased afterload on the right ventricle, as may occur with compression of the umbilical cord.

Arterial Distribution of Fetal Venous Blood

The flow of most superior vena caval blood across the tricuspid valve into the right ventricle had been used to explain the higher blood oxygen saturation in the ascending aorta and its branches, as compared with the descending aorta in the fetus, because the right ventricle ejects most of its blood through the pulmonary trunk and ductus arteriosus into the descending aorta. We have shown that only a small proportion (15–20% or less) of descending aortic blood is derived from passage of ascending aortic blood across the isthmus. It is now evident, however, that preferential streaming of well oxygenated ductus venosus and left hepatic venous blood across the foramen ovale makes an important contribution to the differences in upper and lower body arterial oxygen saturations. This streamlining effect is important not only for oxygen distribution, but also for any substances entering the umbilical veins. Thus, although superior and distal inferior vena caval glucose concentrations are similar, ascending aortic blood shows significantly higher glucose concentrations than descending aortic blood. This can be explained by the higher glucose concentration of umbilical venous blood from placental transfer (18); umbilical venous blood then passes through the ductus venosus and is preferentially distributed through the foramen ovale. Although these venous flow patterns affect oxygen saturation of blood distributed to various organs, regulation of vascular resistances and blood flows to individual organs is the dominant factor influencing tissue oxygen delivery.

Left and Right Ventricular Output

The volume of blood ejected by the heart is determined by four factors: heart rate, preload or filling pressure, afterload or resistance against which the ventricle ejects, and intrinsic myocardial contractile force. Measurements in chronically instrumented fetal lambs by radionuclide-labelled microspheres, as well as by electromagnetic flow transducers applied around the ascending aorta and the pulmonary trunk have shown that the left ventricle ejects only 33–40% of the combined ventricular output, whereas the right ventricle ejects 60–67% (19). The preload on the two ventricles is similar; right and left atrial pressures are almost identical in fetal lambs *in utero*, but inferior vena caval pressure is 0.5–1.5 mmHg higher during all phases of the cardiac cycle. Although the pressures in the pulmonary trunk and aorta are similar in both systole and diastole in lambs up to about 0.9 (135 days) gestation, near-term animals often have a somewhat higher pulmonary trunk pressure, presumably caused by some ductus arteriosus constriction. Under these conditions of similar atrial and arterial pressures, the volume of blood ejected by each ventricle depends on the vascular resistance or afterload against which it ejects. Although pulmonary vascular resistance is very high in the fetus, the right ventricle ejects almost two-thirds of the combined ventricular output; most of this blood passes through the ductus arteriosus to the descending aorta, and two-thirds of the right ventricular blood that traverses the ductus is destined to reach the umbilical-placental circulation, which has a relatively low resistance. Because the volume ejected by the left ventricle is much lower, there must be some functional separation between the ascending and descending aorta at the level of the isthmus in the lamb fetus. In unpublished observations (Heymann and Rudolph) we have found that injection of a bolus of a small amount of acetylcholine into the ascending or descending aorta, with resulting selective vasodilation in the upper or lower body circulation, causes a separation of pressures between the ascending and descending aorta for a few beats. Similar separation of upper and lower body arterial pressures could be produced by selective injection of norepinephrine into one or other arterial circulation. In lambs with electromagnetic flow transducers implanted around the ascending aorta and pulmonary trunk, we found that selective injection of acetylcholine into the descending aorta resulted in an increase of right, but not left, ventricular stroke volume for a few beats. Norepinephrine injected into the descending aorta selectively reduced right ventricular stroke volume for a few beats.

The different ejection characteristics of the left and right ventricles in the fetal lamb are also clearly evident in the blood velocity contours of the pulmonary trunk and ascending aorta (Fig. 2). The velocity in the pulmonary trunk rises

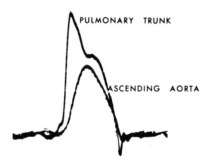

Figure 2. Velocity tracings in the pulmonary trunk and ascending aorta obtained by electromagnetic flow transducer implantation. Note the rapid rise in velocity in the pulmonary trunk as compared with the aortic velocity. Also there is a characteristic notch in the descending limb of the velocity curve. The ascending aortic tracing also shows a sharp incisura at the end of ejection which is caused by back flow. The area under each curve reflects stroke volume; pulmonary trunk flow is about twice that in the aorta.

steeply, compared with the much slower rise in ascending aortic velocity. There is also considerable back flow in the aortic tracing at the end of systole. The area under the velocity curve of the aorta is much smaller than that in the pulmonary trunk, confirming the smaller stroke volume of the left ventricle. The notch on the descending limb of the pulmonary trunk velocity curve is a consistent finding, the cause of which has not been defined. It could be related to a change in velocity associated with the appearance of the wave of blood ejected by the left ventricle at the arteriosus.

Apparently the ventricles of the heart of the fetal lamb are not functioning in a parallel circuit; the aortic isthmus between the origins of the brachiocephalic trunk and the ductus arteriosus is the narrowest segment of the thoracic aorta and presents a functional separation between the ascending and descending aorta. The left ventricle is presented with the high afterload of the high vascular resistance ofthe head, neck, and forelimbs, whilst the right ventricle ejects into the circulation of the lower body with considerably less afterload because umbilical-placental resistance is low. The relative outputs of the two ventricles could readily be altered by selective changes in afterload. Thus, pharmacological agents that decrease systemic vascular resistance without altering umbilical-placental resistance cause a relative increase in left as compared with right ventricular output. Similarly, during the increase of descending aortic resistance resulting from inflation of a balloon, right ventricular output decreases more than that of the left ventricle (10).

Fetal Heart Rate and Cardiac Output

The fetal heart rate shows considerable variation over short periods, as well as beat-to-beat variability. We measured right and left ventricular output continuously with electromagnetic flow transducers and demonstrated a linear correlation between changes in heart rate and changes in left and right ventricular output during spontaneous alterations of heart rate in chronically instrumented fetal lambs at 0.8–0.9 gestation (21). We also found that right atrial pacing resulted in a progressive increase in left ventricular output to a maximum of 15–20% above control values at pacing rates of 270–300 per minute. Slowing the heart by cervical vagal stimulation caused a dramatic fall in left and right ventricular output.

Fetal hypoxaemia is associated with the rapid onset of bradycardia and, with more intense hypoxaemia, a decrease in combined ventricular output (7). The bradycardia is primarily mediated through peripheral chemoreceptor, rather than baroreceptor, stimulation (22). The fall in combined ventricular output could be a result of the bradycardia, or an increase in peripheral vascular resistance (increased afterload), or both. It is most likely associated with the decreased heart rate because abolishing bradycardia by administration of atropine either during or prior to hypoxia prevents the reduction in cardiac output. We have demonstrated a similar effect on left ventricular output (22).

These relationships between fetal cardiac output and heart rate, particularly the limited ability to increase stroke volume when heart rate was decreased (20), suggest that the fetal heart is functioning at near maximal performance and has little reserve. We also proposed that the heart of the normal fetal lamb *in utero* had a limited Starling relationship above resting conditions, and that increases in preload could elicit only small increases in stroke volume. We proposed that, for this reason, increases in cardiac output are largely dependent on increases in heart rate.

Preload and Cardiac Output

The normal end-diastolic pressure of the right and left ventricles in the fetal lamb *in utero* is about 3–5 mmHg above intra-amniotic pressure. We infused 0.9% NaCl solution into fetal lambs while measuring right ventricular output and right ventricular pressure. With increases of right ventricular end-diastolic pressures to 20–25 mmHg there was only a small increase in right ventricular output and work. We suggested that the fetal heart was functioning at or near the top of its function curve (23). Subsequently, several studies have shown that the heart of the fetal lamb demonstrates a Starling relationship at atrial pressures below those normally present (24–27). These studies also confirmed our findings that an increase in filling pressure above normal resting levels has a limited effect in increasing cardiac output. Whether this is due to a limitation in myocardial performance, or is related to a low compliance of the fetal ventricle is unknown. If fetal heart muscle is very stiff, an increase in filling pressure would have little effect in distending the ventricle and changing sarcomere length. Romero *et al.* (28) have reported that the fetal lamb heart demonstrates a much lower compliance than the adult heart. Thus the apparent poor performance of the fetal myocardium could be related to the poor distensibility of the ventricles. This issue still requires resolution.

Afterload and Cardiac Output

Changes in afterload have an important effect on ventricular output in the adult. We showed that the fetal heart is very sensitive to changes in afterload; inflation of a balloon in the fetal descending aorta produced a marked fall in right ventricular stroke volume (20). Also, as mentioned above, short-lived selective reduction or increase in upper or lower body vascular resistances by bolus injections of dilator or constrictor drugs cause a selective increase or decrease in left or right ventricular stroke volumes. The striking effects of changes in afterload or ventricular output have been reported by Gilbert (26) and Thornburg and Morton (27). Gilbert showed that infusion of methoxamine, a potent peripheral vasoconstrictor, resulted in a marked depression of the ventricular function curve. Thornburg and Morton found that right ventricular output, as measured by an electromagnetic flow transducer around the pulmonary trunk, decreased when arterial pressure was raised by peripheral vasoconstriction with phenylephrine, but increased when arterial pressure was reduced by vasodilation with nitroprusside infusion. These findings are important in assessing the role of changes in intrinsic myocardial contractility associated with physiological or pharmacological influences. Thus the decrease in fetal cardiac output during severe hypoxia could result from the associated bradycardia and increased afterload produced by peripheral vasoconstriction, and may not reflect a direct depression of myocardial performance.

Myocardial Contractility

Based on studies with isolated cardiac muscle strips from fetal lambs, the concept was presented that contractility of the heart was lower in fetal than adult animals because the fetal muscle generated less active tension (29). Although actual determinations of intrinsic myocardial contractility have not been made in intact fetal hearts, there is considerable indirect evidence to support this concept. Thus all the studies mentioned above, which demonstrate a limited ability of the fetal heart to increase its output in response to elevations of atrial pressures by infusion of either 0.9% NaCl solution or blood, suggest that the fetal myocardium has a relatively poor contractility.

Following birth, cardiac output increases considerably and left ventricular output is about twice the fetal levels (30) in relation to body weight. When left atrial pressure was raised by rapid infusion of 0.9% NaCl solution, left ventricular output increased to a greater extent (by 35% above resting values) than during fetal life. However, resting cardiac output indexed to body weight fell progressively over the 2 months following birth, but cardiac output increased much more (by about 75%) in response to volume loading. We were puzzled because the resting left ventricular output increased markedly in the normal lamb after birth, yet, in response to volume loading, the fetal heart could produce only a small increase in output. From studies in newborn lambs (30), this response appeared to be exclusively the result of sympatheticoadrenal stimulation after birth. We examined the possible role of the rise in plasma triiodothyronine (T_3) concentrations immediately after birth.

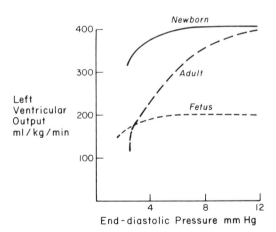

Figure 3. The diagram presents the hypothesis of ventricular function changes after birth. It is suggested the fetus has poor myocardial function with little reserve. The newborn lamb shows a dramatic increase in the resting levels of output, but there is also little reserve available because of high resting demands. The adult function curve shows a steep slope of its ventricular function end-diastolic pressure relationship.

Thyroidectomy in fetal lambs at about 130 days gestation abolished the rise in plasma T_3 concentrations and also prevented the normal rise in left ventricular output and oxygen consumption that occurs after birth (31). If the thyroid gland is removed just prior to delivery, however, plasma T_3 concentrations do not increase, but left ventricular output and oxygen consumption increase normally. Based on these observations, T_3 appears to have an important role in maturation of the fetal myocardial response during the period of gestation near term.

From the studies of fetal, newborn, and adult animals, a concept of cardiac output and myocardial performance is presented in Figure 3. During fetal life, myocardial performance is relatively depressed, and the heart is functioning near the top of its function curve with little reserve available to further increase output. After birth, myocardial contractility is greatly increased but, because of the high demands on the circulation to provide the increased oxygen requirements for metabolism, there is also little reserve available, and thus volume loading results in only a small rise in cardiac output. Beyond the early neonatal period, as oxygen consumption in relation to body weight falls, so does indexed cardiac output decrease, and the function curve characteristic of the adult heart develops. The increase in myocardial contractility manifested after birth requires the prenatal influence of thyroid hormone, but the exact mechanism by which thyroid hormone elicits this change has not been resolved. It could be the result of modification of β-adrenergic receptor numbers, or modulation of their responsiveness to catecholamines.

Acknowledgements

This work was supported by grants from the US Public Health Service, Program Project Grants HL 24056, and HL 23681.

References

1. Rudolph, A. M. and Heymann, M. A. (1967). *Circulat. Res.* **21**, 163–184.
2. Brinkman, C. R. III, Kirschbaum, T. H. and Assali, N. S. (1970). *Bynecol. Invest* **1**, 115–127.
3. Edelstone, D. I. (1980). *J. Develop. Physiol.* **2**, 219–238.
4. Edelstone, D. I., Rudolph, A. M. and Heymann, M. A. (1978). *Circulat. Res.* **42**, 426–433.
5. Greenway, C. V. and Stark, R. D. (1971). *Physiol. Rev.* **51**, 23–65.
6. Gilbert, R. D., Genstler, C. C., Dale, P. S. and Power, G. G. (1981). *J. Develop. Physiol.* **3**, 283–295.
7. Cohn, H. E., Sacks, E. J., Heymann, M. A. and Rudolph, A. M. (1974). *Am. J. Obstet. Gynecol.* **120**, 817–824.
8. Reuss, M. L. and Rudolph, A. M. (1980). *J. Develop. Physiol.* **2**, 71–84.
9. Itskovitz, J., Goetzman, B. W. and Rudolph, A. M. (1982). *Am. J. Physiol.* **242**, H543–H548.
10. Edelstone, D. I., Rudolph, A. M. and Heymann, M. A. (1980). *Am. J. Physiol.* **238**, H656–H663.

11. Itskovitz, J., LaGamma, E. F. and Rudolph, A. M. (1983). *Am. J. Obstet. Gynecol.* **145**, 813-818.
12. Elias, H. and Sherrick, J. C. (1969). "Morphology of the Liver", Academic Press, New York and London.
13. Knisely, M. H., Harding, F. and Debacker, H. (1957). *Science* **125**, 1023-1026.
14. Bristow, J., Rudolph, A. M. and Itskovitz, J. (1981). *J. Develop. Physiol.* **3**, 255-266.
15. Behrman, R. E., Lees, M. H., Peterson, E. N., De Lannoy, C. W. and Seeds, A. E. (1970). *Am. J. Obstet. Gynecol.* **108**, 956-969.
16. Edelstone, D. I. and Rudolph, A. M. (1979). *Am. J. Physoil.* **237**, H724-H729.
17. Reuss, M. L. and Rudolph, A. M. (1981). *Am. J. Obstet. Gynecol.* **141**, 427-431.
18. Charlton, V. and Johengen, M. (1984). *J. Develop. Physiol.* **6**, 431-438.
19. Heymann, M. A., Creasy, R. K. and Rudolph, A. M. (1973). *In:* "Proceedings of the Sir Joseph Barcroft Centenary Symposium: Fetal and Neonatal Physiology" (Comline, K. S., Cross, K. W., Dawes, G. S. and Nathanielsz, P. W., eds) pp. 129-135, Cambridge University Press, Cambridge.
20. Rudolph, A. M. and Heymann, M. A. (1973). *In:* "Proceedings of the Sir Joseph Barcroft Centenary Symposium: Fetal and Neonatal Physiology" (Comline, K. S., Cross, K. W., Dawes, G. S. and Nathanielsz, P. W., eds) pp. 89-111, Cambridge University Press, Cambridge.
21. Rudolph, A. M. and Heymann, M. A. (1976). *Am. J. Obstet. Gynecol.* **124**, 183-192.
22. Itskovitz, J., Goetzman, B. W. and Rudolph, A. M. (1982b). *Am. J. Obstet. Gynecol.* **142**, 66-73.
23. Heymann, M. A. and Rudolph, A. M. (1973). *Circulation*, **48** (suppl. 4), 37.
24. Kirkpatrick, S. E., Pitlick, P. T., Naliboff, J. and Friedman, W. F. (1976). *Am. J. Physiol.* **231**, 495-500.
25. Gilbert, R. D. (1980). *Am. J. Physiol.* **238**, H80-H86.
26. Gilbert, R. D. (1982). *J. Develop. Physiol.* **4**, 299-309.
27. Thornburg, K. L. and Morton, M. J. (1983). *Am. J. Physiol.* **244**, H656-H663.
28. Romero, T., Covell, J. and Friedman, W. F. (1972). *Am. J. Physiol.* **222**, 1285-1290.
29. Friedman, W. F. (1973). *In:* "Neonatal Heart Disease" pp. 21-49, Grune & Stratton, New York.
30. Klopfenstein, H. S. and Rudolph, A. M. (1978). *Circulat. Res.* **42**, 839-845.
31. Breall, J. A., Rudolph, A. M. and Heymann, M. A. (1984). *J. Clin. Invest.* **73**, 1418-1424.
32. Rudolph, A. M. (1983). *Hepatology* **3**, 254-258.

Myometrial Activity—
Control and Effects

P. W. Nathanielsz, J. P. Figueroa, A. El Badry,
S. Sunderji, D. A. Frank, G. Pimentel,
E. R. Poore, and M. D. Mitchell

Department of Reproductive Studies, State University, College of
Veterinary Medicine, Cornell University, Ithaca, New York;
State University of New York, Upstate Medical Center, Syracuse, New York;
Cecil H. and Ida Green Center for Reproductive Biology Sciences,
University of Texas Southwestern Medical School, Dallas, Texas, USA

Different Forms of Myometrial Activity
During Pregnancy

Myometrial activity throughout pregnancy has important implications both for fetal development and the initiation of labour. Tonic, low amplitude myometrial activity, contractures, occur throughout the major portion of pregnancy in several species (12,18,22). This low level myometrial activity is temporally associated with a fall in fetal arterial and venous oxygen tension (PO_2) (12), changes in fetal heart rate (10) alterations in fetal breathing movements (18), a switch in fetal neurophysiological state from rapid eye movements (REM) to non rapid eye movement sleep (NREM) and distortion of the fetus (18). Efficient expulsion of the fetus at term is generally effected by co-ordinated contractions. Therefore a detailed understanding of the hormonal and neural control of both contractures and contractions is a necessary prerequisite for a better understanding of the initiation of labour and delivery. There are several comprehensive reviews on parturition and myometrial activity (31). This present review cannot cover all aspects of the subject and will therefore concentrate on a few important aspects.

The Physiological Development of the Fetus and Newborn
ISBN 0 12 389080 2

Copyright © 1985 by Academic Press, London.
All rights of reproduction in any form reserved.

The Need for Precise Description and
Quantification of Contractures

Myometrial activity has been recorded both by measurement of intra-
uterine pressure (IUP) and electromyogram (EMG). The techniques for
recording EMG and IUP in chronically instrumented pregnant animals have
been refined over several years in many laboratories. Electromyogram recordings
give an index of the electrical drive to contraction. This is both an
advantage and a limitation. Myometrial EMG reflects the input to the
muscle but changes in activation-contraction coupling may modify the effect
of this input. Such changes in coupling may, in large measure, reflect
alterations in gap junction formation. Techniques for maintenance and
recording EMG at various sites have been described in several recent reviews
(8,21,28).

Visual examination of either the EMG record or IUP tracings throughout
pregnancy clearly shows epochs of myometrial activity of various durations. Three
questions arise. Firstly, how do we distinguish signal from noise? Secondly, are
there qualitatively different epochs of activity? Thirdly, how do we quantify the
different signals?

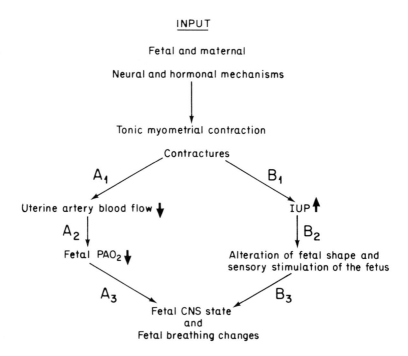

Figure 1. Diagrammatic representation of the mechanisms controlling contractures
and the possible physiological systems that may be affected by contractures.

We have recently used a microcomputer based system for data acquisition and analysis of myometrial EMG. In this investigation it was demonstrated that in late pregnancy, before labour and delivery commences, there are at least two different populations of EMG epoch (5). Uterine EMG took 6–7 days postsurgery to achieve a relatively stable level of activity. When stability had been achieved, the population of epochs with the longer lasting activity had a median duration of 5.9 min. At this time, 83% of EMG activity was in epochs lasting longer than 4 min. We have previously referred to these tonic epochs as contractures (22).

Physiological Effect of Contractures

We have previously reported a temporal relationship in the sheep fetus between contractures and a change in the fetus from low-voltage high frequency fetal electrocorticogram activity to high voltage activity. As a result of these and related studies, we postulated that contractures may affect fetal neurophysiological and neuroendocrine function (22). Figure 1 shows the flow pathways that may be involved in these mechanisms.

Effect of contractures on uterine blood flow

Uterine contractures cause a reduction of maternal uterine blood flow measured with electromagnetic flow probes of up to 20% (1,8). Similar falls have been observed using indicator dilution techniques with 4-aminoantipyrine that depend on the attainment of diffusion equilibrium at "steady-state". These results add further evidence for the effects of contractures on uterine blood flow. A certain caution must accompany the interpretation of experiments using aminoantipyrine. Our recent studies have demonstrated that both 4-aminoantipyrine and antipyrine are powerful inhibitors of both the cycloxygenase (3) and lipoxygenase (unpublished observations). We have observed that the disturbances of eicosanoid production during infusions of 4-aminoantipyrine or antipyrine affect fetal electrocorticographic (ECoG) patterns and fetal breathing movements. This effect of inhibition of prostaglandin synthesis on fetal activity has been described by other workers (14). Studies in the fetal sheep that have been conducted during the infusion of either 4-aminoantipyrine or antipyrine to either fetus or ewe must be interpreted with caution. We have reviewed the literature in relation to variability in uterine perfusion in greater detail elsewhere (24).

Effect of contractures on umbilical blood flow

Walker and co-workers have demonstrated a fall in umbilical blood flow in the sheep at the transition from low to high voltage ECoG activity (32). In this study, myometrial activity was monitored by recordings of IUP. The effect of contractures on umbilical blood flow has not been studied systematically using myometrial EMG as the indicator of contractures. IUP may be a poor marker of contractures since every rise in uterine wall tension (which will be the major factor affecting extrinsic resistance to the uterine circulation) or fetal intra-abdominal pressure (which is caused by the fetal distortion described below) may not be reflected in a change in IUP.

Are small changes in fetal PO_2 sufficient to produce physiological changes in the fetus?

The suggestion we have made that small falls in uteroplacental perfusion (1) and small changes in fetal PO_2 (22) can affect fetal function (12) has caused considerable controversy. The conventional dogma is that there is considerable reserve in placental transfer of oxygen and that uterine blood flow has to fall markedly before the fetus is affected by any change in oxygen delivery. This view is summarized in the following quotation: "Variations of arterial PO_2 and oxygen content do not produce any gross changes in the rate of oxygen consumption of individual organs until the level of oxygenation attains a certain low critical level. For example, the oxygen consumption rate of the fetal brain does not change systematically as the arterial content varies over the 6 to 1 mM range. Therefore it is of interest to note that the flow response to oxygen by heart and central nervous system does not manifest itself only at some critical level of hypoxia" (27). From the figure in the paper and the sense of the statement quoted, the argument is that there is a critical threshold that needs to be exceeded and that the response to hypoxia is not continuous. The implications of such comments depend on interpretation of the words "gross" and "critical". The availability of sensitive continuous monitoring techniques has clearly demonstrated that there is continuous variability at many levels of function in both mother and fetus. The exact thresholds of sensitivity and their physiological implications remain to be determined. Our failure to detect alterations in function should not be interpreted as conclusive proof that significant physiological changes do not occur. We should always bear in mind that the fetus has almost certainly developed sensors as sensitive as those that we as investigators fabricate and use in the laboratory.

Recently it has been demonstrated in the pregnant sheep that short-term uterine artery occlusions resulting in falls of fetal PO_2 from 21.6 to 16.5 mmHg resulted in a cessation of fetal breathing movement in 67 out of 77 occasions in 6 fetuses (10). When considering the physiological significance of these observations it should be noted that the end-point was complete cessation of breathing. Even smaller falls in PO_2 may be sensed by the fetus and produce changes in fetal neurophysiological function that are less easy to monitor. As mentioned below, contractures are associated with distortion of the fetus. Thus the stimulation of the fetus by the combined distortion and PO_2 fall produced by a contracture may well be different from the sensory input associated with a PO_2 fall alone. Contractures are generally temporally associated with an increase in fetal heart rate. The PO_2 falls produced by cuffing the uterine arteries produce fetal bradycardia (10). Using discretely placed stereotaxic lesions in the fetal brain (7) it has been shown that a small area in the Pons plays a central role in controlling the apnoeic response demonstrated by the fetus to hypoxia (13). It is possible that this area is the region of the fetal brain that responds to the small falls in fetal PO_2.

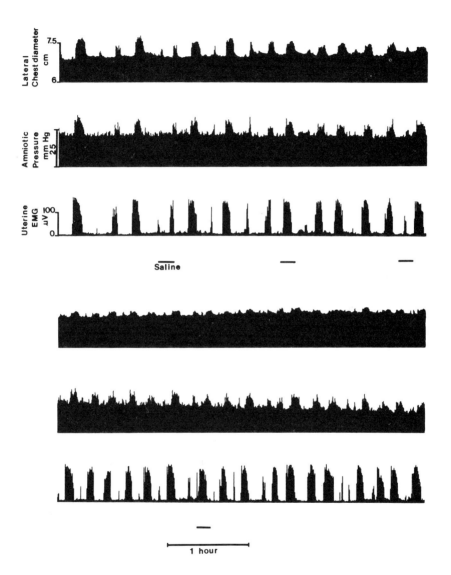

Figure 2. Lateral chest wall diameter (upper trace in both panels), amniotic pressure (middle trace), and intra-uterine pressure measured with a fluid filled balloon (bottom trace) before and after infusion of saline into the amniotic cavity. A total of 3 l saline was administered over the 4 periods marked by the solid bars.

The Effect of Contractures on Intra-uterine Pressure

Pascal's law does not apply to the late gestation uterus. The pressures throughout the uterine cavity are not the same and the uterine contents do not conform to the same laws as a perfect fluid filled cavity. In late pregnancy the volume of amniotic fluid (and allantoic in those species that have an allantoic cavity) falls. The fetus comes into contact with the uterine wall over a large area of its surface. Thus, as the myometrium contracts, the fetus is squeezed (8,18). In preliminary studies we have shown that the distortion of the fetal chest can be decreased by infusing warm physiological saline into the uterus at 115–130 days gestation (Fig. 2). The fetal distortion is greatly decreased as the uterine cavity is distended. One interpretation of this finding is that following the instillation of saline, the uterus is converted from a nonPascalian situation into one in which by reducing physical contact between the fetus and the uterine wall Pascal's law for a fluid filled cavity begins to operate. Further studies of these effects need to interrelate myometrial EMG, uterine wall tension, intra-uterine pressure and fetal distortion.

Factors that Determine the Predominance of Either Contractures or Contractions

The cascade of events that proceeds the activation of the fetal adrenal in the pregnant sheep and the role of cortisol in the conversion of placental progesterone to cortisol is discussed elsewhere in this volume and in several recent reviews. Using the sheep model in which premature labour is induced by the continuous infusion of low doses of $ACTH_{1-24}$ (1 μg/h) (2) or pulsatile injections designed to deliver (4), it has been possible to analyse the sequence of endocrine and myometrial changes that lead to efficient labour and delivery type contractions. In the sheep, estrogens and the eicosanoids are involved.

The role of estrogens in the nonhuman primate has been controversial. The circumstantial evidence of a relationship between amniotic and plasma estrogens to the onset of contractions supports a role for estrogens, but other observations are not so clear cut. We have been able to inhibit the labour and delivery type contractions that follow fetal surgery in the pregnant rhesus monkey by the administration of aromatase inhibitor 4-hydroxyandrostenedione (unpublished observations).

Various recent studies have demonstrated that a delicate balance of eicosanoids is responsible for the regulation of both contractures and contractions (3,15). We have developed an experimental model in which we can induce premature labour with ACTH infusion to the fetus and then by altering prostaglandin synthesis convert contractions back to contractures (6).

Further studies are required to elucidate the precise roles of excitatory and inhibitory factors.

Acknowledgements

This work was supported by grants from the NIH HD-12179 (the sheep studies) and HD 18870 (the monkey studies). We would like to thank Karen Rasche and Susan Haggenmiller for their assistance with the manuscript.

References

1. Cabalum, T. and Nathanielsz, P. W. (1981). *J. Physiol. Lond.* **320**, 104–105P.
2. Cabalum, T. C., Oakes, G. K., Jansen, C. A. M., Yu, H. K., Hammer, T., Buster, J. E. and Nathanielsz, P. W. (1982). *Endocrinology* **110**, 1408–1415.
3. El Badry, A., Figueroa, J. P., Poore, E. R., Sunderji, S., Levine, S., Mitchell, M. D. and Nathanielsz, P. W. (1984). *Am. J. Obstet. Gynecol.* (in press).
4. Evans, C. A., Kennedy, T. G., Patrick, J. E. and Challis, J. R. G. (1981). *Endocrinology* **109**, 1533–1538.
5. Figueroa, J. P., Mahan, S., Poore, E. R. and Nathanielsz, P. W. (1984). *Am. J. Obstet. Gynecol.* (in press).
6. Figueroa, J. P., Poore, E. R., Mitchell, M. D., Fontwit, K. and Nathanielsz, P. W. *In:* "The Physiological Development of the Fetus and Newborn" (Jones, C. T. and Nathanielsz, P. W., eds) pp. 505–509. Academic Press, London and Orlando.
7. Gluckman, P. D. and Parsons, Y. (1984). *In:* "Animal Models in Fetal Medicine" Vol. III. (Nathanielsz, P. W. ed.) pp. 70–119. Perinatology Press, Ithaca, New York.
8. Harding, R. and Poore, E. R. (1984). *Biol. Neonate* **45**, 244–251.
9. Harding, R. and Poore, E. R. (1982). *In:* "Animal Models in Fetal Medicine" Vol. II (Nathanielsz, P. W. ed.) pp. 219–258. Perinatology Press, Ithaca, New York.
10. Harding, R., Poore, E. R. and Cohen, G. L. (1981). *J. Develop. Physiol.* **3**, 231–243.
11. Harding, R., Poore, E. R., Bailey, A., Thorburn, G. D., Jansen, C. A. M. and Nathanielsz, P. W. (1982). *Am. J. Obstet. Gynecol.* **142**, 448.
12. Jansen, C. A. M., Krane, E. J., Thomas, A. L., Beck, N. F. G., Lowe, K. C., Joyce, P., Parr, M. and Nathanielsz, P. W. (1979). *Am. J. Obstet. Gynecol.* **134**, 766–783.
13. Johnston, B. M., Gluckman, P. D. and Parsons, Y. (1984). *In:* "The Physiological Development of the Fetus and Newborn" (Jones, C. T. and Nathanielsz, P. W., eds) pp. 621–625. Academic Press, London and Orlando.
14. Kitterman, J. A., Liggins, G. C., Clements, J. A. and Tooley, W. H. (1979). *J. Develop. Physiol.* **1**, 453–466.
15. Lye, S. J., Carnevale, P., Olson, D. M. and Challis, J. R. G. (1983). *Prostaglandins* **26**, 731–743.
16. Nathanielsz, P. W. (1978). *Ann. Rev. Physiol.* **40**, 411–445.
17. Nathanielsz, P. W., Abel, M. H., Bass, F. G., Krane, E. J., Thomas, A. L. and Liggins, G. C. (1978). *Q. J. Exp. Physiol.* **63**, 221–229.
18. Nathanielsz, P. W., Bailey, A., Poore, E. R., Thorburn, G. D. and Harding, R. (1980). *Am. J. Obstet. Gynecol.* **138**, 653–659.
19. Nathanielsz, P. W., Elsner, C., Magyar, D., Fridshal, D., Freeman, A. and Buster, J. E. (1982). *Endocrinology* **110**, 1402–1407.
20. Nathanielsz, P. W., Figueroa, J. P., Mahan, S. and Poore, E. R. (1984). Myometrial activity throughout pregnancy and its effect on fetal development. Proceedings of the 10th International Congress on Animal Reproduction and Artificial Insemination. University of Illinois, Urbana-Champaign, USA. Symposium No. 2. V-24.
21. Nathanielsz, P. W., Frank, D., Gleed, R., Dillingham, L., Figueroa, J. P. and Poore, E. R. (1984). *In:* "Animal Models in Fetal Medicine" Vol. III. (Nathanielsz, P. W., ed.) pp. 110–161. Perinatology Press, Ithaca, New York.
22. Nathanielsz, P. W., Jack, P. M. B., Krane, E. J., Thomas, A. L., Ratter, S. and Rees, L. H. (1977). *In:* "The Fetus and Birth", CIBA Foundation Symposium No. 47 (new series), pp. 73–91. Elsevier, Amsterdam.
23. Nathanielsz, P. W., Jansen, C. A. M., Lowe, K. C., Fridshal, D., Magyar, D. and Buster, J. E. (1981). *In:* "Changing Patterns of Fetal Placental Steroid Production

in Relation to Preparation for Independent Life", CIBA Foundation Symposium No. 86. (Elliot and Whelan, eds) pp. 66–88. Pitman Ltd., London.

24. Nathanielsz, P. W., Jansen, C. A. M., Yu, H. K. and Cabalum, T. (1984). *In:* "Fetal Physiology and Medicine. The Basis of Perinatology" 2nd Revised Edition. pp. 629–653. Marcel Dekker, New York.

25. Nathanielsz, P. W., Yu, H. K. and Cabalum, T. C. (1982). *Am. J. Obstet. Gynecol.* **144**, 614–618.

26. Novy, M. J. and Walsh, S. W. (1981). *In:* "Fetal Endocrinology". (Novy, M. J. and Resko, J. A., eds) pp. 66–94. Academic Press, New York and London.

27. Peeters, L. H., Sheldon, R. E., Jones, M. D., Makowski, E. L. and Meschia, G. (1979). *Am. J. Obstet. Gynecol.* **135**, 637–646.

28. Sopalek, V. M. and Hodgen, G. D. *In:* "Animal Models in Fetal Medicine" Vol. III. (Nathanielsz, P. W., ed.) pp. 162–183. Perinatology Press, Ithaca, New York.

29. Sunderji, S. G., El Badry, A., Poore, E. R., Figueroa, J. P. and Nathanielsz, P. W. (1984). *Am. J. Obstet. Gynecol.* (in press).

30. Taylor, N. J., Martin, M. C., Nathanielsz, P. W. and Seron-Ferre, M. (1983). *Am. J. Obstet. Gynecol.* **146**, 557–567.

31. Thorburn, G. D., Harding, R., Jenkin, G., Parkington, H. and Sigger, J. N. (1984). *J. Develop. Physiol.* **6**, 31–43.

32. Walker, A. M., Fleming, J., Smolich, J., Stunden, R., Horne, R. and Maloney, A. M. (1984). *J. Develop. Physiol.* **6**, 267–274.

Fetal Signals for Birth

J. R. G. Challis, S. J. Lye, B. F. Mitchell,
D. M. Olson, C. Sprague, L. Norman,
S. G. A. Power, J. Siddiqi and M. E. Wlodek

The Research Institute, St. Joseph's Hospital, The University of Western Ontario,
Departments of Obstetrics and Gynaecology and of Physiology,
MRC Group in Reproductive Biology, London, Ontario, Canada

Introduction

It is now generally accepted that parturition in the sheep is triggered by the fetus through increased activity of the fetal pituitary-adrenal axis (31). Recent studies have extended this concept to suggest that parturition in this species results from the maturation, and possibly sequential maturation, of a series of organ or endocrine systems. This sequence may originate at the level of the fetal brain and hypothalamus, and continue through the fetal pituitary and adrenal resulting in increased cortisol output. The pathway extends to the placenta, endometrium and fetal membranes to effect changes in steroid and prostaglandin (PG) production, and to the myometrium where the response of the muscle cells to increased agonist input is further enhanced. Birth and organ maturation proceed synchronously through provision of a common stimulus, cortisol, from the fetal adrenal gland.

We shall concentrate on two aspects of the fetal signals for birth. We shall describe changes in fetal pituitary-adrenal responsiveness during late gestation in the sheep, and discuss mechanisms by which the mother may influence these events. We shall then describe how trophoblast-derived structures, the fetal membranes, may be important in producing prostaglandins during late gestation, and we shall suggest that controls of PG output may include paracrine influences of steroids produced within the same structures and by the endometrium.

Fetal Pituitary-Adrenal Function

To examine whether fetal pituitary responsiveness changed during late gestation we administered synthetic ovine corticotrophin releasing factor (oCRF) to

The Physiological Development of the Fetus and Newborn
ISBN 0 12 389080 2

Copyright © 1985 by Academic Press, London.
All rights of reproduction in any form reserved.

chronically catheterized fetal sheep during the last third of gestation. In the youngest group of fetuses (110–113 days), bolus injections of oCRF (10 ng/100 ng) had no effect on the concentration of immunoreactive ACTH (IR-ACTH) in plasma. However there was a significant rise in IR-ACTH after 1 μg CRF injection. In older fetuses (126 128 days and 134–136 days) significant rises in plasma ACTH were measured at 100 ng CRF injected, and there was a further dose-related increment in this response at the highest amounts of CRF (Fig. 1 upper panel). At these times plasma ACTH remained elevated for up to 120 min after CRF injection.

In the youngest groups of fetuses there was no change in plasma cortisol at any one of the 3 doses of CRF injected, even at the highest amount to which there had been a rise in IR-ACTH (Fig. 1b). This observation is compatible with others suggesting that the fetal adrenal is relatively unresponsive to ACTH stimulation at this stage of gestation (4), although one cannot preclude the possibility that the IR-ACTH released is without biological activity. In fetuses

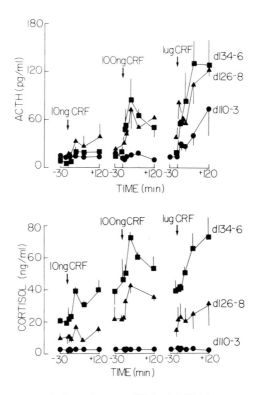

Figure 1. Plasma concentrations (mean ± SEM) of ACTH (upper panel) and cortisol (lower panel) in fetal sheep at 110–113 days (●——●), 126–128 days (▲——▲), and 134–136 days (■——■) of pregnancy before and after injection of 10 ng, 100 ng or 1 μg CRF.

at 124–126 days the changes in plasma ACTH were accompanied by a modest increase in plasma cortisol; greater increments in plasma cortisol were seen in the oldest group of fetuses (136–138 days; Fig. 1 lower panel).

These experiments provided *in vivo* evidence for maturation of both pituitary and adrenal responsiveness in late gestation, and suggested that the enhancement of the pituitary response preceded that of the adrenal. These findings extended results from Wintour *et al.* (34). These *in vivo* studies do not, however, allow us to define the mechanisms for changing pituitary responsiveness. Jones (12) has suggested that CRF may influence the processing of POMC by sheep fetal pituitary tissue *in vitro*, to promote release of $ACTH_{1-39}$. Alternatively it is possible that the number of pituitary CRF receptors increases, or that these receptors become coupled better to adenylate cyclase (1) in late gestation. Further, the concentration of vasopressin in fetal plasma rises in late pregnancy (30), and studies in the rat and in man have shown that CRF synergizes with AVP in stimulating pituitary ACTH (16,27). The changes in adrenal responses seen in this study are consistent with previous observations from *in vivo* and *in vitro* experiments in which an increase in steroidogenic enzyme activities and in functional coupling of the ACTH receptor have been described (4,20).

Relation of ACTH Release and Uterine Activity

In the next series of experiments we began to examine the hypothesis that pulsatile release of ACTH *in vivo* may occur in response to the transient episodes of

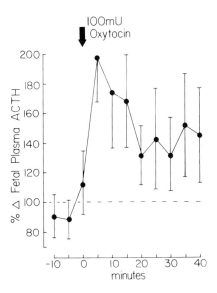

Figure 2. Changes in fetal plasma ACTH concentration (mean ± SEM) during oxytocin-induced uterine contractions and associated fetal hypoxaemia in 10 experiments in 2 late gestation fetuses. The average pre-oxytocin ACTH concentration was taken as 100%, and all other ACTH concentrations were expressed as a percentage of that value.

hypoxaemia that accompany the uterine activity pattern termed contractures by Nathanielsz and colleagues (9). Others had previously established that more severe episodes of hypoxaemia provoked rises in fetal catecholamine and ACTH concentrations (13). Contractures or Type A contractions (18) are characterized by bursts of uterine EMG activity lasting 5–7 min and by an accompanying rise in intra-uterine pressure (IUP) of 3–4 mmHg. A qualitatively similar pattern of uterine activity was stimulated by maternal injection of oxytocin into late pregnant sheep. This stimulus produced dose-dependent changes in IUP and fetal PaO_2 which were themselves directly correlated (19) and an approximate doubling of fetal plasma IR-ACTH concentrations (Fig. 2). If these results can be extrapolated to episodes of spontaneous hypoxaemia, either associated with or in the absence of contractures (10), the possibility exists of a relationship between these episodes and pulses of ACTH release in fetal life (11).

Prostaglandin Production during Late Gestation in Sheep

The rise in fetal adrenal cortisol causes an increase in placental 17 α-hydroxylase activity leading to a decrease in the concentration of progesterone and rise in

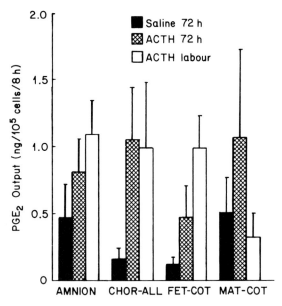

Figure 3. The output of PGE_2 (ng/10^5 cells/8 h) by dispersed cells from sheep amnion, chorioallantoic membrane, fetal and maternal components of the placenta. Tissues were collected from fetuses that had received saline for 72 h (■), or pulsatile ACTH for 72 h (▨) or 100 h (□). The mean time interval to induce premature delivery is 100 h with the amounts of ACTH administered. The increase in mean output of PGE_2 was significant for chorioallantois ($P < 0.05$).

the concentration of unconjugated estrogen in maternal peripheral plasma (6). In several animal species, including sheep, it is established that progesterone inhibits, and estrogen stimulates the output of PGF_2 from the uterus, and current dogma suggests that the changes in maternal steroid concentrations are responsible for a later increase in the concentration of PGF in maternal utero-ovarian venous plasma (31). More recently we have shown that the fetal membranes are a major site of prostaglandin production during late pregnancy in the sheep, and we suggest that steroid hormones, produced within these same structures, may contribute to the stimulus to prepartum generation of PGs.

We have used an experimental model in which ACTH pulses are administered to fetal sheep through late gestation, in the knowledge that parturition occurs reliably in singleton pregnancies within about 100 h (18). The concentration of stimulatory prostaglandins (PGE, PGF) in amniotic fluid rose before the appearance of labour-like uterine activity (24) supporting a role for these PGs in the stimulus to myometrial activity, rather than the prostaglandin changes simply resulting from uterine contractions. We found also that the output of PGE_2 by cells from amnion, choriallantois and the fetal component of the placenta was significantly elevated after 72 h P-ACTH (24; Fig. 3). There was no change in PG output by cells from the maternal component of the placenta. These results suggested remarkable similarities between the sheep and the human. In both species the fetal membranes were major sites of prostanoid output, and there appeared to be a preponderance or directed synthesis towards PGE particularly within amnion (22,29).

Effects of PGI_2 on Sheep Myometrium

The major prostanoid in sheep amniotic and allantoic fluid (5) and in myometrium (14) is PGI_2 (6-keto PGF_1). In allantoic fluid the ratio of 6-keto PGF_1: PGE + PGF decreased at the time of labour. To examine the physiologic role of PGI_2 we bilaterally ovariectomized nonpregnant sheep and recorded changes in uterine electrical and mechanical activity before and after administration of PGI_2 (17). PGI_2 provoked rapid suppression of uterine activity which lasted for 35–55 min although the uterus retained its ability to respond to agonists such as oxytocin or $PGF_{2\alpha}$. This finding suggested the possibility that the level of uterine activity resulted from a balance between stimulatory and inhibitory prostaglandins. It led us to propose a pendulum hypothesis of prostanoid generation, in which it is envisioned that endoperoxide metabolism favours production of PGI_2 for much of pregnancy, thereby promoting uterine quiescence. Towards term, the balance changes in favour of stimulatory PGIs. In dispersed chorioallantoic cells we found that estradiol decreased PGI_2 output by 40%, and similar results were obtained with human decidual cells (25). Thus, at term estrogen might effect a substantial increase in the relative outputs of stimulatory over inhibitory prostanoids.

There are other potential regulatory influences on PG generation which may originate in the fetus. The presence of inhibitors of PG production in human (28) and ovine fetal fluids has been reported (15). In the human, a protein which may originate in the fetal kidney (3) is present in fetal urine and amniotic fluid and stimulates PGE_2 output by amnion cells maintained in monolayer culture. The effect is time- and dose-dependent, and selective for amnion cells (3). Furthermore, studies by Bleasdale *et al.* (2) have delineated that calcium is essential in the activation of protein kinase C as well as the phospholipases A_2 and C which are required for the liberation of arachidonate from phosphatidyl-ethanolamine and phosphatidylinositol respectively. When isolated cells from amnion, chorioallantois and endometrium from sheep were incubated in the presence of the calcium ionophore A23187, the output of prostaglandin F was raised significantly. Further, this effect was attenuated in the presence of a calmodulin antagonist trifluoperazone (TFP). This result suggests that calcium is of similar importance in the stimulus to PG generation in the sheep, and raised the question whether the uptake of calcium might be mediated through binding to calmodulin.

Steroid Production by Sheep Fetal Membranes

In the human we and others have suggested that local production of steroids by intra-uterine tissues may be important in relation to the controls of PG production in late gestation (21,23). In the sheep, we have observed tissue specificity in the distribution of steroid metabolizing enzymes between the fetal membranes (amnion, choriallantois) and endometrium. 3 β-hydroxysteroid dehydrogenase activity was present in chorioallantois and endometrium, but absent from amnion (26). Estrone sulphatase activity was present in all 3 tissues (Table 1). However, aromatase activity was present only in the chorioallantoic membrane, and was absent in amnion and endometrium. It is possible that locally formed estrogen within this membrane may affect several functions. Estrogen may facilitate progesterone withdrawal by inhibiting 3BHD activity and enhance stimulatory PG production. Further, as indicated, locally produced estrogen may be important in suppressing the production of the inhibitory prostaglandin, PGI_2, at term. In addition, in nonpregnant sheep the uterine responsiveness to oxytocin and

Table 1. Relative activities of steroid metabolizing enzymes in sheep fetal membranes at term

	Amnion	Chorioallantois	Endometrium
3β-hydroxysteroid dehydrogenase (P5→P4)*	−	+ + +	+ + +
Aromatase (δ4→E_1)	−	+	−
E_1 sulphatase (E_1S→E_1)	+ + +	+ +	+ + +

*Products measured by RIA in the presence of 100 ng appropriate substrate, and isolated cell preparations (~ 500,000 cells/ml) from the different tissues. Steroid outputs were corrected for endogenous (To) steroid contents of the tissues and for RIA blanks obtained by incubating the substrates in the absence of cells. P_5, pregnenolone; P_4 progesterone; δ4, androstenedione; E_1, estrone, E_1S, estrone sulphate. The plus signs provide a qualitative summary of relative activities.

PGF_2 is significantly increased by estrogen pretreatment (33) presumably as a result of increased synthesis of receptors for these agonists. Garfield *et al.* (7) have shown that the changing steroid milieu at term in sheep is associated with an increase in the number of gap junctions between adjacent myometrial cells, which may facilitate synchrony of uterine activity, and account for the increase in myometrial space constants at this time (32). These findings are in accordance with the stimulatory effects of estrogen on gap junction formation in the myometrium of the rat and other species reported by Garfield and colleagues in an elegant series of experiments (8).

Acknowledgements

This work was supported by the Canadian Medical Research Council (Group grant in reproduction biology, JRGC; Fellowship, SJL; Studentships, SGAP and JS; by a Studentship from NSERC (LJN) and by equipment grants from The Jean and Richard Ivey Fund, and from The Physicians' Services Inc., Foundation of Ontario.

References

1. Bilezikjian, L. M. and Vale, W. W. (1983). *Endocrinology* **113**, 657–662.
2. Bleasdale, J. E., Okazaki, T., Sagawa, W., Di Renzo, G. C., Okita, J. R., MacDonald, P. C. and Johnston, J. M. (1983). *In:* "Initiation of Parturition: Prevention of Prematurity" (MacDonald, P. C. and Porter, J., eds) Report of the 4th Ross Conference on Obstetric Research, pp. 129–137. Columbus, Ohio, Ross Laboratories.
3. Casey, M. L., MacDonald, P. C. and Mitchell, M. D. (1983). *Biochem. Biophys. Res. Commun.* **114**, 1056–1063.
4. Challis, J. R. G., Mitchell, B. F. and Lye, S. J. (1984). *J. Develop. Physiol.* **6**, 93–105.
5. Evans, C. A., Kennedy, T. G. and Challis, J. R. G. (1982). *Biol. Reprod.* **127**, 1–11.
6. Flint, A. P. F., Anderson, A. B. M., Steele, P. A. and Turnbull, A. C. (1975). *Biochem. Soc. Trans.* **3**, 1189–1194.
7. Garfield, R. E., Rabideau, S., Challis, J. R. G. and Daniel, E. E. (1979). *Biol. Reprod.* **21**, 999–1007.
8. Garfield, R. E., Sims, S., Kannan, M. S. and Daniel, E. E. (1978). *Am. J. Physiol.* **235**, C168–C179.
9. Harding, R., Poore, E. R., Bailey, A., Thorburn, G. D., Jansen, C. A. M. and Nathanielsz, P. W. (1982). *Am. J. Obstet. Gynecol.* **142**, 448–457.
10. Harding, R., Sigger, J. N. and Wickham, P. J. D. (1983). *J. Develop. Physiol.* **5**, 267–276.
11. Jones, C. T. (1979). *Horm. Met. Res.* **11**, 237–241.
12. Jones, C. T. (1983). *In:* "Initiation of Parturition: Prevention of Prematurity" (MacDonald, P. C. and Porter, J., eds) Report of the 4th Ross Conference on Obstetric Research, pp. 17–23. Columbus, Ohio, Ross Laboratories.
13. Jones, C. T., Boddy, K., Robinson, J. S. and Ratcliffe, J. G. (1977). *J. Endocrinol.* **72**, 279–292.
14. Jones, R. L., Poyser, N. L. and Wilson, N. H. (1977). *Br. J. Pharmacol.* **59**, 436–437.

15. Leach Harper, C. M. and Thorburn, G. D. (1984). *Can. J. Physiol. Pharmacol.* (in press).
16. Liu, J. H., Muse, K., Contreras, P., Gibbs, D., Vale, W., Rivier, J. and Yen, S. S. C. (1983). *J. Clin. Endocrin. Metab.* **57**, 1087–1089.
17. Lye, S. J. and Challis, J. R. G. (1982). *J. Reprod. Fertil.* **66**, 311–315.
18. Lye, S. J., Sprague, C., Mitchell, B. F. and Challis, J. R. G. (1983). *Endocrinology* **113**, 770–776.
19. Lye, S. J., Wlodek, M. E. and Challis, J. R. G. (1984). *Can. J. Physiol. Pharmacol.* (submitted).
20. Manchester, E. L., Lye, S. J. and Challis, J. R. G. (1983). *Endocrinology* **113**, 777–782.
21. Milewich, L., Gant, N. F., Schwarz, B. E., Chen, G. T. and MacDonald, P. C. (1977). *Obstet. Gynecol.* **50**, 45–48.
22. Mitchell, M. D., Bibby, J., Hicks, B. R. and Turnbull, A. C. (1978). *Prostaglandins* **15**, 377–382.
23. Mitchell, B. F., Cruickshank, M., McLean, D. and Challis, J. R. G. (1982). *J. Clin. Endocrin. Metab.* **55**, 1237–1239.
24. Olson, D. M., Lye, S. J., Skinner, K. and Challis, J. R. G. (1984). *J. Reprod. Fertil.* (in press).
25. Olson, D. M., Skinner, K. and Challis, J. R. G. (1983). *Prostaglandins* **25**, 639–651.
26. Power, S. G. A. and Challis, J. R. G. (1983). *J. Endocrinol.* **97**, 347–356.
27. Rivier, C. and Vale, W. (1983). *Nature* **305**, 325–327.
28. Saeed, S. A., Strickland, D. M., Young, D. C., Dang, A. and Mitchell, M. D. (1982). *J. Clin. Endocrin. Metabol.* **55**, 801–804.
29. Skinner, K. A. and Challis, J. R. G. (1984). *Am. J. Obstet. Gynecol.* (submitted).
30. Stark, R. I., Daniel, S. S., Husain, K. M., James, L. S. and van de Wiele, R. L. V. (1979). *Biol. Neonate* **35**, 235–241.
31. Thorburn, G. D. and Challis, J. R. G. (1979). *Physiol. Rev.* **59**, 863–918.
32. Thorburn, G. D., Harding, R., Jenkin, G., Parkington, H. and Sigger, J. N. (1984). *J. Develop. Physiol.* **6**, 31–43.
33. Windmoller, R., Lye, S. J. and Challis, J. R. G. (1983). *Can. J. Physiol. Pharmacol.* **61**, 722–728.
34. Wintour, E. M., Bell, R. J., Fei, D. T., Southwell, C., Tregear, G. W. and Xiaoming, W. (1984). *Neuroendocrinology* **38**, 86–87.

Birth, its Physiology, and the Problems it Creates

J. Job Faber, Debra F. Anderson, Mark J. Morton, Christine M. Parks, C. Wright Pinson, Kent L. Thornburg and Dale M. Willis

Departments of Physiology and Medicine, School of Medicine, Oregon Health Sciences University, Portland, Oregon, USA

Introduction

The title of this paper, which was given to us, is encompassing in scope. It makes birth accountable for most of the misery in the world and suggests Physiology is to blame for it. Needless to say, we interpret the title in the spirit in which it was given.

Most "problems" arise from failure to maintain the constancy of the milieu interieur. This constancy is normally assured by numerous control mechanisms that make appropriate corrections to deviations from preset "normal" values. Fetal control mechanisms are of two kinds. Some operate during fetal life in the same way they operate later, perhaps with modifications. Regulation of intracellular composition, endocrine regulation of metabolism, autoregulation of peripheral blood flow, and the regulation of cell division and growth are examples. Controls of this kind may be stressed at any time during development but are not specially stressed at birth and for that reason they do not concern us here. But there are also control mechanisms whose function is altered by the changes that occur at birth or whose function is taken over by another organ system at the moment a fetus becomes a neonate.

Long-term Cardiovascular Control

The theory of "integral control" put forward by Guyton *et al.* (12) on the basis of earlier work by Borst and Borst-de Geus (7), has the virtue of internal consistency. In this theory, renal modulation of the excretion of water and salt

The Physiological Development of the Fetus and Newborn
ISBN 0 12 389080 2

Copyright © 1985 by Academic Press, London.
All rights of reproduction in any form reserved.

is governed by systemic arterial pressure. Changes in renal excretion lead to changes in fluid volumes, diastolic filling pressure and cardiac output. Changes in cardiac output lead to autoregulatory responses of the peripheral tissues and hence to changes in peripheral resistance and arterial pressure. The crux of the arrangement is the co-operativity of the heart, the tissues, and the kidney. That interaction ensures the near constancy of systemic arterial blood pressure and cardiac output.

However, fetal fluid volumes are not under the exclusive control of the fetal kidney and the fetal cardiac function curves, unlike their adult counterparts, show little or no increase in stroke work at filling pressures above normal. Thus, the fetal and adult forms of long-term cardiovascular control promise to be different.

Transduction of filling pressure to flow in fetal heart

The earliest work on the Frank-Starling mechanism in chronically instrumented fetal lambs seemed to indicate that "the Frank-Starling relationship is both operative and effective in . . . the narrow, but physiological, range of end-diastolic pressures from 2.5 to 8 mmHg" (16). Later work by Gilbert (11) indicated that the *bi*ventricular output did not increase at right atrial pressures much higher than about 5 mmHg. The latest and most accurate measurements of right ventricular output indicate that the Frank-Starling mechanism operates in the right ventricle only at right atrial pressures below a mean of 3.4 ± 1.2 SD mmHg (Fig. 1). At higher right atrial pressures right ventricular stroke volume is constant at 1.5 ± 0.4 SD ml/min/kg. It was also found that right ventricular stroke volume falls at abnormally high arterial pressures (20). Unlike the right ventricle, the fetal left ventricle has some stroke volume reserve (*ca* 10%) at left atrial pressures above a mean "breakpoint" of 3.0 ± 1 SD mmHg (Fig. 1), and it is, in contrast to the right ventricle, not very sensitive to afterload (21).

The physiologic basis for the difference between adult and fetal Starling curves must be sought in the diastolic distensibility of the fetal ventricles and/or in the distribution of sarcomere lengths and their active length-tension relationships and/or in the geometric arrangement of the muscle fibres in the heart.

In the intact fetus, the left and right sides of the heart operate at the atrial pressures and stroke volumes of the "break points" in their respective function curves (20,21). This presents difficulties for the application of the adult theory of cardiovascular regulation to the fetus. In the fetus increases in cardiac filling pressure are not immediately transformed into substantial increases in ventricular stroke work. One could hypothesize that ventricular growth (hyperplasia and hypertrophy) in the fetus takes the place of the Frank-Starling mechanism in the adult. Such growth controlled by filling pressure could slowly lead to increases in stroke work. But there is no evidence for this hypothesis and its proof by long-term experimentation would be a toilsome effort.

The observation that the fetal ventricles operate at the break points of their function curves presents further difficulties. Feta left ventricular stroke volume rises rapidly after birth (15). The corresponding increase in left ventricular stroke work is not likely to be entirely due to increased preload and may, therefore,

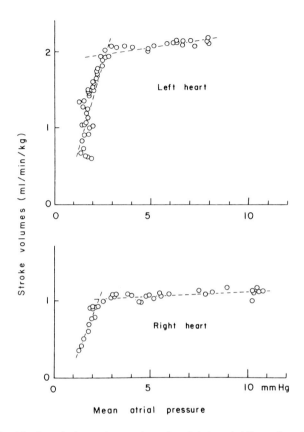

Figure 1. Ventricular stroke volumes (per kg fetal weight) as functions of the corresponding atrial pressures during blockade of the autonomic nervous system. Note lack of stroke volume reserve in right ventricle and limited reserve in left ventricle beyond mean atrial pressures of about 3 mmHg. The 2 curves are from 2 different animals; ordinarily, maximum stroke volume on the right side of the heart exceeds that on the left.

be partly due to increased contractility. That increase in contractility of the neonatal ventricle may be caused by an increase in sympathetic adrenergic support, or by the postnatal increase in arterial oxygen tension and oxygen content. Current experiments in our laboratory favour the latter explanation (Thornburg and Morton, unpublished). If true, it would place the neonatal ventricles at the mercy of the respiratory system.

Hydraulics of flow through the foramen ovale as a determinant of the filling of the left ventricle vs the right ventricle during diastole

Almost the entire venous return is by way of the superior and inferior caval veins, pulmonary blood flow being of the order of 5% of the combined ventricular output. The partition of the inferior caval flow into a right and a left atrial inflow is determined by the fraction of the venous return that flows through the foramen ovale into the left atrium.

It is, by now, well known that the foramen ovale in the fetal lamb is not a window between the right and left atria. The anatomy is clearly described by Amoroso et al. (1). As the title states, the inferior caval vein terminates into two vessels, both of considerable length, of which the left one is called the "foramen ovale". In spite of the precise descriptions by Amoroso et al. (1) and Barcroft (4), we must admit that the great length of this channel was not apparent to us until we made casts of the atrial inflow tracts (3).

The hydraulic energy that drives the blood through the foramen ovale is not only the difference in driving pressure across this channel but also the kinetic energy of the blood in the inferior caval vein. The decrease in the velocity of the blood in the inferior caval vein when placental venous return is lost "probably diminishes the pressure of the jet which impinges on the foramen" (4) and may be more important than the reversal of the pressure difference in the mechanism that closes the foramen after birth. Anderson et al. (3) could find no reliable correlation ($r=0.22$) between foramen ovale flow (mean 157 ± 36 SEM, ml/min/kg) and atrial pressure difference (L-R mean 0.6 ± 0.6 SEM, mmHg) in 7 chronically instrumented fetal lambs whose central shunt flows were measured with a combination of electromagnetic flow meter and microsphere techniques. These authors did, however, find a correlation ($r=0.59$, $P<0.05$) between foramen ovale flow and inferior caval vein flow (mean 305 ± 38 SEM, ml/min/kg), both expressed per kg fetal weight. We recently extended these findings by measuring central shunt flows in 8 additional chronically instrumented fetuses. One of these was studied as before, three were ventilated *in utero* by means of indwelling tracheal tubes and 4 were studied immediately after they had been delivered by their ewes. The purpose of the additional experiments was to measure foramen ovale flows when atrial pressures, inferior caval vein flows and flows in the foramen itself were as different as possible from those found in the fetus. We fitted an equation of the form:

$$Q^{Fo} = a\Delta p + b(Q^{Icv})^c \tag{1}$$

on the assumption that the driving force consisted of a pressure term and a kinetic energy term (8). We used nonlinear regression analysis (6) to determine the least squares fit of the parameters a, b, and c. The best fit was obtained with the regression equation:

$$Q^{Fo} = 24\Delta p + 0.0095(Q^{Icv})^{1.7} \tag{2}$$

on a set of 16 observations of foramen ovale flows (Q^{Fo}) and inferior caval vein flows (Q^{Icv}) and pressure differences (Δp) between right and left atria (Anderson et al., unpublished). Flows were expressed per kg fetal weight, ml/min/kg, to remove spurious correlations between the two flows due to fetal weight alone. Pressures were in mmHg.

The parameter of interest is c, which was close to 2; its 95% confidence limits were 1.3 and 2.1. This is reasonably good when one expects a value of exactly 2 for the square of the linear velocity of the blood in the kinetic energy term of fluid energy (ref. 8, p. 102).

We concluded that before birth foramen ovale flow and, therefore, individual ventricular filling are affected by the square of the blood flow in the inferior caval vein.

Arterial blood pressure

Bilateral nephrectomy abolishes all renal excretion and should, therefore, lead to an arterial hypertension if fluid volumes, cardiac output, and tissue perfusion are indirectly affected by renal excretion of water and salt. Bilateral nephrectomy in fetal sheep did not, however, lead to arterial hypertension in the 18 fetal sheep in which the experiment was tried (5). This finding probably means that fetal fluid volume control is not a renal but a placental function. In that case, control of fetal arterial pressure may be a placental function also (9).

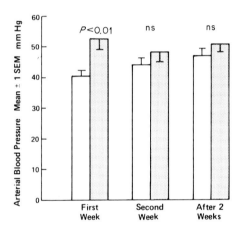

Figure 2. Arterial blood pressures in 11 unilaterally nephrectomized sheep fetuses with stenosed contralateral renal arteries in the weeks after surgery.

As a further test of renal pressure control, we subjected 11 fetal lambs to unilateral nephrectomy and contralateral renal artery stenosis (Anderson and Faber, unpublished). This did not lead to an elevation in plasma renin activity in comparison to 9 sham operated controls and caused a transient arterial hypertension of an average of 13 mmHg only in the first week after surgery; 2 or more weeks after surgery, there were no differences in arterial pressures between the experimental and the sham operated fetuses (Fig. 2). We did not find a correlation between arterial blood pressure and plasma renin activity in the fetuses with renal artery stenosis at any time after surgery.

The preponderance of the evidence so far does not support a renal role in the regulation of fetal arterial blood pressure. It appears that the kidney starts to control pressure only at the moment of birth when it assumes control over fluid volume.

Control of Oxygen Acquisition and Carbon Dioxide Elimination

Regulation of prenatal gas exchange

The mechanisms of placental oxygen acquisition and carbon dioxide elimination are well understood (17,19). However, the control of this acquisition is a complete mystery, in contrast to postnatal respiratory control, for which a broadly satisfactory explanation is available.

The factors that limit prenatal oxygen acquisition include the oxygen already present in the umbilical artery blood, which limits the total amount of oxygen that can be added before the blood is completely saturated. Further factors are the haemoglobin content of the fetal blood and its P_{50}, fetal placental blood flow, and maternal placental oxygen delivery. The oxygen diffusing capacity of the placenta is now known to be at most only a mild limitation for oxygen uptake (17) and the geometric arrangement of the placental microcirculations (10) is not a matter that the fetus or the mother can do much about.

Fetal placental haemoglobin flow is determined by fetal haemoglobin concentration and fetal placental blood flow, which in turn depends on arterial (and venous) blood pressure and fetal placental resistance to flow. We, therefore, artificially restricted fetal placental blood flow in 11 fetal lambs to investigate which, if any, of these determinants of placental haemoglobin flow would respond. Figure 3 shows data from these experiments in which fetal placental blood flow

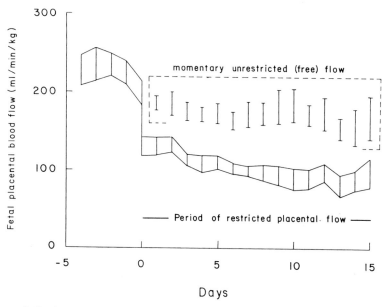

Figure 3. Control placental blood flow (before day 0) and restricted placental blood flow in 11 fetal lambs (mean ± 1 SEM). Bars indicate recorded flows when the restriction on flow was removed for a period of 1 min (mean ± SEM). Only 2 experimental fetuses (not included in this series) succumbed to the procedure in the first week of restriction.

was restricted to two-thirds of the control flow in the week after surgery and kept there, with no allowance for fetal growth (2).

The instrument for flow restriction was an inflatable occluder placed just above the iliac bifurcation of the aorta. Corrections for nonplacental flow were determined before and during flow restriction with microspheres. The average period of flow restriction was 15 days. Arterial PO_2 and pH decreased, and PCO_2 increased. There was no change in fetal arterial blood pressure above the level of the occluder, there was no change in fetal haematocrit and the fetal placental resistance to flow decreased slightly less than it does during normal gestation (2). Fetal growth, measured as an increase in fetal plasma volume, was 2% per day, as opposed to about 4% per day, normally. We conclude from these experiments that fetal placental haemoglobin flow is not defended by some form of negative feedback control since none of its determinants responded to a prolonged reduction.

We do not know whether a reduction in fetal placental oxygen acquisition leads to compensatory changes, such as an increase in maternal placental oxygen delivery. Experiments on pregnant sheep kept at altitude suggest to us that a reduction in fetal oxygen supply leads to an increase in maternal placental blood flow (13,14,18), but other interpretations remain possible.

Regulation of postnatal gas exchange

At birth, gas exchange suddenly begins to be controlled by the respiratory center and its complement of sensors and effectors, a mechanism that has no known relation to prenatal gas exchange. The very surprising feature of the postnatal mechanism of respiratory control is that it is turned off about half of the time before birth. Perhaps it is turned off even most of the time; this depends on whether one accepts prenatal "respiration" as a manifestation of the postnatal control mechanism.

Figure 4 shows results obtained in our laboratory with chronically instrumented fetal sheep with indwelling tracheal catheters. The fetuses were ventilated with various gas mixtures while still *in utero*. At the end of a 10 min period of ventilation with any particular gas mixture, the respirator was stopped and the tracheal pressure record was inspected for spontaneous respiratory activity. An arterial blood sample was obtained at the same time. These experiments were done with the umbilical circulation intact and also with the umbilical circulation completely occluded by means of an inflatable occluder on the cord.

The results obtained on fetuses with and without cord occlusion were very similar (Fig. 4). But when the same fetuses were delivered (under spinal anaesthesia for the ewe), all of them breathed spontaneously at blood gas tensions that produced only occasional respiratory activity before birth (22,23). The conclusion must be that some aspect of birth disinhibits the respiratory centre and allows it to assume control over arterial blood gas tensions. What aspect of birth is the cause of this disinhibition we do not know, except that it is not the cessation of the umbilical circulation, not the initial expansion of the lungs, and not the resultant changes in the gas tensions in the lungs or in the blood.

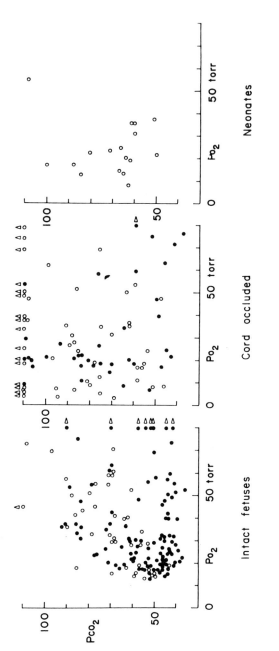

Figure 4. Arterial PO_2 and PCO_2 after 10 min periods of *in utero* ventilation, or after birth. Open circles indicate that respiratory activity was present, closed circles that it was absent. Arrow heads show gas tensions that exceeded the range of tensions on the abscissa or the ordinate. Respiratory activity was always present in neonates (panel on the right) at the same blood gas tensions where it was only occasionally present in fetuses regardless of whether their umbilical circulations were intact (left panel) or occluded (centre panel).

Conclusion

Many variables affect or disturb the milieu interieur before as well as after birth. The constancy of the milieu interieur is nevertheless ensured by various mechanisms that "control" or "regulate". It is now clear that in some cases the fetal mechanism is not merely a miniature of the adult counterpart but is either absent or completely different. It appears that it is specially the mechanisms that change identity at the moment of birth that may lead the neonate into trouble.

Acknowledgements

These studies were performed with the expert assistance of Tom Green, Dana McNaught, and Bob Webber. C. Wright Pinson was supported by a postdoctoral fellowship of the American Heart Association, Oregon Affiliate. The studies were financially supported by grants from the National Heart Lung and Blood Institute (5 RO1 HL29324 and 5 RO1 HL27194) and the National Institute of Child Health and Human Development (5 PO1 HD10034).

References

1. Amoroso, E. C., Barclay, A. E., Franklin, K. J. and Prichard, M. M. L. (1942). *J. Anat.* **76**, 240–247.
2. Anderson, D. F. and Faber, J. J. (1984). *Am. J. Physiol.* (submitted).
3. Anderson, D. F., Bissonnette, J. M., Thornburg, K. L. and Faber, J. J. (1981). *Am. J. Physiol.* **241** (*Heart Circ. Physiol.* **10**), H60–H66.
4. Barcroft, J. (1946). Researches on Prenatal Life, vol. 1. Blackwell Scientific Publications, Oxford.
5. Binder, N. D., Anderson, D. F., Potter, D. M., Thornburg, K. L. and Faber, J. J. (1982). *Biol. Neonate* **42**, 50–58.
6. Boardman, T. J. (1982). Statistical Library Hewlett-Packard, Fort Collins.
7. Borst, J. G. G. and Borst-deGeus, A. (1963). *Lancet* **I**, 677–682.
8. Burton, A. C. (1965). "Physiology and Biophysics of the Circulation". Year Book Medical Publishers, Chicago.
9. Faber, J. J. (1972). *In:* "Respiratory Gas Exchange and Blood Flow in the Placenta". (Longo, L. D. and Bartels, H., eds), DHEW, Bethesda, MD.
10. Faber, J. J. (1977). *Fed. Proc.* **36**, 2640–2646.
11. Gilbert, R. D. (1980). *Am. J. Physiol.* **238** (*Heart Circ. Physiol.* **7**), H80–H86.
12. Guyton, A. C., Coleman, T. G., Cowley, W., Manning, R. D., Norman, R. A. and Ferguson, J. D. (1974). *Circulat. Res.* **35**, 159–176.
13. Huckabee, W. E., Metcalfe, J., Prystowsky, H. and Barron, D. H. (1961). *Am. J. Physiol.* **200**, 274–278.
14. Kaiser, I. H., Cummings, J. N., Reynolds, S. R. M. and Marbarger, J. P. (1958). *J. Appl. Physiol.* **13**, 171–178.
15. Kirkpatrick, S. E., Covell, J. W. and Friedman, W. F. (1973). *Am. J. Obstet. Gynecol.* **116**, 963–972.
16. Kirkpatrick, S. E., Pitlick, P. T. and Friedman, W. F. (1976). *Am. J. Physiol.* **231**, 495–500.
17. Longo, L. D., Hill, E. P. and Power, G. G. (1972). *Am. J. Physiol.* **222**, 730–739.

18. Metcalfe, J., Meschia, G., Hellegers, A., Prystowsky, H., Huckabee, W. and Barron, D. H. (1962). *Q. J. Exp. Physiol.* **47**, 74–92.
19. Power, G. G., Hill, F. P. and Longo, L. D. (1972). *Am. J. Physiol.* **222**, 740–746.
20. Thornburg, K. L. and Morton, M. J. (1983). *Am. J. Physiol.* **244** (*Heart Circ. Physiol.* **13**), H656–H663.
21. Thornburg, K. L., Morton, M. J., Anderson, D. F. and Faber, J. J. (1982). *Physiologist* **25**, 254.
22. Willis, D. M., Anderson, D. F., Thornburg, K. L. and Faber, J. J. (1981). *Clin. Res.* **29**, 98A.
23. Willis, D. M., Anderson, D. F., Thornburg, K. L. and Faber, J. J. (1982). *Fed. Proc.* **41**, 1491.

Prostaglandins and the Regulation of Myometrial Activity: A Working Model

G. D. Thorburn

Department of Physiology, Monash University,
Clayton, Australia

Introduction

The uterus remains relatively quiescent throughout pregnancy but, at term, it explodes into activity to effect the delivery of the fetus. Our interest in prostaglandins stems from their putative role as a major activator of the uterine muscle (myometrium). It is thought that, with regard to the myometrium, prostaglandins have two major functions. Firstly, to act as an external stimulant of uterine activity and secondly, a possible modulation of the contractile processes. There is, however, a paucity of information on the mechanisms by which prostaglandins influence myometrial activity. In this presentation I would like to propose a working hypothesis for the role of prostaglandins in the regulation of myometrial activity and to discuss it in the light of the evidence which is presently available.

A model for the contractile response pathway

The model system that I shall use is based on that proposed by Nishizuka (27,28) for human platelets (Fig. 1). This system is commonly used for exploring hormone action since many extracellular messengers, e.g. thrombin, are known to cause both aggregation and the exocytosis of dense granules containing serotonin and ATP (the release reaction). Thrombin-stimulated release of serotonin is initiated by the interaction of thrombin with a membrane receptor. This interaction stimulates phospholipid turnover within the membrane and is associated with the selective phosphorylation of two endogenous proteins which are essential for the aggregation and release of serotonin from platelets.

The Physiological Development of the Fetus and Newborn
ISBN 0 12 389080 2
Copyright © 1985 by Academic Press, London.
All rights of reproduction in any form reserved.

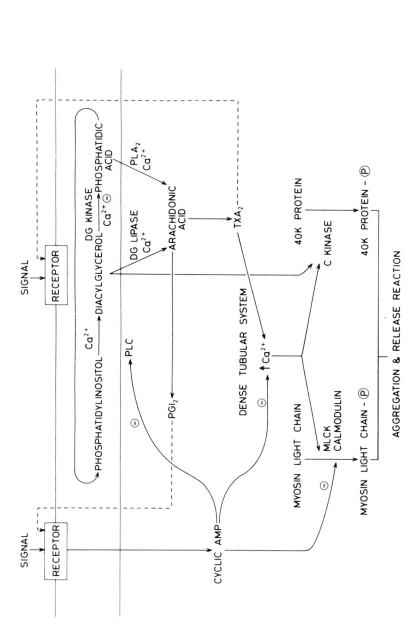

Figure 1. The contractile-response pathway in platelets, as proposed by Nishizuka (27,28).

Elucidation of the mechanism of signal transmission across the cell membrane is essential for the formulation of a model of hormone action. A wide variety of hormones, neurotransmitters and other chemical substances stimulate the turnover of phospholipid in their target tissues. Most of the lipid in the cell membrane is found in the phospholipid fraction, with phosphatidylcholine (PC), phosphatidylethanolamine (PE), phosphatidylserine (PS) and phosphatidylinositol (PI) being the major phospholipids. A number of phospholipases (PL) are found in cells: PLA_1 and PLA_2 hydrolyse the phospholipid fatty acid ester bond at the 1-acyl, or 2-acyl position, respectively; PLD hydrolyses the phospholipid base group; and PLC, the polar head group.

The sequence of events between stimulation with thrombin and secretion involves the activation of PLC, which in platelets has a substrate specificity for PI. Diacyl glycerol and inositol phosphate are the initial products of PI breakdown (Fig. 1). The diacylglycerol can be metabolized in two different ways which both generate arachidonic acid. Following thrombin stimulation of the platelet, phosphatidic acid (PA) turnover occurs principally as a result of the action of diacylglycerolkinase, an enzyme which is dependent upon Mg^{2+} and ATP and which phosphorylates diacylglycerol. The PA that is generated may activate PLA_2 and cause the release of arachidonic acid from other phospholipids. PA may also release its own arachidonic acid through the action of PA-specific PLA_2 (4). The second pathway by which diacylglycerol can yield free arachidonic acid depends upon the action of diacylglycerol lipase. This enzyme cleaves the fatty acid ester bond at sn-1 and produces a 2-arachidonyl monoglyceride, which releases free arachidonic acid upon hydrolysis at sn-2 by monoglyceride lipase (2). The arachidonic acid released is metabolized to thromboxane A_2 (TXA_2) or prostacyclin (PGI_2). Billah et al. (3) have proposed that membrane-active agents, like thrombin, induce a conformational change in the membrane allowing exposure of the PI to the cytosolic enzyme PLC for production of diacylglycerol and arachidonate release. It is noteworthy that, in platelets, the generation of diacylglycerol and/or PA is sufficient to affect membrane properties relating to shape changes, fusogenesis or aggregation. The activation of PLA_2 and the subsequent biosynthesis of prostaglandins (PG) facilitates the release reaction and further aggregation.

An increase in the cytoplasmic concentration of Ca^{2+} has been implicated in the release reaction and aggregation in platelets. Stimulation of PI turnover increases intracellular Ca^{2+} availability and a number of mechanisms have been proposed: PI turnover is involved in Ca^{2+} gate opening (23); and phosphatidic acid, and inositol-1,4,5-triphosphate, breakdown products of PI, are active Ca^{2+} ionophores and may participate in Ca^{2+} mobilization (19). Similarly, TXA_2 acts as a Ca^{2+} ionophore in platelets. High intracellular Ca^{2+} concentrations are required for the activation of 2 pathways which facilitate platelet aggregation and the release reaction. In the first of these Ca^{2+} activates the calmodulin-dependent, myosin light chain kinase (MLCK) which in turn phosphorylates the 20 000 dalton (20K) protein, myosin light chain (8) causing contraction of actomyosin filaments and platelet aggregation. In the second of these pathways, diacylglycerol, in the presence of Ca^{2+} and a phospholipid membrane factor, preferably phosphatidyl serine or phosphatidic acid activates C-kinase which phosphorylates a 40 000 dalton (40K) protein. Nishizuka (27,28) has suggested that the phosphorylation of this protein is involved in serotonin release.

In most tissues there appears to be two major receptor mechanisms for controlling cellular functions. One class, which we have already discussed, induces PI turnover and immediate Ca^{2+} mobilization. The second class of receptors is related to cyclic AMP. In most systems, such as platelets and smooth muscle, the receptors that induce PI turnover promote activation of cellular functions, whereas the receptors that produce cyclic AMP usually antagonize such activation (27,28). It has been well established that cyclic AMP exerts its actions through activation of cyclic AMP-dependent protein kinase (A-kinase). In human platelets, it has been shown that PI breakdown, diacylglycerol formation, 40K protein phosphorylation and the release reaction were all inhibited in a parallel manner by dibutyryl cyclic AMP as well as prostaglandin E_1 (17). Their results indicated that cyclic AMP inhibited PI turnover by inhibiting PLC activity.

In platelets, PGI_2 inhibits the release reaction by stimulating cyclic AMP production. Nishizuka (27) proposed that this effect is mediated by the interaction of PGI_2 with a membrane bound receptor. In this model, cyclic AMP activates A-kinase to inhibit PLC activity, thus acting as a negative feedback control. As a result, PG synthesis decreases resulting in lower intracellular Ca^{2+} concentrations. In platelets cyclic AMP also enhances the cellular sequestration of Ca^{2+} into membrane vesicles (18). Cyclic AMP dependent kinase (A-kinase) may also enhance the inhibitory phosphorylation of phospholipases (20) and inhibit the Ca^{2+}-dependent cyclooxygenase (12). Cyclic AMP has also been implicated in the inactivation of MLCK by phosphorylation in smooth muscle (9) and the extrusion of Ca^{2+} from the cell.

The analogy to smooth muscle becomes immediately apparent (Fig. 2). A signal (e.g. oxytocin) activates PLC which causes turnover of PI with the formation of diacylglycerol, PA and inositol phosphate. The generation of these moieties and the Ca^{2+} mobilization, resulting from the stimulation of PI turnover, may be sufficient to induce activation of MLCK and C-kinase resulting in muscle contraction. Stimulation of PLA_2 causes further release of arachidonic acid providing more substrate for PG production. The PG would then cause mobilization of Ca^{2+} from the sarcoplasmic reticulum (7) and the formation of gap junctions (11). This process acts to amplify the contractile response to the signal.

The inhibition of PI turnover and the readjustment of intracellular calcium concentrations, which result in muscle relaxation, proceed by cyclic AMP-dependent processes. PGI_2 stimulates receptor-linked cyclic AMP production. De Lanerolle et al. (9), as a result of their studies on canine tracheal smooth muscle, have proposed that high concentrations of cyclic AMP activate A-kinase, which phosphorylates myosin light chain kinase (MLCK) converting it into an inactive form. Dephosphorylation of myosin by phosphatases and muscle relaxation follows (Fig. 2). Their experiments indicate that it may be possible to relax smooth muscle, by a mechanism involving MLCK phosphorylation, even in the presence of high intracellular Ca^{2+}. Such a mechanism may be most important when the muscle

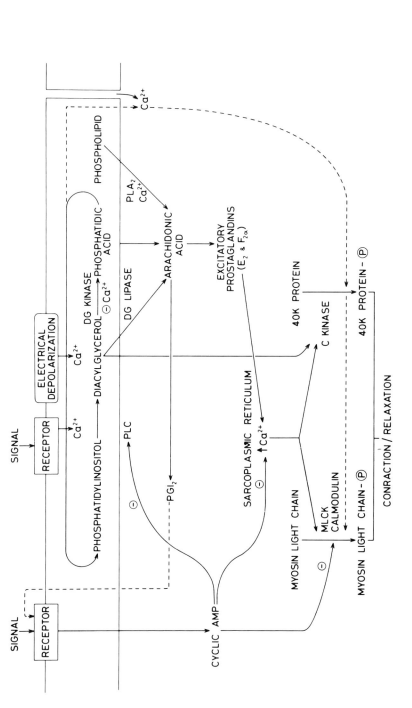

Figure 2. The analogous contractile-response pathway for the contraction and relaxation of myometrial smooth muscle.

is being maximally stimulated and when it may be advantageous to have a mechanism of relaxing the muscle in which Ca^{2+} concentration is still high. Similarly, as in the platelet, cyclic AMP may enhance the cellular sequestration of Ca^{2+} into membrane vesicles (18). A-kinase may also enhance the inhibitory phosphorylation of phospholipases (20). It is thought β-mimetics act on this second type of receptor to stimulate cyclic AMP production and the inhibition of uterine activity.

Control of myometrial activity

Two patterns of myometrial EMG actively will be considered in this analogy: 1. nonlabour contractures, which are of low intensity and occur at a frequency of $1-4\,h^{-1}$; and 2. labour-associated contractions, which are characterized by increased frequency and amplitude and decreased duration of bursts.

Progesterone

There is considerable evidence which is indicative that progesterone is involved in the suppression of ovine myometrial electrical activity during pregnancy and that progesterone withdrawal is associated with parturition. In sheep, progesterone is maintained at luteal phase levels during early pregnancy before increasing to higher concentrations around day 90. Progesterone concentrations remain elevated until decreasing in the few days before parturition (1,33). The uterus is relatively quiescent during pregnancy and its responsiveness to signals which stimulate the contractile pathways (e.g. oxytocin) is low until near delivery. Marked uterine activity commences only 12–24 h before delivery at a time when the plasma levels of progesterone are decreasing.

The effects of progesterone withdrawal on ovine uterine activity have been examined using the 3β-HSD inhibitor, trilostane (16). Trilostane, in doses of 100 mg administered intravenously, reduced progesterone levels and enhanced PG synthesis, as indicated by the metabolite levels of $PGF_{2\alpha}$. Concomitantly, myometrial EMG activity and the number of intra-uterine pressure (IUP) elevations increased over this period. Ewes which aborted prematurely did so at a time when PGFM levels were maximal. No consistent change in plasma estradiol levels was observed after trilostane treatment. It appears that this extent of progesterone withdrawal may be adequate to cause $PGF_{2\alpha}$ release and parturition.

In a further series of experiments, $PGF_{2\alpha}$ was infused extra-amniotically, into pregnant ewes at approximately 125 days gestation (16). Both fetal and maternal plasma, and amniotic fluid PGFM concentrations were increased to values in excess of those observed at term. There was, however, no sustained increase in EMG activity or IUP during the 84 h of the $PGF_{2\alpha}$ infusion. Maternal plasma progesterone concentrations were maintained at pre-infusion levels during this treatment. When trilostane (100 mg) was injected intravenously, during the extra-amniotic administration of $PGF_{2\alpha}$, there was a precipitous decline in maternal plasma progesterone concentrations and parturition was initiated within 48 h in 3 of the 4 animals treated. These experiments clearly indicate that the myometrium of pregnant ewes, presumably as a result of progesterone, is insensitive to $PGF_{2\alpha}$ and the removal of the progesterone block increases the sensitivity of the myometrium to $PGF_{2\alpha}$ stimulation.

The mechanism by which progesterone suppresses the contractile-response pathway has yet to be elucidated. I suggest, however, that progesterone acts at a level of the PI turnover by inducing the synthesis of a phospholipase inhibitor (lipomodulin). Bleasdale et al. (6) have suggested that in human fetal amniotic membrane, the 40K protein may be lipomodulin, a glucocorticoid-dependent protein, which inhibits phospholipase activity (5,10,15). Bleasdale et al. (6) further suggested that C-kinase may phosphorylate lipomodulin thus removing its inhibitory action on phospholipase activity. I propose that progesterone may act in a similar way to the glucocorticoids by interacting with a cytosolic receptor which induces a lipomodulin-like protein in the myometrium (Fig. 3). This protein inhibits phospholipase activity and thus interferes with signal transmission and the formation of prostaglandins in the myometrium. A similar mechanism may apply to the endometrium (decidua), placenta and fetal membranes.

As mentioned previously, the withdrawal of progesterone by either lutectomy in goats or the use of 3β-HSD inhibitors in sheep, result in increased myometrial EMG activity. Similarly, the progesterone receptor antagonist, RU486, induces uterine activity and abortion in humans (14). These effects may be mediated by decreased concentrations of progesterone-induced lipomodulin. The inhibition of the contractile response pathway would thus be removed.

Prostaglandins

According to our model, arachidonic acid is generated as a result of the activity of PLC and PLA_2 provided the level of activity of cyclooxygenase (PG synthetase) enzyme complex is adequate, the arachidonic acid is converted into endoperoxides which are then converted to various prostanoids (PGE_2, $PGF_{2\alpha}$, PGI_2 and TXA_2) depending on the relative activity of the synthetic enzymes in the tissue. PG synthesis can, therefore, be blocked at a number of sites. As mentioned in the previous section, phospholipase activity can be blocked by lipomodulin, a 40K protein induced in neutrophils by glucocorticoids (15). In this model, it has been proposed that progesterone may induce the synthesis of a similar 40K inhibitory protein which, for convenience, we have called lipomodulin. Cyclooxygenase activity can be blocked by the nonsteroidal anti-inflammatory drugs such as aspirin, indomethacin and meclofenamic acid (MFA).

Returning to the model, prostaglandins have a number of actions on the myometrium. Firstly, they can act on the excitatory membrane receptor to stimulate PI turnover and the subsequent cascade of events leading to Ca^{2+} mobilization and uterine contraction. Secondly, the excitatory prostaglandins ($PGF_{2\alpha}$ PGE_2) generated in the myometrial cell following the release of arachidonic acid can mobilize more Ca^{2+} from the sarcoplasmic reticulum (7) and increases cell-to-cell coupling by the formation of gap junctions (11). Prostaglandins are highly diffusible, and may diffuse through the cell membrane to act on other cells, thus enhancing cell-to-cell coupling. These secondary actions

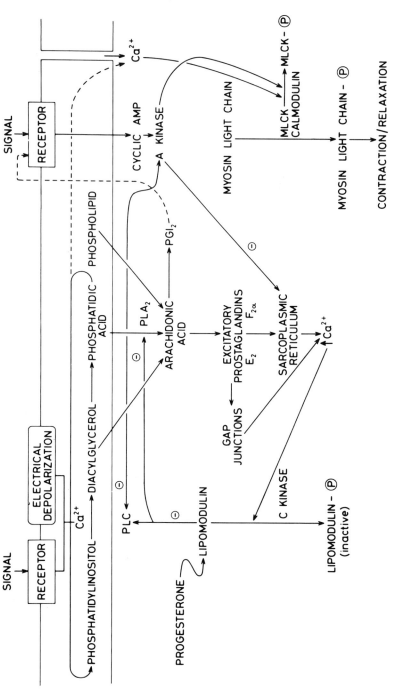

Figure 3. The proposed mechanism for progesterone-induced lipomodulin control of myometrial EMG activity. See text for a complete description.

would act to amplify the initial signal and increase the contractile force by increasing the number of active cells and by increasing the force generated by each cell. Finally, the model proposes the generation of PGI_2 which acts on the inhibitory membrane receptor to stimulate cyclic AMP production and muscle relaxation. Thus, PGs may play an intimate role in both myometrial contraction and relaxation. One might also predict that inhibition of PG synthesis may also interfere with muscle relaxation.

From the above discussion we might expect that the inhibition of PG synthesis (at the cyclooxygenase level) would prevent the amplification effect of PGs without interfering with their effect on the contractile response. Furthermore, one would expect a contractile response to oxytocin in the presence of cyclooxygenase blockers, but the response would be impeded because of the lack of amplification to the signal normally provided by PGs. This is supported by the observation of Windmoller *et al.* (35), who showed that the response of estrogen-treated ovine uterus to oxytocin was sustained in the presence of MFA, a PG synthetase inhibitor (35, see Fig. 7). Mitchell and Flint (24) administered MFA to ewes to prevent dexamethasone-induced delivery. MFA did not effect the parturition-associated changes in the concentration of progesterone and estrogen in the maternal plasma. The data obtained by Mitchell and Flint (24) from ewes treated with dexamethasone and MFA, is of particular interest because the contractures are unusually frequent (5/h). There are pressure spikes within the bursts suggesting desynchronous uterine activity resulting from poor propagation. Following removal of the MFA, classical labour-associated uterine contractions appeared rapidly over the next hour. It would seem that despite the low progesterone concentration, the propagation of impulses is impaired and that PGs may play a vital role in facilitating cell-to-cell coupling since the removal of the block on PG synthetase causes a rapid change in the contractile pattern.

Recent *in vitro* studies have shown that the contractile force generated per action potential during labour was approximately 15 times that recorded from tissues obtained from ewes prior to day 60 of pregnancy (29,34). The increase in the contractile force may have resulted from an increase in the total number of cells active (an expression of cell-to-cell coupling) or possibly from an increase in force generated by each cell. In these experiments (29), the space constant (λ) (an index of current spread between cells) increased during the latter part of pregnancy but showed a further increase during labour, the increase could result from an increase in the membrane resistance (Rm) of the muscle cells or an increase in cell-to-cell coupling or both. An increase in cell-to-cell coupling may be the physiological correlate of the increase in the number of gap junctions reported in sheep myometrium at term (11). The membrane time constant (τ_m) was unchanged during pregnancy but increased markedly during labour (29,34). The increase τ_m during labour was considered to be due to an increase in membrane resistance (Rm) and such a change may result from the altered lipid pattern in the cell membrane associated with the marked phospholipid turnover which results in the major PG release at that time.

Referring back to the data of Mitchell and Flint (24), it would appear that despite PG synthesis being blocked, there is an increase in the frequency of the nonlabour type contraction. In this animal, with high estrogen, low progesterone levels, we might expect an increase population of oxytocin receptors. The increased frequency of the contractures may be associated with the action of oxytocin on an estrogen-dominated uterus. Sigger (personal communication) has shown that the systemic administration of oxytocin can induce a nonlabour type contraction (contracture). Following removal of the MFA, classical labour-associated uterine contractions appear rapidly over the next hour or so (24, see Fig. 1). It would seem that despite the low progesterone concentration, the propagation of impulses is impaired which is consistent with our thesis that PGs play a vital role in facilitating cell-to-cell coupling possibly by means of increasing gap junctions, increasing propagation in the myometrium and increasing the number of active cells. $PGF_{2\alpha}$ and PGE_2 have been shown to inhibit Ca^{2+} uptake by the sarcoplasmic reticulum vesicles $in\ vitro$ (7) and the increased PG concentrations in the myometrial cell would be expected to increase intracellular Ca^{2+} and increase the force of contraction in individual cells; inhibition of PG synthesis would interfere with these actions which would help to explain the contracture type pattern. The pattern of uterine activity seen under MFA treatment in the pregnant ewe (24) closely resembles that observed in the nonpregnant, estradiol plus MFA treated ewe (22, see Fig. 5) and that observed during pregnancy in the ewe (13), all of which we feel may be explained by low myometrial PG synthesis. Earlier it was proposed that PGI_2, through the generation of cyclic AMP, may stimulate relaxation of the myometrium. We might anticipate therefore, that inhibition of PG synthesis may interfere with this process. The contracture type pattern may therefore result in part from interference with the normal relaxation mechanisms.

It is of considerable interest that Parkington (29,34) has found that the uterus obtained from ewes in early labour is quiescent. She found the tissue obtained from most ewes in labour were not active spontaneously (7 out of 9), however single action potentials and contractions could be evoked by electrical stimulation of these muscle pieces. It has been suggested that the major prostaglandins produced by the myometrium at that time is PGI_2 which is known to inhibit estrogen-induced uterine activity in overiectomized ewes whilst still leaving myometrial responsive to oxytocin and $PGF_{2\alpha}$ (21). Furthermore, PGI_2 has been shown to increase in amniotic fluid and fetal and maternal plasma in the 24 h preceding parturition (25). As mentioned earlier, the intrinsic changes of the electrical properties of the myometrium at that time (increase in membrane resistance, increasing number of gap junctions) are likely to improve the propagation of impulses through the tissue and to increase the number of cells activated by each period of electrical activity, thereby increasing the force generated. These changes may well be mediated by the increased PG production of the myometrium at that time since they don't occur when PG synthesis is inhibited (24). During labour, when oxytocin and exogenous PGs provide maximal stimulation and contractions become more frequent, the large amounts of endogenous PGI_2 produced would stimulate the rapid accumulation of cyclic AMP which would phosphorylate MLCK and relax the myometrium in the face of still high levels of Ca^{2+}, thus allowing the uterus to respond again quickly to a further stimulus.

Estrogens

Estrogens increase uterine activity (22,30,31). Administration of estradiol-17β to nonpregnant ewes resulted in a cyclical pattern of uterine activity; periods of high activity alternating with periods of low activity or quiescence (2–3 h) (22). Vena cava levels of PGFM were significantly elevated during periods of high activity compared with low activity periods. The administration of MFA to these estrogen-treated animals not only abolished the periods of high activity and the periods of low activity or quiescence but also produced a pattern of activity in which short (3–5 min) bursts of IUP and associated EMG activity occurred with a periodicity of between 5 and 40 min. This pattern strongly resembles that seen during pregnancy in the sheep (13,26) and in the MFA-treated pregnant animals (24). As mentioned earlier, this pattern of activity may be associated with low levels of PG synthesis, removal of the inhibition resulting in a normal labour-associated (contracture) pattern of uterine activity. In pregnancy, the contracture type pattern is first seen at a time when placental estrogen output is rising (50–60 days gestation) (32). Windmoller et al. (35) have suggested that this pattern of uterine activity is associated with high estrogen levels presumably when PG synthesis is low. This suggests, that in the pregnant sheep, this pattern of activity is due to increased myometrial levels of estrogen in the presence of high levels of progesterone which inhibits endogenous myometrial PG synthesis and make it less responsive to exogenous PGs and oxytocin. The withdrawal of the progesterone block allows a reversal of the inhibition permitting the labour-associated contractions to emerge.

Earlier work suggested that estrogens may increase "PG synthetase" (cyclooxygenase) activity and this may certainly account for the high level of PG synthesis in these tissues. Furthermore, estrogens may increase the activity of phospholipase in the cell thus increasing the overall reactivity of the cell to contractile response signals, in addition to increasing the level of PG synthesis. This action of estrogen would therefore counteract the putative inhibitory role of progesterone on the phospholipases. A number of studies have shown that it is not the absolute concentration of progesterone or estrogen, but ratio of these hormones that determines the effect on uterine activity. I propose that the level of phospholipase activity in the myometrial cell may be determined by the relative activity of these two steroid hormones.

Concluding Remarks

A model of the hormonal regulation of myometrial activity and specifically, the involvement of prostaglandins in the contractile-response pathway has been described in this presentation. The model is comprised of 4 interrelated processes: (i) the interaction of a signal (e.g. oxytocin, $PGF_{2\alpha}$) with a myometrial cell membrane receptor or electrical depolarization of the membrane; (ii) calcium-stimulated phosphatidyl inositol turnover within the membrane and the release of arachidonic acid; (iii) the synthesis of PGE_2 and $PGF_{2\alpha}$, which results in an increase in intracellular calcium concentration and cell-to-cell coupling;

(iv) calcium-dependent phosphorylation of myosin light chain and muscle contraction.

Relaxation of myometrium is achieved by a cyclic AMP-dependent process. The endogenous arachidonic acid released during contraction may be metabolized to PGI_2 which stimulates receptor-linked cyclic AMP production. Cyclic AMP activates A-kinase which catalyses the phosphorylation of MLCK and PLC, inhibiting their activity. The sequestration of calcium into sarcoplasmic reticulum and the extrusion of calcium from the cell are also stimulated by cyclic AMP. Under the condition characteristic of mid-pregnancy, i.e. high progesterone and low circulating contractions of estrogen and prostaglandin, lipomodulin synthesis is induced and suppresses phospholipase activity (both PLC and PLA_2). Signal transmission across the membrane is inhibited and the cell is unresponsive to oxytocin and endogenous PGs. At labour, progesterone concentrations decrease resulting in decreased lipomodulin production.

The myometrium is therefore released from the inhibitory influence of progesterone-induced lipomodulin. Concomitantly, increased estrogen concentrations increase the number of oxytocin and PG receptors on the myometrial cell membrane, may increase phospholipase and cyclooxygenase activity in the myometrium, and enhance the release of oxytocin from the posterior pituitary. This would increase the number of oxytocin receptors and at least in the latter phase of delivery increase the circulating levels of oxytocin. The myometrium would also be exposed to prostaglandins derived from the endometrium directly and from the placenta via the lungs (although a majority of the $PGF_{2\alpha}$ is metabolized in the lungs, a significant proportion would reach the myometrium via the arterial circulation).

These changes in the endocrine milieu of the myometrium at labour would act to amplify the contractile-response to signal, and thus cause the high activity pattern observed at labour.

Acknowledgements

I acknowledge the generous support of Dr Greg Rice and Ms Cathy Leach Harper in the preparation of this manuscript and for providing such stimulating discussion. I also wish to thank my secretary, Mrs Alison Woods, for her untiring help and the typing of the manuscript and Mrs Jill Poynton for the preparation of the figures.

References

1. Bassett, J. M., Oxborrow, T. J., Smith, I. D. and Thorburn, G. D. (1969). *J. Endocrinol.* **45**, 449–457.
2. Bell, R. L., Kennerly, D. A., Stanford, N. and Majerus, P. W. (1979). *Proc. Nat. Acad. Sci. USA* **76**, 3238–3241.
3. Billah, M. M., Lapetina, E. G. and Cuatrecasas, P. (1980). *J. Biol. Chem.* **255**, 10227–10231.

4. Billah, M. M., Lapetina, E. G. and Cuatrecasas, P. (1981). *J. Biol. Chem.* **256**, 5399–5403.
5. Blackwell, G. J., Carnuccio, R., Di Rossa, M., Flower, R. J., Langham, C. S. J., Parente, L., Persico, P., Russell-Smith, N. C. and Stone, D. (1982). *Br. J. Pharmacol.* **76**, 185–194.
6. Bleasdale, J. E., Okazaki, T., Sagawa, N., Di Renzo, G. C., Okita, J. R., MacDonald, P. C. and Johnston, J. M. (1983). *In:* "Initiation of Parturition: Prevention of Prematurity" Report, 4th Ross Conf. Obstetric Res. pp. 129–137.
7. Carsten, M. E. and Miller, J. D. (1979). *Proc. 26th Ann. Meet. Soc. Gynecol. Invest.* Abstr. 142.
8. Daniel, J. L., Holmsen, H. and Adelstein, R. S. (1977). *Thrombos. Haemostas.* **38**, 984.
9. de Lanerolle, P., Nishikawa, M., Yost, D. A. and Adelstein, R. S. (1984). *Science* **223**, 1415–1417.
10. Flower, R. F. and Blackwell, G. J. (1979). *Nature* **278**, 456.
11. Garfield, R. E., Rabideau, S., Challis, J. R. G. and Daniel, E. E. (1979). *Biol. Reprod.* **21**, 999–1007.
12. Gorman, R. R., Wierenga, W. and Miller, O. V. (1979). *Biochem. Biophys. Acta* **572**, 95–104.
13. Harding, R., Poore, E. R., Bailey, A., Thorburn, G. D., Jansen, C. A. M., Nathanielsz, P. W. (1982). *Am. J. Obstet. Gynecol.* **142**, 448–457.
14. Herrman, W., Wyss, R., Riondel, A., Philibert, D., Teutsch, G., Sakiz, E. and Baulieu, E.-E. (1982). *C. R. Acad. Sci. Paris.* **294**, 933–938.
15. Hirata, F. (1981). *J. Biol. Chem.* **256**, 7730–7733.
16. Jenkin, G. and Thorburn, G. D. (1984). *Can. J. Physiol. Pharmacol.* (in press).
17. Kaibuchi, K., Takai, Y., Ogawa, Y., Kimura, S., Nishizuka, Y., Nakamura, T., Tomomura, A. and Ichihara, A. (1982). *Biochem. Biophys. Res. Commun.* **104**, 105–112.
18. Käser-Glauzman, R., Jakabova, M., George, J. N. and Luscher, E. F. (1977). *Biochem. Biophys. Acta* **446**, 429–440.
19. Knight, D. E., and Scrutton, M. L. (1984). *Nature* **304**, 66–68.
20. Laychock, S. G. and Putney, J. W. (1982). *In:* "Cellular Regulation of Secretion and Release", (Conn, P. M., ed.) pp. 53–105. Academic Press, New York and London.
21. Lye, S. J. and Challis, J. R. G. (1982). *J. Reprod. Fertil.* **66**, 311–315.
22. Lye, S. J., Sprague, C. L. and Challis, J. R. G. (1983). *Can. J. Physiol. Pharmacol.* **61**.
23. Michell, R. H. (1975). *Biochem. Biophys. Acta* **415**, 81–147.
24. Mitchell, M. D. and Flint, A. P. F. (1978). *J. Endocrinol.* **76**, 101–109.
25. Mitchell, M. D., Anderson, A. B. M., Brunt, J. D., Clover, L., Ellwood, D. A., Robinson, J. S. and Turnbull, A. C. (1979). *J. Endocrinol.* **83**, 141–148.
26. Nathanielsz, P. W., Bailey, A., Poore, E. R., Thorburn, G. D. and Harding, R. (1980). *Am. J. Obstet. Gynecol.* **138**, 653–659.
27. Nishizuka, Y. (1983). *In:* "Endocrinology", (Shizume, K., Imura, H. and Shimizu, N., eds) pp. 15–24. Excerpta Medica, Amsterdam.
28. Nishizuka, Y. (1983). *Phil. Trans. R. Soc. London* B **302**, 101–112.
29. Parkington, H. C. (1984). *J. Reprod. Fertil.* (in press).
30. Porter, D. G. and Lye, S. J. (1983). *J. Reprod. Fertil.* **67**, 227–234.
31. Rawlings, N. C. and Ward, W. R. (1978). *J. Reprod. Fertil.* **54**, 1–8.
32. Sigger, J. N., Harding, R. and Bailey, A. (1984). *Aust. J. Biol. Sci.* (in press).
33. Thorburn, G. D. and Challis, J. R. G. (1979). *Physiol. Rev.* **59**, 863–918.
34. Thorburn, G. D., Harding, R., Jenkin, G., Parkington, H. and Sigger, J. N. (1984). *J. Develop. Physiol.* **6**, 31–43.
35. Windmoller, R., Lye, S. J. and Challis, J. R. G. (1983). *Can. J. Physiol. Pharmacol.* **61**, 722–728.

Different Patterns of Reflex Heart Rate Control during Stress in Fetal and Neonatal Lambs: Implications for Ventricular Function

Adrian M. Walker, J. P. Cannata,
B. C. Ritchie and J. E. Maloney

Monash University Centre for Early Human Development,
Queen Victoria Medical Centre, Melbourne, Australia

Introduction

Analysis of heart rate control during acute stresses of hypoxaemia or hypotension reveals different patterns of autonomic nervous system activation before and after birth (1,2). In fetal lambs, both parasympathetic and sympathetic tone (quantified using selective autonomic blockade) increase in an antagonistic pattern, preventing tachycardia. In neonatal lambs, vagal tone is withdrawn, supplementing increased sympathetic tone in a synergistic pattern, and contributing to tachycardia. Simultaneous activation of the opposing autonomic pathways appears to be a characteristic fetal response to stress, being found also in acute fetal haemorrhage (3) and in the chronically growth retarded and hypoxaemia fetal lamb (4). This study questions how the sympathetic and parasympathetic components of these nervous patterns influence ventricular function during hypoxaemia.

Methods

Using methods which we have described previously (1,2) fetal and newborn lambs were chronically implanted with carotid arterial and jugular venous catheters and ECG electrodes, using sterile surgical procedures performed using general anaesthesia (halothane and oxygen). Calibrated electromagnetic flow transducers (Micron, 5–10 mm lumen diameter) were placed around the right ventricular

The Physiological Development of the Fetus and Newborn
ISBN 0 12 389080 2

Copyright © 1985 by Academic Press, London.
All rights of reproduction in any form reserved.

outflow tract for measurement of right ventricular output (RVO) or around the
aortic root for measurement of left ventricular output minus coronary flow (LVO).
Four fetal lambs were employed for measurement of RVO; 12 fetal lambs and
9 newborn lambs entered the study of LVO.

Studies began after 2 or more days postoperative recovery, spanning 110–143
days gestation and 5–28 days after birth. Ewes stood quietly in a cage; newborn
lambs were quietly awake, supported in a sling which allowed their feet to contact
the cage floor. We followed a basic protocol composed of three 20-min periods;
a control period in which the ewe or lamb breathed air in a vented polythene
head bag; an hypoxic period in which the O_2 concentration in the head bag was
reduced to approximately 10%; and a recovery period in which the animal was
returned to breathing air.

Continuous recordings of blood flow, blood pressure, EKG and heart rate were
made throughout (Hewlett Packard 7758A chart recorder, Tandberg 100 magnetic
tape recorder). Pre-ejection period (PEP) was measured from the tape recordings
as the interval between the QRS complex of the ECG and the beginning of systolic
ejection indicated by the upstroke of the aortic flow signal. Arterial blood samples
(0.4 ml) were taken in each period for measurement of PO_2, PCO_2 and pH
(Radiometer E 5021a). Experiments were conducted under three conditions
(a) no drug (b) parasympathetic muscarinic blockade (atropine 0.2–0.3 mg/kg) and
(c) sympathetic (β-adrenergic) blockade (propanolol 1 mg/kg).

Results

A moderate level of fetal and neonatal hypoxaemia was achieved during
10% O_2 breathing. Values (mean ± SEM) of fetal arterial PO_2, PCO_2 and pH were
22 ± 1 torr, 48 ± 1 torr and 7.34 ± 0.01 units during airbreathing, and 14 ± 1 torr,
48 ± 1 torr and 7.33 ± 0.01 units respectively during hypoxia; in newborn lambs,
these values were 91 ± 2 torr, 39 ± 1 torr and 7.38 ± 0.01 units during airbreathing,
and 39 ± 1 torr, 37 ± 1 torr and 7.41 ± 0.02 units during hypoxia.

Table 1. Effects of hypoxia on LVO (% change) and
HR (% change) of fetal and neonatal lambs before
and after propranolol injection

	No drug	Propranolol
Fetal lambs		
HR	± 4	-14 ± 3**
LVO	-7 ± 3*	-15 ± 3**
n	15	14
Neonatal lambs		
HR	50 ± 10**	10 ± 6
LVO	22 ± 4**	5 ± 3
n	11	5

n = no. of experiments; *indicates $P < 0.05$; **$P < 0.01$

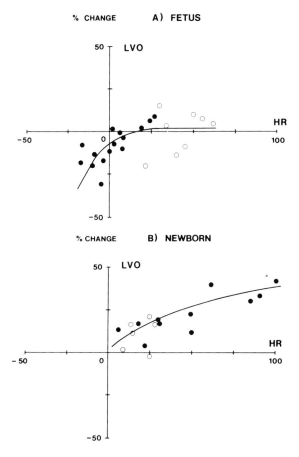

Figure 1. Illustrates the relationship between changes of aortic flow (LVO) and heart rate (HR) during hypoxaemia in control experiments (●) and in the presence of parasympathetic blockade with atropine (○). A. In fetal lambs, LVO is sensitive to falls of HR in the control experiments (●) but is not increased during unopposed tachycardia in the presence of atropine (○). B. In neonatal lambs LVO is augmented by tachycardia in both conditions.

Fetal lambs showed no significant change of HR and a small depression of LVO (average -7%) in response to hypoxaemia, after propranolol injection both HR and LVO were significantly reduced (Table 1). Neonatal lambs responded to hypoxaemia with increased HR and LVO; these changes were prevented by β-adrenergic blockade. PEP in fetal lambs fell during hypoxaemia (from 49 ± 2 to 44 ± 1 ms) consistent with inotropic stimulation, but no reduction occurred after propranolol injection. Newborn lambs also showed shortening of PEP during hypoxaemia (from 47 ± 1 to 38 ± 1 ms); after β-blockade this response was less (55 ± 2 and 50 ± 3 ms respectively).

RVO in fetal lambs increased by $9 \pm 4\%$ ($n = 10$) during hypoxaemia; heart rate was not changed. After atropine the increase of RVO was similar $12 \pm 3\%$ ($n = 10$), and heart rate now increased significantly by $34 \pm 8\%$ ($n = 10$). Similarly, LVO in fetal lambs did not increase during hypoxaemia in the control experiments, nor in the presence of atropine when large increases of heart rate occurred (Fig. 1A). This was in contrast to neonatal lambs in which tachycardia was effective in augmenting LVO in hypoxaemia both in the unblocked state and in the presence of vagal blockade (Fig. 1B).

Discussion

These experiments provided evidence of increased activity in both divisions of the autonomic nervous system, each with the potential to change significantly fetal heart rate. However, because increased sympathetic activity was matched by increasing vagal inhibition of the heart, fetal heart rate was not accelerated.

There have been many studies of fetal combined ventricular output, which is unchanged or decreased in mild hypoxaemia (5,6). However in the fetal circulation right and left ventricular outputs can change independently and there are only limited data relating to changes in the respective ventricular outputs in hypoxaemia (7). Our data show that fetal LVO is not increased during hypoxaemia; fetal RVO is slightly increased by approximately 10%.

The important role of sympathetic activation during hypoxaemia in supporting ventricular output in the fetus, and augmenting it in the neonate is illustrated by selective blockade. After the application of β-adrenergic blockade in the fetus, unopposed parasympathetic activation during hypoxaemia resulted in falls of HR and LVO, whereas these were unchanged in the control response. In the neonate, significant increases of heart rate and cardiac output occurring in hypoxaemia were reduced by propranolol injection. Shortening of the PEP consistent with increased inotropy during hypoxaemia was abolished by propranolol injection in the fetus and significantly reduced in the neonate, signifying an important role of the β-adrenergic system in augmenting LV inotropy before and after birth.

As spontaneous HR changes are positively correlated with ventricular output changes in the normoxaemic fetus (8), the ineffectiveness of tachycardia in augmenting fetal cardiac output in hypoxaemia conditions probably reflects an imbalance between myocardial O_2 supply and demand. Fetal myocardial metabolism remains aerobic during moderate hypoxaemia, and myocardial oxygen consumption is maintained by increased myocardial blood flow (9). If the fetus is unstable to increase myocardial blood sufficiently to meet extra oxygen requirements associated with tachycardia (10), oxygen availability may impose a limit on ventricular performance, even in mild hypoxaemic or hypotensive stress. If so, parasympathetic activation would provide an important benefit to the fetus by minimizing myocardial oxygen consumption for a given level of cardiac output.

References

1. Walker, A. M., Cannata, J. P., Dowling, M. H., Ritchie, B. C. and Maloney, J. E. (1983). *Biol. Neonate* **35**, 1980208.
2. Walker, A. M., Cannata, J. P., Ritchie, B. C. and Maloney, J. E. (1983). *Biol. Neonate* **44**, 358–365.
3. MacDonald, A. A., Rose, J., Heymann, M. A. and Rudolph, A. M. (1980). *Am. J. Physiol.* **239**, H789–H793.
4. Llanos, A. J., Green, J. R., Creasy, R. K. and Rudolph, A. M. (1980). *Am. J. Obstet. Gynecol.* **136**, 808–813.
5. Cohn, H. E., Sacks, E. J., Heymann, M. A. and Rudolph, A. M. (1974). *Am. J. Obstet. Gynecol.* **120**, 817–824.
6. Reuss, M. L., Parer, J. T., Harris, J. L. and Krueger, T. R. (1982). *Am. J. Obstet. Gynecol.* **142**, 410.
7. Green, J. R., Creasy, R. K., Heymann, M. A. and Rudolph, A. M. (1977). *Gynecol. Invest.* **8**, 36.
8. Rudolph, A. M. and Heymann, M. A. (1974). *Am. J. Obstet. Gynecol.* **124**, 183.
9. Fisher, D. J., Heymann, M. A. and Rudolph, A. M. (1982). *Am. J. Physiol. (Heart Circ. Physiol.* **11***)* H657–H661.
10. Cohn, H. E., Piasecki, G. J. and Jackson, B. T. (1980). *Am. J. Obstet. Gynecol.* **138**, 1190.

Distribution of Cardiac Output in the Fetal Pig During Late Gestation

Alastair A. Macdonald, Michael A. Heymann,
Anibal J. Llanos, Erkki Pesonen and Abraham M. Rudolph

Cardiovascular Research Institute, Departments of Pediatrics and Obstetrics
Gynecology and Reproductive Sciences, University of California,
San Francisco, USA; Department of Anatomy, Royal (Dick) School of
Veterinary Studies, University of Edinburgh, Scotland

Introduction

Fetal development varies between species with respect to the time scale involved and the amount of growth required before birth (*cf.* rat, guinea-pig, polar bear). Differences may therefore be expected in a number of aspects of the physiology of the fetus. Whereas many studies have examined the cardiovascular physiology of the sheep fetus (1,2), relatively little is known about the same system in other species. We report observations made on the fetal pig.

Materials and Methods

Physiological studies were made on 45 fetuses aged between 85 and 113 days gestation (term = 114 ± 1 day) of whom 38 fetuses were from 11 sows of mixed Duroc, Hampshire, Chester White breeding, and 7 fetuses were from 3 Hormel miniature swine. The sows were sedated (15 mg Valium® i.m.: diazepam). Anaesthesia was induced with thiopental sodium (i.v.) and deep surgical anaesthesia maintained by a halothane (Fluothane®), nitrous oxide, oxygen mixture. We inserted polyvinyl catheters (ID 0.77 mm OD 1.22 mm) via the saphenous artery and medial saphenous vein of the sow until the tips lay in the descending aorta and caudal vena cava respectively. We operated on those fetuses lying adjacent to a vertical 15 cm incission made through the maternal flank. A 15-20 mm incission was made in the uterus and placenta on the antimesometrial border of the cornua. Polyvinyl catheters (ID 0.28 mm OD 0.61 mm or ID

The Physiological Development of the Fetus and Newborn
ISBN 0 12 389080 2

Copyright © 1985 by Academic Press, London.
All rights of reproduction in any form reserved.

0.38 mm OD 0.89 mm or ID 0.76 mm OD 1.22 mm) were inserted via an internal carotid artery and external jugular vein of each fetus until the tips lay in the brachiocephalic artery and cranial vena cava respectively. A second incission was made in the uterus and placenta of 12 fetuses and one or both hind limbs exteriorized. Polyvinyl catheters (ID 0.28 mm OD 0.61 mm or ID 0.38 mm OD 0.89 mm) were introduced via a femoral artery and vein until the tips lay in the descending aorta and caudal vena cava respectively. A polyvinyl catheter (ID 1.27 mm OD 2.29 mm) was placed in the amniotic cavity and the incisions sutured. The catheters were exteriorized on the left flank. We injected 1 000 000 IU of penicillin G and 500 mg of kanamycin into the maternal venous catheter and one quarter of these amounts into the amniotic catheters.

The fetuses were studied 24–36 h after surgery. We measured fetal arterial blood and amniotic pressures with Statham P23Db pressure transducers and report arterial pressures with respect to an amniotic fluid pressure of zero. The cardiotachometer was triggered by the fetal arterial pressure signal. We drew 0.3–0.5 ml samples of arterial blood into dry heparinized glass syringes. The haematocrit was measured with a microcentrifuge; pH, PO_2 and PCO_2 were measured with a Radiometer blood gas analyser and the appropriate electrodes.

Organ blood flow and the distribution of combined ventricular output were measured in 7 fetuses aged between 97 and 113 days using the radionuclide-labelled microsphere technique (3,4). Care was taken to inject enough microspheres to ensure that more than 400 were trapped in the smaller organs. We injected 15 μm nuclide-labelled microspheres into the cranial and caudal venae cavae of the fetus and drew 3.5–10 ml reference blood samples over 1.25–1.75 min from the descending aorta and carotid artery. Upper body blood flow was measured in 4 miniature pig fetuses. A volume of blood equivalent to that removed as reference samples was returned to the fetus.

We applied a perturbation to the circulation of 12 fetuses by withdrawing between 7 and 20 ml from the arterial catheter. In 4 of these instances blood flow was measured before and after blood loss.

Studies were terminated 36 h after surgery, the sow killed with an overdose of sodium pentobarbital and uterus and contents removed. Fetal organs and tissues were incinerated and counted for radioactivity in a 512-channel pulse height analyser (Searle Analytic). Fetal blood flow to the tissue vascular beds was calculated with the aid of an IBM 370 computer, using the counts in the tissue and reference samples, and the withdrawal rate of the reference sample (4). As a check on adequate mixing of the microspheres, right and left kidneys and hemisections of the cerebrum were counted separately. Observations are presented as means $\pm$ SEM. We assessed the significance of differences between groups of observations by analysis of variance and paired t test. Anatomical studies were made on the hearts of 25 pig fetuses of mixed Landrace, Large White breeding aged between 85 and 113 days gestation. The tissues were fixed in buffered formalin or glutaraldehyde, and studied as 10–15 μm sections by light microscopy or as dissected, sputter-coated specimens by means of a scanning electron microscope (Phillips 505).

Results

Resting maternal pH, PO_2, PCO_2 and haematocrit values were 7.50 ± 0.01, 97 ± 5 mmHg 34 ± 2 mmHg and 36 ± 2 respectively ($n = 8$). Equivalent fetal values were 7.47 ± 0.01, 23 ± 1 mmHg, 40 ± 1 mmHg and 29 ± 1 ($n = 45$). Resting fetal mean arterial pressure increased from 37 ± 1 mmHg at 85 days to 56 ± 1 mmHg at 113 days. Conversely heart rate slowed with advancing gestation from 214 ± 5 beats/min at 85 days to 171 ± 4 beats/min at 113 days. Haemorrhage produced a decrease in blood pressure from 47 ± 3 to 36 ± 3 mmHg and an increase in heart rate from 206 ± 5 to 228 ± 8 beats/min ($n = 12$; $P < 0.01$).

Combined ventricular output increased from 320 ml/min at 97 days to 1015 ml/min at 113 days, closely paralleling the increase in weight of the products of conception: average combined ventricular output and stroke volume were 615 ± 62 ml/min/kg and 3.2 ± 0.4 ml/kg of fetal body weight respectively. The placenta received between 22% and 33% of combined ventricular output (mean $= 28 \pm 2$%) the mean umbilical arterial blood flow being 168 ± 16 ml/min/kg fetal body weight. The skeletal muscle, bone and skin of the fetus was supplied with between 20% and 34% (mean $= 25 \pm 2$%) of combined ventricular output. The proportion of combined ventricular output to the brain ranged between 3.5% and 6% (mean $= 4.7 \pm 0.4$%), the left and right cerebral hemispheres receiving blood flows of respectively 93 ± 19 and 96 ± 20 ml/min/100 g of cerebral tissue. Blood flow to the left and right kidneys was 182 ± 20 and 173 ± 20 ml/min/100 g of kidney weight respectively. Blood flow to the myocardium represented between 1.9% and 5.4% of combined ventricular output (mean $= 4.2 \pm 0.5$%), and varied between 127 and 401 ml/min/100 g. Blood flow to the liver via the hepatic arteries ranged between 11 and 73 ml/min/100 g, whereas the stomach received between 36 and 82 ml/min/100 g, and the small and large intestine received between 49 and 123 ml/min/100 g. Blood flow to the pancreas and spleen ranged from 44 to 195 ml/min/100 g and 27 to 928 ml/min/100 g respectively, and blood supply to the thyroid and thymus ranged from 40 to 430 ml/min/100 g and from 26 to 82 ml/min/100 g respectively. The proportion of combined ventricular output received by the lungs increased from 16% at 97 days to 26% just prior to birth. Blood flow values to tissues in the upper bodies of miniature pigs were comparable.

Haemorrhage of approximately 8% fetal blood volume reduced fetal blood pressure and increased heart rate; cardiac output increased in 3 of 4 fetuses. An increased proportion of combined ventricular output was supplied to the placenta ($\Delta = 7 \pm 1$%), heart ($\Delta = 1.8 \pm 0.7$%), cerebellum and brain stem ($\Delta = 0.21 \pm 0.07$%), intestines ($\Delta = 0.75 \pm 0.07$%), spleen ($\Delta = 0.73 \pm 0.16$%) and thyroid ($\Delta = 0.07 \pm 0.02$%). Blood flow to the lungs decreased by 13 ± 5%. The myocardium received less than 2% of cranial vena cava blood flow; between 2% and 15% of caudal vena cava blood flows through the foramen ovale to supply the myocardium. Increased blood flow to the fetal lung reduced the myocardial supply from the cranial vena cava to zero, whereas between 1% and 5% of caudal vena cava blood supply was maintained.

A wedge of right atrial tissue with a convex leading edge is so arranged as to divide the blood flow from the caudal vena cava into two streams, one of which passes through the foramen ovale and is funnelled into the left atrium. Blood flow from the coronary sinus is discharged into the lumen of the right atrium in close proximity to, but beyond the division of the caudal vena cava flow. The opening of the cranial vena cava lies opposite the caudal vena cava and coronary sinus openings. Pulmonary veins discharge into the left atrium close to the base of the funnelled foramen ovale flow.

Discussion

The similarity of blood flow measured in left and right kidneys, and in left and right cerebral hemispheres indicated that the radioactive microspheres had been evenly mixed in the blood stream. Combined ventricular output was slightly higher than in the near-term sheep fetus, and the proportion received by the placenta was lower than that in the sheep (2). Blood flow to the brain showed little sign of having been compromised by fetal surgery and was similar to that found in the neonatal piglet (5). The blood flow to the lung seemed to be sensitive to quite small changes in systemic blood volume and pressure. Further studies are required to confirm the suggested increase in blood flow and increased sensitivity seen towards term, however. The topography of the vascular inlets to the atria suggest mechanisms of blood flow direction that preempt much cranial vena cava flow from reaching the left atrium, particularly when pulmonary and/or coronary arterial blood flow and venous return are increased.

Acknowledgements

The excellent technical assistance of Christine Roman, Louise Wang, Colin MacFarlane, Bruce Payne, Derek Penman, Carl McWatters and Les Williams is gratefully acknowledged. Financial support was received from the Fulbright-Hays program (AAM) and Program Project Grant HL 06285 from the US Public Health Service.

References

1. Dawes, G. S. (1968). "Foetal and Neonatal Physiology". Year Book Medical Publishers, Chicago.
2. Heymann, M. A., Iwamoto, H. S. and Rudolph, A. M. (1981). *Ann. Rev. Physiol.* **43**, 371–383.
3. Rudolph, A. M. and Heymann, M. A. (1967). *Circulat. Res.* **21**, 163–184.
4. Heymann, M. A., Payne, B. D., Hoffmann, J. I. E. and Rudolph, A. M. (1977). *Prog. Cardiovasc. Dis.* **20**, 55–79.
5. Laptook, A. R., Stonestreet, B. S. and Oh, W. (1983). *Pediat. Res.* **17**, 77–80.

Dynamics of Fetal Organ Blood Flow Redistribution and Catecholamine Release during Acute Asphyxia

Arne Jensen, Wolfgang Künzel and Manfred Hohmann

Department of Obstetrics and Gynaecology,
University of Giessen, West Germany

Introduction

Hypoxia and asphyxia cause a redistribution of fetal organ blood flow in favour of the brain, heart and adrenal glands at the expense of almost every other organ (11,2,8,9). This circulatory centralization is caused by sympathetic reflex mechanisms which are partly mediated by peripheral arterial chemoreceptor activation (1,6,4) and are accompanied by a release of vasoactive substances into the fetal circulation (3,15,20,7,12,14,11). The skin blood flow is very sensitive to sympathetic stimulation, and it has been suggested from clinical (10) and experimental studies (18,13) that low transcutaneous PO_2 values during delivery may be caused by fetal peripheral vasoconstriction, indicating a circulatory centralization early during labour.

Since the dynamics of fetal blood flow changes during acute severe asphyxia have not yet been reported the present study was designed to investigate the process of centralization during arrest of uterine blood flow for 4 min.

Method

Nine unanaesthetized fetal lambs at a mean gestational age of 130 ± 2 days (term is at 147 days) were studied. Uterine blood flow was arrested for 4 min by a balloon occluder around the lower descending maternal aorta in 5 chronic and 4 acute experiments. Five fetuses died during the recovery period.

Catheters were inserted under maternal spinal (2 ml Tetracaine 1%, w/v) and fetal local (Xylocaine 1%, w/v) anaesthesia as previously described (13), using

The Physiological Development of the Fetus and Newborn
ISBN 0 12 389080 2
Copyright © 1985 by Academic Press, London.
All rights of reproduction in any form reserved.

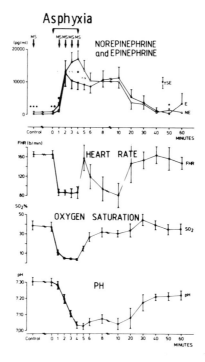

Figure 1. Changes during 4 min asphyxia (⊢————⊣, shaded) by arrest in uterine blood flow in 9 unanaesthetized fetal lambs at a mean gestational age of 130±2 days.

aseptic techniques. Reference samples were withdrawn from a carotid (catheter passed through a cranial thyroid artery to avoid occlusion) and femoral artery. Chronically instrumented lambs were allowed to recover for 3 days before the experiment, while acutely prepared lambs were studied *in utero* 2 h after the operation.

Blood flow measurements were made by injection of radioactively labelled microspheres (15 μ diameter) into the fetal inferior vena cava during a control period and after 1, 2, 3 and 4 min asphyxia (Fig. 1). The reference sample method (19) was modified in that multiple injections were made during asphyxia with continuous withdrawal of reference blood, simultaneously replaced by maternal blood. Thus, the methodological error due to the variance of 4 separate sampling procedures was reduced to a quarter and observations at intervals of 1 min were possible. Fetal heart rate and blood pressure, amniotic fluid pressure and maternal blood pressure were recorded on a polygraph (Hellige, West Germany). The fetal arterial pressures were corrected for amniotic fluid pressure. Blood samples were drawn from the femoral artery to measure blood gases, acid-base balance and catecholamine concentrations (Radioenzymatic assay (5), modified by Schömig and Dietz).

For statistical evaluation the Wilcoxon Rank Test was applied; the results are given as means ± SEM.

Results

Changes after 1 min asphyxia

Arrest of uterine blood flow caused an almost immediate fall in O_2 saturation and heart rate, with concomitant rises in norepinephrine and epinephrine concentrations (Fig. 1), but no significant changes in pH or arterial blood pressure were measured. There were significant falls in blood flows to the fetal scalp, lungs, kidneys, choroid plexus, liver, thyroid gland, body skin, pancreas, brown adipose tissue, thymus, skeletal muscles, stomach, gut and spleen between −54% and −99% of control values, not related to changes in catecholamine concentrations. The flow changes to the heart (+22%), adrenals (−24%), and brainstem (+1) were not significant. The concentrations of epinephrine and norepinephrine exerted a logarithmic ($P < 0.001$) and linear ($P < 0.01$) relation to the arterial O_2 saturation, respectively.

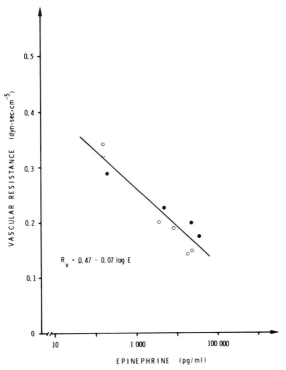

Figure 2. The relation between plasma concentrations of epinephrine and the vascular resistance in the brainstem after 2 min asphyxia in fetal lambs as in Fig. 1. $r = -0.93$; $P < 0.001$.

The blood flows to the heart ($P<0.01$), cerebrum ($P<0.05$) and midbrain ($P<0.01$) were linearly related to the O_2 saturation. There was also a linear relation between epinephrine concentrations and vascular resistance in the brainstem ($P<0.05$). The ratio between the hormones (NE?E) revealed a log-linear relation to the blood flows to the cerebrum ($P<0.05$) and the brainstem ($P<0.05$), but not to the adrenals. The brain blood flow was not dependent on changes in PCO_2, base excess, pH or blood pressure.

Changes after 2 and 3 min asphyxia

After 2 and 3 min asphyxia the O_2 saturation was between 4 and 5% and the pH steadily declined, accompanied by a progressive rise of blood pressure as well as norepinephrine concentrations, while the heart rate remained unchanged. Epinephrine concentrations increased exponentially during the first 2 min, well correlated (Fig. 2) with the vascular resistance in and flow ($P<0.05$) to the brainstem and cerebrum ($P<0.05$), and, unlike norepinephrine, failed to increase thereafter, resulting in a significant difference between both hormones at 4 min ($P<0.05$). The mean ratio between norepinephrine and epinephrine concentrations (NE/E) diminished from 11:1 at control to 1:1 at 2 min.

There were progressively increasing blood flows to the heart and brainstem, but cerebral blood flow was reduced, rendering the total brain flow unchanged throughout the asphyxial period (Fig. 3). The blood flow to the adrenals rose in animals that survived, whereas it decreased in animals which died. In most

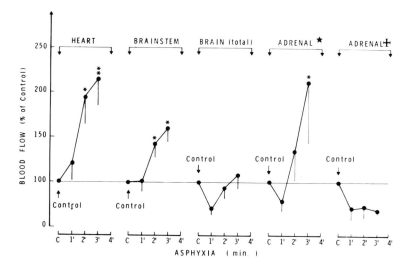

Figure 3. Blood flow changes during 3 min asphyxia in fetal lambs as in Fig. 1. Note, the slow increase in blood flow (i.e. after 2 min) to the heart, brainstem and to the adrenals of the surviving animals. The flow to the adrenals of subsequently deteriorating fetuses failed to increase at all. ↑ ±SEM, Wilcoxon rank test. * $P \le 0.05$. ** $P \le 0.01$. ★ Survivors ($n=4$). ✛ Nonsurvivors ($n=5$).

organs that were already poorly perfused after 1 min, vasoconstriction was continued or increased after 2 and 3 min, including the placenta, kidneys and scalp. However, in the liver and diaphragm (unlike the skeletal muscle) vasoconstriction was transient, blood flows increasing after 3 and 4 min, respectively.

Changes after 4 min asphyxia

There were no significant differences in organ blood flow during the first 3 min asphyxia between surviving animals and nonsurviving animals, except for a poorer skin perfusion ($P<0.01$) after 3 min in the latter group. After 4 min asphyxia, however, the blood flows to the cardiac ventricles, cerebrum, medulla, adrenals and skin were significantly reduced ($P<0.05$) in those fetuses that died, although the blood pressure was no different as compared with surviving animals, but the heart rate was lower ($P<0.05$).

Summary and Conclusions

1. Acute asphyxia in unanaesthetized fetal lambs caused a rapid vasoconstriction in many peripheral organs, suggesting neuronal reflex mechanisms. The blood flow increase to the heart, brainstem and adrenals (survivors) was delayed, suggesting blood borne mechanisms.
2. The blood flow to the brain during asphyxia was not correlated with changes in blood pressures, PCO_2, pH or base excess. The vascular resistance in the brainstem after 2 min was closely related to epinephrine concentrations, but not to the arterial O_2 saturation.
3. Fetal survival seems to be related to blood flow to the adrenals. Fetal death was preceded by a sudden increase in vascular resistance in the heart, cerebrum, brainstem and adrenals.
4. The immediate and sustained vasoconstriction of the choroid plexus during asphyxia is suggested to be reflex in nature and may lead to hypoxic damage of the endothelium with subsequent plexus and intraventricular haemorrhages.
5. The high sensitivity of the cutaneous perfusion to asphyxia and the fact that the skin blood flow as well as the adrenal blood flow and the decreased fetal heart rate were the only variables predicting subsequent fetal deterioration supports recent demands (11,12,10,14) for introduction of skin blood flow measurements into human fetal monitoring during high risk deliveries.

Acknowledgements

The authors would like to thank Mrs S. Jelinek and Mrs Achenbach for their technical assistance and Dr R. Dietz and Dr A. Schömig for the catecholamine analysis. We are further gratefully indebted to Dr B. Winkler, Professor Dr W. Schaper, Max Planck Institute for Heart Research, Bad Nauheim (FRG), Professor Dr Sattler and Dr Lewe, Zentrale Abteilung, Strahlenzentrum, Giessen University (FRG) for supporting our blood flow measurements. Arne Jensen's work was supported by Deutsche Forschungsgemeinschaft, Je 108/2-2.

References

1. Bernthal, T. G. and Schwind, F. J. (1945). *Am. J. Physiol.* **143**, 361–372.
2. Cohn, H. E., Sacks, E. I., Heymann, M. A. and Rudolph, A. M. (1974). *Am. J. Obstet. Gynecol.* **120**, 817–824.
3. Comline, R. S. and Silver, M. R. (1965). *J. Physiol.* **178**, 211–238.
4. Critchley, I. A. I. H., Ellis, P. and Ungar, A. (1980). *J. Physiol.* **298**, 71–78.
5. Da Prada, M. and Zürcher, G. (1976). *Life Sci.* **19**, 1161–1174.
6. Dawes, G. S., Lewis, B. V., Milligan, I. E., Roach, M. R. and Talner, N. S. (1968). *J. Physiol.* **195**, 55–81.
7. Iwamoto, H. S. and Rudolph, A. M. (1981). *Circulat. Res.* **48**, 183–188.
8. Jensen, A., Bamford, O. S., Dawes, G. S., Hofmeyr, G. J. and Parkes, M. J. (1984). *In:* "The Physiological Development of the Fetus and Newborn", (Jones, C. T. and Nathanielsz, P. W., eds) pp. 605–610. Academic Press, London and Orlando.
9. Jensen, A., Hohmann, M. and Künzel, W. (1983). *Arch. Gynecol.* **235** (1–4), 646–647.
10. Jensen, A. and Künzel, W. (1980). *Gynecol. Obstet. Invest.* **II**, 249–264.
11. Jensen, A., Künzel, W. and Hohmann, M. (1982). *Pflügers Arch. Europ. J. Physiol.* **394**, (suppl.) R20.
12. Jensen, A., Künzel, W. and Kastendieck, E. (1982). *J. Perinat. Med.* **10**, suppl. 2, 109–110.
13. Jensen, A., Künzel, W. and Kastendieck, E. (1983). *In:* "Continuous Transcutaneous Blood Gas Monitoring", (Huch, R. and Huch, A., eds) pp. 591–602, Reproductive Medicine Series, Vol. 5 No. 8, Marcel Dekker, Inc. New York, USA.
14. Jensen, A., Künzel, W. and Kastendieck, E. (1985). *J. Develop. Physiol.* (submitted).
15. Jones, C. T. and Robinson, R. O. (1975). *J. Physiol.* **248**, 15–23.
16. Jones, M. D., Jr., Sheldon, R. E., Peeters, L. L., Meschia, G., Battaglia, F. C. and Makowski, E. L. (1977). *J. Appl. Physiol. Resp. Env. Exc. Physiol.* **43**, 1080–1084.
17. Koizumi, K. and Kollai, M. (1981). *J. Autonom. Nerv. Syst.* **3**, 483–501.
18. Künzel, W., Kastendieck, E., Kurz, C. S. and Paulik, R. (1980). *J. Perinat. Med.* **8**, 85–91.
19. Rudolph, A. M. and Heymann, M. A. (1967). *Circulat. Res.* **21**, 163–184.
20. Rurak, D. W. (1978). *J. Physiol.* **277**, 341–357.

Regulation of Human Myometrial Gap Junctions: *in vitro* Studies

R. H. Hayashi,[1] R. E. Garfield,[2] and M. J. K. Harper[3]

[1]Department of Obstetrics and Gynecology, UCLA Medical Center,
Torrance, California, USA
[2]Departments of Neurosciences and Obstetrics and Gynecology,
McMaster University, Hamilton, Ontario, Canada
[3]Department of Obstetrics and Gynecology, University of Texas,
San Antonio, Texas, USA

Introduction

Gap junctions develop between muscle cells of the myometrium during term and preterm labour in various animals (1) and humans (2). The presence of the junctions corresponds to the time when the myometrium is active and the occurrence of these cell-to-cell contacts is thought to be responsible for changing the myogenic properties of the muscle cell such that electrical events propagate between cells to synchronize contractility. If gap junctions are necessary for labour than an understanding of the conditions which either stimulate or inhibit their presence is of considerable clinical significance.

The mechanisms which promote the existence of myometrial gap junctions is not completely understood. In animals, changes in the levels of steroid hormones and prostaglandins, which precede and accompany labour, are thought to control the synthesis and enlargement of the junctions (6). In the human myometrium there is no evidence for the regulatory mechanisms and the steroid hormone changes which take place before and during labour are not as distinct as those of most animals (3). However, in all species including humans, increased synthesis and release of prostaglandins are apparent and these compounds appear to be involved in the onset and progression of labour (3). There is also evidence that prostaglandins interact with the steroid hormones to regulate gap junctions in the rat uterus (4) and it is possible that the prostaglandins are the primary control mechanism in the human uterus.

The Physiological Development of the Fetus and Newborn
ISBN 0 12 389080 2
Copyright © 1985 by Academic Press, London.
All rights of reproduction in any form reserved.

Studies of treatments which may prevent or initiate gap junctions are prohibitive in humans. However, previous studies of animal tissues have shown that gap junctions develop spontaneously *in vitro* and this model has been used to investigate agents which either promote or inhibit the junctions (1). In the present study, we quantitated gap junctions in myometrial tissues from nonlabour women before and after various *in vitro* treatments.

Materials and Methods

The methods used in this study were similar to those used previously for animal (1) and human tissues (2).

Tissues

Uterine tissues (*ca* 3cm × 2cm × 1cm) were excised from the lower uterine segments of the caesarean openings from women not in labour undergoing term elective operations. Informed consent to remove the tissue and participate in the study was obtained.

Immediately after removal of the tissues they were placed in icecold Krebs-Ringers solution and within 20 min divided into pieces (*ca* 1cm × 1mm × 0.5mm) with the muscle oriented in the long axis. Each piece was stretched 1.5 times the excised length on stainless steel pins. Some tissues were then fixed for electron microscopy (control, zero time). Other tissues from the same uterine segment were fixed after incubation in a CO_2 incubator at 37°C for various times and treatments. The incubation media used was MEM (Minimum Essential Medium, Gibco) without fetal calf serum. The media was collected at selected times and processed for prostaglandin analysis by RIA using procedures previously published (5).

All tissues were fixed by immersion in buffered 2% glutaraldehyde solution and prepared for electron microscopy and gap junctions quantitated as described previously (1,2). The tissues were examined and photographed (*ca* 40 photos/tissue) in a Philips Model 301 electron microscope.

Statistical analysis

The paired Student's *t* test was used to compare differences between control tissues and segments of the same tissues after treatments.

Results

Time course and effects of indomethacin

Figure 1 shows the gap junction area in tissues from 8 women before and following incubation for up to 48 h. All tissues contained very few gap junctions before incubation. Tissues from 3 women (MC, ET and RD) progressively developed more junctions and contained very high values after 48 h. There was little gap junction development in tissues from 5 women (VW, KB, MB, LO and VS) over the 48 h incubation period. Tissue from one postdated woman (41 weeks, VS) contained the lowest area of junctions after 48 h *in vitro*.

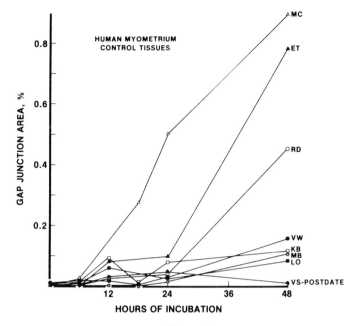

Figure 1.

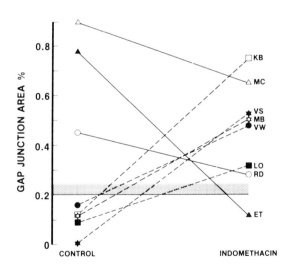

Figure 2.   MEANS±SD

			P
0.33±0.34	All data	0.45±0.21	ns
0.10±0.06	Low controls	0.52±0.15	<0.002
0.71±0.23	High controls	0.35±0.27	ns

P<0.001

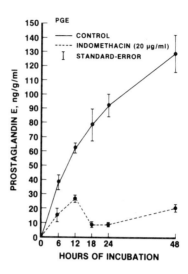

Figure 3.

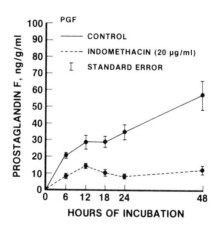

Figure 4.

Comparison of the gap junction areas in control and indomethacin-treated (20 μg/ml) tissues at 48 h is shown in Fig. 2. There was no significant difference ($P > 0.05$) between the mean control junction values (0.33 ± 0.34 SEM) and the mean values from all the indomethacin-treated tissues (0.45 ± 0.21). However, indomethacin resulted in a significant increase ($P < 0.05$) in all 5 tissues from women in which the control tissues developed very few junctions over 48 h (ie below 0.2%). Indomethacin reduced but not to significant levels, the gap junction area in 3 tissues from the 3 women where the control tissues had many junctions at 48 h.

Prostaglandins in the media

The levels of prostaglandins E (PGE) and F (PGF) in the media collected at various times from dishes containing the control and indomethacin-treated tissues is shown in Figs 3 and 4. The levels of PGE and PGF in the media surrounding control tissues increased progressively with time. At 48 h there was about 3 times as much PGE as PGF. The levels of both prostaglandins were significantly reduced by indomethacin.

Discussion

Our results show that gap junctions develop slowly in some of the tissues *in vitro*. Tissues removed from women prior to labour contained very few gap junctions but segments of some of the same tissues contained more after incubation. These results are similar to animal tissues studied *in vitro* (1). Tissues from some women had less capacity to form gap junctions, and might be explained on the basis that the development and presence of gap junctions *in vitro* or *in vivo* is the result of maturational events in preparation for labour and that the tissues used in this study were from women at different stages of the maturation process.

It is obvious that the placenta, decidua, fetal membranes and fetus are not necessary for gap junctions to form as our tissues were primarily muscle. However, these tissues may modulate the presence of the junctions through the production of prostaglandins and other regulatory molecules or mediate action of the steroid hormones.

Our results show that the tissues released PGE and PGF into the incubation media (Figs 2 and 3) and that the amount of prostaglandins was reduced by indomethacin treatments. Previously we have found in human and animal tissues that labour and delivery occur when about 0.2–0.3% of the plasma membrane area is occupied by gap junctions (2,6). In this study we show that indomethacin increases gap junctions in segments of those same control tissues which developed less than 0.2% of membrane area (Fig. 2). This may mean that a product of the cyclo-oxygenase pathway prevents gap junction development and that a shift in the synthesis of the cyclo-oxygenase inhibitory product is one of the steps involved in the maturational process.

Other studies in animals also show that indomethacin increases gap junction area (4).

Our study has important implications in the management of labour. Inhibition of prostaglandin synthesis may stimulate the presence of gap junctions as well as preventing the formation of products which may stimulate the muscle to contract. However, further studies are needed to fully define the mechanisms for control of myometrial gap junctions and their involvement in labour.

Acknowledgements

This work was supported by grants from the Medical Research Council of Canada and NIH grants (HD14048 and HD10202).

References

1. Garfield, R. E., Merrett, D. and Grover, A. K. (1980). *Am. J. Physiol.* **239**, C217.
2. Garfield, R. E. and Hayashi, R. H. (1981). *Am. J. Obstet. Gynecol.* **140**, 254.
3. Csapo, A. I. (1981). *In:* "Principles and Practice of Obstetrics and Gynecology", (Iffy, L. and Kaminetzky, H. A., eds) pp. 761–799. John Wiley and Sons, Inc. New York.
4. MacKenzie, L. W., Puri, C. P. and Garfield, R. E. (1983). *Prostaglandins* **26**, 925.
5. Harper, M. J. K., Valenzuela, G. and Hodgson, B. J. (1978). *Prostaglandins* **15**, 43.
6. Puri, C. P. and Garfield, R. E. (1982). *Biol. Reprod.* **27**, 967.

Perinatal Endocrine Responses in Piglets: Effects of Prematurity and Acidaemia

Marian Silver, Abigail L. Fowden, R. S. Comline,
Jean Knox and S. R. Bloom*

Physiological Laboratory, Cambridge, UK and
*Hammersmith Hospital, London, UK

Introduction

In common with many other species, the fetal piglet shows the characteristic gradual prepartum rise in plasma cortisol which begins 10–15 days before term (*ca* 115 days), with a very rapid increase in cortisol during labour itself (1,2). A smaller though comparable intrapartum rise in fetal plasma cortisol was also seen in prematurely induced labour in the sow (3), although prepartum plasma cortisol levels were low. Such piglets did not survive more than 24 h and it seemed probable that other fetal maturational events had been circumvented by the premature induction of labour by maternal luteolysis. For example, the amount of available adrenaline which may be released at parturition is dependent, in part, upon enhanced glucocorticoid secretion. Another hormone associated with stress is glucagon, although information about its release before or during birth is limited (4). In the present experiments perinatal changes in plasma glucagon and catecholamines have been examined in chronically catheterized piglets and in their unoperated littermates.

Methods

Intravascular catheters were inserted into 12 sows and 1–2 piglets per litter at 95–102 days of gestation as described previously (1,3). The animals were sampled daily until labour was induced with cloprostenol (Estrumate, ICI 200 μg im) either near term (109–111 days, Group I) or prematurely at 104–105 days (Group II).

The Physiological Development of the Fetus and Newborn
ISBN 0 12 389080 2

Copyright © 1985 by Academic Press, London.
All rights of reproduction in any form reserved.

Where possible the catheterized piglets were monitored throughout the 24 h induction period as well as during delivery; after birth they were sampled by cardiac puncture or by catheter, together with their unoperated littermates at intervals of 0, 30, 60 and 120 min. Blood pH, O_2 saturation and packed cell volume were measured routinely and the plasma apportioned for cortisol, glucagon and catecholamine assay using methods described previously (3,5,6). Due to limitations on sample size (1–1.5 ml) glucagon was measured on prepartum and birth samples only. All results are expressed as mean values ± SEM.

Results

Hormone levels in late gestation

Between 95–103 days of gestation (Group II), mean levels of adrenaline were significantly lower than the corresponding nonadrenaline values (Fig. 1), whereas in the older fetuses (Group I) both adrenaline and noradrenaline concentrations were higher and more variable. The mean plasma adrenaline in Group I during the pre-induction period (1.14 ± 0.22 ng/ml) was significantly higher than the value for Group II (0.55 ± 0.12 ng/ml, $P < 0.05$, $n = 15$). Mean noradrenaline levels in the two groups were similar.

Fetal plasma glucagon concentrations remained low in both groups of fetuses during the last 10–15 days of gestation (mean 9.3 ± 1.3 pmol/l, $n = 10$). Elevated glucagon levels were observed after surgery (37.7 ± 10.2 pmol/l) but these had fallen to basal concentrations within 48 h.

Induction of labour

During the 24 h between the injection of cloprostenol and the delivery of the first piglet fetal blood gases, pH and catecholamine levels were similar to pre-induction values in the majority of piglets whether premature or near-term, although fetal plasma cortisol had risen significantly 8–12 h before delivery, as found previously (3). In the 1–2 h before birth fetal plasma cortisol concentrations were high (Fig. 1), whereas plasma catecholamines had not changed significantly from pre-induction levels, apart from the rise in noradrenaline at 30 min before delivery in Group I ($+1.3 \pm 0.41$ ng/ml, $P < 0.02$). At birth the incremental changes over pre-induction values for both noradrenaline ($+2.4 \pm 0.23$ ng/ml) and adrenaline ($+1.5 \pm 0.29$ ng/ml) were significant in Group I ($P < 0.01$, $n = 6$), while in Group II only the rise in noradrenaline was significant ($+1.4 \pm 0.43$ ng/ml, $P < 0.05$, $n = 4$). The perinatal changes in maternal catecholamines were not related to fetal levels.

Changes after birth

In Group II a higher proportion of piglets (33%) had a pH of 7.25 or below at delivery compared to Group I (18%). Neonatal acidaemia was associated with every high catecholamine and glucagon levels (2–30 ng/ml noradrenaline; 1–9 ng/ml adrenaline; 36–148 pmol/l glucagon). There was a significant inverse

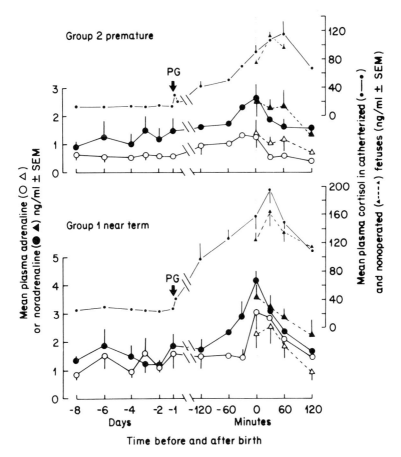

Figure 1. Mean changes in plasma catecholamines and cortisol in catheterized (●○) and non-catheterized (▲ △) piglets in which blood pH > 7.25. Cloprostenol was given at ↓ . (Details of dose and gestational age groups in text).

relationship between blood pH (X) and the total catecholamine levels (Y) at birth in both Group I (Y = −58.31X + 432.77, r = −0.75, n = 48, P < 0.01) and in Group II (Y = −26.95X + 201.96, r = −0.60, n = 28, P < 0.01): the difference between the slopes was statistically significant (P < 0.01). There was also a significant inverse relationship between pH and plasma glucagon concentrations at birth (r = 0.74, n = 21, P < 0.01) but no difference in the glucagon response to acidaemia could be detected between premature and term piglets.

When data from piglets with neonatal pH > 7.25 were excluded, the catheterized and unoperated piglets in each group had similar cortisol and catecholamine levels during the postnatal period (Fig. 1). Comparison of the 2 groups at birth using the combined data from catheterized and unoperated piglets showed that mean plasma cortisol (79.4 ± 3.8 ng/ml) and adrenaline (1.18 ± 0.33 ng/ml) concentrations in the premature group were significantly lower than the corresponding values (134.2 ± 10.4 and 2.54 ± 0.48 ng/ml respectively) for Group I piglets ($P < 0.01$ and 0.05, $n = 21$), whereas mean noradrenaline values for the 2 groups did not differ significantly. There was a significant correlation between neonatal plasma cortisol and the corresponding adrenaline level ($r = 0.518$, $P < 0.05$, $n = 21$), but not between cortisol and noradrenaline.

No differences in the levels of plasma glucagon were found between catheterized and unoperated fetuses or between premature and term piglets at birth in those animals with a neonatal blood $pH > 7.25$. There was, however, a wide range of plasma glucagon levels even in apparently unstressed piglets. The overall mean value of 28.0 ± 8.7 pmol/l was significantly higher than the pre-induction value of 9.4 ± 1.4 pmol/l ($P < 0.05$, $n = 22$).

Discussion

The present findings have confirmed that adrenocortical activity in the fetal piglet is markedly increased throughout labour even when parturition is induced prematurely (3). However, the intra- and postpartum cortisol levels obtained in premature piglets were significantly lower than those seen near term. The catecholamine response at birth in the former was comparatively small and adrenaline levels were not maintained postnatally by comparison with more mature piglets. Similar findings have been reported for premature delivery in lambs (7). The correlation between plasma cortisol and adrenaline concentrations at birth in the piglet is comparable with observations on premature and full-term foals where a similar relationship was detected (6).

Fetal catheterization *per se* had no detectable effect on the postnatal changes in any of the hormones measured. The main parameter which appeared to affect catecholamines, glucagon and to a lesser extent plasma cortisol concentrations at birth, was the degree of acidaemia at delivery. In other species notably horse, human and sheep, a correlation between plasma catecholamine levels and blood pH has been demonstrated in the fetus and neonate (6,8,9). It seems unlikely, however that acidaemia is the primary cause of sympatho-adrenal stimulation. All the evidence from both fetal and newborn animals points to hypoxia as the most effective stimulus for catecholamine release (9) and hence a low blood pH at birth is probably indicative of some intrapartum hypoxia. However, during the course of second stage labour in the sow the catheterized fetuses remained well oxygenated and in good condition until close to delivery which confirms previous observations in this and other species (3,10).

Glucagon release at birth has been reported in other species and catecholamines have been implicated in this response (4,10). The rise in fetal glucagon following surgery and also after arginine injection in the fetal pig (unpublished observations) suggest that the α-cells are active *in utero*. Certainly these cells can be identified at an earlier stage of gestation than pancreatic β-cells (11). The role of glucagon in the fetus and at delivery is not known nor is it certain to what extent catecholamine release at birth is important for postnatal survival. It has been suggested that adrenaline increases lung liquid absorption at birth (12) while both glucagon and catecholamines are almost certainly involved in the mobilization of energy reserves during the immediate postnatal period.

Acknowledgements

This work was funded by the Agricultural and Food Research Council.

References

1. Silver, M., Barne, R. J., Comline, R. S., Fowden, A. L., Clover, L. and Mitchell, M. D. (1979). *Anim. Reprod. Sci.* **2**, 305–322.
2. Randall, G. C. B. (1983). *Biol. Reprod.* **29**, 1077–1084.
3. Silver, M., Comline, R. S. and Fowden, A. L. (1983). *J. Develop. Physiol.* **5**, 307–321.
4. Sperling, M. A. (1977). *Rec. Prog. Pediat. Endocr.* **12**, 21–32.
5. Bloom, S. R. and Long, R. G. (1982). "Radioimmunoassay of Gut Regulatory Peptides". W. B. Saunders, London.
6. Silver, M., Ousey, J., Dudan, F., Fowden, A. L., Knox, J., Cash, R. S. G. and Rossdale, P. D. (1984). *Eq. Vet. J.* (in press).
7. Eliot, R. J., Lein, A. H., Glatz, T. H., Nathanielsz, P. W. and Fisher, D. A. (1981). *Endocrinology* **108**, 1678–1682.
8. Lagercrantz, H. and Bistoletti, P. (1977). *Pediat. Res.* **11**, 889–993.
9. Jones, C. T. (1980). *In* "Biogenic Amines in Development." (Parvez, H. and Parvez, S., eds) pp. 63–86. Elsevier/North Holland.
10. Comline, R. S. and Silver, M. (1975). *Brit. Med. Bull.* **31**, 25–31.
11. Comline, R. S., Rowden, A. L., Robinson, P. M. and Silver, M. (1980). *J. Physiol.* **307**, 11–12P.
12. Walters, D. V. and Olver, R. E. (1978). *Pediat. Res.* **12**, 239–242.

Cardiorespiratory Effects of Calcium Channel-blocker Tocolysis in Pregnant Rhesus Monkeys

C. A. Ducsay, M. J. Cook, J. C. Veille and M. J. Novy

Department of Perinatal Physiology,
Oregon Regional Primate Research Center, Beaverton, Oregon,
and Department of Obstetrics and Gynecology,
Oregon Health Sciences University, Portland, Oregon, USA

Introduction

It is now recognized that the coupling of excitation and contraction in myometrium is regulated by the intracellular free calcium concentration even though the molecular basis of this interaction remains controversial (1). Calcium entry blockers inhibit the influx of extracellular calcium through specific channels in the cell membrane (2). They are potent smooth muscle relaxants and are widely used clinically in the treatment of cardiovascular disorders. Because of the pivotal role of calcium in myometrial contraction, the potential use of the calcium-blocking agents (e.g. nifedipine, verapamil) in the management of preterm labour has generated considerable interest.

Nifedipine inhibits spontaneous and oxytocin-induced myometrial contractions *in vitro* and is a potent inhibitor of drug-induced myometrial contractions *in vitro* and is a potent inhibitor of drug-induced myometrial activity in the early postpartum period in women (3). Additional studies in pregnant sheep (4) and pregnant rabbits (5) have also demonstrated a significant tocolytic effect of calcium channel blockers. While it is clear that calcium antagonists are potentially useful uterine relaxing agents, their efficiency, specificity and possible adverse maternal and fetal cardiovascular side-effects remain to be elucidated. Previous studies on uterine contractility and co-existing maternal and fetal cardiovascular effects have been carried out in pregnant rabbits (5) and sheep (4), but not in subhuman primates. We report the effects of nifedipine on uterine activity and on maternal

The Physiological Development of the Fetus and Newborn
ISBN 0 12 389080 2

Copyright © 1985 by Academic Press, London.
All rights of reproduction in any form reserved.

and fetal cardiorespiratory parameters in chronically catheterized pregnant rhesus monkeys.

Materials and Methods

Twelve individual studies were conducted in 7 chronically catheterized rhesus monkeys between days 127 and 137 of gestation. Surgical procedures were performed by methods previously described in detail (6). Briefly, polyvinyl catheters were implanted in the fetal carotid artery and jugular vein, maternal femoral artery and vein and in the amniotic fluid cavity. Electrocardiogram electrodes were also attached to the fetus. Each animal was placed in a primate restraining chair 48 h after surgery. Fetal heart rate and uterine activity (amplitude, frequency and hourly contraction area) were monitored continuously by methods previously described (7).

Nifedipine (Pfizer Laboratories) in alcohol:phosphate buffer was administered intravenously to the mother as intermittent bolus injections (15–85 μg/kg) or as a continuous infusion by Harvard infusion pump (3 μg/kg/min) for 1 h during spontaneous uterine activity. Maternal femoral arterial and fetal carotid arterial blood samples were drawn at frequent intervals to monitor pH and PO_2 while arterial pressures were monitored continuously during periods of nifedipine administration.

Results

The results from 7 bolus injection studies are listed in Table 1. Administration of nifedipine as a bolus resulted in a dramatic and statistically significant decline in mean amplitude of contraction as well as contraction area. Contraction frequency followed a similar trend, which was not statistically significant. None of the cardiorespiratory parameters monitored were significantly affected by nifedipine administration (Table 1). However, trends toward fetal hypoxia and acidosis were observed.

Table 1. Effect of maternal bolus injections of nifedipine on uterine activity and cardiorespiratory parameters

	Control	Nifedipine[†]	n
Contraction frequency (number/h)	28.3±2.3	24.3±3.4	7
$\bar{x}$ amplitude (mmHg)	28.4±3.0	16.9±1.4**	7
Contraction area (mmHg s/h)	19,207±2633	8,200±2002**	7
$\bar{x}$ maternal blood pressure (mmHg)	116.0±4.0	112±5.3	5
$\bar{x}$ fetal blood pressure (mmHg)	44.0±1.9	42.2±2.2	5
Fetal heart rate (beats/min)	230.0±4.5	213.5±12.8	5
Fetal arterial pH	7.348±0.020	7.319±0.028	5
Fetal arterial PO_2	24.2±1.1	23.5±1.9	5

[†]Means±SEM 1 h after administration.
(ANOVA, **$P<0.01$, compared to control)

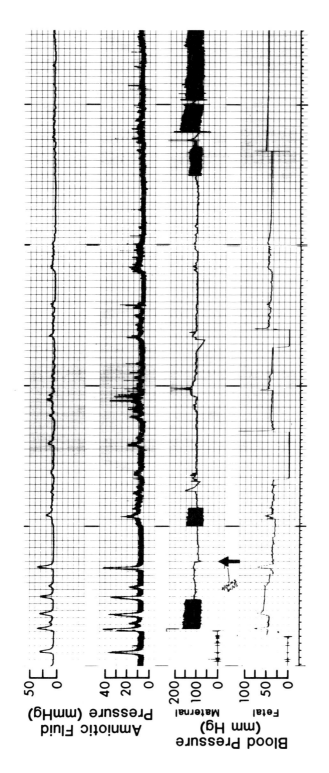

Figure 1. Maternal and fetal arterial pressures and intraamniotic fluid pressure changes during maternal IV nifedipine administration (400 μg bolus injection indicated by arrow). Note: Gaps in fetal and maternal pressure recording are due to sampling. Time intervals in min.

A representative example of the effect of a bolus nifedipine injection is illustrated in Fig. 1. An instantaneous decline in maternal arterial pressure occurred following nifedipine administration (indicated by arrow). This effect was transient as maternal arterial pressure returned to control levels by 1 h. Little change was observed in fetal arterial pressure after bolus administration of nifedipine (Table 1, Fig. 1). Uterine activity (as measured by intraamniotic fluid pressure) declined after nifedipine administration (Fig. 1) and in this particular animal, the uterus remained quiescent throughout the night.

Continuous nifedipine infusion (3 μg/kg/min) for 1 h had similar effects on uterine activity. A significant decline in contraction area was observed after nifedipine infusion. A similar trend was observed in contraction frequency and mean contraction amplitude, but was not significant (Fig. 2a). Fetal arterial PO_2 was also significantly affected by nifedipine treatment (Fig. 2b). At the end of the 60 minute infusion, values declined from a control value of 21.7 to 14.2 mmHg. A dramatic decline was also observed in fetal pH during the nifedipine infusion (Fig. 2b). Fetal arterial pressure appeared to decline during the infusion, but the effect was not significant.

Comments

Results from the present study indicate that nifedipine has a marked tocolytic effect on the uterus of the pregnant rhesus monkey. There is some concern, however, that maternal nifedipine administration has an adverse effect on fetal cardiorespiratory parameters.

Both bolus injections and continuous infusions of nifedipine resulted in a trend toward fetal hypoxaemia and acidosis (Table 1 and Fig. 2b). These effects were statistically significant when the drug was administered by continuous infusion (Fig. 2b). Initially we attributed the decline in fetal arterial pH and PO_2 after bolus nifedipine injections, to the transitory hypotensive effect in the mother. During continuous nifedipine infusion, no decline in maternal pressure was observed. However, the fetal side-effects were more pronounced after 1 h than previously observed during bolus administration of the drug.

The high degree of protein-binding of nifedipine in plasma would tend to minimize placental transfer (3). However, in view of the deleterious effects on fetal cardiorespiratory parameters without apparent alteration of maternal blood pressure or maternal arterial blood gases, a direct effect on the fetus or the uterine vasculature cannot be ruled out.

Another possible explanation is a dose-response effect. In the studies in which the animals received a bolus injection of nifedipine, a maximum dose of 500 μg was injected, while the infusion animals received a total of approximately 1000 μg of nifedipine during the 1 h infusion period. Pharmacokinetic studies have indicated that the half-life of nifedipine is approximately 2–3 h (8). If nifedipine is indeed reaching the fetus, the increased dosage and duration of administration could be responsible for the increased severity of the deleterious effects observed in these fetuses.

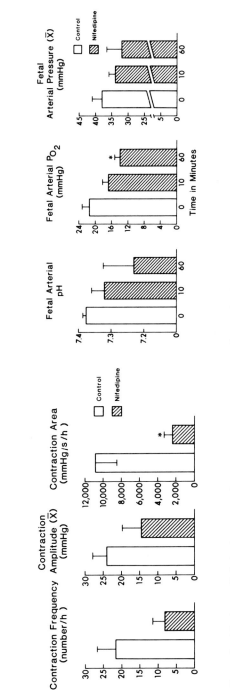

Figure 2a: Uterine activity before and after a 1 h nifedipine infusion (3 µg/kg/min). $P<0.05$; $n=5$.

Figure 2b: Fetal cardiorespiratory parameters measured at 0, 10, and 60 min after the start of a 1 h nifedipine infusion (3 µg/kg/min). $P<0.05$; $n=5$.

The tocolytic effect of nifedipine was significant in all of the animals in this study. The drug was administered during periods of spontaneous uterine activity which we have previously described (7). When administered as a bolus injection, the tocolytic effect was instantaneous whereas the continuous infusion required 10–20 min before a decrease in uterine activity became evident. The duration of the tocolytic effect after bolus injections of nifedipine varied inversely with the intensity of the uterine activity prior to administration of the drug. When the initial activity exceeded 10 000 mmHg/s/h, the effect of nifedipine lasted for approximately 1 h after the infusion was stopped. Tocolysis was much longer in duration, often lasting several hours, when the uterine activity was less than 10 000 mmHg/s/h prior to infusion.

In a small human clinical trial, nifedipine was found to be an effective tocolytic agent (9). In all 10 patients, delivery was postponed for at least 3 days, with no apparent adverse effects on fetal outcome. However, fetal blood gases were not assessed in this study. Calcium antagonists appear to offer a new means of regulating uterine activity. The results of the present study, however, indicate the need for further clarification of the effect of nifedipine on fetal cardiorespiratory parameters. Simultaneous measurements of drug levels in maternal and fetal blood are needed to determine whether fetal effects are related to transplacental passage of calcium blocking agents.

Acknowledgements

Supported in part by grant RR00163 from the National Institutes of Health, grant HD06159 from the National Institute of Child Health and Human Development, and from the Autzen Foundation.

References

1. Carsten, M. E. and Miller, J. D. (1983). *In:* "Initiation of Parturition: Prevention and Prematurity", (MacDonald, P. C. and Porter, J. eds) pp. 168–171, Ross Laboratories, Columbus.
2. Church, J. and Zoster, T. T. (1980). *Can. J. Physiol. Pharmacol.* **58**, 254–259.
3. Forman, A., Andersson, K. E. and Ulmsten, U. (1981). *Semin. Perinatol.* **5**, 288–294.
4. Holbrook, H., Court, D., Parer, J. T. and Creasy, R. K. (1984). Proc. 31st Ann. Meeting Soc. Gynecol. Invest., March 21–24, San Francisco, CA, p. 210 (Abstr. No. 352P).
5. Holbrook, H., Lirette, M. and Katz, M. (1984). Proc. 31st Ann. Meeting Soc. Gynecol. Invest., March 21–24, San Francisco, CA, p. 209 (Abstr. No. 350P).
6. Walsh, S. W., Norman, R. and Novy, M. J. (1979). *Endocrinology* **104**, 1805–1813.
7. Ducsay, C., Cook, M. J., Walsh, S. W. and Novy, M. J. (1983). *Am. J. Obstet. Gynecol.* **145**, 389–396.
8. Pedersen, O. L. and Mikkelsen, E. (1978). *Eur. J. Clin. Pharmacol.* **14**, 375–381.
9. Ulmsten, U., Andersson, K. E. and Wingerup, L. (1981). *Arch. Gynecol.* **229**, 1–5.

Progesterone Metabolism During Induction of Delivery by Infusion of Cortisol to the Ovine Fetus

G. Jenkin, G. Jorgensen, G. D. Thorburn, P. W. Nathanielsz and J. E. Buster

Department of Physiology, Monash University, Victoria, Australia;
Cornell University New York State College of Veterinary Medicine, Ithaca,
New York; and Harbour UCLA Medical Centre, Torrance, California, USA

Introduction

Parturition, in sheep, is preceded by an increase in the concentration of cortisol in fetal plasma and a decrease in the maternal plasma concentration of progesterone (1,2). Under normal circumstances, progesterone withdrawal at delivery modifies the responsiveness of the myometrium, converting the uterus from a relatively refractory to a reactive organ which will respond to the stimulatory action of prostaglandin released in response to the preparturient rise in estrogen (3). Administration of progesterone during late pregnancy fails, however, to delay normal or dexamethazone induced parturition unless supraphysiological doses of progesterone are administered (3,4). Since an increase in placental 17α-hydroxylase, C-17,20 lyase and aromataze activity has been demonstrated at the time of spontaneous parturition, or of parturition induced by exogenous glucocorticoid administration (5,6,7), it is possible that exogenous administration of progesterone, at this time, will provide additional substrate for estrogen biosynthesis necessitating the administration of supraphysiological amounts of progesterone to suppress delivery. Such a possibility would provide an explanation for the observation of Liggins and associates (3) that, although the decrease in plasma progesterone observed during dexamethazone induction of delivery was prevented by supraphysiological exogenous progesterone administration, there was no significant increase in plasma progesterone concentrations above control levels even when 200 mg progesterone was administered daily.

The Physiological Development of the Fetus and Newborn
ISBN 0 12 389080 2

Copyright © 1985 by Academic Press, London.
All rights of reproduction in any form reserved.

We have compared the fate of exogenously administered progesterone, during induction of delivery by infusion of cortisol to the fetus, with that of endogenous progesterone during induction of delivery alone or after administration of medroxyprogesterone acetate (MPA), a synthetic progestagen which is not metabolized *in vivo* to estrogen or to 20α-hydroxyprogesterone (20α-OHP).

Methods

Maternal and fetal vascular catheters were implanted into sheep at 124–128 days gestation as described previously (8). Cortisol was infused into the fetal jugular vein, commencing 6 days after surgery. The quantity of cortisol infused was increased every 24 h from 2.8 mg/24 h for the first 24 h, followed by 5.6 mg/24 h for 24 h, 11.2 mg/24 h for 24 h and subsequently 22.4 mg/24 h, until delivery of the fetus, or until the experiment was terminated. Six fetuses were infused with cortisol alone. Four fetuses were infused with cortisol as above but the ewe was also injected every 12 h with 100 mg progesterone, commencing 24 h before the start of cortisol infusion. Seven ewes were injected intramuscularly with 250 mg MPA 24 h before the start of infusion of cortisol to the fetus. Fetal and maternal blood samples were assayed for steroid hormones by radioimmunoassay (9,10).

Results and Discussion

Premature induction of delivery in fetuses infused with cortisol was brought about in 123.5 ± 7.7 (mean ± SEM) h after the start of cortisol infusion. The ewes injected with progesterone, during infusion of cortisol to their fetuses, did not deliver. Only one ewe injected with MPA delivered within 2SDs of the mean time of delivery of the fetuses infused with cortisol alone. Two further ewes, injected with MPA, delivered live lambs 147.7 and 175 h after the start of cortisol infusion while the remaining ewes in this group failed to deliver during the course of the experiment which was terminated between 10 and 15 days after the start of cortisol infusion.

Maternal plasma progesterone and 20α-OHP concentrations before cortisol infusion were 10.51 ± 0.49 ng/ml (mean ± SEM; $n=33$) and 11.32 ± 0.61 ng/ml ($n=38$) respectively. The concentration of progesterone decreased in both cortisol infused and in MPA treated ewes in a similar fashion during cortisol infusion, to 2.16 ± 2.80 ng/ml ($n=7$) and 4.88 ± 3.70 ng/ml ($n=9$) respectively, on the sixth day of cortisol infusion. Plasma progesterone increased significantly above pre-infusion levels in those ewes that were injected with progesterone ($P<0.05$) reaching a concentration 19.46 ± 1.50 ng/ml ($n=32$) during treatment. Plasma 20α-OHP concentrations decreased to undetectable levels in cortisol infused and MPA treated ewes but did not change significantly from pre-infusion concentrations in progesterone treated ewes (mean concentration during treatment 15.32 ± 0.86 ng/ml, $n=32$).

Fetal plasma progesterone and 20α-OHP concentrations before cortisol infusion were 1.06 ± 0.08 ng/ml ($n=23$) and 24.07 ± 1.35 ng/ml ($n=36$) respectively and decreased to basal levels in all 3 groups of animals studied during cortisol infusion.

A concomitant increase in maternal and fetal 17α-hydroxyprogesterone, dehydroepiandrosterone, estrone and estrone sulphate occurred during cortisol infusion alone and during cortisol infusion after MPA treatment, indicating that the infusion of cortisol to the fetus had induced placental 17α-hydroxylase, C17–20 lyase and aromatase activity to switch metabolism of the endogenous progesterone from 20α-OHP to estrogen. The induction of placental 17α-hydroxylase, C17–20 lyase and aromatase was not suppressed by progesterone treatment, since the increase in maternal and fetal dehydroepiandrosterone, estrone and estrone sulphate was similar to that observed in the other two groups of animals studied. There was, however, no difference between the increase in maternal and fetal estrone and estrone sulphate concentrations in animals treated with progesterone or with MPA. The finding that the plasma concentration of these steroids continued to increase when parturition was prevented by progestagen treatment is further evidence that the maintained plasma concentrations of progesterone or MPA did not suppress placental estrogen biosynthesis. Thus, although administration of progestagen to the ewe prevented the induction of delivery by infusion of cortisol to the fetus, it appears that the exogenous progesterone administered in this study was unable to gain access to those placental cells which are responsible for estrogen biosynthesis, but was metabolized instead in the periphery to 20α-OHP which was elevated in this group of animals. The endogenous progesterone, produced by the placenta was, however, redirected away from progesterone and towards estrogen biosynthesis which was secreted into the maternal and fetal compartment.

In a previous study by Gurpide and colleagues (11) it was suggested that the majority of progesterone production by the placenta was directed towards the maternal circulation and that practically all fetal progesterone and 75% of fetal 20α-OHP was derived from maternal circulating progesterone. In our study placental impermeability to progesterone is suggested by the fall observed in the fetal concentrations of this steroid in the face of maintained maternal concentrations during exogenous progesterone treatment of the ewe. The majority of progesterone entering the fetal compartment would be rapidly metabolized to 20α-OHP by the active 20α-reductase in the fetal liver (12) and fetal red blood cells (13). However, the fall in concentration of fetal 20α-OHP during cortisol infusion to the fetus, indicated that neither progesterone, nor 20α-OHP itself, was transferred from the mother to the fetus to any great extent. We have shown that placental tissue, incubated *in vitro*, is able to metabolize progesterone to 20α-OHP in late pregnancy as well as to C18 steroids at the time of parturition. However, preliminary experiments in which [H^3]20α-OHP was infused into either the maternal or fetal vascular compartment to constant specific activity, support the concept that the placenta is relatively impermeable to this steroid since very little [H^3]20α-OHP was transferred from the mother to the fetus, during infusion to the mother. Although there was considerable metabolism of [H^3]20α-OHP when infused to the fetus there was some transfer of this steroid from the fetus to the mother as judged by the elevated concentration of [H^3]20α-OHP observed in the uterine vein during infusion to the fetus.

These experiments demonstrate that, when progesterone is administered to sheep during induction of delivery by infusion of cortisol to the fetus, it is unable to enter the steroidogenic pathway leading to estrogen biosynthesis and is metabolized in periphery to 20α-OHP. Extensive metabolism of endogenous progesterone to estrogen, which is then secreted into both the maternal and fetal compartments, occurs, however, during infusion of cortisol to the fetus even when parturition is inhibited by exogenous progestagen administration to the ewe. Thus, if exogenous progesterone administration is to prevent labour, it must be administered in sufficient quantities to overcome the stimulatory effects of the rising estrogen concentrations brought about by the cortisol induction of placental 17α-hydroxylase, C-17,20 lyase and aromataze.

Furthermore, circulating maternal progesterone and 20α-OHP appear unable to gain access to the fetal compartment even when present in high concentrations in maternal plasma during administration of progesterone to the ewe.

References

1. Bassett, J. M. and Thorburn, G. D. (1969). *J. Endocrinol.* **44**, 285–286.
2. Bassett, J. M., Oxborrow, T. J., Smith, I. D. and Thorburn, G. D. (1969). *J. Endocrinol.* **45**, 449–457.
3. Liggins, G. C., Grieves, S. A., Kendall, J. Z. and Knox, B. S. (1972). *J. Reprod. Fertil.* **16**, (suppl.) 85–103.
4. Bengtsson, L.Ph. and Schofield, B. M. (1963). *J. Reprod. Fertil.* **5**, 423–431.
5. Anderson, A. B. M., Flint, A. F. P. and Turnbull, A. C. (1975). *J. Endocrinol.* **66**, 239–246.
6. Steele, P. A., Flint, A. P. F. and Turnbull, A. C. (1976). *J. Endocrinol.* **69**, 239–246.
7. Mann, M. R., Curet, L. B. and Colás, A. E. (1975). *J. Endocrinol.* **65**, 117–125.
8. Jenkin, G., Jorgensen, G., Thorburn, G. D., Buster, J. E. and Nathanielsz, P. W. (1984). *Can. J. Physiol. Pharmacol.* (in press).
9. Elsner, C. W., Magyar, D. M., Fridshal, D., Eliot, J., Klein, A., Glatz, T., Nathanielsz, P. W. and Buster, J. E. (1980). *Endocrinology* **107**, 801–808.
10. Nathanielsz, P. W., Elsner, C., Magyar, D., Fridshal, D., Freeman, A. and Buster, J. E. (1982). *Endocrinology* **110**, 1402–1407.
11. Gurpide, E., Tseng, J., Escarcena, L., Fahning, M., Gibson, C. and Fehr, P. (1972). *Am. J. Obstet. Gynecol.* **113**, 21–32.
12. Anderson, A. B. M., Pierrepoint, C. G., Griffiths, K. and Turnbull, A. C. (1970). *J. Endocrinol.* **48**, 665–666.
13. Nancarrow, C. D. and Seamark, R. F. (1968). *Steroids* **12**, 367–380.

Some Aspects of Pre- and Afterload on the Fetal Stroke Volume and Heart Rate

J. Morgenstern and R. Leblanc

Department of Obstetrics and Gynecology,
Biomedical Technique Unit, University of Düsseldorf,
Federal Republic of Germany

The data were derived from 7 chronically instrumented (*) fetal lambs with weights from 2900–3200 g and gestational ages from 128–134 days. Up to 16 cardiovascular parameters were simultaneously measured during 58 different episodes, each lasting from 0.5–1.5 h, depending on the different digitizing rate between 3 and 9 ms, and on-line stored on digital tapes. A total monitoring time of about 60 h with 350 000 heart beats are evaluated.

Right and left ventricular outputs were measured continuously *in utero* from 2–8 days after implantation of electromagnetic flow-transducers around the main pulmonary trunk and ascending aorta. The arterial blood pressure was measured in the aortic arch, pulmonary artery and in the descending aorta simultaneously with 2 different transducer types each. Programme systems for beat-to-beat evaluation of each parameter have been developed.

Though we think that data reduction by simply calculating mean values etc. does not exhibit any clinical valuable information, the values shown in Table 1 for this $n = 13\,200$ heart beats were derived.

Except for the first 4 rows, the set-up of each row refers to one parameter and its values for the left (above) and right ventricle. Thus e.g. the mean values for the SV are 3.09 ± 0.17 ml and 5.59 ± 0.26 ml, respectively. On average the right ventricle ejects blood during nearly the same time period (VET), but shows a 1.88 times higher amplitude A and develops a 2.54 times higher contractility index S compared to the left side. This results in a 1.8 times higher CO in favour of the right ventricle.

*The surgeries were performed by A. M. Rudolph, MD and M. A. Heymann, MD, Cardiovascular Research Institute, San Francisco, USA

The Physiological Development of the Fetus and Newborn
ISBN 0 12 389080 2

Copyright © 1985 by Academic Press, London.
All rights of reproduction in any form reserved.

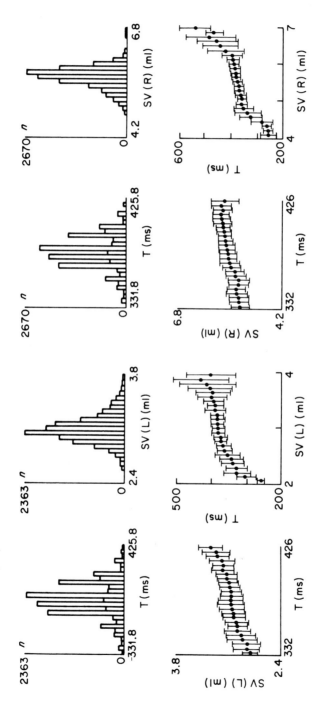

Figure 1. T and SV histograms and corresponding mean values for the left (L) and right (R) ventricle.

Table 1

		mean	SD	max	min	
FHR	bpm	159	11	267	84	fetal heart rate
T	ms	379	16	465	291	heart period
P	mmHg	4.0	1.9	12.0	0.3	inf. vena cava
PA	mmHg	49.8	2.5	59.9	41.9	art. end diast.
SV	ml	3.09	0.17	3.84	2.36	stroke
		5.59	0.26	6.69	4.51	volume
S	l/s*s	10.5	0.8	14.8	7.1	slope increas.
		26.8	1.6	33.9	19.8	flow signal
PEP	ms	37.3	2.7	48.4	20.5	pre-ejection
		35.8	2.4	45.1	26.1	period
VET	ms	149	3	166	131	ventricular
		150	2	162	137	ejection time
A	ml/min	1768	65	2104	1512	max. stroke
		3318	84	3682	2961	amplitude
CO	ml/min	491	36	843	62	cardiac
		887	45	1308	516	output

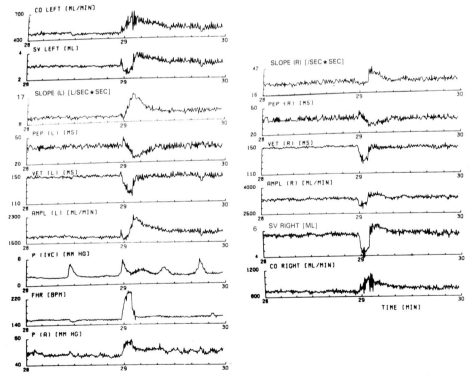

Figure 2. A 2 min cutout with a FHR acceleration (middle trace) at the 29th min from beginning. The top 6 traces are derived from the left and the bottom 6 from the right ventricle.

The heart period T, which covers the physiological range and the SVs were summarized in frequency distributions (Fig. 1, top). Within each group the corresponding mean values with SD were calculated and plotted below (Fig. 1, bottom). Depending on which parameter was grouped the corresponding mean values look different. While e.g. T was grouped from 319 ms to 408 ms in 25 classes, the corresponding SV mean values change from 3.33±0.07 ml to 3.88±0.12 ml and 5.14±0.11 ml to 5.72±0.06 ml for the left and right side as shown in Fig. 1 (bottom, 1 and 3 plot). Grouping on the other side the SV values, the mean values in relation to T changed from 2.43 ml to 3.77 ml and 4.25 to 6.75 ml (Fig. 1, bottom, 2 and 4 plot).

However it may be that the fetal heart has a limited ability to increase stroke volume (1) in this episode.

From all episodes a 1.5 h lasting one, taken at the fourth day after surgery with only spontaneous changes was taken and within this a single but typical FHR acceleration (Fig. 2, middle trace) selected and analysed in more detail. Above the FHR trace the mean pressure in the inferior vena cava P(ivc) and below the

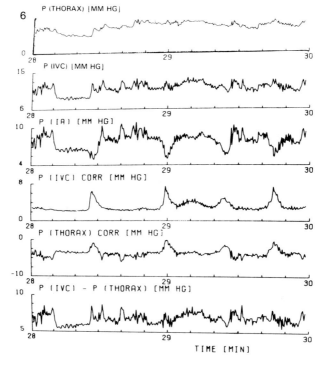

Figure 3. Original and for intra-amniotic pressure P(ia) corrected pressure traces for the same cutout as Fig. 2 with: P(thorax) intrathoracic, P(ivc) inferior vena cava. Bottom trace shows the result of trace 4 minus 5.

arterial end diastolic blood pressure (Pa) is shown. The top 6 traces refer to the left ventricle, while the bottom 6 are those for the right ventricle. While the FHR increases from 155 beats/min at resting level to 242 beats/min the values for the two SVs start from 2.95 ml and 5.63 ml and decrease to 2.50 ml and 4.32 ml, respectively. After these low SV values, both increase far above resting level to 3.73 ml and 6.20 ml. Thus the total amount of increase for the left ventricle is 1.23 ml and for the right ventricle, 1.88 ml, which related to the resting levels is about 40% and 33%. To underline this huge amount of SV increase, we found that the SV area below resting level compared to the SV area above resting level are as 1 to 5.3 and 1 to 4.9. The fetal cardiovascular control system seems to compensate the relatively low SV during a relatively short time of 6.34 s and 6.69 s by a 5 times bigger total SV lasting for about 39.6 s and 17.3 s, respectively.

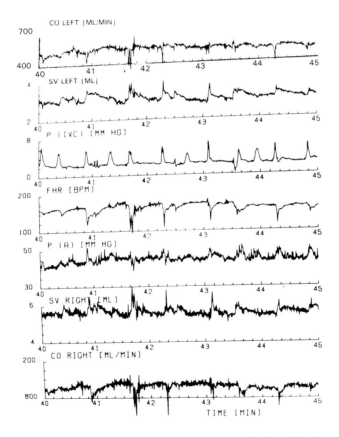

Figure 4. A 5 min cutout with several FHR decelerations. For the other traces refer to the text for Fig. 2.

These facts could be followed visually in the course of both CO traces. While the FHR values have already returned to the resting level, the CO values are still well above. Thus in this part, changes in CO are not based on FHR but on SV changes. In further details not the VET but the amplitude A is responsible for the increase in SV. Since in this episode all parameters show similar variation coefficients (2) of round about 5%, it is clear from Fig. 2, that nearly all parameters show a high variation, from 30–160%, after the event.

The P(ivc)—which might express the preload—was corrected by subtracting the intra-amniotic pressure P(ia). The fact, that the changes in P(ivc) from about 1.5 to 6 mmHg did neither affect the FHR nor the SV, was very surprising. We therefore analyzed the low pressure signals shown in Fig. 3. Since even this analysis does not give an indication that the event is reflected in one of these signals, we may conclude that it is not based primarily on the preload.

The P(a), as a measure of the afterload, which increases from resting level of 47.1 ± 0.95 mmHg to 56.4 ± 1.2 mmHg at maximum and decreases via 51.5 ± 0.86 mmHg at minute 29.25 to 49.8 ± 1.4 mmHg shows a clear correlation to the event.

It is worth mentioning that S for the left ventricle increases while SV(l) decreases and S for the right starts increasing when SV(r) increases from minimum.

About 10 min later, within the same episode, several FHR decelerations with SV accelerations occurred (Fig. 4). These, on the other hand, are closely correlated to the increasing values of P(ivc) and not that clear to the changing afterload.

From these more or less depictive findings we do not dare to conclude that FHR accelerations with decreasing and later increasing SV values are based on the interaction with afterload, while FHR decelerations with increasing SV values are accompanied by increasing preload.

References

1. Rudolph, A. M., Heymann, M. A. (1972). *Am. J. Obstet. Gynecol.* **124**, 183.
2. Morgenstern, J., Abels, T., Bender, K., Somville, T. (1985). *In*: 2nd International Conference "Fetal and Neonatal Physiological Measurements", Butterworth, London (to be published).

High Frequency Heart Rate Variability in the Fetal Lamb

G. J. Hofmeyr*, O. S. Bamford,
G. S. Dawes and M. J. Parkes

The Nuffield Institute for Medical Research,
University of Oxford, Oxford, UK

Introduction

In fetal lambs, during high voltage electrocortical activity the heart rate is increased (1,2). Dalton *et al.* (3) found that the heart rate varied consistently during breathing episodes in one or other direction in individual lambs. van der Wildt (2) found that during low voltage electrocortical activity the heart rate increased during breathing episodes, and more so after vagotomy.

Beat-to-beat fetal heart rate variability increases during breathing episodes in sheep (2,3) and man (4), and was not found to be associated with electrocortical state *per se* in the former (2,3).

During isocapnic hypoxia in sheep, beat-to-beat variation is greatly increased in spite of the absence of breathing (3,5). A similar increase occurs during adrenaline infusion (3). We have undertaken experiments to define further the association between fetal heart rate, activity states and hypoxia.

Methods

Fetal lambs were cannulated under general anaesthesia (3). In 4 fetuses the pons was transected under direct vision at the level of the inferior colliculus after removal of the cerebellum. Experiments were performed at 120–138 days' gestation, 4 or more days after operation. Fetal heart rate was measured as previously described (3) except that an AIM-65 microprocessor and a new measurement of short-term variability were used. Indices of beat-to-beat variation in common use compare each pulse interval with the preceding valid interval.

*Witwatersrand University Council overseas research fellow.

The Physiological Development of the Fetus and Newborn
ISBN 0 12 389080 2

Copyright © 1985 by Academic Press, London.
All rights of reproduction in any form reserved.

Therefore progressive changes in heart rate such as occur during decelerations are measured as beat-to-beat changes even in the absence of true short term variation. To minimize this error we have calculated the difference between each pulse interval and the mean of the preceding and subsequent intervals, averaged over 2 min epochs. In simulated runs this measurement was 15% lower than the 2-interval beat-to-beat difference for heart rates with high short-term and low long-term variation, and 61% lower for those with low short-term and high long-term variability. This measurement should be distinguished from others by a term such as "beat-to-beat deviation", but for the purposes of this paper we shall refer to the generally understood short-term variability.

Statistical comparisons in the hypoxia, naloxone and catecholamine experiments were paired for comparable breathing and electrocortical activity. Calculations were by the paired t test unless otherwise stated.

Results

Activity states

The mean heart rate in 8 intact fetuses (Fig. 1) was about 12% higher during high than low voltage electrocortical activity, with or without breathing. The

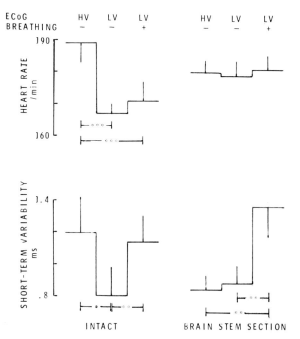

Figure 1. Comparison of heart rate and short-term variability between activity states in 8 intact fetuses and 4 with upper pontine brain stem section. (Mean values and standard error.) • =$P<0.05$; •• =$P<0.02$; ••• =$P<0.01$

small increase in heart rate during breathing episodes was not statistically significant. In 4 fetuses after brain stem section the heart rate was not significantly associated with fetal activity. When the fetuses were considered individually the heart rate was significantly greater during consecutive high than low voltage electrocortical episodes in one fetus, and during breathing episodes within low voltage electrocortical activity in two.

The short term variation in 8 intact fetuses was greater by about 60% during high voltage electrocortical activity and low voltage with breathing, compared with low voltage without breathing. There was no significant difference between high voltage without and low voltage electrocortical activity with breathing. When these states were compared in individual fetuses, there was a significant increase (mean 60%) during low voltage electrocortical activity with breathing in 3 and a decrease (mean 34%) in another 3 $(P<0.05)$.

After brain stem section there was no association between short-term variation and electrocortical state in the absence of breathing, but the increase during breathing episodes persisted.

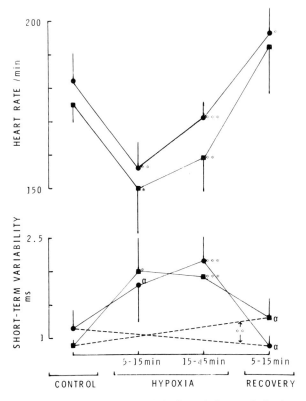

Figure 2. Heart rate and short-term variability before, during and after isocapnic hypoxia in 5 fetuses without (●) and 4 with (■) naloxone infusion. (Mean values and standard error.) Difference from control: α=trend; = $P<0.05$; = $P<0.02$; = $P<0.01$

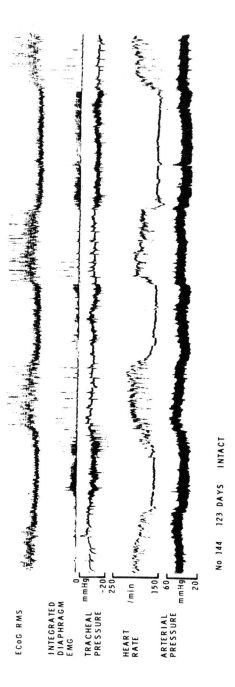

ECoG RMS

INTEGRATED
DIAPHRAGM
EMG

TRACHEAL   mmHg ⌐ 0
PRESSURE   ⌐ -20
                     ⌐ 250

HEART   /min
RATE   ⌐ 150

ARTERIAL   ⌐ 60
PRESSURE   mmHg ⌐ 20

No 144   123 DAYS   INTACT

Figure 3. A 70-min recording from an intact fetus to illustrate the association between electrocortical state and heart rate and variability.

Hypoxia

During isocapnic hypoxia (PO_2 21 ± 1.5 reduced to $12 \pm .5$ mmHg mean $\pm$ SEM by maternal inhalation of 8.5% O_2 mixture) in 5 intact fetuses the mean heart rate fell (see Fig. 2). During recovery it was increased above the control value. Short-term variability was greatly increased during hypoxia, and fell during recovery to slightly below the control value. Naloxone infusion (Norcan, DuPont, 0.8 mg followed by 1.6 mg/h) did not significantly alter the heart rate or short-term variation or their response to hypoxia (PO_2 18 ± 1.3 to 12 ± 1.1 mmHg) except that after hypoxia the short-term variation remained above the control value. The difference between control and recovery values was significantly different from that measured without naloxone ($P < 0.02$, unpaired t test).

Catecholamine infusions

Both adrenaline and noradrenaline (1.3 μg/min infused into the inferior vena cava to reproduce levels occurring during hypoxia[6]) infusion caused a large increase in short-term variation (1.2 ± 0.25 increased to 4.9 ± 1.7 and 0.93 ± 0.2 to 3.8 ± 0.7 ms respectively), which did not return to control values within the subsequent 15 min (2.1 ± 0.3 and 1.6 ± 0.2 ms).

Discussion

The increased heart rate and short-term variability during high voltage electrocortical activity may reflect cyclical alteration in autonomic tone accompanying electrocortical changes. If so, this autonomic cyling is either abolished or dissociated from electrocortical state by brain stem section. The effect of breathing upon short-term variability, however, is not dependent upon suprapontine mechanisms. Our finding of greater short-term variation during high than low voltage electrocortical activity without breathing differs from previous studies (2,3). The reason may be that much of the time in low voltage electrocortical state without breathing occurs shortly after changes from high voltage when falling heart rate may contribute to the short-term variability measured by indices using comparisons between pairs of pulse intervals only.

Opioid peptides are thought to decrease heart rate variability. During hypoxia certain peptides such as β-endorphin and β-lipotropin increase 3–4 fold (7). Their effect upon short-term variability during hypoxia, if any, is clearly overridden by some other factor, possibly catecholamines. Persistently elevated opioids may, however, be responsible for the abrupt decrease to or below control values in short-term variability after hypoxia, as this was significantly impaired by naloxone infusion and did not occur after catecholamine infusion without hypoxia. The mechanism may be similar to the depression of movements and heart rate variability and accelerations observed in human fetuses during recovery from a period of manipulation for attempted external cephalic version (8).

Conclusions

We conclude that cycles of high and low heart rate are either abolished or dissociated from electrocortical cycles by brain stem section; that the effect of breathing upon short-term variability is not dependent upon suprapontine mechanisms; and that opioid peptides may cause the abrupt fall of short-term variability after hypoxia.

Acknowledgements

We thank the MRC for a grant to Professor Dawes, and the Royal College of Obstetricians and Gynaecologists, South African Regional Council for a grant to Dr Hofmeyr.

References

1. Ruckebusch, Y., Gaujox, M. and Eghbali, B. (1977). *Neurophysiol.* **42**, 226–237.
2. van der Wildt, B. (1982). Doctoral thesis, University of Nijmegen, Holland.
3. Dalton, K. J., Dawes, G. S. and Patrick, J. E. (1977). *Am. J. Obstet. Gynecol.* **127**, 414–424.
4. Campogrande, M., Alemanno, M. G. Viora, E. and Bussolini, S. (1982). *J. Perinat. Med.* **10**, 203–208.
5. Stänge, L., Rosén, K. G., Hökegård, K.-H., Karlsson, K., Rochlitzer, F., Kjellmer, I. and Joelsson, I. (1977). *Acta Obstet. Gynecol. Scand.* **56**, 205–209.
6. Jones, C. T. and Ritchie, J. W. K. (1978). *J. Physiol.* **285**, 381–393.
7. Wardlaw, G. L., Stark, R. I., Daniel, S. and Frantz, A. G. (1981). *Endocrinology* **108**, 1710–1715.
8. Hofmeyr, G. J. and Sonnendecker, E. W. W. (1983). *Br. J. Obstet. Gynaecol.* **90**, 914–918.

Effects of Feeding and Haemorrhage on the Femoral Circulation of Developing Swine

Alice C. Yao, Phyllis M. Gootman,*
Patricia Pierce and Steven M. DiRusso

Departments of Pediatrics and Physiology*, Downstate Medical Center,
State University of New York, USA

Introduction

In the term newborn infant, lower limb blood flow decreased within 30 min after feeding, followed by an increase (above control) at 2–3 h (1). These results suggest a redistribution of peripheral blood flow to favour increased splanchnic circulatory demand. Since clinically, the splanchnic circulation is not readily accessible, measuring limb blood flow has provided an indirect method for investigations of cardiovascular (CV) responses to feeding. In order to verify the results obtained in clinical studies, in this paper, we present the femoral vascular responses of neonatal swine to feeding and feeding following haemorrhage. This study was carried out as part of a larger investigation concerning the effects of feeding on regional blood flows including the superior mesenteric circulation (2,3).

Methods

Piglets, 3 h–4 weeks old (fasted 2–12 h), were lightly anaesthetized with 0.25% halothane in O_2, immobilized with decamethonium-Br and artificially ventilated. Blood gases and pH were maintained within normal limits. The right femoral (Fem) artery was catheterized for blood sampling and aortic pressure (AoP) monitoring. Fem blood flow (F), measured with an electromagnetic flow probe on the left Fem artery, was recorded continuously with EKG and AoP. Fem vascular resistance (R) was calculated from the ratio of mean AoP (MAP) to mean Fem F. Postprandial measurements were compared to control values and the

The Physiological Development of the Fetus and Newborn
ISBN 0 12 389080 2

Copyright © 1985 by Academic Press, London.
All rights of reproduction in any form reserved.

compared to zero change to determine statistical significance of the observed change by a paired sample *t* test and cross-comparisons were made using analysis of variance with repeated measures; $P \leq 0.05$ was accepted as statistically significant. Values are expressed in mean $\pm$ SEM.

Group I: Feeding (26 ml/kg of commercially formulated milk: Similac) was accomplished by gavage via a tube in the stomach in piglets aged ≤ 2 days ($n = 6$) and 2–4 weeks ($n = 16$) old. Physiologic measurements were continuously recorded for 2 h after feeding.

Group II: Piglets, ≤ 2 days ($n = 5$) and 2–4 weeks ($n = 8$) old, were bled by withdrawing 15% of the estimated blood volume (4) from the femoral arterial catheter. After a stabilization period of 30–45 min, posthaemorrhage baseline recordings were obtained and the feeding protocol was carried out as in Group I.

Results

Group I: There were no significant changes in heart rate (HR) or MAP following feeding in all piglets studied (Table 1). Figure 1 shows that no significant Fem F

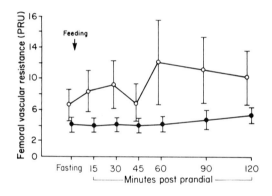

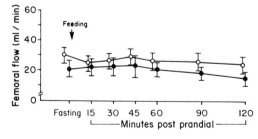

Figure 1. Postprandial changes in femoral arterial flow (lower panel) and femoral vascular resistance (upper panel) of developing swine. In swine 2–4 weeks old, the decreases in femoral flows were statistically significant at 15, 30, 90 and 120 min ($P < 0.05$). There was a trend towards increased femoral vascular resistance, significant at 15, 30, 90 and 120 min ($0.01 < P < 0.05$). ●≤2 days old, ○2–4 weeks old, ⚊ mean ± SEM.

Table 1. Control and maximal postprandial changes in mean aortic pressure (MAP) and heart rate (HR)

Measurement	Group	Age ≤2 days		2-4 weeks	
		Control	Postprandial	Control	Postprandial
MAP (mmHg)	I	65.0±4.7	63.3± 4.6	90.9± 2.5	87.2± 2.9
	II	57.8±3.8	54.6± 2.6	80.6± 3.2	85.0± 2.8
HR (bpm)	I	198.2±7.7	207.9± 9.2	210.9±11.2	200.1± 7.6
	II	219.4±8.9	196.4±11.2	241.7±10.6	210.9±10.9

Group I feeding only, Group II feeding following haemorrhage, P values, NS.

Table 2. Control data before and after haemorrhage (Group II)

Age	Fem F (ml/min)	Fem R (PRU)	MAP (mmHg)	PP (mmHg)	HR (bpm)
≤2 days Before	16.1± 4.6	6.9±2.8	61.7±4.7	42.0±2.6	204.0± 8.8
After	11.0± 3.6	7.9±2.5	57.8±3.8	37.6±3.0	219.4± 8.9
2-4 weeks Before	37.1±10.6*	5.7±2.8[+]	87.6±5.2*	55.6±3.8**	210.3±12.1**
After	23.0± 6.1	9.7±4.4	80.6±3.2	42.9±1.8	241.7±10.6

Student t test, pre-*vs* posthaemorrhage values *$P<0.05$, **$P<0.01$, [+]$P=0.07$, MAP, mean aortic pressure, PP, pulse pressure, HR, heart rate.

or FEM R changes occurred postprandially in piglets ≤2 days old. On the other hand, in swine 2-4 weeks old Fem F decreased (15-25%) significantly ($P<0.05$) for 15-120 min. There was a trend towards increased Fem R (30-39%); per cent change was statistically significant from control.

Group II: In all animals after haemorrhage, Fem F, MAP and pulse pressure (PP) decreased while Fem R and HR increased (Table 2). The changes were statistically significant in animals 2-4 weeks old. After feeding there was a trend towards decreased HR and MAP (see Table 1) in the younger piglets. There were no significant changes in Fem F and Fem R (Fig. 2). In piglets 2-4 weeks of age, PP significantly increased (21-24%) after feeding (42.9±1.8 to 54.9±4.8 mmHg) without significant changes in HR or MAP (Table 1). As shown in Fig. 2, there was a trend toward an increase in Fem F and a decrease in Fem R 45-90 min postprandially. Fem F significantly increased 40-45% at 45-60 min while Fem R significantly decreased 23-29% at 45-90 min postprandially.

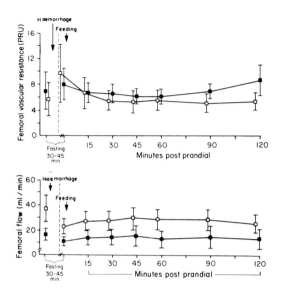

Figure 2. Postprandial changes in femoral arterial flow (lower panel) and femoral vascular resistance (upper panel) after haemorrhage (15% estimated blood volume, (4)) showing a trend towards an increase in blood flow and a decrease in vascular resistance in piglets 2-4 weeks old. The percent changes from control were statistically significant (see text). ■ ≤2 days old, ○ 2-4 weeks old, $\bar{\mathbf{I}}$ mean±SEM.

Discussion

This study demonstrated that in piglets ≤2 days old, there were no significant responses of the Fem vasculature to feeding or feeding following haemorrhage. However, in piglets 2-4 weeks old, Fem vasoconstriction occurred following feeding, suggesting a redistribution of regional blood flow flavouring the splanchnic circulation; mesenteric vasodilation has been reported by us to occur postprandially (2,3). After haemorrhage of 15% of the blood volume, feeding again did not elicit changes in the Fem vascular bed in piglets ≤2 days old. On the other hand, Fem F increased in those 2-4 weeks old. This increased Fem F was the reverse of the postprandial responses observed in piglets of the same age without haemorrhage. This data suggests that the older swine were able to compensate for the stress of haemorrhage. The increase in PP and regional arterial flows, e.g. mesenteric (3), with feeding support this explanation. Although these results are not directly comparable to the human study because of species differences and the acute experimental state, it is interesting to find that in the piglets 2-4 weeks of age, Fem F decreased with feeding, a response similar to that reported for term newborn infants (1). The lack of significant Fem vascular response in the ≤2 day olds may be comparable to the lack of limb blood flow changes in some premature infants with feeding (5). These results probably also reflect the absence of tonic sympathetic vasoconstrictor tone to the femoral vasculature in very young piglets (6,7).

Thus feeding alone, or feeding following haemorrhage, did not induce a significant change in the Fem vascular bed of piglets ≤ 2 days old. In those 2–4 weeks old, Fem vasoconstriction occurred to feeding, as shown by significant falls in Fem F with a tendency towards increased Fem R. In relation to findings of postprandial increased mesenteric blood flow (2,3), our results support those reported in the clinical literature suggesting a redistribution of blood flow from the peripheral to the splanchnic region. Following haemorrhage, the 2–4-week-old piglets were able to continue to respond to feeding in the presence of reflex circulatory responses to hypotension. Fem F increased as part of an overall circulatory response to feeding. Thus in the older piglets, the CV controlling system is capable of responding to at least two dissimilar pertubations.

Acknowledgements

This work was supported by a USPHS grant HL-20864 from the HLBI of NIH awarded to PMG.

References

1. Yao, A. C., Wallgren, C. G., Sinha, S. N. and Lind, J. (1971). *Pediatrics* **47**, 378–382.
2. Yao, A. C., Gootman, P. M., Pierce, P. J. and DiRusso, S. M. (1984). *Am. J. Physiol.* (in revision).
3. Yao, A. C., Gootman, P. M., Pierce, P. J. and DiRusso, S. M. (1984). *Pediat. Res.* **18**, 218A.
4. Buckley, B. J., Gootman, N., Nagelberg, J. S., Griswold, P. G. and Gootman, P. M. (1984). *Am. J. Physiol.* (in press).
5. Raziuddin, K., Kim, M. H. and Yao, A. C. (1984). *J. Pediat. Gastroenterol. Nutr.* **3**, 89–94.
6. Buckley, N. M., Brazeau, P., Frasier, I. D. and Gootman, P. M. (1981). *Am. J. Physiol.* **240**, H505–H510.
7. Buckley, N. M., Brazeau, P. and Gootman, P. M. (1983). *Fed. Proc.* **42**, 1643–1647.

The Effects of Leukotriene Inhibition on the Perinatal Pulmonary Circulation in the Lamb

Scott J. Soifer, Michael D. Schreiber, Robert D. Loitz, Christine Roman and Michael A. Heymann

Cardiovascular Research Institute, and
Departments of Pediatrics, Physiology, and Obstetrics, Gynecology, and
Reproductive Sciences, University of California, San Francisco,
California, USA

The mechanisms through which the increased pulmonary vascular resistance and the decreased pulmonary blood flow in the fetus is maintained and the mediators of hypoxic pulmonary vasoconstriction in older animals are unknown. The cyclo-oxygenase metabolites of arachadonic acid including prostaglandin (PG) E_2, prostacyclin, PGI_2, and PGD_2 decrease pulmonary vascular resistance and increase pulmonary blood flow in fetal and newborn sheep and goats (1,2,3). Other cyclo-oxygenase metabolites including PGF_2 and thromboxane A_2 increase pulmonary vascular resistance and decrease pulmonary blood flow (2,4). Leukotrienes, the slow reacting substance of anaphylaxis, are the products of $5'$-lipoxygenation of arachadonic acid. Leukotrienes C_4 and D_4 induce smooth muscle contraction and pulmonary hypertension in several animal species (5,6,7). Selective antagonism of leukotriene action by FPL 57231 (Fisons, plc, Loughborough, UK) attenuates hypoxic pulmonary vasoconstriction in adult sheep (8). In order to evaluate the possible role of leukotrienes in the perinatal control of pulmonary blood flow and vascular resistance, the circulatory effects of leukotriene inhibition were studied in late gestational fetal and newborn lambs.

Methods

Fetal studies

Seven mixed-breed western pregnant ewes were operated on under epidural anaesthesia, at 138 days gestation, to expose the fetus. Using local anaesthesia,

The Physiological Development of the Fetus and Newborn
ISBN 0 12 389080 2

Copyright © 1985 by Academic Press, London.
All rights of reproduction in any form reserved.

polyvinyl catheters were placed in the fetal inferior and superior vena cavae, descending and ascending aorta, main and left pulmonary arteries and the amniotic cavity. All catheters were secured in a pouch on the ewe's flank. Two days were allowed for recovery.

Heart rate, amniotic, venous, systemic and pulmonary arterial pressures were measured. Pulmonary blood flow was measured by the inferior vena caval injection of 15 micron radionuclide labelled microspheres with a reference sample withdrawn from the main pulmonary artery (9). Pulmonary vascular resistance was calculated.

Pulmonary blood flow, the other haemodynamic variables and descending aortic blood gases were measured during the preinfusion period. In 5 fetuses, FPL 57231 was dissolved in sterile water and infused into the left pulmonary artery at 1.2 to 2.4 mg/kg/min for 60 min. Measurements of the haemodynamic variables were repeated at the end of the infusion. Two other fetuses received an equal volume infusion of sterile water without drug. At the end of the study, the fetus and ewe were killed by an overdose of sodium pentobarbital. Fetal organs were removed for microsphere analysis. The differences in the haemodynamic variables and blood gases between the preinfusion and infusion periods were compared by a paired t test. $P < 0.05$ was considered statistically significant.

Newborn studies

Six newborn lambs, 3–7 days of age, were operated on under local anaesthesia. Polyvinyl catheters were placed in the inferior vena cava, and ascending and descending aorta. A no. 5 French thermodilution catheter was advanced from the internal jugular vein to the pulmonary artery to measure right atrial, pulmonary arterial and capillary wedge pressures. Cardiac output was measured intermittently. The absence of intracardiac shunting was determined by modified indicator dilution techniques. Arterial blood gases were measured. Pulmonary and systemic vascular resistances were calculated. All lambs received FPL 57231 prior to the onset of hypoxia. Five of the lambs also received FPL 57231 during hypoxia. The lambs were studied, resting in an animal sling.

Infusion of FPL 57231 prior to hypoxia

Two hours after surgery, the haemodynamic variables were measured during normoxia. FPL 57231 was then infused at 1 mg/kg/min. After 10 min, the haemodynamic variables were measured. While the infusion continued, isocarbic hypoxia was induced by placing a loosely fitting bag over the lamb's head and decreasing the inspired oxygen concentration by the addition of nitrogen and carbon dioxide to the gas mixture to produce stable pulmonary hypertension. The haemodynamic variables were measured after 10 min. The infusion was stopped and the lamb was returned to normoxia: 2–24 h were allowed for recovery.

Infusion of FPL 57231 during hypoxia

The haemodynamic variables were measured during normoxia. Isocarbic hypoxia was then induced. The haemodynamic variables were measured. During hypoxia,

FPL 57231 was infused at 2 mg/kg/min into the inferior vena cava. The haemodynamic variables were measured after 10 min of infusion. The infusion was stopped and the lamb returned to its mother. The differences in the haemodynamic variables and blood gases between the experimental conditions were analysed by analysis of variance.

Results

Fetal studies

During the infusion of FPL 57231, there was a 7-fold increase in pulmonary blood from 160.5 ± 136.9 to 1156.6 ± 265.2 ml/100g/min (mean $\pm$ SD) ($P < 0.05$) and an 11-fold decrease in pulmonary vascular resistance from 0.47 ± 0.30 to 0.04 ± 0.02 mmHg/ml/100g/min ($P < 0.05$). Pulmonary arterial pressure decreased from 55.2 ± 5.9 to 45.4 ± 8.6 mmHg and systemic arterial pressure from 55.1 ± 7.0 to 45.5 ± 9.5 mmHg. Heart rate increased from 175.2 ± 19.2 to 240.0 ± 50.0/min ($P < 0.05$). These haemodynamic changes occur despite deterioration in fetal descending aortic blood gases. PO_2 was not changed by the infusion. PCO_2 increased from 49.4 ± 1.1 to 56.6 ± 6.6 mmHg and pH decreased from 7.38 ± 0.01 to 7.28 ± 0.06 ($P < 0.05$). Infusion of sterile water vehicle produced no haemodynamic effect.

Newborn studies (Table 1)

Hypoxia produced significant haemodynamic effects. There was a 73% increase in pulmonary arterial pressure (PAP) ($P < 0.05$) and a 62% increase in pulmonary vascular resistance (PVR) ($P < 0.05$). During normoxia, the infusion of FPL 57231 produced no significant haemodynamic effects. When hypoxia was induced and the infusion of FPL 57231 continued, pulmonary arterial pressure increased by only 7% and pulmonary vascular resistance decreased by 10%. Pulmonary arterial pressure and vascular resistance were significantly lower than during hypoxia without FPL 57231 ($P < 0.05$).

Table 1

	PAP (mmHg)	PVR (mmHg/l/kg/m)	SAP (mmHg)	CO (l/kg/min)
Infusion of FPL 57231 prior to hypoxia				
Normoxia	18.4 ± 2.7	47.1 ± 4.8	68.3 ± 5.8	0.4 ± 0.1
Normoxia + Drug	17.9 ± 2.2	49.0 ± 6.6	65.7 ± 9.2	0.4 ± 0.1
Hypoxia + Drug	19.6 ± 3.6	42.4 ± 5.9	63.9 ± 9.3	0.5 ± 0.1
Infusion of FPL 57231 during hypoxia				
Normoxia	17.5 ± 2.9	43.1 ± 8.8	68.5 ± 10.5	0.4 ± 0.1
Hypoxia	$30.3 \pm 4.7*$	$70.3 \pm 15.5*$	71.0 ± 12.4	0.5 ± 0.1
Hypoxia + Drug	19.8 ± 3.6	44.0 ± 7.6	64.5 ± 11.1	0.5 ± 0.1

Mean $\pm$ SD. $*P < 0.05$

With the infusion of FPL 57231 during hypoxia, there was a 35% decrease in pulmonary arterial pressure ($P < 0.05$) and a 37% decrease in pulmonary vascular resistance ($P < 0.05$). Pulmonary arterial pressure and vascular resistance were similar to normoxia. Cardiac output (CO), heart rate and systemic arterial pressure (SAP) were unchanged. Arterial blood gases during normoxia with or without FPL 57231 were similar, as were the arterial blood gases during hypoxia with or without FPL 57231.

Discussion

This study shows that an infusion of FPL 57231 markedly increases pulmonary blood flow and decreases pulmonary vascular resistance in fetal lambs. These changes are similar in magnitude to those seen with the initiation of ventilation. FPL 57231 attenuates hypoxic pulmonary vasoconstriction in the newborn lamb. Whether these effects are primarily due to leukotriene antagonism, or to inhibition or activation of other substances, or to direct vascular effects of the compound is not known.

Administration of leukotrienes to guinea pig perfused lungs and rats peritoneal mononuclear cells results in an increased production of the cyclo-oxygenase metabolites PGE2, PGI2 and thromboxane A2 (10,11). Some of the smooth muscle constricting effects of leukotrienes can be antagonized by blocking the formation of thromboxane A2. Hypoxic pulmonary vasoconstriction in the adult sheep cannot be blocked by the cyclo-oxygenase inhibitor, indomethacin, but can by the leukotriene antagonist FPL 57231 (8). FPL 55712 (Fison, plc), another leukotriene inhibitor, is a potent inhibitor of thromboxane synthetase in human platelets (12). Whether FPL 57231 shows similar effects is not known. Continued research on the interaction between the cyclo-oxygenase and lipoxygenase pathways is needed.

The market increase in pulmonary blood flow in the fetal lamb produced by FPL 57231 was associated with deteriorating arterial blood gases with hypercarbia and acidosis. FPL 57231 induces pulmonary vasodilation which leads to a marked increase in pulmonary blood flow, inadequate return of blood to the placenta and acidosis. Constriction of the ductus arteriosis or an increase in cardiac output cannot explain these changes. Constriction of the ductus arteriosis by aspirin produces a large increase in pulmonary arterial pressure and a small increase in pulmonary blood flow (13). In this study, there was no evidence for ductal constriction as pulmonary arterial pressure decreased, and the difference between the mean pulmonary and descending aortic pressures were unchanged during the infusion. FPL 55712 also has little effect on isolated ductal strips in concentrations used in this study (14).

FPL 57231, a leukotriene antagonist, produced a marked increase in pulmonary blood flow in fetal lamb and attenuation of hypoxic pulmonary vasoconstriction in newborn lambs. Leukotrienes are present in tracheal fluid of fetal lambs near term and have been isolated from lung lavage fluid from newborns with pulmonary hypertension (15). Leukotrienes may play an important role in the pulmonary vascular changes which occur at birth.

Acknowledgements

This work was supported in part by the American Lung Association and US Public Health Service Program Project Grant HL 24056. Dr Soifer is recipient of New Investigators Award HL 29941 from the NHLBI.

References

1. Cassin, S., Tyler, T., Leffler, C. *et al.* (1979). *Am. J. Physiol.* **236**, H828–H834.
2. Lock, J. E., Olley, P. M. and Coceani, F. (1980). *Am. J. Physiol.* **238**, H631–H638.
3. Soifer, S. J., Morin, F. C. and Heymann, M. A. (1982). *J. Pediat.* **100**, 458–463.
4. Cartwright, D., Soifer, S., Mauray, F. and Clyman, R. (1983). *Pediat. Res.* **17**, 306A.
5. Hand, J. M., Wall, J. A. and Buckner, C. K. (1981). *Eur. J. Pharm.* **76**, 439–442.
6. Hanna, C. J., Bach, M. K., Pare, P. D., and Schellenberg, R. R. (1981). *Nature* **290**, 343–344.
7. Yokochi, K., Olley, P. M., Sideris, E. and Hamilton, F. (1981). *In:* "Leukotrienes and Other Lipoxygenase Products", (Samuelesson, B. and Paoletti, R. eds) pp. 211–214, Raven Press, New York.
8. Ahmed, T. and Oliver, W. (1983). *Am. Rev. Resp. Dis.* **127**, 566–571.
9. Heymann, M. A., Payne, B. D., Hoffman, J. I. E. and Rudolph, A. M. (1977). *Prog. Cardiovasc. Dis.* **20**, 55–79.
10. Folco, G., Hansson, G. and Granstrom, E. (1981). *Biochem. Pharmacol.* **30**, 2491–2493.
11. Feuerstein, N., Folgh, M. and Ramwell, P. M. (1981). *Br. J. Pharmacol.* **72**, 389–391.
12. Welton, A. F., Hope, W. C., Tobias, L. D. and Hamilton, J. G. (1981). *Biochem. Pharmacol.* **30**, 1378–1382.
13. Heymann, M. A. and Rudolph, A. M. (1976). *Circulat. Res.* **38**, 418–422.
14. Coceani, F., Jhamondas, V. M., Bodach, E., Labur, J. *et al.* (1982). *Can. J. Physiol. Pharmacol.* **60**, 345–349.
15. Stenmark, K. R., James, S. L., Voelkel, N. F. and Toews, W. H. (1983). *New Engl. J. Med.* **309**, 77–80.

Studies on the Physiology and Pathophysiology of Preterm and Term Foals

P. D. Rossdale and J. C. Ousey

Beaufort Cottage Stables, Newmarket, Cambridgeshire, UK

Introduction

Equine prematurity is characterized by foals of low birthweight, delivered in the period 300–320 days gestation (0.88–0.94 of term: mean 340 days) (1). Premature foals exhibit weak reflex responses and other neurological signs, hyperextension of the "fetlock" joints and, sometimes, have an undernourished appearance, a silky coat and red tongue. From two surveys of limited numbers, the incidence of prematurity among Thoroughbreds appears to be about 10% (1,2) of which there is approximately 20% mortality (2). Full-term foals showing signs of prematurity, often associated with evidence of placental pathology, are described as dysmature (1).

Aims

An experimental and field investigation into the physiology and pathophysiology of premature and dysmature foals has been performed since 1978, in order to further understanding of the pathogenesis of these conditions and thereby to provide an improved basis for diagnosis and therapy.

Materials and Methods

A herd of 16 mixed breed ponies has been used in each breeding season for experimental protocols. The majority of mares were induced to foal with oxytocin or a synthetic prostaglandin $F_2\alpha$ analogue (fluprostenol: Equimate, ICI). The decision to induce was determined, in part, by gestational age and partly by electrolyte concentrations (calcium, sodium and potassium) in mammary secretions. Details of delivery and sampling protocol are described elsewhere (3).

The Physiological Development of the Fetus and Newborn
ISBN 0 12 389080 2

Copyright © 1985 by Academic Press, London.
All rights of reproduction in any form reserved.

P. D. Rossdale and J. C. Ousey

Results

Forty-five foals were delivered in the 1981–1983 foaling seasons. They were of differing states of maturity which have been subsequently classified into 3 groups (4): premature, mature and intermediate ("twilight"). Significant differences were found between premature and mature (full term) foals in adrenal activity (5), glucose metabolism (6), renin angiotensin aldosterone (RAA) function (7) and haematological parameters (8).

Premature foals have low levels of plasma cortisol during the first 2 h postpartum and fail to respond to endogenous ACTH or to the administration of exogenous $ACTH_{1-24}$, compared with full-term foals. Total white blood cell count and neutrophil:lymphocyte ratio which have been shown to be a convenient clinical measurement which reflects changes in adrenocortical activity in the foal.

Endogenous ACTH concentrations fell in the 30 min following delivery of full-term foals but showed a peak in those delivered prematurely. Higher concentrations of plasma glucose and insulin, and a marked response of insulin concentrations following glucose infusion, were found in full-term, compared with premature, foals. Plasma renin substrate was higher in premature, compared with full-term, foals immediately following delivery; and blood gas and acid base status was initially less optimal and tended to decline in individuals born prematurely.

Some individuals displayed characteristics of both groups. For example, 3 individuals had a small rise in plasma cortisol postpartum, in contrast to the considerable increase found in full term foals and little or no increase in premature foals.

Concentrations of mammary secretion electrolytes showed some correlation with the adaptive responses of the foal. Calcium and potassium levels exceeding 10.0 and 30.0 mmol/l respectively and sodium levels of less than 35 mmol/l were associated with the delivery of foals that appeared physiologically to be full term following induction. In contrast, calcium and potassium were less than 3.0 and 10.0 mmol/l respectively and sodium greater than 100 mmol/l were associated with foals which appeared to be physiologically premature.

Discussion

This work has established that, even within the normal range of full-term gestation (320–360 days), induced delivery produces foals at varying stages of maturity. The investigation has shown that premature foals may be structurally mature but functional maturity of various physiological systems, particularly adrenocortical activity, is incomplete. Full-term mature foals are well adapted to extra-uterine existence and can respond to various challenge tests, such as $ACTH_{1-24}$, glucose and insulin.

The exact relationship between electrolyte concentrations of mammary secretion and foal maturity has not been established but it appears, from our data, that the events are parallel rather than directly related. However, once "full-term" concentrations are achieved in mammary secretions of multiparous mares, the foetus is mature and ready for birth. Primiparous mares may be an exception and this aspect is currently under further investigation.

Having established the physiological inadequacies of premature foals, current work is in progress to develop effective protocols of therapy. Administration of long acting $ACTH_{1-24}$ (Depot Synacthen: Ciba Laboratories) and cortisol (Efcortelan; Glaxo Laboratories) have been shown to improve the general condition and, in particular, the haematological values of premature foals. An osmotic minipump (Alzet; Scientific Marketing Associates, London) implanted subcutaneously has been used to deliver a dose of 0.5 mg cortisol/h and, in combination with 1 mg Depot Synacthen administered in 3 divided doses during the first 24 h appeared to improve adrenocortical activity.

Acknowledgements

The project has been financed, in part, by the Wellcome Trust, the Horserace Betting Levy Board and the Animal Health Trust. Invaluable collaborative support has been provided by Drs Silver and Fowden of the Physiological Laboratory, Cambridge, and Dr Broughton Pipkin of the Queens Medical Centre, University Hospital, Nottingham.

References

1. Rossdale, P. D. (1976). *Proc. Roy. Soc. Med.* **69**, 631–632.
2. Laing, J. A. and Leech, F. B. (1975). *J. Reprod. Fertil.* **32** (suppl.) 307–310.
3. Rossdale, P. D., Ousey, J. C., Silver, M., Dudan, F. E., Jeffcott, L. B., Leadon, D. P., Cash, R. S. G., Fowden, A. L., Broughton Pipkin, F. and Reddy, R. (1984). *Equine Vet. J.* **16**, 275–278.
4. Rossdale, P. D., Ousey, J. C., Silver, M. and Fowden, A. L. (1984). *Equine Vet. J.* **16**, 300–302.
5. Silver, M., Ousey, J. C., Dudan, F. E., Fowden, A. L., Knox, J., Cash, R. S. G. and Rossdale, P. D. (1984). *Equine Vet. J.* **16**, 278–286.
6. Fowden, A. L., Silver, M., Ellis, L., Ousey, J. C. and Rossdale, P. D. (1984). *Equine Vet. J.* **16**, 286–291.
7. Broughton Pipkin, F., Ousey, J. C., Wallace, C. and Rossdale, P. D. (1984). *Equine Vet. J.* **16**, 292–297.
8. Jeffcott, L. B., Rossdale, P. D. and Leadon, D. P. (1982). *J. Reprod. Fert.* **32** (suppl.) 537–544.

The Relationship between Cerebral, Cardiovascular and Metabolic Functions during Labour in the Lamb Fetus

K. G. Rosén, H. Lilja,* K.-H. Hökegård* and I. Kjellmer

Departments of Physiology, Pediatrics I and Obstetrics and Gynecology,*
University of Göteborg, Göteborg, Sweden

Asphyxia, a well known cause of perinatal mortality and morbidity, has been the subject of numerous studies both experimentally and clinically. The experimental model has applied different means of inducing fetal asphyxia such as administration of gas mixtures with low oxygen to the mother, reduction of maternal placenta blood flow and occlusion of the umbilical vessels. Depending on the aim of the study all these models could give relevant information. However, it would be desirable to be able to follow the natural course of asphyxia in an experimental model during labour in order to mimic the main threat to intact survival of the fetus at term.

Previous work from our group have been focussed on the evaluation of waveform changes in the fetal ECG as a mean for fetal surveillance (1–3). The main response consists of a progressive increase in T wave amplitude, quantified by the T/QRS ratio and related to the anaerobic breakdown of myocardial glycogen. Thus, appearing as a sign of negative myocardial energy balance. The aim of the present study was to compare different means of fetal surveillance with special emphasis on ST waveform analysis of the fetal ECG during spontaneous labour in the chronically catheterized fetal lamb.

Methods

The data presented are 2 case reports both ending in intra-uterine death due to fetal asphyxia. The fetuses were operated on 28 and 11 days prior to labour with

The Physiological Development of the Fetus and Newborn
ISBN 0 12 389080 2

Copyright © 1985 by Academic Press, London.
All rights of reproduction in any form reserved.

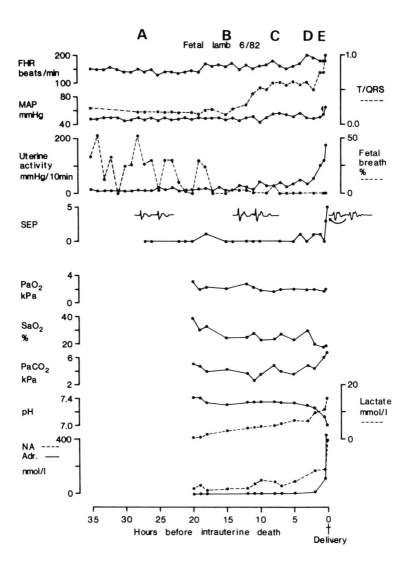

Figure 1. Recordings from a mature fetal lamb in spontaneous labour. MAP = mean arterial pressure. SEP = somato-sensory evoked potentials. The SEP was quantified according to a scoring system (4). Grade 0 = unaffected response, grade 1-2 = 30-50% reduction in amplitude indication slight asphyxia, grade 3 = more than 50% reduction in amplitude with no secondary component indicating a more severe asphyxia. Grade 5 shows no response at all and indicates cerebral death. Examples of ipsi and contralateral responses are given in the graph.

catheters placed in the carotid artery, for blood pressure recording and blood sampling, and in the trachea for detection of fetal breathing (F.br.) activity. The fetal ECG was recorded as a precordial lead. Fetal heart rate was recorded from the arterial puls. Fetal cortical activity was obtained from somatosensory evoked EEG potentials (SEP) by means of a tactile stimulator on the left nostril and EEG electrodes screwed into the bond over the supra sylvian gyrus on both sides. A microprocessor system was used for SEP averaging. The metabolic status was judged from blood gases, oxygen saturation, pH, lactate and plasma levels of noradrenaline and adrenaline. Uterine activity was recorded as the sum of maximal uterine pressures measured during a 10 min period.

Results

Case 1, 143 days gestation

The recordings made during 35 h of labour are presented in Fig. 1. The outcome was fetal death at time of delivery due to progressive increase in severity of asphyxia. Seventeen hours prior to death SaO_2 fell to 24% and a primary apnoea appeared. No F.br. was thereafter recorded until gasping during the last hour and the time for "last gasp" was 5 min before death. FHR was largely unaltered (140–150 beats (min) until the last 3 hours where a tachycardia (200 beats/min) was seen. Bradycardia and fall in blood pressure appeared during the last 5 min. Significant ST waveform changes occurred during the last 12 h of labour with a progressive increase in T wave amplitude in parallel with an increase in uterine activity and the degree of hypoxia.

The fetal brain showed a remarkable capacity to maintain its functional integrity and not until the last 30 min a rapid deterioration occurred with brain death 6 min before the last heart beat.

Metabolically PO_2 showed a relative hypoxaemia with values of 1.7–2.0 kPa. SaO_2 fell progressively from 39 to 19%. No acidosis appeared until the last 2 hours. Lactate increased progressively from 0.5 to 14.07 mmol/l. Noradrenaline was elevated at 11 h to levels around 80 nmol/l and showed a very marked increase to 386 nmol/l before death. Adrenaline was elevated at 7 h and rose to 438 nmol/l.

Case 2, 125 days gestation (Fig. 2)

The cardiovascular variables revealed compensatory changes with a tachycardia, FHR between 190 and 270 beats/min, and elevated blood pressure from 45 to 70 mmHg. The T/QRS ratio increased from 0.30 to 0.80 between 14 and 9½ hours before fetal death. Thereafter a T/QRS level of 0.60 was reached. Circulating catecholamines was elevated throughout the recording period with an increase from 9.65 to 60.69 nmol/l (noradrenaline) and from 1.40 to 16.86 nmol/l (adrenaline). Fetal breathing activity was reduced for the last 8 hours with a primary apnoea occurring during the last 4 hours. Last gasp appeared 13 min before fetal death. Cortical activity as indicated from SEP was unaffected until the last 45 min with marked changes appearing at time of circulatory collapse.

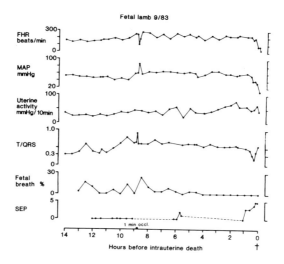

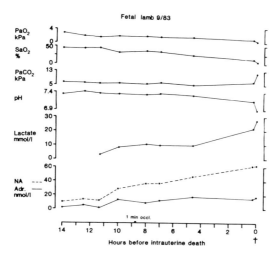

Figure 2. Recordings from an immature fetus of 126 days gestation. The same functions as in Fig. 1 are shown.

Discussion

Although there are differences when comparing man and sheep concerning pattern of uterine contractions and pressures recorded some information could be gained from recordings made in the lamb fetus during parturition. One parameter that appeared to differ was the fetal heart rate pattern as bradycardia with contractions (early or late decelerations) was not noted until the time of circulatory collapse within minutes of fetal death.

The number of parameters studied, including different aspects of cardiovascular, metabolic and cerebral activity, gives an opportunity to record a sequence of changes emerging during intra-uterine asphyxia lasting for hours. The 2 cases presented give a similar pattern of changes. This pattern is most clearly identified in the most mature fetus (case 1, 143 days gestation).

The fetus was unaffected during the initial recording period (A). At B, oxygen saturation started to fall and the fetus reacted with an apnoea (primary) and tachycardia. With the increase in uterine activity noted at C, signs of fetal asphyxia was substantial with the liberation of noradrenaline, elevated blood lactate and high peaked T waves with T/QRS ratios ≥ 0.60 as a sign of myocardial glycogenolysis. With a further increase in uterine activity, D, SaO_2 fell and the fetus was no longer able to compensate for an acidosis and pH started to fall. A further increase in FHR and T/QRS was noted but the cardiovascular and cortical activity was intact. The last 60 min was characterized by a surge in catecholamines, thereby trying to keep the circulation going in spite of the marked asphyxia.

The end result was an ability of the fetus to maintain an intact SEP until the last 30 min thereafter the response deteriorated with cerebral death 6 min before the last heart beat. The complete loss of evoked potentials was simultaneous with time of "last gasp".

The immature fetus of 126 days gestation was able to react to the threat of labour but with some quantitative differences i.e. less marked catecholamine surge, but the end result was an intact cortical activity until the last hour and cerebral death 12 min before cardiac arrest.

Among methods for fetal surveillance fetal breathing was affected early and a primary apnoea dominated. In the lamb fetus a tachycardia occurred in parallel with an increase in T/QRS ratio and it appears as if ST waveform changes of the fetal ECG could serve as relevant indicator of the fetal reaction to asphyxia. Biochemically a metabolic acidosis occurred late and were well preceded by changes in oxygen saturation, lactate and catecholamines.

Acknowledgements

This study was supported by grants from the Swedish Medical Research Council (Grants nos 5654, 2591, 5234), the "Expressen" prenatal Research Foundation and Allmänna Barnbördshusets Minnesfond.

References

1. Rosen, K. G. and Kjellmer, I. (1975). *Acta Physiol. Scand.* **93**, 59–66.
2. Hökegård, K.-H., Eriksson, B. O., Kjellmer, I., Magno, R. and Rosen, K. G. (1981). *Acta Physiol. Scand.* **113**, 1–7.
3. Greene, K. R., Dawes, G. S., Lilja, H. and Rosen, K. G. (1982). *Am. J. Obstet. Gynecol.* **144**, 950–958.
4. Rosen, K. G., Hrbek, A., Karlsson, K., Kjellmer, I., Olsson, T. and Riha, M. (1976). *Biol. Neonate* **30**, 95–101.

Reopening of the Ductus Arteriosus in Premature Lambs and Human Newborns

Ronald I. Clyman, Donnie Campbell,
Michael A. Heymann and Francoise Mauray

Department of Pediatrics, Mt Zion Hospital and Medical Center
and the Cardiovascular Research Institute and Department of Pediatrics,
University of California, San Francisco, USA

We have previously found that once the ductus arteriosus of the full term, neonatal lamb constricts, it behaves like an ischaemic tissue (1). It is no longer responsive to the constricting effect of oxygen and indomethacin nor to the dilating action of Prostaglandin E_2 (PGE_2). This loss of ductus responsiveness is directly related to the degree of ductus constriction and to the subsequent reduction in luminal blood flow (1).

Although the ductus arteriosus in full-term lambs may lose its functional reactivity once it has constricted *in vivo*, this does not necessarily appear to be the case for premature human infants. Table 1 demonstrates the effectiveness of indomethacin in constricting the ductus arteriosus in premature infants with a large left-to-right shunt, who were cared for in the intensive care nursery at Mt Zion Medical Center from 1979–1983. Overall, 87% of the infants who were treated with oral indomethacin (0.4 mg/kg over 36 h) closed their ductus arteriosus. There was no difference in the initial closure rate by gestational age or birthweight. However, 23% of those who initially closed their ductus with indomethacin, developed a large left-to-right shunt 9–10 days after the initial treatment. The incidence of reopening was inversely related to the birthweight: 33% of the infants with birthweights < 1000 g reopened their ductus following initial closure, while only 8% of infants > 1500 g reopened their ductus. Interestingly, the ducti that reopened after initial closure still seemed to be reactive and responsive to indomethacin. Of those who were treated again with indomethacin, 76% closed their ductus a second time. Therefore, we conducted the following study to

The Physiological Development of the Fetus and Newborn
ISBN 0 12 389080 2

Copyright © 1985 by Academic Press, London.
All rights of reproduction in any form reserved.

Table 1. Effects of indomethacin in infants with symptomatic PDA shunts

Birthweight	Initial closure	PDA reopened	Closed when retreated
570–1000 g	30/36 (83%)	10/30 (33%)	8/10 (80%)
1001–1500 g	51/56 (91%)	13/51 (25%)	9/13 (69%)
1501–2500 g	26/31 (84%)	2/26 (8%)	2/2 (100%)
Total	107/123 (87%)	25/107 (23%)	19/25 (76%)

The 3 columns of data represent the initial closure rate when treated with indomethacin, the incidence of recurrent of a symptomatic shunt in infants who initially closed their ductus after indomethacin, and the closure rate in infants whose ductus reopened following retreatment with indomethacin.

examine the factors that determine when the ductus arteriosus loses its ability to dilate and contract after its initial closure.

Methods

We used 36 fetal and 42 neonatal lambs, between 120 and 147 days gestation, 148 days is full term in our lambs. The 42 neonatal lambs were delivered by caesarean section, treated with a surfactant mixture, paralysed with pancuronium bromide, and ventilated with an infant ventilator (2). Lambs were kept alive for at least 3 h after delivery, with the mean survival time of 6.6 ± 0.5 h (mean $\pm$ SEM, $n = 42$).

Catheters were inserted (via peripheral vessels) into the pulmonary, right brachial and femoral arteries, the left ventricle, and the superior and inferior vena cavae. Cardiac output and left-to-right shunt through the ductus arteriosus were measured by injecting radiolabelled microspheres into the left ventricle and counting the number of microspheres in the reference sample and the number of microspheres that passed through the ductus and lodged in the lungs (2). Microsphere measurements were made at 1 h after delivery and were repeated at 1 or 2 h intervals as long as the animals survived. Haemodynamic measurements made during the last 2–3 hours before sacrifice were averaged to determine the degree of ductus constriction and reduction in luminal blood flow.

Following the series of microsphere measurements, the animals were killed in order to see how the effects of *in vivo* ductus constriction altered the responsiveness of the ductus *in vitro*. The ductus was divided into 1 mm thick rings and suspended in an organ culture bath between 2 hooks (one of which was connected to a force transducer so that isometric tensions could be measured) (2,3).

Each of the rings was initially incubated in a low PO_2 environment (PO_2 20–25 torr) in a buffered salt solution until a steady tension developed. The rings were then successively contracted with oxygen (PO_2 680 torr) and indomethacin ($2 \mu g/ml$) (in order to inhibit endogenous prostaglandin production) (4). Once these oxygen and indomethacin contracted rings reached a steady tension, a cumulative dose-relaxation response to PGE_2 was performed.

Results

Table 2 shows the degree of ductus arteriosus constriction that occurred *in vivo* in the 27 premature newborn lambs and the 15 near-term newborn lambs. We defined the degree of ductus constriction that occurred *in vivo* as either *tightly constricted* or *moderately constricted*. *Tightly constricted* ductuses had both a left-to-right shunt that was less than 10% of the systemic blood flow and a calculated

Table 2. Characteristics of neonatal lambs with moderate and tight degrees of ductus constriction *in vivo*

Degree of ductus constriction *in vivo*	$\dot{Q}_{ductus}/\dot{Q}_{systemic}$ (%)	R_{ductus} (torr/l/min/kg)	$\frac{R_{ductus}}{r_{systemic}}$ (%)	Survival (h)
Moderate				
120–134 d ($n=20$)	45±5	115±26	32±7	5.7±0.6
135–147 d ($n=5$)	36±7	127±50	36±15	6.2±1.5
Tight				
120–134 d ($n=7$)	7±2	3508±1158	1439±579	10.3±1.0
135–147 d ($n=10$)	7±1	3944±836	1227±308	6.0±0.9

Values represent mean±SEM. Haemodynamic values for each lamb obtained by averaging the measurements made during the last 2–3 h prior to sacrifice. See text for definitions of tight and moderate constriction.

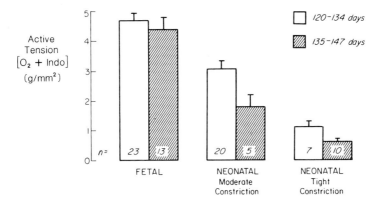

Figure 1. Contractility *in vitro* following different degrees of ductus constriction *in vivo*. Values represent mean±SEM. Moderate and tight constriction is defined in text for newborn lambs. Fetal ductuses came from animals that were never ventilated. All rings first were allowed to equilibrate in a low PO_2 environment (20–25 torr); steady state low PO_2 tensions were: fetal (120–134 d) = 3.14±0.37 g/mm², fetal (135–147 d) = 4.38±0.29 g/mm²; moderate constriction (120–134 d) = 3.00±0.23 g/mm², moderate constriction (135–147 d) = 2.86±0.45 g/mm²; tight constriction (120–134) = 2.34±0.33 g/mm², tight constriction (135–147 d) = 2.70±0.33 g/mm². The oxygen + indomethacin tension is the different between the steady state tensions at low PO_2 and the tensions after the rings have contracted with high PO_2 (680–700 torr) and indomethacin.

ductus resistance that was greater than 1000 torr l/min/kg. Moderately constricted ductuses had a left-to-right shunt that was greater than 10% of the systemic flow and a resistance of less than 300 torr l/min/kg.

Immature lambs produced significantly weaker degrees of ductus constriction than the more mature lambs. Only 26% of immature lambs developed a tightly constricted ductus, whereas 67% of more mature animals were able to do so.

Figure 1 compares the ability of rings of isolated ductus arteriosus from 36 fetal lambs (that were never ventilated) and the 42 newborn lambs to actively contract when exposed to a high oxygen environment and indomethacin *in vitro*. With increasing degrees of ductus constriction *in vivo* ductuses from both age groups steadily lost their ability to contract actively to oxygen and indomethacin.

Despite the fact that fetal ductuses from both age groups had similar contractile responses to oxygen and indomethacin, there was a significantly greater loss of ductus contractility in the more mature animals at each degree of *in vivo* constriction.

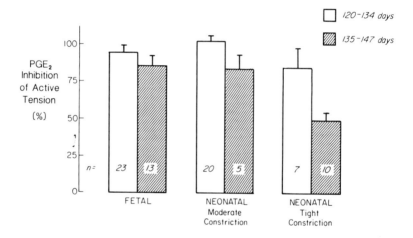

Figure 2. PGE_2 relaxation *in vitro* following different degrees of ductus constriction *in vivo*. Details as for Fig. 1.

Figure 2 compares the ability of PGE_2 to relax maximally the ductus arteriosus *in vitro*. With tight constriction of the ductus arteriosus *in vivo*, ductuses from mature newborn lambs lose their ability to respond to PGE_2. In contrast, there is no decrease in the ability of PGE_2 to relax the ductus of immature animals following *in vivo* constriction.

Discussion

In the first hours after birth, increasing degrees of ductus arteriosus constriction *in vivo* lead to an increasing loss of the ductus' ability to respond to contracting or relaxing agents any further. Premature lambs are more likely to have reactive ductuses after their initial postnatal constriction than are more mature lambs for at least two reasons: 1) premature lambs do not constrict their ductuses as tightly as more mature lambs; and, 2) there is a persistence of ductus responsiveness in premature lambs (when compared with more mature lambs), for the same amount of ductus constriction.

This persistence of ductus responsiveness in premature lambs following ductus constriction may account for the high reopening rate in preterm infants after successful indomethacin-induced closure. It is also consistent with our finding that 76% of the preterm infants who did reopen their ductus, were still responsive to indomethacin treatment.

Acknowledgements

This work was supported by grants from the United States Public Health Service Program Project HL24056 and SCOR HL27356.

References

1. Clyman, R. I., Mauray, F., Roman, C., Heymann, M. A. and Payne, B. (1983). *Circulation* **68**, 433–436.
2. Clyman, R. I., Jobe, A., Heymann, M. A., Ikegami, M., Roman, C., Payne, B. and Mauray, F. (1982). *J. Pediat.* **100**, 101–107.
3. Clyman, R. I., Mauray, F., Wong, L., Heymann, M. A. and Rudolph, A. M. *Biol. Neonate* **34**, 177–181.
4. Clyman, R. I., Mauray, F., Roman, C., Heymann, M. A. and Payne, B. (1983). *J. Pediat.* **102**, 907–911.

Is there a Relationship between the Presence of Gap Junctions and Myometrial Growth?

L. W. MacKenzie and R. E. Garfield

Departments of Neuroscience and Obstetrics & Gynecology,
McMaster University Health Sciences Centre, Hamilton, Ontario, Canada

Introduction

Gap junctions are present between myometrial cells of the pregnant uterus of various species only immediately prior to, during and for a brief time following term and preterm labour (1). The myometrium increases in size throughout gestation to accommodate the growing fetus. The growth of the myometrium, however, stops just prior to normal parturition when gap junctions begin to appear between myometrial cells. Control over the presence of gap junctions in pregnant myometrium remains incompletely understood, but may reflect effects of hormonal changes that precede labour. Gap junctions are also present between myometrial cells of nonpregnant animals after estradiol treatment and we have recently provided evidence suggesting that prostaglandins are also involved in regulating the presence of the junctions (2). Moreover, estradiol stimulates the normal growth of the uterus (3).

Intercellular communication is believed to be involved in the normal, controlled growth of tissues. Direct pathways between cells via gap junctions, are believed to be required for cell-to-cell communication by providing the basis for electrical and metabolic coupling between cells (4). Alterations in the structure and/or function of gap junctions between cells may be responsible for normal or abnormal growth of tissues including cancers (7). It is possible that myometrial growth, in response to the steroid hormones, is related to the presence of gap junctions between the muscle cells.

In this study we have evaluated the relationship between myometrial gap junctions and growth of the uterus in nonpregnant rats after various hormonal treatments and in pregnant animals on different days of gestation.

The Physiological Development of the Fetus and Newborn
ISBN 0 12 389080 2

Copyright © 1985 by Academic Press, London.
All rights of reproduction in any form reserved.

Materials and Methods

Immature and mature (nonpregnant and pregnant) female Wistar rats were used in these studies. All mature nonpregnant rats were bilaterally ovariectomized as previously described (2) and allowed to recover for 3 weeks before hormonal treatments began. Immature and ovariectomized mature animals were treated subcutaneously daily with estradiol (50 and/or 500 μg/day suspended in 0.1 sesame oil) for 1–6 days.

Nonpregnant rats were killed daily over their respective treatment periods. Pregnant rats were also killed on various days of gestation, parturition and 24 hours postpartum. Uteri from the animals were quickly removed and either used for gap junction quantitation or dry weight estimations using methods previously described (2,5,6).

Results

Administration of estradiol (50 and 500 μg/day) for 1–6 days to immature rat results in a similar increase in normalized uterine dry weight (Figs 1A and B) reaching maximum values after 3 days of treatment. Figure 1 also shows the area of gap junctions in myometrial tissues from immature rats treated with both doses of estradiol. Gap junctions occupied a low percentage of membrane area in tissues from rats treated with 50 μg/day estradiol. However, when estradiol was administered at 500 μg/day, the area of membrane occupied by gap junctions was significantly increased after the fourth injection. Furthermore, concomitant treatment with either low or high doses of estradiol plus indomethacin or sodium meclofenamate potentiated the effects of estradiol in stimulating the presence of myometrial gap junctions. The rapid growth phase of the immature uterus following estradiol treatments occurred when the myometrial membrane area of gap junctions was extremely low. Significant increases in gap junction area was observed only after growth of the uterus plateaus (Fig. 1).

Treatment of ovariectomized mature rats with estradiol (500 μg/day) also resulted in an increase in normalized uterine dry weight with maximum weight occurring after the first injection (Fig. 2). Myometrial gap junctions were also present in ovariectomized mature rats treated with estradiol (Fig. 2). The percentage of membrane area occupied by junctions was extremely low after the first injection, but thereafter significantly increased throughout the remainder of the treatment period. The myometrial membrane area of gap junctions was further increased by simultaneous injections of estradiol plus indomethacin similar to that observed in immature rats. A relationship between uterine growth and the presence of myometrial gap junctions in ovariectomized mature rats after estradiol treatment was observed. The presence of gap junctions between myometrial cells following hormone treatments occurred only after growth of the uterus (Fig. 2).

Uterine dry weights were also measured from pregnant rats on various days of gestation, parturition and one day postpartum. Normalized dry weights increased with gestational age reaching maximum weight just prior to parturition followed by a significant decrease 24 h postpartum (Fig. 3). Myometrial tissues

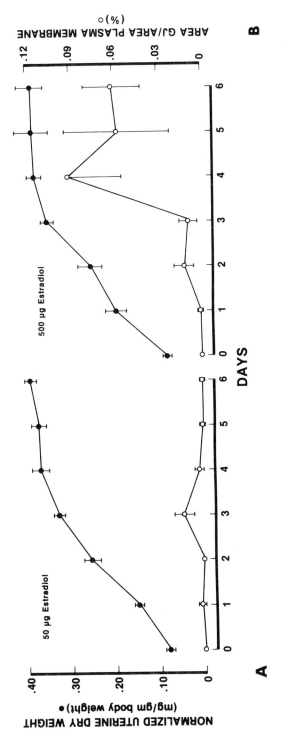

Figure 1. Effect of estradiol doses of (a) 50 μg/day and (b) 500 μg/day on normalized uterine dry weight (●) and on the area of gap junctions in myometrial tissues (○) in immature rats.

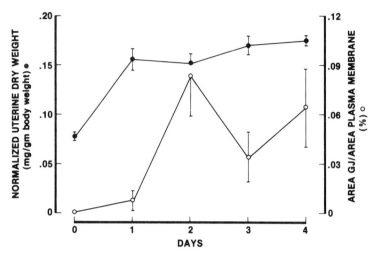

Figure 2. Effect of estradiol (500 μg/day) on normalized uterine dry weight (●) and the area of gap junctions in myometrial tissues (○) in ovariectomized mature rats.

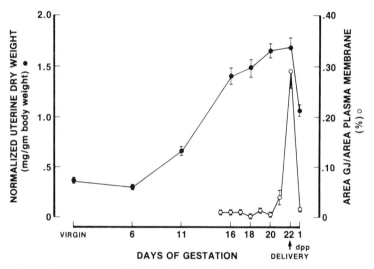

Figure 3. Normalized dry weight (●) and the urea of gap junctions in myometrial tissues (○) at various stages of gestation, parturition and 24 h postpartum in pregnant rats.

examined for the presence of gap junctions revealed that the junctions were undetectable or occupied a very low percentage of the muscle membrane area throughout gestation (Fig. 3). The membrane area of gap junctions began to increase immediately prior to labour, reached maximum levels during delivery and then significantly decreased postpartum (Fig. 3). The increase in membrane area of gap junctions occurred only after uterine growth.

Discussion

The observations reported in this study clearly show that uterine growth in immature and nonpregnant ovariectomized mature rats treated with estradiol and in untreated pregnant animals occurs when the membrane area of myometrial gap junctions is extremely low. Gap junctions occupy a significant area of myometrial membrane only after the rapid phase of myometrial growth ceases. These results may be explained on the basis that the absence of gap junctions and intercellular communication may be necessary for growth and proliferation of myometrial cells and similar to the phenomenon of contact inhibition observed in other cell systems. Furthermore, uterine growth in response to estradiol or the stimulation during pregnancy may in part be necessary for the presence of gap junctions. Uterine growth by itself, however, does not appear to be a sufficient stimulus for the development of junctions because growth ceases after treatments with low (50 μg/day) and high (500 μg/day) doses of estradiol whereas significant levels of gap junctions are present only in response to the higher dose of the hormone. Moreover, myometrial gap junctions are present during preterm labour when the uterus is growing indicating that maximum growth is not necessary for the appearance of the junctions.

Our findings support the hypothesis that the presence or absence of gap junctions may control growth or proliferation of cells. The absence of gap junctions between some types of cells is believed to be responsible for normal cellular proliferation. Alterations in structure or function of gap junctions may also result in abnormal growth of tissues including cancers (4). The results of our study therefore, may have significant implications not only for the control of uterine growth but for control of growth in other tissues including steroid hormone dependent cancer.

Steroid hormones are thought to stimulate uterine growth by working through receptor systems within the cells (3). Furthermore, steroid hormones together with prostaglandins appear to regulate the presence of myometrial gap junctions (2). We have recently shown that indomethacin stimulate uterine growth (6) and myometrial gap junctions in rats treated with estradiol (2). At present we do not understand the relationship between prostaglandins, uterine growth and the presence of myometrial gap junctions, but it appears to be complex and requires further investigation for clarification. Prostaglandins have also been implicated in normal and abnormal growth of tissues. It is possible that prostaglandins play a role in growth through their effects on the presence of gap junctions.

In conclusion, uterine growth may occur in part because of lack of gap junctions and the presence of gap junctions may be partially dependent upon myometrial growth.

Acknowledgements

This work was supported by grants from the Medical Research Council of Canada.

References

1. Garfield, R. E. and Hayashi, R. H. (1981). *Am. J. Obstet. Gynecol.* **140**, 254.
2. MacKenzie, L. W., Puri, C. P. and Garfield, R. E. (1983). Prostaglandins **26**, 925.
3. Clark, J. H., Peck, Jr., E. J., Hardin, J. W. and Ericksson, H. (1976). *In:* "Receptors and Hormone Action", (O'Malley, B. W. and Birnbaumer, L., eds), pp. 1–31, Academic Press, New York and London.
4. Loewenstein, W. R. (1981). *Physiol. Rev.* **61**, 829.
5. Garfield, R. E., Sims, S. M., Kannan, M. S. and Daniel, E. E. (1978). *Am. J. Physiol.* **235**, C168.
6. Puri, C. P., MacKenzie, L. W., Garfield, R. E. and Wiest, W. G. (1984). *Biol. Reprod.* **30**, 1027.

Chemical Sympathectomy *in utero* in the Sheep

C. B. Tan, D. P. Alexander and H. G. Britton

Department of Physiology and Biophysics, St Mary's Hospital Medical School, London, UK

In the sheep fetus there is increasing sympathetic nervous control of the vascular system with advancing gestation and evidence for a significant role of the sympathetic nervous system in the regulation of metabolism in the neonatal period. The sympathetic nervous system may also have developmental functions in the fetus. We have examined therefore the effects of chronic sympathectomy in the sheep fetus during the last third of gestation. Chemical sympathectomy was carried out with 6-hydroxydopamine (6-OHDA).

Preliminary experiments with the acutely exteriorized fetal sheep showed that administration of 6-OHDA by the intravenous route was more manageable and perhaps more effective than the intraperitoneal route. A suitable dosage for intravenous administration was established and it was shown that the rate of administration was critical for fetal survival since even in the youngest fetuses the initial administration of 6-OHDA was associated with very large increments in blood pressure. All subsequent experiments were carried out on chronically cannulated conscious sheep. Catheters were inserted in the carotid artery and jugular vein of the fetus under halothane anaesthesia at approximately 115 days conceptual age. Typically, after a 5 day recovery period, 6-OHDA was infused into the jugular vein in an estimated dosage of 50 mg/kg body weight. The infusion which lasted about 60 min was adjusted to keep the arterial pressure below 100 mmHg. Repeat infusions were given at weekly intervals at the same estimated dosage. The average animal received 2–3 infusions (range 1–4 infusions). At term, the fetuses were sacrificed, or were delivered either naturally or by Caesarean section and observed for periods up to 72 h. Measurements made on the animals included tissue noradrenaline content, liver glycogen, blood pressure, pH and PCO_2, PO_2, plasma electrolytes, glucose, fructose, free fatty acids, α-amino nitrogen, protein, urea, creatinine, noradrenaline, insulin, glucagon, growth hormone, and antidiuretic hormone.

The Physiological Development of the Fetus and Newborn
ISBN 0 12 389080 2

Copyright © 1985 by Academic Press, London.
All rights of reproduction in any form reserved.

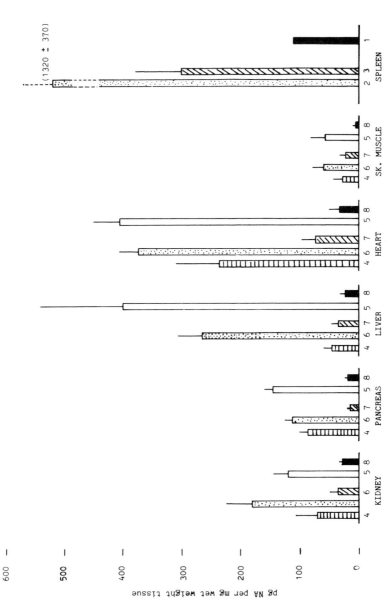

Figure 1. Tissue noradrenaline concentrations measured by radio-enzymatic assay using phenylethanolamine-*N*-methyl transferase. The number of animals is given below each column. The bars indicate the standard errors of the mean. ▦ "young" untreated fetuses (113–120 days conceptual age); ▨ "old" untreated fetuses (131–150 days conceptual age); ☐ untreated lambs (1–3 days old); ▨ "old" 6-OHDA treated fetuses (131–142 days conceptual age); and ■ 6-OHDA treated lambs (1½ h–3 days old).

Tissue noradrenaline levels established that sympathectomy was virtually complete in all animals (Fig. 1). However, the total body and individual organ weights, blood pressure and heart rate, and all other measured parameters were within the normal range in the fetuses at term, with the exception of the plasma insulin which was significantly lower. (Untreated animals 16.8 ± 2.7 (SEM) mU/l, $n = 9$; treated animals 6.3 ± 2.6 (SEM) mU/l, $n = 7$). The sympathectomized animals also showed no cardiovascular disturbances during and after birth. Further, the newborn lambs were vigorous and their behaviour was normal apart from shivering which was pronounced even in the warm laboratory. The free fatty acids were slow to rise and appeared to plateau at 200–400 μmol/l ($n = 4$) at about 2 h after birth. However, on the following day (24 h) the values (650–1000 μmol/l, $n = 4$) were comparable with controls. Liver glycogen fell less in the treated animals than in the controls (Table 1). Insulin and glucagon had risen at 24 h in the untreated animals but there was little change in the treated animals (untreated animals insulin 64 ± 19 (SEM) mU/l, $n = 6$; glucagon 33 ± 17 (SEM) pmol/l, $n = 3$; treated animals insulin 9.4 ± 6 (SEM) mU/l $n = 5$, glucagon 16 ± 5 (SEM) pmol/l, $n = 5$). Two of the treated animals were given a glucose challenge at 24 h and showed a diminished insulin response compared with controls. However, one animal tested at 72 h showed a normal response. In the treated animals, the fall in plasma growth hormone in the first 24 h after birth was not as marked as previously reported (1).

Table 1. Liver glycogen levels in untreated and 6-OHDA treated fetuses and newborn lambs

	mg glycogen/gm wet tissue weight (mean $\pm$ SEM)
Untreated fetuses (131–150 days conceptual age)	49.3 ± 9.0 ($n = 4$)
5-OHDA Treated fetuses (131–143 days conceptual age)	51.4 ± 6.6 ($n = 6$)
Untreated newborn lambs (1–3 days old)	19.0 ± 2.9 ($n = 5$)
6-OHDA Treated newborn lambs (1½ h–3 days old)	38.8 ± 7.2 ($n = 7$)*

(*This value is significantly more than in the untreated newborn animals, $P < 0.04$).

It is concluded that tonic sympathetic activity appears to be remarkably unimportant to the fetus at term, at birth or in the newborn period. However, mobilization of free fatty acids and liver glycogen appear to be impaired. It is probable from the marked shivering that brown fat could not be stimulated. The fact that the blood glucose showed the usual postnatal rise contrasts with the impaired mobilization of liver glycogen. The eventual rise of free fatty acids to high levels suggests that mobilization by nonneural factors had become important. The low insulin levels in the treated animals at 24 h after birth may have been significant in this respect.

A contemporaneous study (2,3) showed that multiple intramuscular or intraperitoneal injections of 6-OHDA may also be used to destroy the sympathetic nervous system in fetal sheep. In this work the depletion was demonstrated after birth by reduction in monoamine histofluorescence of the tissues and by hypersensitivity to the pressor effects of catecholamines. At 1–5 days postpartum summit metabolism was shown to be reduced. These workers also comment on the apparent normality of the lambs at birth.

Acknowledgements

We are grateful to Professor P. S. Sever, St Mary's Hospital Medical School, London for assays of tissue noradrenaline, to Professor S. R. Bloom and Dr K. Mashiter, Royal Postgraduate Medical School, London for assays of glucagon and insulin respectively, Dr M. L. Forsling, Middlesex Hospital Medical School, London for antidiuretic assay; and to Dr H. L. Buttle, National Institute for Dairying, Shinfield, Reading for assay of growth hormone. We thank the Wellcome trust for financial support.

References

1. Bassett, J. M. and Alexander, G. (1971). *Biol. Neonate.* **17**, 112–125.
2. Alexander, G. and Stevens, D. (1980). *J. Develop. Physiol.* **2**, 119–137.
3. Lumbers, E. R., Stevens, A. D., Alexander, G. and Stevens, D. (1980). *J. Develop. Physiol.* **2**, 139–149.

Human Twin Pregnancy in the Study of Endocrine Factors responsible for Parturition

R. J. Norman, M. Marivate and S. M. Joubert

Departments of Chemical Pathology and Obstetrics and Gynaecology,
MRC Unit for Preclinical Diagnostic Research, University of Natal,
Durban, South Africa

Introduction

The study of twin pairs has proved an invaluable model in the study of the relative contribution of genetic and environmental influences in the aetiology of disease in postnatal life. Strangely, this successful approach has not been widely utilized during intra-uterine existence.

In the sheep, Liggins (1,2) demonstrated that infusion of ACTH to one fetus caused premature delivery of both twins. Subsequently he showed that membrane-associated phospholipidase A_2 activity was selectively increased in the infused conceptus (3). Similar information is lacking in the human twin pregnancy despite several case reports recording the relatively rare occurrence of a prolonged interval between the births of first and second twins (4,5,6).

We report a summary of our studies performed in human twin pregnancies relating to parturition and development suggesting that there may be considerable benefits in the application of this model.

Patients and Methods

Of the 160 twin pregnancies seen at the antenatal clinic during the period of study, 60 were delivered by caesarean section either as an elective procedure for standard obstetrical reasons or as emergencies when the patients were already in labour (7). A 10 ml volume of umbilical vein blood was drawn into a syringe for measurement of prostaglandins and 3 ml of arterial cord blood for measurement

The Physiological Development of the Fetus and Newborn
ISBN 0 12 389080 2

Copyright © 1985 by Academic Press, London.
All rights of reproduction in any form reserved.

of other hormones. Amniotic fluid was obtained at the same time by amniocentesis
(8). Twins were designated as I and II in relation to their proximity to the pelvic
outlet. Chemical analyses were performed as described previously (7,8,9,10,11).

Results

Umbilical arterial cortisol

Arterial cord blood levels of cortisol in twin I were significantly higher than those
of twin II in the group in active labour (twin I, 184±85 nmol/l; twin II,
148±86 nmol/l, $P<0.02$) and also higher than those in twin I in the group
delivered before the commencement of labour (twin I in active labour,
184±85 nmol/l; twin I in the group before the onset of labour, 146±65 nmol/l,
$P<0.05$). There were no differences between cortisol concentrations of twins
I and II before labour or during the latent phase. Cortisone levels were not
different between twins in any group.

Other adrenal steroids

Androstenedione levels in arterial cord blood of the first twin were significantly
increased in the latent phase of labour in comparison to twin II and this different
was maintained in the active phase (Table 1). Levels of dehydroepiandrosterone

Table 1. Steroid concentrations in umbilical arterial plasma in twins

Before labour	Twin I	Twin II	n	P
Pregnenolone	72.7±9.6	73.4±10.7	25	NS
DHEAS	5.7±0.4	5.3±0.4	31	NS
Pregnenolone sulphate	7.3±1.1	7.3±0.8	21	NS
Progesterone	1123.1±46.2	1154.2±29.6	26	NS
Androstenedione	6.7±1.2	8.8±2.6	22	NS
Latent phase				
Pregnenolone	57.5±16.3	53.0±16.3	6	NS
DHEAS	7.0±1.3	6.3±1.1	7	NS
Pregnenolone sulphate	13.0±4.4	12.3±2.4	4	NS
Progesterone	501.1±112.5	886.8±131.5	7	$P<0.05$
Androstenedione	9.9±1.7	4.7±0.7	7	$P<0.01$
Active labour				
Pregnenolone	68.6±12.6	50.6±7.1	14	NS
DHEAS	5.5±0.6	4.7±0.5	20	NS
Prenenolone sulphate	7.4±0.8	6.1±0.7	13	NS
Progesterone	1057.8±180.0	1076.8±125.0	16	NS
Androstenedione	11.7±3.4	4.3±0.7	12	$P<0.02$

(mean±SEM) pregnenolone, progesterone, androstenedione concentrations in nmol/l; DHEAS and
pregnenolone sulphate concentrations in μmol/l; n=number of pairs; P=significance levels;
NS=nonsignificant at 5% levels.

sulphate (DHEAS), pregnenolone, pregnenolone sulphate and progesterone were similar between twin pairs at all stages of labour.

Umbilical venous prostaglandin concentrations

Prostaglandins E (PGE), F_{2alpha} (PGF) and 13,14, dihydro-15-keto F_{2alpha} (PGFM) were not different between twins in the prelabour and latent phase groups. In active labour, PGE levels were higher in the leading fetus (twin I, 862 ± 493 pmol/l; twin II, 595 ± 305 pmol/l, $P < 0.02$). PGFM values were also increased in active labour but there was no selective difference in twin pairs.

ACTH and prolactin

There were no statistically significant differences in any group with respect to ACTH or prolactin in arterial cord blood. Neither of these compounds showed an increase in labour.

Constituents in amniotic fluid

Amniotic fluid glucocorticoids (essentially cortisol), the lechithin:sphingomyelin and phosphatidyl ethanolamine:sphingomyelin ratios and all the prostaglandins were significantly increased in the first sac in comparison to the second sac during active labour (8,10). No differences in any of these constituents were found before the onset of contractions.

Discussion

Measurements of cortisol in the umbilical artery of twin pairs at birth in the current study show that a selective increase is found in the leading twin during the active phase of labour. This increase is quite independent of twin II despite the sharing of a common physical, metabolic and endocrine environment. No differences were seen before the onset of labour or during the latent phase suggesting that no dramatic increases in cortisol turnover occur in the human fetus in the immediate prepartum period. The fact that cortisone concentrations were not different between twins as well as the excellent fetal condition at birth of all the twins in the active labour group is strong evidence that maternal and fetal stress were not significant factors in the increased cortisol levels. These results confirm and extend those of Gensser et al. (12) who measured immunoreactive cortisol in cord blood from 20 twin pairs delivered vaginally after spontaneous labour. Despite a much higher prevalence of fetal distress in the second twin a paired comparison revealed consistently higher cord blood concentrations in the first neonate.

The reasons for the raised cortisol levels remains uncertain. Measurement of various other steroid in the cord blood does not suggest an increased supply of cortisol precursors to the adrenal gland. Immunoreactive ACTH and prolactin showed no differences between groups. An increased sensitivity to ACTH of the adrenal gland of the leading fetus has been shown to be unlikely by a study of the cortisol and DHEAS response of the neonatal adrenal to exogenous ACTH (13). The selective rise in PGE in the leading fetus during active labour is of interest, however, in light of the effect of this prostanoid on adrenal cortisol secretion in the lamb (14). As demonstrated by the increased prostaglandins in amniotic fluid of the first sac, there is a selective activation of the prostaglandin biosynthetic capacity of the membranes in this area. It is possible that the placental passage of PGE is responsible for the increase in fetal cortisol, but this must await further evidence. What does appear likely is an increased local prostaglandin production in late pregnancy in the region of the cervix as shown by the relationship between cervical maturity and response of maternal PGFM levels after vaginal examination (15).

Increased umbilical arterial concentrations of androstenedione were seen in the latent and active phases of labour in twin I. These are probably of fetal adrenal origin because of the arteriovenous differences in the levels of the hormone (16). The consequences of this increase might include enhanced estrogen production by the placenta as a result of aromatization of androstenedione. Placental prostaglandins promote aromatization while estrogens increase prostaglandin production setting in motion a train of events that could lead to a positive feedback of two groups of compounds known to promote uterine contractility. It is possible that androstenedione may be an important fetal adrenal compound in the initiation of labour.

Further studies in twin pregnancy may provide similar information vital for the understanding of normal mechanisms operating to control fetal development and human parturition.

References

1. Liggins, G. C. (1972). *In:* "Foetal and Neonatal Physiology", Proc. Sir Joseph Barcroft Centenary Symp., pp. 562–578. Cambridge University Press, Cambridge, UK.
2. Liggins, G. C. (1974). *In:* "Size at Birth", Ciba Foundation Symp 27, pp. 164–185. Elsevier, Excerpta Medica, Amsterdam.
3. Grieves, S. A. and Liggins, G. C. (1976). *Prostaglandins* **12**, 229–241.
4. Williams, B. and Cummings, G. (1953). *J. Obstet. Gynaecol. Brit. Emp.* **60**, 319–321.
5. Abrams, R. H. (1957). *Obstet. Gynecol.* **9**, 435–438.
6. Druker, P., Finkel, J. and Savel, L. E. (1960). *Am. J. Obstet. Gynecol.* **80**, 761–763.
7. Norman, R. J., Deppe, W. M., Coutts, P. C. and Joubert, S. M. (1983). *Br. J. Obstet. Gynaecol.* **90**, 1033–1039.
8. Norman, R. J., Joubert, S. M. and Marivate, M. (1983). *Br. J. Obstet. Gynaecol.* **90**, 51–55.
9. Norman, R. J., Deppe, W. M., Joubert, S. M. and Marivate, M. (1984). *Br. J. Obstet. Gynaecol.* **91**, 776–780.
10. Norman, R. J., Bredenkamp, B. L. F., Joubert, S. M. and Beetar, C. (1981). *Prostaglan. Med.* **6**, 309–316.
11. Norman, R. J. and Joubert, S. M. (1982). *S. Afr. Med. J.* **61**, 939–841.
12. Gensser, G., Ohrlander, S. and Eneroth, P. (1977). *In:* "Fetus and Birth", Ciba Foundation Symp 47, pp. 401–420. Elsevier, Excerpta Medica, Amsterdam.

13. Norman, R. J., Maharaj, T., Adhikari, M. and Joubert, S. M. (1984). *S. Afr. Med. J.* **66**, 90-92.
14. Louis, T. M., Challis, J. R. G., Robinson, J. C. and Thorburn, G. D. (1976). *Nature* **264**, 797-799.
15. Norman, R. J., Martin, R. and Marivate, M. (1982). *S. Afr. Med. J.* **61**, 833-834.
16. Mathur, R. S., Landgrebe, S., Moody, L. O., Powell, S. and Williamson, H. O. (1980). *J. Clin. Endocrin. Metab.* **51**, 1235-1238.

Is there a Topographical Distribution of Prostaglandin E_2 Receptors in the Human Pregnant Uterus?

J. M. Adelantado, J. Humphreys,
A. Lopez Bernal and A. C. Turnbull

Nuffield Department of Obstetrics and Gynaecology,
John Radcliffe Hospital, Headington, Oxford, UK

Introduction

The mechanism(s) underlying human parturition remain(s) a mystery. The human uterus can be considered as a functional unit consisting of two parts: the corpus and the cervix, each with different anatomic and physiological characteristics. A successful outcome of labour involves co-ordinated uterine contractions and the synchronized effacement and dilatation of the cervix and it is now well accepted that the cervix plays an active role during parturition and that cervical dilatation is the result of a ripening process within this tissue (1).

Prostaglandins appear to be involved in both uterine contraction and cervical dilatation (2) and the clinical use of these compounds, particularly prostaglandin E_2 (PGE_2) for the induction of labour is well established (3). Although no mode of action of prostaglandins is far from clear, it is believed that they interact with specific receptors situated on the cell membrane (4). Our preliminary studies (5) suggest that PGE_2 is bound in a specific, saturable manner by membrane preparations of human myometrium and in the present study we have examined the topographical distribution of PGE_2 binding sites in the pregnant uterus at term in an attempt to clarify the possible mechanism of action of this compound.

Materials and Methods

Tissue

Samples of human myometrium and of uterine cervix were obtained after hysterectomies in premenopausal nonpregnant women and at elective caesarean

The Physiological Development of the Fetus and Newborn
ISBN 0 12 389080 2

Copyright © 1985 by Academic Press, London.
All rights of reproduction in any form reserved.

section in pregnant women at term. A whole uterus was obtained after caesarean hysterectomy performed at 39 weeks gestation before the onset of labour. The samples were frozen in solid carbon dioxide and kept at $-70°C$ until assay.

Chemicals

[5,6,8,11,12,14,15(u)-^{3}H] Prostaglandin E_2 (160 Curies/mmol) was obtained from Amersham International PLC, Amersham. Unlabelled prostaglandins were obtained from Upjohn Co, Kalamazoo, Michigan, USA. All other chemicals were of the highest purity available from Sigma Chemical Co (Poole, Dorset) and Fisons (Loughborough). Protein was estimated by the Coomassie blue method with a kit from Bio-Rad Laboratories (Richmond, California, USA).

Preparation of membrane fractions

Tissues were defrosted and washed in ice-cold Tris-HCl buffer 10 mmol, pH 7.4 containing 250 mmol sucrose, 1 mmol $CoCl_2$ 1 mmol dithiothreitol and 1% (w/v) gelatin (Tris-HCl buffer). The tissues were homogenized in a ground-glass homogenizer of a ratio of 1 g titre/3 ml buffer. Unless otherwise stated all procedures were performed at 0–4°C. The homogenates were first centrifuged at 1000**g** for 15 min. The resultant supernatant was centrifuged at 50 000**g** for 60 min. The 30 000**g** supernatant was discarded and the 50 000**g** pellet was resuspended in Tris-HCl buffer to give a protein concentration of approximately 1 mg/ml. The resultant crude membrane suspension was used for assays.

Prostaglandin binding assay

Incubations were carried out at 22°C in duplicate in polypropylene tubes containing 0.1 ml of crude membrane preparation and varying concentration (0.1–2.5 μM) of ^{3}H-PGE$_2$ with and without a 1000-fold excess of nonradioactive PGE$_2$ in a final volume of 0.15 ml. At the end of the incubation period the content of each tube was filtered under reduced pressure through a Whatman GF/B glass microfibre filter disc. The filters were washed twice with 4 ml ice-cold buffer and dried in a heat chamber at 60°C. They were then transferred to scintillation vials and the radioactivity counted spectrophotometrically. Specific binding was calculated as the difference between total binding and nonspecific binding (binding in the presence of nonradioactive PGE$_2$). The results were plotted by the method of Scatchard. Protein concentration was measured using bovine serum albumin as standard. In control experiments the metabolism of PGE$_2$ by the tissue preparations after incubation was checked on ethyl acetate extracts by high pressure liquid chromatography on a Bondapack fatty acid column (Waters Instruments) eluted with acetonitrile and water. In all cases a single radioactive peak corresponding to unmetabolized ^{3}H-PGE$_2$ was obtained.

Results

Prostaglandin E$_2$ binding by membrane preparations of nonpregnant uterus

These experiments are summarized in Table 1 and they revealed that the corpus uteri has a single class of high affinity sites whose concentration decreases towards the cervix. Cervical tissue was found to contain a single class of low affinity sites.

Table 1. Prostaglandin E$_2$ binding by membrane preparations of human nonpregnant uterus

Tissue	Concentration of binding sites (fmol/mg protein)	Apparent K$_d$ (nmol)
Corpus uteri ($n=4$)	850 ± 320	2.1 ± 0.3
Cervix uteri ($n=4$)	300 ± 75	27 ± 9

Results are mean ± SD

Prostaglandin E$_2$ binding by membrane preparations of gestational uterus

Samples of myometrial tissue were classified into 7 groups according to their proximity to the fundus (A) or to the cervix (G). On average the distance between 2 alternate sampling sites was 3 cm. The results presented in Table 2 show that in Scatchard the binding PGE$_2$ had two components of different affinity. A high affinity component was distributed throughout the corpus uteri but was not present in the cervix. A second component of less affinity was also evident in the corpus uteri and it became increasingly dominant towards the cervix. Cervical binding had the lowest affinity and the highest capacity (Table 2).

Table 2. Prostaglandin E$_2$ binding by membrane preparations of human pregnant uterus

Sampling site	First component		Second component	
	Kd_1 (nmol)	fmol/mg protein	Kd_2 (nmol)	fmol/mg protein
A (fundus)	2.6 ± 1.4	237 ± 96	5.3 ± 1.7	283 ± 13
B	2.5 ± 1.3	267 ± 118	4.1 ± 1.0	334 ± 170
C	1.7 ± 0.5	245 ± 72	5.5 ± 2.9	388 ± 160
D	1.5 ± 0.3	265 ± 140	9.4 ± 4.5	541 ± 137
E	1.5 ± 0.5	270 ± 120	8.0 ± 1.1	536 ± 107
F	2.5 ± 1.2	86 ± 50	23.9 ± 2.5	265 ± 63
G (cervix)	ND	ND	54.8 ± 28.8	1015 ± 583

Results are mean ± SD, $n=4$

Comments

This study has shown that the bindings of PGE_2 to membrane preparations of human uterus is heterogeneous and consists of a high affinity and a low affinity component. The concentration of high affinity sites is uniformly distributed throughout the corpus uteri but is absent from the cervix and the concentration of binding sites is higher in nonpregnant myometrium than in pregnant myometrium at term. Cervical tissue in both nonpregnant and pregnant samples has the lowest affinity binding and the concentration of low affinity sites is higher in pregnant than nonpregnant cervix. The distribution of high affinity sites parallels the smooth muscle content of the uterus (6).

These two classes of binding sites could be explained by a phenomenon of negative co-operativity (6) but it is more likely that they represent two different sites of physiological and/or pharmacological action of prostaglandins. This second interpretation is supported by clinical evidence which suggests that when PGE_2 is given systemically the most prominent uterus response is contraction, whereas local intravaginal application of PGE_2 results in cervical dilatation. It is proposed that the high affinity component mediates the oxytocic effect of PGE_2 whereas the low affinity component may be involved in the compliance of the pregnant uterus and the process of cervical ripening and dilatation.

References

1. Liggins, G. C. (1983). *Clin. Obstet. Gynaecol.* **26**, 47–55.
2. Huszar, G. (1981). *Sem. Perinatol.* **5**, 216–235.
3. MacKenzie, I. Z. and Embrey, M. P. (1977). *Br. Med. J.* **2**, 1381.
4. Wakeling, A. E. and Wyngarden, L. J. (1974). *Endocrinol.* **5**, 55.
5. Adelantado, J. M., Lopez Bernal, A., Demers, L. and Turnbull A. C. (1983). *Acta Endocrinol.* **103** (Suppl. 256), 163.
6. Hoffmann, G. E., Rao, Ch. V., Barrows, G. H. and Sanfilippo, J. S. (1983). *J. Clin. Endocrinol. Metab.* **57**, 360.

Calcium Requirement for Prostaglandin Synthesis by Human Amnion

D. M. Olson, J. R. G. Challis, A. Opavsky,
Z. Smieja, D. Kramar and K. Skinner

Departments of Paediatrics, Obstetrics and Gynaecology and of Physiology,
The Research Institute, St Joseph's Hospital, MRC (Canada) Group in
Reproductive Biology, The University of Western Ontario,
London, Ontario, Canada

Parturition in the human is associated with an increase in amniotic fluid prostaglandin (PG) E and F levels during cervical dilatation (1,2) and an increase in the concentrations of PGs in the amnion, decidua and myometrium during late gestation and labour (3). The source of these prostaglandins most certainly includes the fetal membranes (amnion, chorion).

The fetal membranes are richly endowed with esterified arachidonic acid, the precursor for all prostaglandins, and the enzymes necessary for the de-esterification of arachidonic acid and its subsequent conversion to prostaglandins (4–7). It has been reasoned that changes in the amount or activity of enzymes which release arachidonic acid or convert it to primary PGs may be responsible for the sharp increase in PG production in women at term. The 2 principal lipases which catalyse the release of arachidonic acid, phospholipases A_2 and C, are Ca^{2+}-dependent enzymes (8), and, therefore, the possibility exists that the intracellular availability of Ca^{2+} may play a crucial regulatory function in prostaglandin biosynthesis. We tested this possibility in cells dispersed from term human amnion.

Dependence of Prostaglandin Synthesis upon Extracellular Ca^{2+}

Cells dispersed from amnions obtained by elective caesarean section at term before the onset of labour (CS) or after spontaneous vaginal delivery at term (SL) were

The Physiological Development of the Fetus and Newborn
ISBN 0 12 389080 2

Copyright © 1985 by Academic Press, London.
All rights of reproduction in any form reserved.

incubated for 3 h in Krebs' solution containing increasing levels of $CaCl_2$, and the output of PGE_2 was determined by radioimmunoassay (Fig. 1A). The output of PGE_2 at all $CaCl_2$ concentrations was greater for SL cells than for CS cells. In each case, the production of PGE_2 was lowest when $CaCl_2$ was absent from the medium (plus 0.1 mmol EGTA). Restoration of $CaCl_2$ to the medium increased PGE_2 output approximately 2-fold at concentrations as low as 0.25 mmol. Further increases in extracellular $CaCl_2$ levels had no further stimulatory effects on PGE_2 production. These results suggested that PGE_2 synthesis in human amnion is partially dependent upon extracellular Ca^{2+}.

To test further whether PGE_2 synthesis is dependent upon extracellular Ca^{2+}, we attempted to attenuate PG output by use of the potential-sensitive Ca^{2+}-ion channel blocker, D-600 (methoxyverapamil) (Fig. 1B). Increasing concentrations of D-600 (10^{-7}–10^{-5} M) in the extracellular medium in the presence of 2.5 mmol $CaCl_2$ decreased PGE_2 output by both CS and SL amnion cells up to 50–60% of control levels in 3 h incubations. This was the same level of inhibition achieved in these cells by eliminating $CaCl_2$ in the incubation medium in the absence of D-600. Interestingly, addition of the Ca^{2+} ionophore, A23187 (10^{-5} M), restored PGE_2 production in incubations containing D-600 (10^{-5} M) and $CaCl_2$ (2.5 mmol).

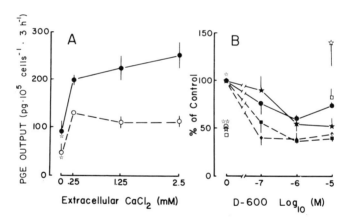

Figure 1. Dependency of PGE_2 output by human amnion cells upon extracellular Ca^{2+}. (A) Effects of extracellular $CaCl_2$ concentration: ● mean±SEM from 3 separate SL women; ○ mean±SEM from 4 separate CS women. *$P<0.01$ compared with all other $CaCl_2$ concentrations. (B) Effect of D-600 concentration in presence of extracellular $CaCl_2$ (2.5 mmol). Cells were preincubated (10 min) with varying levels of D-600 prior to addition of $CaCl_2$. Each solid symbol represents the mean±SEM of 3 replicate cell cultures from an individual patient. Solid lines indicate the responses from SL women and dashed lines indicate CS women. *$P<0.01$ from the mean responses for all other concentrations of D-600. Open symbols at zero D-600 represent PGE_2 output in the absence of Ca^{2+} (0.1 mmol EGTA). **$P<0.0001$ compared with values in presence of Ca^{2+} (paired *t* test). Open symbols at 10^{-5} mD-600 represent responses from 1 CS and 1 SL woman in the presence of A23187 (10^{-5} M) plus D-600 plus Ca^{2+}. Courtesy of the National Research Council of Canada (9).

Mechanism of Ca²⁺ Action

At least 3 separate mechanisms may exist for Ca^{2+} regulation of prostaglandin biosynthesis. The first is that Ca^{2+} may directly stimulate phospholipases A_2 and C (8). This mechanism, however, is plagued by the problem that for each phospholipase, optimal activation occurs with Ca^{2+} concentrations in the millimolar range; levels which may not be achieved intracellularly. Another mechanism may be via activation of protein kinase C which in turn would phosphorylate (deactivate) lipomodulin or macrocortin, a phospholipase inhibitor (8,10). This pathway requires only micromolar concentrations of Ca^{2+}. Protein kinase C activity has been identified in human amnion tissue (8). Activation of protein kinase C is enhanced by diacylglycerol, and, interestingly, diacylglycerol levels in amnion increase 2-fold with the onset of labour in women (11). Whether protein kinase C has a specific function in the regulation of prostaglandin production in human amnion remains to be shown.

The third mechanism by which Ca^{2+} may be acting is through the intracellular Ca^{2+} mediator, calmodulin. It has been proposed that calmodulin may enhance the activities of phospholipases A_2 and C in a number of tissues (12,13) as well as inhibit the activity of 15-hydroxy prostaglandin dehydrogenase, the principal prostaglandin metabolizing enzyme (14). Calmodulin is activated by Ca^{2+} in the micromolar range.

We examined the possibility that calmodulin may be involved in amnion PG synthesis by studying the effects of inhibitors of calmodulin action, trifluoperazine and calmidazolium. The addition of trifluoperazine (TFP, 10^{-5} M) to CS amnion cells (Fig. 2) inhibited the output of PGE_2 in relation to cells without additions for up to 3 h. The Ca^{2+} ionophore, A23187 (10^{-5} M) promoted PGE_2 output, but when A23187 and TFP were coincubated, PGE_2 output was decreased, suggesting that calmodulin is involved in the intracellular mechanism of Ca^{2+} action. The same pattern of responses was observed also in SL amnion cells. In 3 experiments, there was no difference in cell viability after 3 h of incubation

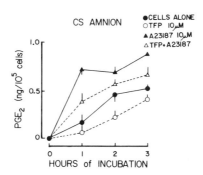

Figure 2. Effect of trifluoperazine (TFP) on PGE₂ output by CS amnion cells. Each point is the mean±SEM of 4 replicate cell cultures from a single patient. Typical of 4 experiments.

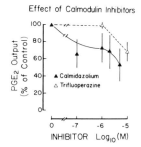

Figure 3. Effect of calmodulin inhibitors upon PGE₂ output. Each point is the mean±SEM of 3 women.

for cells incubated with TFP (10^{-5} M) ($93.0\pm0.7\%$) or without TFP ($93.1\pm3.8\%$). However, since TFP may affect also the activity of calmodulin-sensitive enzymes and calmodulin-insensitive enzymes (see 15), we compared the effect of another inhibitor of calmodulin, calmidzaolium (15), with TFP (Fig. 3). In 3 h incubations of SL amnion cells from the same 3 patients, a dose-related inhibition of PGE₂ output for both calmidazolium and TFP was observed. The calmidazolium effect was evident at concentrations approximately an order of magnitude lower than TFP concentrations. No effect on cell viability by either inhibitor was noted.

These results suggest an apparent involvement of calmodulin in the process of prostaglandin synthesis in human amnion. The identification and subcellular location of calmodulin within the amnion and whether it activates phospholipases directly or indirectly (16,17) or whether it acts at another level of prostaglandin biosynthesis remain to be determined.

Acknowledgements

Supported by NIH National Research Service Award F32-HD06327-01A2 and the St Joseph's Hospital Research Institute (DMO), MRC (Canada) Group in Reproductive Biology (JRGC) and an Ontario Graduate Scholarship (KS).

References

1. Salmon, J. A. and Amy, J. J. (1973). *Prostaglandins* **4**, 523–533.
2. Keirse, M. J. N. C. and Turnbull, A. C. (1973). *J. Obstet. Gynaecol. Brit. Commonwealth* **80**, 970–973.
3. Willman, E. A. and Collins, W. P. (1976). *J. Endocrinol.* **69**, 413–419.
4. Schultz, F. M., Schwarz, B. E., MacDonald, P. C. and Johnston, J. M. (1975). *Am. J. Obstet. Gynecol.* **123**, 650–653.
5. Grieves, S. A. and Liggins, G. C. (1976). *Prostaglandins* **12**, 229–241.
6. DiRenzo, G. C., Johnston, J. M., Okazaki, T., Okita, J. R., MacDonald, P. C. and Bleasdale, J. E. (1981). *J. Clin. Invest.* **67**, 847–856.

7. Okazaki, T., Casey, M. L., Okita, J. R., MacDonald, P. C. and Johnston, J. M. (1981). *Am. J. Obstet. Gynecol.* **139**, 373–381.
8. Bleasdale, J. E., Okazaki, T., Sagawa, N., DiRenzo, G., Okita, J. R., MacDonald, P. C. and Johnston, J. M. (1983). *In:* "Initiation of Parturition: Prevention of Prematurity", (MacDonald, P. C. and Porter, J., eds) pp. 129–137, Ross Laboratories, Columbus, Ohio.
9. Olson, D. M., Opavsky, M. A. and Challis, J. R. G. (1983). *Can. J. Physiol. Pharmacol.* **61**, 1089–1092.
10. Hirata, F. (1981). J. Biol. Chem. **256**, 7730–7733.
11. Okita, J. R., MacDonald, P. C. and Johnston, J. M. (1982). *Am. J. Obstet. Gynecol.* **142**, 432–435.
12. Craven, P. A. and DeRubertis, F. D. (1983). *J. Biol. Chem.* **258**, 4814–4823.
13. Moskowitz, N., Shapiro, L., Schook, W. and Puszkin, S. (1983). *Biochem. Biophys. Res. Commun.* **115**, 94–99.
14. Wong, P. Y. K., Lee, W. H., Chao, P. H. W. and Cheung, W. Y. (1980). *Proc. N.Y. Acad. Sci.* 179–189.
15. Gietzen, K. (1983). *Biochem. J.* **216**, 611–616.
16. Withnall, M. T. and Brown, T. J. (1982). *Biochem. Biophys. Res. Commun.* **106**, 1049–1055.
17. Ballou, L. R. and Cheung, W. Y. (1983). *Proc. Nat. Acad. Sci. USA* **80**, 5203–5207.

The Effect of Nifedipine Administration on the Fetus and the Myometrium of Pregnant Sheep during Oxytocin Induced Contractions

M. M. Roebuck, B. M. Castle, L. Vojcek[1],
A. Weingold[2], G. S. Dawes[3] and A. C. Turnbull

Nuffield Department of Obstetrics and Gynaecology, John Radcliffe Hospital,
Oxford, UK
[1]Department of Obstetrics and Gynaecology,
University Medical School of Debrecen, Hungary
[2]George Washington University Medical Center, Washington DC, USA
[3]Nuffield Institute for Medical Research, Oxford, UK

Nifedipine (Bayer) is used for the treatment of human adult hypertension (1). It is under consideration for similar use in pregnancy and to arrest uterine activity. We have used 15 pregnant sheep 132–140 days pregnant to investigate the effects of this slow Ca^{2+} channel blocking agent on the fetus and the myometrium during both quiescent pregnancy and oxytocin induced contractions.

Nifedipine is prepared in a 60% ethanol solution, control infusions of 0.18 g/kg/l ethanol had no significant effect on the ewe or fetus. During maternal intravenous infusion, nifedipine reaches constant plasma concentrations in the ewe after 20 min and in the fetus after 30 min.

The maternal heart rate increased 25% associated with a 16% fall in diastolic blood pressure during the infusion of 20 μg/kg maternal weight/min nifedipine. There was no significant change in maternal systolic blood pressure, carotid artery PO_2, PCO_2 or pH (2). The fetal carotid arterial PO_2 fell from a mean 22 ± 0.6 by 2.3 mmHg ($P<0.02$); there was no change in PCO_2 or pH. There was a fall in mean fetal carotid arterial pressure of 4–5 mmHg from a mean of 51.7 ± 2.6 together with a 48% increase in heart rate from a mean of 158 ± 6.4 beats/min. Nifedipine had no effect on the incidence or amplitude of fetal high voltage

The Physiological Development of the Fetus and Newborn
ISBN 0 12 389080 2

Copyright © 1985 by Academic Press, London.
All rights of reproduction in any form reserved.

Ewe 48   134 days pregnant

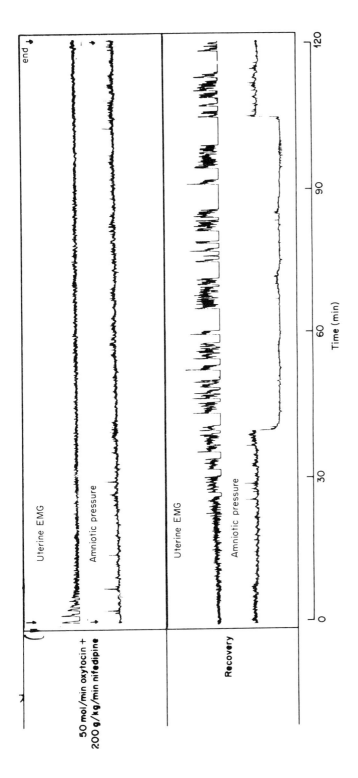

Figure 1. Recording of uterine electromyographic and amniotic pressure changes in the pregnant sheep uterus. There was a control period of 2 h then 50 mU oxytocin/min was infused for 2 h and this was followed by infusion of 50 mU oxytocin/min with 20 mg/kg nifedipine/min for 2 h.

electrocortical activity nor on fetal breathing movements as measured by tracheal-amniotic pressure changes (2).

The mean incidence of bursts of uterine electromyographic (emg) activity in 10 ewes 132–142 days pregnant was 2.62 ± 1.2/h, their duration 7.9 ± 1.8 min, and the interval between was 24.5 ± 6.2 min. Amniotic fluid pressure changes coinciding with uterine emg activity lasted 6.2 ± 1.4 min with an amplitude of 7.04 ± 2.4 mmHg.

The intravenous infusion of 50 mU/min oxytocin to the pregnant sheep for 4 h changed the pattern of uterine emg activity to a frequency ot 34.4 ± 7.25/h lasting 1.42 ± 0.25 min separated by intervals of 0.85 min. Contractions, measured by amniotic fluid pressure changes lasted 1.16 ± 0.99 min with an amplitude of 145 ± 3 mmHg. Regular uterine activity was achieved within 20 min of starting the oxytocin infusion and normal activity was restored at 5 ± 3 h after the end of the infusion (Fig. 1).

The intravenous infusion of 20 μg/kg maternal weight/min nifedipine (Bayer) during the final 2 h of oxytocin administration to 5 pregnant ewes altered the pattern of uterine emg activity to a continuous discharge with $21.3 \pm 10\%$ of the amplitude of the oxytocin induced activity (Fig. 1). No changes in amniotic fluid pressure could be detected after 15 min of nifedipine infusion. Recovery of normal uterine activity was faster 3 ± 1 h ($P < 0.001$) after the end of the infusions. Ethanol (60 ml of 60% in 2 h) had no significant effect on the oxytocin induced uterine activity.

Two hours of the intravenous infusion of 50 mU/min oxytocin increased maternal carotid artery plasma prostaglandin FM concentrations (3) from 140 ± 56 pg/ml to 375 ± 177 pg/ml. Continued oxytocin or oxytocin with Nifedipine infusions did not change the plasma concentration of prostaglandin FM. The concentrations of the 11,16-bicyclic analogue of 13,14-dihydro-15-keto PGE (4) in the maternal carotid plasma were unchanged by either oxytocin or nifedipine infusions.

Oxytocin infusion had no effect on maternal arterial pressure, heart rate or blood gases. The infusion of 20 μg/kg/min nifedipine for 2 h, in the presence of oxytocin, increased the heart rate from 123 ± 7 to 180 ± 16 beats/min and lowered the diastolic pressure by 15%; there were no changes in systolic pressure or arterial blood gases and pH.

There was no change in the incidence or duration of fetal electrocortical activity with either oxytocin or oxytocin with nifedipine infusions to the pregnant ewe. Oxytocin infusions caused no change in fetal carotid arterial PO_2 from a mean of 20 ± 1.7 mmHg, PCO_2 from 48.86 ± 2.45 mmHg, pH from 7.328 ± 0.0075, heart rate from 163 ± 10 beats/min or mean blood pressure from 54 ± 1.8 mmHg. The maternal infusion of 20 μg/kg/min nifedipine for 2 h during the administration of oxytocin caused a fall in fetal carotid artery pH from a mean of 7.32 ± 0.02 to 7.296 ± 0.033, a fall in mean arterial blood pressure from 56.8 ± 4 to 52.2 ± 2.8 mmHg and an increase in heart rate from 167.2 ± 18.6 to 243 ± 4.6 beats/min. There was no significant change in PaO_2 or $PaCO_2$.

The Ca^{2+} antagonist nifedipine is being considered as a drug for use in arresting uterine activity, particularly pre-term labour. Our results suggest that nifedipine at 20 μg/kg/min is effective in stopping oxytocin induced contractions in the pregnant sheep. However, it is not without effects on the fetus which might make interpretation of fetal monitoring difficult.

Acknowledgements

We would like to thank the MRC, Bayer UK Ltd., and the Nuffield Medical Fund for funding the project and Jan Humphries for expert technical assistance.

References

1. Guazzi, M., Olivari, M. T., Polese, A., Florentini, C., Magrini, F. and Moruzzi, P. (1977). *Clin. Pharmacol. Ther.* **22**, 528–532.
2. Roebuck, M. M., Castle, B., Vojcek, L., Weingold, A., Hofmeyr, G. J., Dawes, G. S. and Turnbull, A. C. (1984). Society for the Study of Fetal Physiology XI Annual Conference, Oxford.
3. Mitchell, M. D. and Flint, A. P. F. (1978). *J. Endocrinol.* **76**, 111–121.
4. Demers, L. M., Brennecke, S. P., Mountford, L. A., Brunt, J. D. and Turnbull, A. C. (1983). *J. Clin. Endocrin. Metab.* **57**, 101–106.

The Effect of the Prostaglandin Synthetase Inhibitor 4-Aminoantipyrine on Myometrial Activity during ACTH-induced Labour

J. P. Figueroa, E. R. Poore, M. D. Mitchell,
K. Fontwit and P. W. Nathanielsz

Reproductive Studies, State University of New York,
College of Veterinary Medicine, Cornell University, Ithaca, New York, USA;
Cecil H and Ida Green Center for Reproductive Biology Sciences,
The University of Texas Southwestern Medical School, Dallas, Texas, USA

Introduction

Prostaglandins (PG) have been implicated in the control of myometrial activity during pregnancy in sheep. During most of pregnancy tonic epochs of myometrial contractility have been demonstrated using either electromyography (EMG) or intra-uterine pressure (IUP) measurements (4–6). Recently we demonstrated that the prostaglandin synthetase inhibitor 4-amino-antipyrine (4AA) reduced both frequency and total integrated myometrial EMG activity of tonic uterine contractures (3). We have investigated the effect of 4AA on labour and delivery contractions during induction of premature labour.

Materials and Methods

Four pregnant Rambouillet Columbia ewes mated on one occasion only were used. At 116–127 days gestation fetal and maternal instrumentation was performed as previously described (11,12). Vascular catheters were placed in the fetal jugular vein, carotid artery and maternal uterine vein and stainless steel EMG leads were sewn into the myometrium. In the 3 pregnancies carrying twin fetuses, both fetuses were catheterized.

The Physiological Development of the Fetus and Newborn
ISBN 0 12 389080 2

Copyright © 1985 by Academic Press, London.
All rights of reproduction in any form reserved.

At least 5 days after surgery, synthetic adrenocorticotrophin (ACTH$_{1-24}$; Cortrosyn, Organon; 1 μg/h) was infused continuously into the fetal jugular vein to induce premature labour. All 7 fetuses were infused with ACTH. Following 62–104 hours of ACTH infusion when the EMG and IUP trace showed well established labour and delivery contractions, 4AA was administered to the fetal jugular vein while the ACTH infusion was continued. A 300 mg bolus of 4AA was administered to the fetal jugular vein followed by infusion of 15 mg/min for 3 h. Uterine EMG activity was monitored using an Apple II microprocessor based

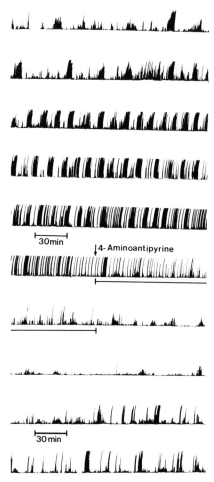

Figure 1. Myometrial EMG recorded continuously beginning 67 h after the commencement of infusion of ACTH, 1 μg/h to both fetuses in a twin pregnancy in a sheep. ACTH infusion was begun at 128 days gestation. After 83.5 h of ACTH infusion, 4-amino-antipyrine was infused into the fetuses at 15 mg/min following a bolus of 300 mg. Reprinted with permission from Perinatology Press (14).

system. Fetal carotid artery and maternal uterine vein blood was taken for PG measurement before commencement of the 4AA infusion and at 60, 120, 180, 420, 480 and 660 min during and after the infusion.

Measurement of fetal and maternal plasma prostaglandin E_2 (PGE_2) 6-keto prostaglandin $F_{1\alpha}$ ($6KPGF_{1\alpha}$) the major metabolite of prostacyclin and 13,14 dihydro 15-keto prostaglandin $F_{2\alpha}$ (PGFM) were performed by radioimmunoassay (8-10).

Comparison of means within the experimental groups was performed by Analysis of Variance and Student's t test with the Bonferroni modification for multiple comparisons.

Results

Fetal blood gases and pH were within the normal range at the start and throughout the ACTH infusion and during the 4AA infusion.

The criteria for commencement of the 4AA were that the myometrial EMG showed only short-lived contractions lasting less than 2 min and that IUP increases were more than 15 mmHg. Administration of 4AA converted EMG and IUP patterns from labour and delivery contractions to contractures (Fig. 1).

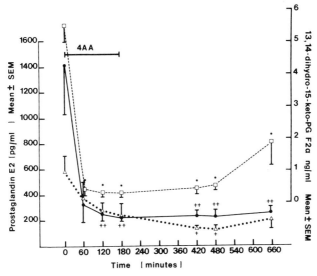

Figure 2. Fetal carotid (●) and maternal uterine vein (▵) plasma prostaglandin E_2 (PGE_2) and (▢) 13,14-dihydro-15-keto-prostaglandin $F_{2\alpha}$ (PGFM) concentrations (mean±SEM) immediately before, during and after the infusion of 4-amino-antipyrine (4AA) for 180 min into the fetal jugular vein during premature labour induced by the infusion of synthetic $ACTH_{1-24}$ (1 μg/h) to the fetus. +At 420 and 480 min after the 4AA infusion, uterine vein PGE_2 had fallen significantly ($P < 0.008$). + +At 120, 180, 420, 480, and 660 min after the 4AA infusion fetal PGE_2 concentrations had fallen significantly ($P < 0.008$). *PGFM concentrations are significantly lower than base-line throughout the sampling period ($P < 0.008$).

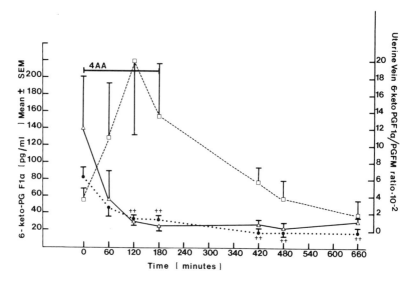

Figure 3. Fetal carotid (●) and maternal uterine vein (▵) plasma 6-keto-prostaglandin $F_{1\alpha}$ (6KPGF$_{1\alpha}$) concentrations and (□) ratio of maternal uterine vein 6KPGF$_{1\alpha}$ to 13,14-dihydro-15-keto-prostaglandin $F_{2\alpha} \times 10^{-2}$ (mean±SEM) immediately before, during and after the infusion of 4-aminoantipyrine for 180 min to the fetus during premature labour induced by the infusion of synthetic ACTH$_{1-24}$ (1 µg/h) to the fetus. The fetal carotid 6-keto-PGF$_{1\alpha}$ concentrations had fallen significantly by 120 min ($++P<0.008$).

Infusion of 4AA resulted in a rapid fall in plasma PGE_2 concentrations in both the fetal and maternal plasma. This fall was significant by 120 min in fetus ($P<0.008$) and 420 min in the ewe ($P<0.008$) (Fig. 2). In the uterine venous blood, PGFM concentrations fell from a mean of 550 pg/ml to 430 pg/ml at 180 min. This fall was significant by 60 min ($P<0.01$) (Fig. 2). Fetal 6KPGF$_{1\alpha}$ fell significantly by 120 min ($P<0.01$) (Fig. 3). There was an 84% fall in mean maternal 6KPGF$_{1\alpha}$ concentration. Due to the large inter-animal variation this fall was not statistically significant. Figure 3 shows the 6KPGF$_{1\alpha}$ to PGFM ratio in maternal uterine vein. The ratio increased in all 4 ewes. This change was not statistically significant due to the wide variation between animals.

Discussion

In more than 20 pregnancies at 120–130 days gestation using this ACTH regime (1,2,4,6,13), contractures gave way to contractures after 65–100 h, contractions then continued to delivery. Myometrial contractures can be decreased by 4AA or increased by administration of arachidonic acid, the major substrate for prostaglandin synthesis, to the pregnant ewe. In both situations the extent of contracture activity was directly proportional to the maternal uterine vein PGFM (3, and unpublished observations). This present investigation shows that PGs are also implicated in the control of labour and delivery contractions. The delicate balance of the various eicosanoids required to maintain contraction activity appears to differ from that present during contractions. It has been suggested that prostacyclin is an inhibitor of myometrial activity (7). Our data would support this view since the change from contractions to contractures occurs at the time of an increase in the $6KPGF_{1\alpha}$ to PGFM ratio.

Acknowledgement

This work was supported by a grant from the NIH-HD 12274. We are grateful to Karen Rasche for the preparation of this manuscript.

References

1. Buster, J. E., Cabalum, T., Jansen, C. A. M. and Nathanielsz, P. W. (1981). *J. Physiol.* **325**, 69–70P.
2. Cabalum, T. C., Oakes, G. K., Jansen, C. A. M., Yu, H. K., Hammer, T., Buster, J. E. and Nathanielsz, P. W. (1982). *Endocrinology* **110**, 1402–1407.
3. El Badry, A., Figueroa, J. P., Poore, E. R., Sunderji, S., Levine, S., Mitchell, M. D. and Nathanielsz, P. W. (1984). *Am. J. Obstet. Gynecol.* **5**, 474–479.
4. Harding, R., Poore, E. R., Bailey, A., Thorburn, G. D., Jansen, C. A. M. and Nathanielsz, P. W. (1982). *Am. J. Obstet. Gynecol.* **142**, 448–457.
5. Jansen, C. A. M., Krane, E. J., Thomas, A. L., Beck, N. F. G., Lowe, K. C., Joyce, P., Parr, M. and Nathanielsz, P. W. (1979). *Am. J. Obstet. Gynecol.* **134**, 776–783.
6. Jansen, C. A. M., Yu, H. K., Cabalum, T., Buster, J. E. and Nathanielsz, P. W. (1982). Society for Gynecologic Investigation. Abstract No. 289.
7. Lye, S. J. and Challis, J. R. G. (1982). *J. Reprod. Fertil.* **66**, 311–315.
8. Mitchell, M. D. (1978). *Prostaglan. Med.* **1**, 13–21.
9. Mitchell, M. D. and Flint, A. P. F. (1978). *J. Endocrinol.* **76**, 111–121.
10. Mitchell, M. D., Flint, A. P. F. and Turnbull, A. C. (1976). *Prostaglan.* **11**, 319–329.
11. Nathanielsz, P. W., Abel, M. H., Bass, F. G., Krane, E. J., Thomas, A. L. and Liggins, G. C. (1978). *Quart. J. Exp. Physiol.* **63**, 211–219.
12. Nathanielsz, P. W., Bailey, A., Poore, E. R., Thorburn, D. and Harding, R. (1980). *Am. J. Obstet. Gynecol.* **138**, 653–659.
13. Nathanielsz, P. W., Jansen, C. A. M. and Buster, J. E. (1983). *Endocrinology* **113**, 2216–2220.
14. Nathanielsz, P. W., Poore, E. R., Brodie, A., Taylor, N. F., Pimentel, G., Figueroa, J. P. and Frank, D. (1984). In: "Research in Perinatal Medicine", Vol. I, (Nathanielsz, P. W. and Parer, J. T., eds) Perinatology Press, Ithaca, New York.

Regional Changes in Uterine Catecholamines with Pregnancy as measured by High Pressure Liquid Chromatography with Electrochemical Detection

S. J. Arkinstall and C. T. Jones

The Nuffield Institute for Medical Research,
University of Oxford, Oxford, UK

Introduction

Mammalian uterus receives a rich adrenergic innervation consisting of long neurones originating in lumbar and mesenteric ganglia, and short neurones from peripheral sympathetic ganglia at and around the uterovaginal junction. These predominantly innervate blood vessels and the musculature respectively (1,2,3). Fluorescence histochemistry and fluorometric determinations revealed that noradrenaline is the major transmitter associated with these neurones (1,3). Using the same techniques it was reported that pregnancy caused a fall in neuronal histofluorescence and noradrenaline content in rabbit and guinea-pig uterus such that myometrium surrounding the fetus (perifetal) experiences an early and near total withdrawal of sympathetic influence whereas cervical innervation appears unaltered until late gestation when it too is almost devoid of noradrenaline. Myometrium adjacent to oviducts (tubal) receives an intact innervation throughout pregnancy (1,2,3,4). Similar pregnancy related noradrenaline depletion was observed in human isthmic myometrium (5) and sheep cervix (6). Conversely, rat uterine noradrenaline content was reported to increase with pregnancy (7). However, the fluorescence histochemistry and fluorometric assay used in these and other studies is unable to distinguish adequately between catechol compounds and so confidently quantitate tissue levels. This has led to discrepancies. For

The Physiological Development of the Fetus and Newborn
ISBN 0 12 389080 2

Copyright © 1985 by Academic Press, London.
All rights of reproduction in any form reserved.

instance high concentrations of adrenaline have been found in the uterus of rat (8), sheep (9) and rabbit (7), and in human uterus at levels above those of noradrenaline (7), while others have reported the uterus to be devoid of adrenaline (1,2). In the same way, dopamine has been detected in (10,11) and reported absent from uteri of various species (1,3). Such adrenaline and dopamine stores within uterine smooth muscle would be potential regulators of myometrial contractility (12,13) and it is therefore of some importance to accurately measure tissue levels of such putative peripheral neurotransmitters.

Methods

All laboratory animals were virgin or primigravida. Human uterus however was obtained from females with 1–3 previous pregnancies. Myometrial samples from rat, rabbit, guinea-pig, sheep and human were homogenized in 2 vol of ice cold 0.4 M perchloric acid containing 2 mmol sodium metabisulphite and a known amount of 3,4 dihydroxybenzylamine (DHBA) as internal standard. Catecholamines were extracted from neutralized supernatent with alumina at pH 8.6, eluted with 0.1 M perchloric acid containing 0.1 mmol sodium metabisulphite and 0.05 ml injected directly onto a Sphenisorb ODS (25 cm × 5 mm id, 5 μmol particle size) analytical column. Catechols were detected using a glassy-carbon working electrode at +0.72 V.

The mobile phase was 1.0% (w/v) citric acid monohydrate, 1.0% (w/v) sodium dihydrogen phosphate dihydrate, 1% (w/v) disodium hydrogen phosphate, 1 mmol EDTA, 0.048% (w/v) 1-octane sulphonic acid and 5% (v/v) methanol adjusted to pH 2.80–2.81 flowing at 1.0 ml/min.

Results

In no species at any gestational age was adrenaline detected (i.e. < 15 pmol/g). Noradrenaline was consistently the major catechol, although dopamine and its catabolite 3,4 dihydroxyphenylacetic acid (DOPAC) were present in guinea-pig and particularly sheep uterus at relatively high concentrations. L-DOPA was present in all tissues at around 20–100 pmol/g, but no species, regional or pregnancy related changes were observed.

In all species uterine noradrenaline concentration fell progressively with pregnancy and was regionally specific with a more rapid and extensive decline in perifetal myometrium which becomes almost devoid of transmitter by term (Fig. 1). Figure 2 shows progressive regional changes in guinea-pig uterine noradrenaline concentrations with pregnancy and is typical of changes observed in other species. In rat, rabbit and guinea-pig total uterine noradrenaline content fell some 40–50% by term ($P < 0.02$).

High concentrations of dopamine and DOPAC were detected in nonpregnant guinea-pig and particularly sheep uterus where, in some regions dopamine levels approached those of noradrenaline. In sheep these values remained largely unchanged near term except in perifetal tissue (Table 1). In guinea-pig however, both dopamine concentration and total content fell with pregnancy while DOPAC

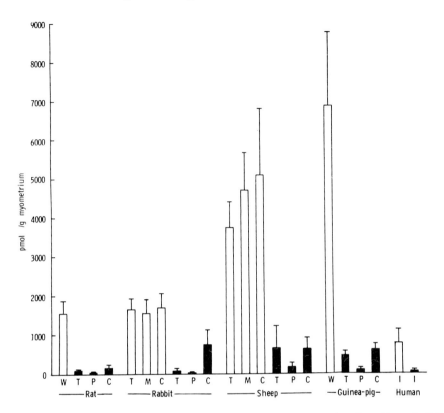

Figure 1. Noradrenaline concentrations in nonpregnant (open bars) and term (solid bars) uterus. Regions depicted are whole uterus, W; tubal myometrium, T; mid-uterine region, M; perifetal myometrium, P; cervix, C; isthmic myometrium, I. Vertical bars represent SD of the mean of 4–7 determinations.

content increased reflecting a large fall in dopamine/DOPAC ratio (Table 2). The near term mean dopamine concentrations reflected higher values in cervical and tubal myometrium (often >25 pmol/g), with perifetal tissue completely devoid of dopamine.

Discussion

Uterine sympathetic activation causes either relaxation or contraction depending on species and hormonal state. Thus, rabbit uterus under progesterone dominance responds to both exogenous and neuronal noradrenaline with relaxation and while under estrogen dominance with contractions (14). Guinea-pig uterus has been reported both to contract (15) and relax (16) in response to sympathetic stimulation, while an increased contractile state is most commonly reported for sheep and human uterus (5,9,12). Adrenergic stimulation in guinea-pig uterus

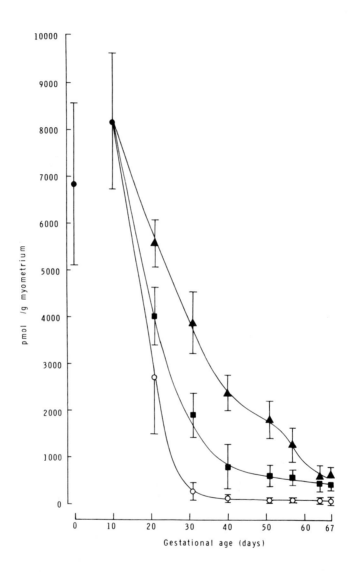

Figure 2. Changes in noradrenaline concentration in guinea-pig whole uterus, ●; perifetal myometrium, ○; tubal myometrium, ■; and cervix, ▲ with pregnancy in uterine horns bearing 2 or 3 fetuses. Full term is 67 days. Vertical bars represent SD of the mean of 2–5 determinations. Perifetal and tubal myometrium were significantly less than nonpregnant values at 20 days ($P<0.01$) and the cervix by 30 days ($P<0.01$). Tubal and cervical concentrations were greater than perifetal values at all times after 30 days ($P<0.01$).

Table 1. Concentration of dopamine and DOPAC (pmol/g) in non pregnant and 125–135 day pregnant sheep uterus. Full term is 147 days. Values given are mean ± SD of 6 determinations

	Dopamine	DOPAC
Nonpregnant		
Tubal	1307 ± 619	5256 ± 1868
Mid	2164 ± 1028	5417 ± 2328
Cervical	521 ± 205	2262 ± 1233
125–135 day		
Tubal	904 ± 475	2471 ± 1432
Perifetal	707 ± 555*	1517 ± 329*
Cervical	451 ± 325	1341 ± 643

*Significantly less than equivalent nonpregnant region ($P < 0.02$).

Table 2. Total mean dopamine concentration (pmol/g), dopamine content (pmol/uterus) and dopamine/DOPAC ratio in nonpregnant and pregnant guinea-pig uterus. Full term is 67 days. Values are the mean ± SE of 6–8 determinations

Gestational age	Dopamine Concentration (pmol/g)	Dopamine Content (pmol/uterus)	Dopamine/DOPAC
Nonpregnant	292 ± 122	315 ± 118	1.15 ± 0.13
10 day	281 ± 43	306 ± 31	1.10 ± 0.17
21 day	*161 ± 53	322 ± 100	0.95 ± 0.55
31 day	*63 ± 23	256 ± 55	*0.35 ± 0.25
40 day	*33 ± 17	242 ± 74	*0.11 ± 0.07
51 day	*13 ± 6	213 ± 96	*0.06 ± 0.03
57 day	*5 ± 4	*95 ± 75	*0.03 ± 0.03
64 day	*5 ± 4	*30 ± 42	*0.02 ± 0.02

*Significantly less than nonpregnant ($P < 0.01$).

also indirectly myometrial contractility by increasing sensitivity to oxytocin (17). Thus, the physiological role of the sympathetic innervation in myometrial contractility appears complex.

Changes in uterine noradrenaline with pregnancy presented here are in general agreement with previous studies using less specific histochemical and fluorometric techniques (1,2,3,5,6). Histological (18) and ultrastructural (19) signs of neuronal breakdown in term perifetal myometrium suggest that the fall in noradrenaline concentration reported here and elsewhere (1,2,3,5,6) is at least partly due to sympathetic neuronal degeneration. However, since steroid hormones have been implicated in the control or noradrenaline metabolism in uterine short adrenergic neurones (1,20,21) the changing hormonal milieu associated with pregnancy is likely to contribute towards and observed withdrawal of sympathetic influence from the uterus.

Previously it was reported that rat total uterine noradrenaline content was increased during pregnancy (7). Using HPLC other catechol compounds were found only at low levels and so nonspecific assay techniques do not explain this discrepancy. Since it was proposed that rat uterine adrenergic innervation is unique, constituting mainly long sympathetic neurones insensitive to steroid action (1,3,21), the observed decline must be related to some other factor(s) accompanying pregnancy such as stretch-induced neuronal breakdown (3).

It is reported that perifetal adrenergic innervation is not fully recovered 6 months postpartum (3). Thus, the low noradrenaline concentrations in human isthmus in comparison with other species (Fig. 1) may be due to incomplete postpartum recovery.

However the exceedingly low noradrenaline concentrations during late pregnancy will probably limit considerably or even abolish the ability of adrenergic innervation to elicit contractile responses in this region. Further, the observed β-adrenergic (relaxatory) super-sensitivity in the late pregnant uterus (5,16) is likely to result from reduced uptake and breakdown of catecholamines, and potentially an increased β-receptor coupling and/or number due to the absence of sympathetic transmitter (22). The resultant perifetal myometrial quiescence would be of importance if expulsive uterine contractions which may be initiated in tubal regions (3), are to be transmitted in a synchronized manner down towards the cervix.

An important difference between measurements made here and those elsewhere (7,8,9) is the absence of detectable adrenaline in any uterine tissue studied. Interest in adrenaline stems from its capacity to relax the pregnant uterus (12) and hence be a potentially important agent regulating myometrial quiescence. Although present studies do not eliminate a possible highly localized but limited storate site, they indicate that adrenaline is unlikely to be a regulator of myometrial contractility.

In the past, peripheral dopamine was assumed to be only a precursor of noradrenaline. There is now evidence however that it functions as a neuro-transmitter and/or co-transmitter in some peripheral tissues (23). The high concentrations of dopamine found in guinea-pig and particularly sheep uterus is in contrast to previous studies using fluorometric techniques (1,3). In some peripheral tissues of rat and human the dopamine catabolites DOPAC and homovanillic acid are present in high concentrations and it was suggested that this reflects release of dopamine in preference for use in noradrenaline synthesis (11). If it is assumed that dopamine present within guinea-pig and sheep uterus is the result of local synthesis, the high concentrations of DOPAC present within these tissues may reflect catabolism of dopamine following its release as a neurotransmitter. If this interpretation is correct, the precipitous fall in dopamine/DOPAC ratio in guinea-pig uterus with pregnancy (Table 2) may indicate increased activity of a dopaminergic innervation on release of dopamine as cotransmitter.

References

1. Sjoberg, N.-O. (1967). *Acta Physiol. Scand.* **305** (suppl.).
2. Rosengren, E. and Sjoberg, N.-O. (1968). *Acta Physiol. Scand.* **72**, 412–424.

3. Thorbert, G. (1978). *Acta Obst. Gynecol. Scand.* **79** (suppl.).
4. Thorbert, G., Alm, P., Owman, Ch., Sjoberg, N.-O. and Sporrong, B. (1978). *Acta Physiol. Scand.* **103**, 120–131.
5. Nakanishi, H., McLean, J., Wood, C. and Burnstock, G. (1969). *J. Reprod. Med.* **11**, 20–33.
6. More, J. and Nedjar, K. (1984). *Histochem.* **80**, 59–62.
7. Cha, K.-S., Lee, W.-C., Rudzik, A. and Miller, J. W. (1965). *J. Pharmacol.* **148**, 9–13.
8. Wurtman, R. J., Axelrod, J. and Kopin, I. J. (1963). *Endocrinology* **73**, 501–503.
9. Rexroad, C. E. and Barn, C. R. (1978). *Biol. Reprod.* **19**, 297–305.
10. Swedin, G. and Brudin, J. O. (1968). *Experientia* **24**, 1015–1016.
11. Lackovic, Z., Rezja, M. and Neff, N. H. (1982). *J. Neurochem.* **38**, 1453–1458.
12. Zuspan, F. P., Cibils, L. A. and Pose, S. V. (1962). *Am. J. Obstet. Gynecol.* **84**, 841–851.
13. Urban, J., Radwan, J., Laudanski, T. and Akerlund, M. (1982). *Br. J. Obstet. Gynecol.* **89**, 451–455.
14. Miller, M. D. and Marshall, J. M. (1965). *Am. J. Physiol.* **209**, 859–865.
15. Isaac, P. F. and Pennefather, J. N. (1969). *Eur. J. Pharmacol.* **5**, 384–390.
16. Elmer, M., Alm, P. and Thorbert, G. (1980). *Acta Physiol. Scand.* **108**, 209–213.
17. Russe, W. M. and Marshall, J. M. (1970). *Biol. Reprod.* **3**, 13–22.
18. Gardmark, S., Owman, C. and Sjoberg, N.-O. (1971). *Am. J. Obst. Gynecol.* **109**, 997–1002.
19. Sporrong, B., Alm, P., Owman, Ch., Sjoberg, N.-O. and Thorbert, G. (1978). *Cell. Tiss. Res.* **195**, 189–193.
20. Falck, B., Owman, Ch., Rosengren, E. and Sjoberg, N.-O. (1969). *Endocrinology* **84**, 958–959.
21. Falck, B., Gardmark, S., Nybell, G., Owman, Ch., Rosengren, E. and Sjoberg, N.-O. (1974). *Endocrinology* **94**, 1475–1479.
22. Harden, T. K. (1983). *Pharmacol. Rev.* **35**, 5–32.
23. Goldberg, L. I. (1972). *Pharmacol. Rev.* **24**, 1–29.

Placental Electrolyte Transfer with particular reference to Sodium

C. P. Sibley, B. S. Ward,
Jocelyn D. Glazier and R. D. H. Boyd

Departments of Obstetrics and Gynaecology, Paediatrics and Physiology,
University of Manchester at St Mary's Hospital, Manchester, UK

"Does the placenta behave like an inert membrane between the maternal and fetal circulations, or does it contribute energy in the transfer of material from mother to fetus, thereby becoming a secretory organ? Before this problem can be solved, it is probable that the transfer rate of many physiologic substances across the placenta will have to be investigated."

Flexner and Gellhorn (1)

Ion Transfer by Diffusion?

It is widely believed that small ions, notably sodium and chloride, cross the placenta only by simple diffusion and ultrafiltration through water filled channels (e.g. 2). The high unidirectional flux for sodium across the haemochorial placenta (3), the absence of substantial maternofetal plasma concentration differences for chloride or sodium (4) and the absence of any reports of inhibition or stimulation of transplacental sodium or chloride flux by inhibitors or hormones all lend support to this point of view. The argument is especially cogent with regard to the haemochorial placenta which tends to mimic a capillary wall in its permeability to hydrophilic nonelectrolytes, unlike the epitheliochorial sheep placenta which more closely resembles the cell membrane (5).

However, in both haemochorial and epitheliochorial placentas certain strands of evidence are not entirely easy to reconcile with this view. There are 3 general categories of experiment:

(i) Evidence that sodium and chloride movement across the limiting membrane of the syncytiotrophoblast of haemochorial placentae does involve specific carriers.

The Physiological Development of the Fetus and Newborn
ISBN 0 12 389080 2

Copyright © 1985 by Academic Press, London.
All rights of reproduction in any form reserved.

(ii) Evidence that the movement of other ions of comparable size to sodium and chloride across both haemochorial and epitheliochorial placentae is not at all, or not entirely, by diffusion.

(iii) Direct evidence for active sodium transport across certain *in vitro* systems.

The Syncytial Microvillous Membrane

Although water filled channels can be demonstrated partially traversing the syncytiotrophoblast in the perfused guinea-pig placenta following elevation of umbilical venous outflow pressure (6), we are not aware of direct evidence for water filled channels permeating the entire distance across the syncytiotrophoblast of haemochorial placentae. Until such are demonstrable it seems prudent to assume that all substances, including sodium, that cross the placenta must traverse the maternally facing microvillous "cell" membrane of the syncytium and also its basal membrane. The maternally facing syncytial membrane has been quite extensively studied in the human. Thus transmembrane potential has been measured using intracellular micro-electrodes (7), syncytial membrane has been reconstituted as micro-vesicles (8), and the efflux of radio ion into the surrounding medium has been measured after preloading individual villi with 86 rubidium as a marker for potassium (9).

Micro-electrodes demonstrate the presence of a membrane potential of 40 mV, inside negative, suggesting that, as with other animal cells, sodium is actively extruded across the syncytial cell membrane (7). Micro-vesicles allow entry of sodium, but only if chloride is present and, if present, that chloride entry is not blocked by frusemide (10). This is evidence of sodium and chloride co-transport. Pre-loaded whole villi allow rubidium out of the cell at an increased rate if the villus is placed in hypertonic medium but this increase does not occur if sodium or chloride is excluded from the external medium; again evidence for sodium and chloride co-transport, on this occasion linked to potassium efflux. Both micro-electrode studies and investigations of whole villi also support the existence of a second potassium channel whose permeability depends on calcium ions (9,11).

There is thus compelling evidence for carrier-mediated, specific ion transport across the maternally facing syncytial brush border; *transmembrane* transport. It is difficult however to prove that this membrane is indeed obligatorily involved in *transplacental* transport and not by-passed through hitherto undiscovered transsyncytial shunts. Studies across the entire width of the placenta *in vivo* provide some support for transport indeed involving carriers.

Transplacental Ion Movement *in vivo*

Flexner (1) demonstrated unidirectional sodium flux across the placentae of several species and inferred that the ratio of net to unidirectional flux was wide, ranging from about 1:3 in the sow to 1:1000 in the human; both near term. He pointed out that the result of the experiments did not provide evidence either for or against "secretion" of sodium (1).

At first sight, the existence of a maternofetal electrical potential difference (PD) (reviewed in (12)) in most species studied except the rabbit (13) and the human at term (14) does provide *prima facie* evidence in favour of active transplacental ion transport, but the elegant studies of Faber and co-workers have discredited this line of reasoning. They measured the distribution of exogenous ions such as sulphate, lithium and bromide in species with a substantial maternofetal PD, the guinea-pig (in which they also studied rubidium) (15) and the sheep (16). In no instance did the ions take up a maternofetal steady state ratio importantly different from one, as might have been predicted if there were a transplacental PD of 15–30 mV or more; the *in vivo* value. In the face of this it is difficult to suppose that a maternofetal PD is the same as a transplacental PD. Positive evidence for active transplacental ion transport *in vivo* has to be sought elsewhere than in the maternofetal PD alone.

There are 3 other *in vivo* approaches that must be considered. First, even the haemochorial placenta maintains concentration differences for calcium ions (17), for phosphate ions (4), and, perhaps less securely, for potassium (4). It is a little hard, though not impossible, to see how concentration gradients for some small molecules can be maintained if there are water filled channels sufficiently wide to allow sodium and chloride to pass without a carrier mechanism. Secondly, there is clear evidence for carrier mediated, competitively inhibitable, transfer of at least one small ion, iodide, both in the sheep, in which steady state transplacental flux of radio iodide but not of sodium or chloride is markedly inhibited by thiocyanate (18), and in the guinea-pig (19). Finally, the placenta seems able to maintain a widened potassium concentration difference across the haemochorial placenta of the rat in response to fetal need. Dancis (20) reared pregnant rats with and without a diet sufficiently deficient in potassium to render the mother hypokalaemic. The concentrations of potassium in fetal and maternal plasma in the hypokalaemic and control rats are shown in Table 1.

Table 1. Effect of diet on potassium concentrations in plasma of rats (20)

Diet	No. of animals	Maternal plasma level	Fetal plasma level
		mEq/l	
Control	11	4.61±0.25	5.5±0.15
K deficient	6	2.3±0.18	6.0±0.27

Thus the maintenance of concentration differences is evidence for transplacental active transport; inhibition of iodide flux points towards carrier-mediated ion movement; and protection from hypokalaemia supposes the control of movement of at least potasisum ions. What can *in vitro* systems tell us?

In vitro Systems

The obvious approach would be to study ion transfer across the perfused placenta but this has provided little positive evidence of active or controlled transfer of most ions; though it does for calcium (21). Either there is none for other ions or it is masked by the known increase in "leakiness" on placental perfusion (22). There is evidence in perfused placentae for ouabain inhibition of potassium movement but it is not clear that *transplacental* potassium movement is involved (23). Two other *in vitro* placental systems have however shown evidence of active ion movement.

One is the wall of the blastocyst, in itself the precursor of placental trophoblast. It has been extensively studied. The rabbit blastocyst investigated using radiosodium to measure ion flux and micro-electrodes to record PD demonstrates definite active sodium accumulation (reviewed in 24). The permeability characteristics of the blastocyst changes rapidly in early gestation (25) and the period studied is far distant in time, in terms of embryonic development, from the placenta of late gestation. Nevertheless the "placenta" of this species which, near term, is one of the leakier placentae at an early stage demonstrates active and inhibitable sodium transport.

The other *in vitro* system that we ourselves have been studying is the pig placenta. This species has a diffuse epitheliochorial placenta covering almost the entire inner surface of the uterus surrounding each fetus (26). A membranous layer can be stripped off the myometrium (see Fig. 1) and mounted in an Ussing type chamber between two fluid-filled compartments (27,28,29). The tissue as

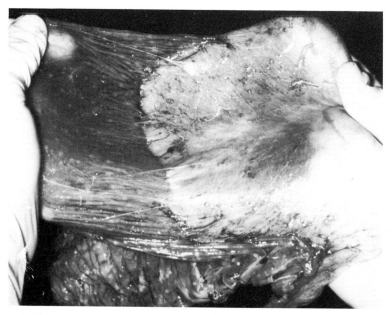

Figure 1. Manual separation of placenta (on left) from myometrium after excision of uterus from anaesthetized Large White/Landrace sow. Gestational age approximately 100 days. Note membranous nature of placenta and areolae (white spots) just visible on placental surface.

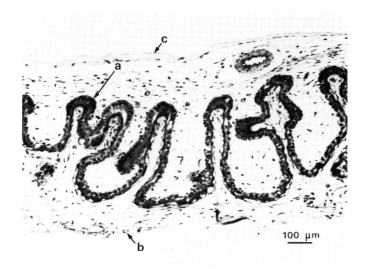

Figure 2. Cross-section of pig placenta at 101 days gestation, obtained immediately following caesarean hysterectomy. a. epitheliochorial membrane; b. surface of attachment to myometrium; c. amniotic epithelium. (Reprinted with permission from Ref. 7.)

mounted by us (Fig. 2) consists of two layers of loose connective tissue separated by two interdigitated single cell layers, the chorion and the maternal epithelial layers. On the fetal side there is in addition a thin cellular amniotic or allantoic layer depending from where in the uterus the placenta has been stripped. At intervals of a few mm over the placenta small white spots or areolae can be identified with the naked eye (30). They are just visible in Fig. 1.

We find that discs of placentae mounted in an Ussing chamber generate a PD which is, in contrast to previous reports using early gestation placentae (27), positive on the fetal rather than the maternal side. Mean short circuit current, open circuit PD and resistance measured using 8 cm² placental discs 90 min after voltage clamping are shown in Table 2. The placentae were taken from anaesthetized Large White/Landrace sows of 95–105 days gestation (term 115 days) much later than the specimens studied by McCance (27). It can be seen that there is a significant PD, short circuit current and resistance recorded from such placentae. Placentae from mini-pigs similarly mounted show a net

Table 2. Mean values 90 min after voltage clamping on 8 cm²discs of placenta mounted in Ussing chamber and bathed with oxygenated Kreb's bicarbonate ringer

PD (fetal side +)	Short circuit current	Resistance
4.2 ± 0.5 mV	$6.8 \pm 0.75 \mu A/cm^2$	$635 \pm 40 \Omega/cm^2$
($n=50$)	($n=50$)	($n=50$)

Table 3. Maximum change in short circuit current Iscc and pd ($t_{90}=0$) mean±SEM n=number of chambers (8 cm^2 discs of placentae from Large White/Landrace sows 95–105 days gestation)

Addition	Change in Iscc ($\mu A/cm^2$)	Change in pd mV
dbcAMP (10^{-3} M) $n=8$	$+3.1\pm1$**	$+1.1\pm0.5$**
None (control) $n=10$	-0.6 ± 0.8	-1.0 ± 0.4
dbcAMP (10^{-3} M) + Ouabain (10^{-4} M) $n=6$	-4.2 ± 0.8**	-2.4 ± 0.3**
None (control)	-0.4 ± 0.3	-0.5 ± 0.2
Adrenaline (10^{-5} M) $n=14$	$+3.0\pm0.6$**	$+1.0\pm0.2$**
None (control) $n=10$	-0.1 ± 0.4	-0.6 ± 0.3

(t test *vs* control; **$P<0.01$)

sodium flux towards the fetal chamber after addition of dibutyryl cyclic AMP (10^{-3} M) (31). A similar stimulation of short circuit current and PD is shown in Table 3 for placentae from Large White/Landrace pigs after addition of dibutyryl cyclic AMP or adrenaline to the fetal compartment.

Other sympathomimetics also stimulate PD and short circuit current with an activity sequence isoprenaline > noradrenaline > adrenaline > phenylephrine. Isopraneline gives a 50% maximal stimulation of short circuit current at 6×10^{-9} M; for phenylephrine the concentration is 4×10^{-5} M. We conclude from this sequence that the stimulatory effect of sympathomimetics is likely to be due to activation of a β-receptor. It is of interest that fetally facing β-receptors have been previously described in other placentae (32,33). The fetal concentration of circulating noradrenaline in the pig (34) after cord occlusion is comparable to the fetal level necessary to stimulate the placenta *in vitro*.

As also shown in Table 3, there is inhibition of dibutyryl cyclic AMP stimulation by ouabain at 10^{-4} M. These observations led Firth (35) to examine our material histochemically for sodium potassium ATPase. To our astonishment this enzyme is almost entirely localized to the fetal cells of the previously mentioned areolae or white spots. There is in addition weak staining in the glands of uterine epithelium opposite the areolae; elsewhere no activity.

On the basis of present evidence we conclude that sodium transport across the isolated pig placenta near term is, after stimulation, active in the direction mother to fetus and we further speculate that stimulation takes place through activation of β-receptors. Sodium potassium ATPase activity appears to be localized only to certain placental areas; the areolae.

Very much more remains to be done to confirm these findings and other interpretations are still possible. It is impossible at present to be sure that the active ion transport is performed by the placental rather than the amniotic or allantoic layers of the tissue, though on both histological grounds and distribution of ATPase an ion transporting role for the amniotic or allantoic layer appears unlikely. Excluding this possibility is particularly important in view of reports of marked ion concentration differences between plasma and allantoic fluid in this species (36).

Acknowledgements

We are grateful to the Wellcome Trust for financial support.

References

1. Flexner, L. B. and Gellhorn, A. (1943). *Am. J. Obstet. Gynecol.* **43**, 965–974.
2. Faber, J. J. and Thornburg, K. L. (1983). "Placental Physiology". p. 94. Raven Press, New York.
3. Flexner, L. B., Cowie, D. B., Hellman, L. M., Wilde, W. S. and Vosburgh, G. J. (1948). *Am. J. Obstet. Gynecol.* **55**, 469–480.
4. Faber, J. J. and Thornburg, K. L. (1981). *Placenta* **S2**, 203–214.
5. Faber, J. J. (1977). *Fed. Proc.* **36**, 2640–2646.
6. Kaufmann, P., Schroder, H. and Leichtweiss, H.-P. (1982). *Placenta* **3**, 339–348.
7. Yano, J., Okada, Y., Tsuchiya, W., Kinoshita, M., Tominaga, T. and Nishimura, T. (1981). *Acta. Obstet. Gynecol. Jpn.* **33**, 137–141.
8. Bissonnette, J. M. (1982). *Placenta* **3**, 99–106.
9. Boyd, C. A. R. (1983). CIBA Symp. No. 95, pp. 300–314. Pitman Publishing Ltd, London.
10. Boyd, C. A. R., Chipperfield, A. R. and Lund, Elizabeth, K. (1980). *J. Physiol.* **307**, 86.
11. Yano, J., Okada, Y., Tsuchiya, W., Kinoshita, M. and Tominaga, T. (1982). *Biochem. Biophys. Acta* **685**, 162–168.
12. Canning, Jane F. and Boyd, R. D. H. (1984). *In:* "Fetal Physiology and Medicine", (Beard and Nathanielsz, eds) Marcel Dekker, New York.
13. Mellor, D. J. (1969). *J. Physiol.* **204**, 395–405.
14. Mellor, D. J., Cockburn, F., Lees, M. M. and Blagden, A. (1969). *J. Obst. Gynaecol. Brit. Commonwealth* **76**, 993–998.
15. Binder, N. D., Faber, J. J. and Thornburg, K. L. (1979). *J. Physiol.* **282**, 561–570.
16. Thornburg, K. L., Binder, N. D. and Faber, J. J. (1979). *Am. J. Physiol.* **236**, C58–65.
17. Schauberger, C. W. and Pitkin, R. M. (1979). *Obstet. Gynecol.* **53**, 74.
18. Boyd, R. D. H., Canning, Jane F., Stacey, T. E. and Ward, R. H. T. (1981). *J. Physiol.* **312**, 23–24.
19. Logothetopoulos, J. and Scott, R. F. (1956). *J. Physiol.* **132**, 365–371.
20. Dancis, J. and Springer, D. (1970). *Pediat. Res.* **4**, 346–351.
21. Twardock, A. R. and Austin, M. K. (1970). *Am. J. Physiol.* **218**, 540–545.
22. Hedley, R. and Bradbury, M. W. B. (1980). *Placenta* **1**, 277–285.
23. Bailey, D. J., Bradbury, M. W. B., France, V. M., Hedley, R., Naik, S. and Parry, H. (1979). *J. Physiol.* **287**, 45–56.
24. Benos, D. J. and Biggers, J. D. (1981). In: "Fertilization and Embryonic Development *in vitro*", (Mastroianni, L. and Biggers, J. D., eds) pp. 283–297. Plenum Press, New York.
25. Benos, D. J. and Biggers, J. D. (1983). *J. Physiol.* **342**, 23–33.
26. Crombie, P. R. (1972). The morphology and ultrastructure of the pig placenta throughout pregnancy. Ph.D Thesis, University of Cambridge.
27. Crawford, J. D. and McCance, R. A. (1960). *J. Physiol.* **151**, 458–471.
28. Moore, W. M. O., Ward, B. S. and Shields, R. A. (1974). *Am. J. Obstet. Gynecol.* **120**, 932–936.
29. Bazer, F. W., Goldstein, M. H. and Barron, D. H. (1981). *In:* "*In vitro* Fertilization". (Mastroianni, L. and Biggers, J. D., eds) pp. 299–321. Plenum Press, New York.

30. Hunter, J. (1861). "1781 Essays and Observations". (Professor Owen, ed.) London.
31. Boyd, R. D. H., Glazier, Jocelyn, D., Moore, W. M. O., Sibley, C. P. and Ward, B. S. (1984). *J. Physiol.* **349**, 43.
32. Whitsett, J. A., Johnson, C. L., Noguchi, A., Darovec-Beckerman, C. and Costello, M. (1980). *J. Clin. Endocrinol. Metab.* **50**, 27-32.
33. Boyd, C. A. R., Chipperfield, A. R. and Steele, L. W. (1979). *J. Develop. Physiol.* **1**, 361-377.
34. MacDonald, A. A., Colenbrander, B., Versteeg, D. H. G., Heilecker, A. and Wenning, C. J. G. (1984). *Roux Arch. Dev. Biol.* **193**, 19-23.
35. Firth, J. A. (1984). *Phys. Soc. Proc.* (July) 79.
36. Goldstein, M. H., Bazer, F. W. and Barron, D. H. (1980). *Biol. Reprod.* **22**, 1168.
37. Michael Kalliope, Ward, B. S. and Moore, W. M. O. (1983). *Placenta* **4**, 369-378.

Control of Fluid and Electrolyte Balance during Fetal Life

Jean E. Robillard, Kenneth T. Nakamura and Nancy A. Ayres

Department of Pediatrics and the Cardiovascular Research Center,
University of Iowa, Iowa City, Iowa, USA

Introduction

Prematurity is complicated by the fact that the physiologic mechanisms that should regulate and control the adaptation of premature infants to extra-uterine life are still in a fetal stage of development. Hyponatraemia, severe oliguria and renal failure are now diagnosed more and more frequently in preterm infants. The development of experimental models to study the fetal kidney *in utero* (1,2) has improved our knowledge of the functional maturation of the premature nephron.

Recent investigations (3–6) have focussed on the humoral mechanisms regulating sodium and water homeostasis by the fetal kidney. More specifically, the responsiveness of the fetal kidney to vasopressin (5) as well as the role of the renin-angiotensin-aldosterone system (3), the prostaglandin system (6), and the kallikrein-kinin system (5) in modulating renal sodium excretion have been investigated.

Renal-Sodium Homeostasis during Fetal Life

Recent studies (7–9) have demonstrated that the percentage of filtered sodium excreted (fractional excretion of sodium) is elevated early in gestation and decreases as gestation advances. In chronically catheterized fetal lambs, the fractional excretion of sodium decreases from 11% at 130 days of gestation to 5% near term (term being 145 days) (8). Merlet-Benichou *et al.* (7,9) have also observed in fetal guinea-pigs that the relative clearance of sodium and of other solutes are always higher in the fetus than in the newborn animal. Moreover, it was found that the urinary Na^+/K^+ ratio decreases as a function of gestation (7–9). Renal

The Physiological Development of the Fetus and Newborn
ISBN 0 12 389080 2

Copyright © 1985 by Academic Press, London.
All rights of reproduction in any form reserved.

tubular immaturity (10), large extracellular fluid volume (11), and relative tubular insensitivity to circulating aldosterone (12) have been suggested as possible factors to explain the high rate of urinary sodium excretion during fetal life.

Based on morphological evidence, it has been suggested that the relatively high fractional sodium excretion during fetal life is secondary to an inadequate tubular surface area for reabsorption (10). Also, since there is anatomic glomerular preponderance during fetal development (10), it has been postulated that a functional glomerulotubular imbalance may be partly responsible for the decreased tubular function in fetal lambs (8). More recently, Merlet-Benichou *et al.* (9) demonstrated in fetal guinea-pigs that there is a period of functional glomerular preponderance in the early stages of superficial nephron maturation followed by a phase of tubular catch-up.

The large extracellular fluid volume found normally during fetal life has been suggested as a potential factor controlling sodium reabsorption by the fetal kidney. It has been demonstrated that contraction of fetal extracellular fluid space following fetal peritoneal dialysis significantly decreases fractional excretion of sodium (11).

The role of aldosterone in controlling sodium reabsorption by the fetal kidney has been investigated. It has been shown that there is a decrease in urinary $(U/P)Na^+:K^+$ ratio values as the fetus matures and that this decrease is associated with a concomitant increase in fetal plasma aldosterone concentration (Fig. 1) (3). Merlet-Benichou *et al.* (7) have suggested that the rise in sodium reabsorption observed during maturation and postnatally is probably secondary to an increase in plasma aldosterone concentration. Moreover, it has been demonstrated that administration of exogenous aldosterone does stimulate distal renal tubular reabsorption of sodium and increase potassium excretion in fetal lambs (12–14). It has been suggested that the increase in the sensitivity of the renal tubule to aldosterone during development may be related to aldosterone induction of Na-K-ATPase and that the inductive process is probably mediated via glucocorticoid receptors (15).

Since prostaglandins (PGE_2 and PGI_2) have potent natriuretic properties (16) and that experiments in chronically catheterized fetal lambs have demonstrated that urinary excretion of prostaglandins is elevated during fetal life (4,6), it was proposed that prostaglandins may have an important role in modulating sodium homeostasis during development. However, contrary to what is found in adult animals (16), Matson *et al.* (6) have demonstrated that inhibition of prostaglandin synthesis produces an increase in fetal urinary sodium and chloride excretion despite a decrease in fetal renal blood flow. It was then suggested that endogenous prostaglandins generated by the fetal kidney have an opposite effect on fetal tubular sodium chloride transport than the one found in most adult animals. It has been previously observed that most prostaglandins synthesized in the kidney are natriuretic and that indomethacin, a cyclo-oxygenase inhibitor, reduces sodium excretion after sodium loading in adult animals (16).

Recent studies have suggested that the renal kallikrein-kinin system participates directly in the control of electrolytes and water excretion (17). During fetal life it has been demonstrated that urinary kallikrein excretion rate corrected for kidney

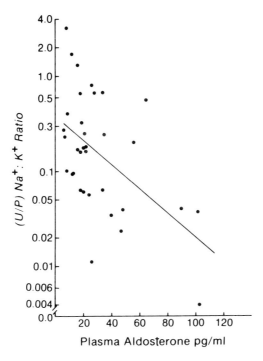

Figure 1. Relationship between plasma aldosterone concentration and (U/P)Na+:K+ ratio during fetal life. (U/P)Na+:K+ = Ratio of (U/P)Na+ over (U/P)K+. (From Ref. 3.) Log y = $-0.3587 - 0.0134 \cdot x$. $r = -0.53$. $P < 0.005$.

weight increases as gestation progressed and after birth (4). It has been observed that the rise in fetal urinary kallikrein excretion rate closely followed the increase in plasma aldosterone concentration, and a significant negative correlation was found between urinary kallikrein excretion rate and urinary sodium excretion.

Renal Water Metabolism during Fetal Life

In mammals, urine produced by the fetal kidney is hypotonic when compared to plasma values (18,19) and remains hypotonic until very late in gestation (19). In fetal lambs there is a significant increase in urine osmolality after 130 days of gestation (term, 145 days) and this rise is secondary to a parallel increase in urinary urea and nonurea solute (19). It is interesting to observe that the changes in urine composition during the last part of gestation are not accompanied by major changes in the electrolyte composition of fetal plasma. On the other hand, it was found that the percentage of filtered water excreted (V/GFR) and free water clearance corrected for GFR (CH_2O/GFR) decrease significantly after 130 days of gestation, suggesting a true increase in free water reabsorption by the fetal kidney in late gestation.

Factors that control the developmental aspects of renal tubular reabsorption of water during fetal life have been reviewed (20). The antidiuretic hormone, vasopressin, has been shown to be present in the posterior pituitary of fetal animals (21) and as early as the 11th week of gestation in the human (22). Moreover, it has been shown that during human and ovine parturition there is a release of vasopressin by the fetus (23,24). Furthermore, it has been demonstrated that both volume and osmoreceptor controls of vasopressin secretion are fully functional in the last trimester of gestation in the lamb fetus (25,26). On the other hand, it was found that the fetal nephron is less sensitive to vasopressin than the adult and that the capacity of the fetal kidney to concentrate increases with gestation (5,27) (Fig. 2). The increase in fetal urine osmolality during vasopressin infusion was 3 times less than in adult animals for the same plasma concentration of circulating AVP (Fig. 2). It can thus be speculated that there is an end-organ hyporesponsiveness to vasopressin during fetal life. It has been suggested that the smaller vasopressin stimulation of cyclic-AMP during development (28) may be an important factor contributing to the limited renal concentrating ability in immature animals. Moreover, one can speculate that prostaglandin E_2, found in high concentration in fetal lamb urine (6), may inhibit the action of vasopressin to promote water flow across the distal portion of the fetal nephron.

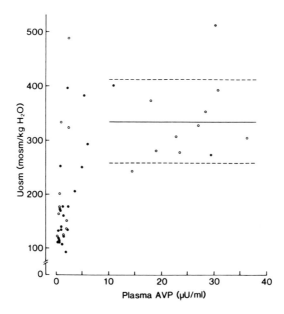

Figure 2. Relationship of plasma AVP to urine osmolality. Regression line for P_{AVP} values below 6 μU/ml was expressed by the formula $U_{osmol} = 135 + (35 \cdot P_{AVP})$. Coefficient of correlation for this relationship ($r = 0.50$) was statistically significant ($P < 0.005$). Broken lines represent ± 1 standard deviation from mean U_{osmol} value (solid line) for P_{AVP} levels above 6 μU/ml. (From Ref. 5.)

The structural immaturity of the medulla characterized by short loops of Henle (29) and the relatively increased blood flow to the medulla (30), have been suggested as major limiting factors for the build up of a cortical to papilla interstitial osmotic gradient by the fetal kidney. Zink and Horster (31) have shown that the ability of the loop of Henle to reabsorb sodium chloride and generate an hypotonic urine—a condition essential to create an osmotic gradient that permits the concentrating mechanisms to operate—is still immature in Wistar rats between 12–25 days postnatally. On the other hand, it has been demonstrated that an intrarenal solute and osmolar gradient is present in fetal lamb kidneys by early mid-gestation (32), suggesting that quantitatively the counter current multiplier system is fully functional in near-term fetal animals. Moreover, since the blood flow in the immature kidney is distributed to a greater extent to the juxtamedullary glomeruli, whose efferent arterioles supply the vasa recta of the medulla, it is possible that a high flow of blood through the vasa recta may disperse the intrarenal solute gradient normally found in the medulla of more mature animals. Taken together, these studies demonstrate that the medullary interstitium of the fetus does not become as hypertonic as that of the newborn or adult. On the other hand, it is shown that the fetal kidney may participate in the maintenance of fetal osmolar and volume homeostasis.

In summary, it has been demonstrated that the ability of the kidney to conserve sodium and to concentrate urine is limited during fetal life and the mechanisms regulating fluid and electrolyte balance during fetal life have been reviewed.

Acknowledgements

The present work was supported by United States Public Service Grants HD-11466 and HL-14388, and Iowa Heart Association Grant 83-G-32. K. T. Nakamura is the recipient of a National Research Service Award, HD-06438. N. A. Ayres is supported by training agent grant T-32-HL-07413.

References

1. Gresham, E. L., Rankin, J. H. G., Makowski, E. L., Meschia, G. and Battaglia, F. C. (1972). *J. Clin. Invest.* **41**, 149–156.
2. Robillard, J. E., Kulvinskas, C., Sessions, C., Burmeister, L. and Smith, F. G., Jr. (1975). *Am. J. Obstet. Gynecol.* **122**, 601–606.
3. Robillard, J. E., Ramberg, E., Sessions, C., Consamus, B., VanOrden, D., Weismann, D. and Smith, F. G., Jr. (1980). *Develop. Pharmacol. Ther.* **1**, 201–216.
4. Robillard, J. E., Lawton, W. J., Weismann, D. N. and Sessions, C. (1982). *Kidney Int.* **22**, 594–601.
5. Robillard, J. E. and Weitzman, R. E. (1980). *Am. J. Physiol.* **238**, F407–F414.
6. Matson, J. R., Stokes, J. B. and Robillard, J. E. (1981). *Kidney Intern.* **20**, 621–627.
7. Merlet-Benichou, C. and deRouffignac, C. (1977). *Am. J. Physiol.* **232**, F178–F185.
8. Robillard, J. E., Sessions, C., Kennedey, R. L., Robillard, L. H. and Smith, F. G., Jr. (1977). *Am. J. Obstet. Gynecol.* **128**, 727–734.

9. Merlet-Benichou, C., Pegorier, M., Muffat-Joly, M. and Augeron, C. (1981). *Am. J. Physiol.* **241**, F618–F624.
10. Fetterman, G. H., Shuplock, N. A., Philipp, F. J. and Gregg, H. S. (1965). *Pediat.* **35**, 601–619.
11. Robillard, J. E., Sessions, C., Burmeister, L. and Smith, F. G., Jr. (1977). *Pediat. Res.* **11**, 649–655.
12. Siegel, S. R., Oakes, G. and Palmer, S. (1981). *Pediat. Res.* **15**, 163–165.
13. Robillard, J. E., Nakamura, K. T., McWeeny, O., Wear, S. and Lawton, W. (1985). *Pediat. Res.* (in press).
14. Lingwood, B., Hardy, K. J., Coghlan, J. P. and Wintour, E. M. (1978). *J. Endocrinol.* **76**, 553–554.
15. Aperia, A., Larsson, L. and Zetterstrom, R. (1981). *Am. J. Physiol.* **241**, F356–F360.
16. Dunn, M. J. (1979). *In:* "Hormonal Function and the Kidney", (Brenner, B. M. and Stein, J. H., eds) pp. 89–114. Churchill Livingstone, New York.
17. Carretero, O. and Scicli, A. G. (1980). *Am. J. Physiol.* **238**, F247–F255.
18. Alexander, D. P. and Nixon, D. A. (1961). *Br. Med. Bull.* **17**, 112.
19. Robillard, J. E., Matson, J. R., Sessions, C. and Smith, F. G., Jr. (1979). *Pediat. Res.* **13**, 1172–1176.
20. Robillard, J. E., Weitzman, R. E., Fisher, D. A. and Smith, F. G., Jr. (1982). *In:* "The Kidney During Development", (Spitzer, A., ed.) pp. 205–213, Masson, New York.
21. Vizsolyi, E. and Perks, A. M. (1969). *Nature* **223**, 1169–1171.
22. Levina, S. E. (1968). *Gen. Comp. Endocrinol.* **11**, 151–159.
23. Chard, T., Hudson, C. N., Edward, C. R. W. and Boyd, N. R. H. (1971). *Nature* **234**, 352–354.
24. Stark, R. I., Daniel, S. S., Husain, K. M., James, L. S. and Wiele, R. L. V. (1979). *Biol. Neonate* **35**, 235–241.
25. Robillard, J. E., Weitzman, R. E., Fisher, D. A. and Smith, F. G., Jr. (1979). *Pediat. Res.* **13**, 606–610.
26. Weitzman, R. E., Fisher, D. A., Robillard, J. E., Erenberg, A., Kennedy, R. and Smith, F. G. (1978). *Pediat. Res.* **12**, 35–38.
27. Daniel, S. S., Stark, R. I., Husain, M. K., Baxi, L. V. and James, L. S. (1982). *Am. J. Physiol.* **242**, F740–F744.
28. Schlondorff, D., Weber, H., Trizna, W. and Fine, L. G. (1978). *Am. J. Physiol.* **234**, F16–F21.
29. Speller, A. M. and Moffat, D. B. (1977). *J. Anat.* **123**, 487–500.
30. Jose, P. A., Logan, A. G., Slotkoff, L. M., Lilienfield, L. S., Calcagno, P. L. and Eisner, G. M. (1971). *Pediat. Res.* **5**, 335–344.
31. Zink, H. and Horster, M. (1977). *Am. J. Physiol.* **233**, F519–F524.
32. Moore, E. S., Kaiser, B. A., Simpson, E. H. and McMann, B. J. (1982). *In:* "The Kidney During Development: Morphology and Function" (Spitzer, A., ed.) pp. 223–231. Masson, New York.

Vasopressin and Plasma Renin Activity following Disturbances in Blood Pressure, Osmolality and/or Blood Volume in the Fetus

Salha S. Daniel, Raymond I. Stark, Alan B. Zubrow, Pamela J. Tropper and L. Stanley James

Columbia University, College of P. & S., Division of Perinatology, Departments of Anaesthesia, Pediatrics and Obstetrics and Gynecology, New York, USA

The third trimester fetal lamb has been shown to be capable of releasing vasopressin (VP) and renin (PRA) into the circulation in response to hypovolaemia and hypotension (1–4). Vasopressin is also released by the fetus in response to changes in plasma osmolality and can contribute to osmolar homeostasis through its effect on the fetal kidney (5–7). The present experiments were designed to examine the relative importance of blood pressure, volume and osmolality on the release of VP and PRA in the fetus.

Methods

A total of 24 chronically instrumented fetal lambs 120–131 days gestation were studied. In group I (8 animals), 15–20% fall in mean arterial blood pressure was produced by intravenous infusion of sodium nitroprusside for 1 h. In group II, fetuses received an intravenous infusion of 4 ml/kg, 4.5% sodium chloride over 30 min. Mothers in group III were given 500 ml of 20% mannitol intravenously over 1 h in order to produce moderate fall in blood volume (BV) in the fetus (4).

Blood and urine samples collected before and following the various experimental treatments were analysed for VP, PRA osmolality and sodium concentration. Fetal arterial blood pressure and heart rate were monitored throughout.

Results in each group were analysed using the Student's t test for paired samples. In addition the findings on all samples were subjected to correlation analyses.

The Physiological Development of the Fetus and Newborn
ISBN 0 12 389080 2
Copyright © 1985 by Academic Press, London.
All rights of reproduction in any form reserved.

Results and Conclusions

None of the experimental procedures was associated with changes in fetal pHa, $PaCO_2$ or PaO_2.

Changes in mean arterial pressure, plasma osmolality and sodium concentration in the 3 groups are presented in Table 1. There was no change in plasma osmolality or sodium concentration as a result of hypotension in group I; no change in arterial blood pressure occurred as a result of infusion of hypertonic saline (group II) or mannitol infusion to the ewe in group III.

Levels of plasma VP and PRA before and following experimental procedures in the 3 groups are shown in Fig. 1. The levels were highest following induced

Table 1. Mean arterial pressure, plasma osmolality and sodium concentration (Mean±SEM) before (C) and following (Exp) experimental procedure

Group	I		II		III	
	C	Exp	C	Exp	C	Exp
MBP (mmHg)	48.1 ± 1.62	38.6** ± 1.92	48.4 ± 2.59	47.6 ± 2.02	49.2 ± 3.16	49.2 ± 4.21
Osm(mOsm/kg)	294.3 ± 2.27	296.3 ± 1.38	293.6 ± 2.44	302.2** ± 2.27	291.6 ± 2.89	299.2* ± 2.11
Na(mEq/l)	142.5 ± 1.45	142.9 ± 1.26	142.1 ± 1.36	146.2** ± 1.18	140.6 ± 1.12	145.0** ± 1.32

*$P<0.05$ compared to control
**$P<0.01$ compared to control

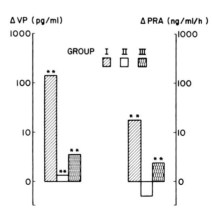

Figure 1. Mean change in fetal plasma vasopressin (VP) and renin activity (PRA) following fetal hypotension (I), hyperosmolality (II) and hypovolaemia (III). **$P<0.01$.

hypotension while the smallest effect was seen following intravenous infusion of hypertonic saline. ΔVP as a result of the various procedures was generally larger than ΔPRA. A good positive correlation was found between log VP and log PRA during the control periods and in groups I and III. Correlations were also found between log PRA and MBP ($-$ve) and between log VP and POSM ($+$ve).

Hypotension and mannitol infusion both caused a decrease in urine output and in free water clearance (Table 2 and Fig. 2). The decrease was larger following hypotension which also caused a significant decrease in sodium excretion. Group II which received hypertonic saline, had a transient rise in urine output, and a small increase in U_{OSM} and C_{H_2O}. There was a good correlation between log VP and urine output ($-$ve), and osmolality ($+$ve). Log PRA correlated well with $U_{Na/k}$ but only weakly with urinary excretion (8).

Table 2. Urine output (V), osmolality (U_{osm}), sodium excretion (UV_{Na}), and free water clearance (C_{H_2O}) before (C) and following (Exp) experimental procedures (mean $\pm$ SEM)

Group	I		II		III	
	C	Exp	C	Exp	C	Exp
V(ml/kg/min)	0.23 $\pm$ 0.026	0.04** $\pm$ 0.015	0.16 $\pm$ 0.015	0.22** $\pm$ 0.005	0.20 $\pm$ 0.023	0.10** $\pm$ 0.009
U_{Osm}(mOsm/kg)	153 $\pm$ 15.8	328** $\pm$ 31.5	118 $\pm$ 7.3	162* $\pm$ 25.3	163 $\pm$ 17.7	218* $\pm$ 18.7
UN_a(μEq/kg/min)	7.6 $\pm$ 0.82	4.0** $\pm$ 0.70	2.5 $\pm$ 0.79	3.6 $\pm$ 1.09	3.6 $\pm$ 1.44	3.7 $\pm$ 0.75
C_{H_2O}(ml/kg/min)	0.10 $\pm$ 0.029	-0.01** $\pm$ 0.003	0.06 $\pm$ 0.012	0.08* $\pm$ 0.005	0.10 $\pm$ 0.006	0.03** $\pm$ 0.004

*$P<0.05$ compared to control
**$P<0.01$ compared to control

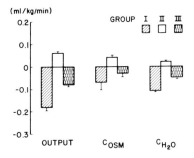

Figure 2. Change in urine output, osmolar (C_{OSM}) and free water clearances (C_{H_2O}) following fetal hypotension (I), hyperosmolality (II) and hypovolaemia (III) (Mean $\pm$ SEM).

These experiments show that hypotension is a potent stimulus for the release of VP and PRA in the fetus. Plasma volume, osmolality and sodium concentration also have an effect but at the level of disturbances produced, the change in VP and PRA was smaller. These experiments also show that the fetal kidney contributes to the maintenance of fluid and osmotic homeostasis. These results indicate that although placental exchange plays the major role, release of VP and PRA by the fetus can contribute to the finer tuning of fetal fluid homeostasis. Because of the good correlation between PRA and MBP and rather weak correlations between PRA and either P_{Na} or urinary excretion, it is speculated that this system is involved mainly with blood pressure regulation.

References

1. Kelly, R. T., Rose, J. C., Meis, P. J., Hargrave, B. Y. and Morris, M. (1983). *Am. J. Obstet. Gynecol.* **146**, 807–812.
2. Leake, R. D., Stegner, H., Palmer, S. M., Oakes, G. K. and Fisher, D. A. (1983). *Pediat. Res.* **17**, 583–586.
3. Mott, J. C. (1975). *Br. Med. Bull.* **31**, 44–50.
4. Lumbers, E. R. and Lewes, J. L. (1979). *Biol. Neonate* **35**, 23–32.
5. Robillard, J. E. and Weitzman, R. E. (1980). *Am. J. Physiol.* **238**, F407–444.
6. Daniel, S. S., Stark, R. I., Husain, M. K., Baxi, L. V. and James, L. S. (1982). *Am. J. Physiol.* **242**, F740–744.
7. Wintour, E. M., Congiu, M., Hardy, K. J. and Hennessy, D. P. (1982). *Q. J. Exp. Physiol.* **67**, 427–435.
8. Stevens, A. D. and Lumbers, E. R. (1981). *J. Develop. Physiol.* **3**, 101–110.

The Effect of Maternal
Water Deprivation on
Ovine Fetal Blood Volume

R. J. Bell and E. M. Wintour

Department of Physiology and the Howard Florey Institute of
Experimental Physiology and Medicine, University of Melbourne,
Parkville, Victoria, Australia

In a previous study (1), it was established that there is a gestational trend in the release of antidiuretic hormone (ADH) by the ovine fetus in response to the osmotic stress induced by maternal water deprivation. The fetal plasma ADH concentration, [ADH] was significantly greater, at a given plasma osmolality, in mature (126–144 days gestation) than immature (107–119 days) fetuses. Hypovolaemia secondary to haemorrhage is an effective stimulus for ADH release by the ovine fetus (2). The aim of this study was to assess whether hypovolaemia compounds the stimulus to ADH release by the ovine fetus during maternal water deprivation.

The study was carried out using the chronically cannulated fetuses of cross-bred merino ewes of known mating dates. The procedures for fetal cannulation and the maintenance of cannulae have been described previously (3). Surgery was performed between 90 and 110 days (term = 147 ± 5 days). The animals were maintained after surgery in individual metabolism cages with food and water available *ad lib.* No experiments were performed until at least 10 days after surgery and then only if fetal urinary osmolality was within the normal range (4).

The normal pattern of increase in fetal blood volume secondary to growth in the last third of pregnancy was established by measuring fetal blood volume weekly in a series of 4 control animals. Changes in fetal blood volume were then measured in a series of 6 animals undergoing 12 episodes of maternal water deprivation. At the start of each experiment fetal blood volume was determined on a control day (day 1). The ewe then underwent complete water deprivation for 24 h and was then given 500 ml water daily for the following 3 days. Fetal blood volume

The Physiological Development of the Fetus and Newborn
ISBN 0 12 389080 2

Copyright © 1985 by Academic Press, London.
All rights of reproduction in any form reserved.

was measured on the day of maximal maternal dehydration (day 5) after which water was returned to the ewe *ad lib*.

Fetal blood volume was determined using a dilution technique [with ^{125}I-labelled Human Serum Albumin (HSA) (Amersham) as the indicator] to measure plasma volume and the haematocrit was used to convert plasma volume to blood volume taking into account the correction factors for trapped plasma and whole body haematocrit (5); 1.0 ml of a sterile solution of ^{125}I-labelled-HSA (0.1 μCi) was injected into the fetal venous cannula after initially collecting a 2.5 ml sample of fetal blood to determine background counts; 2.5 ml samples of fetal arterial blood were collected at 10, 20, 30 and 40 min from the time of injection. The volume of each sample was replaced with sterile normal saline at the time of collection. The plasma was separated from the cells by centrifugation and 1.0 ml samples of plasma and triplicate 1.0 ml samples of a standard solution (prepared by diluting 1.0 ml of the [125]-I-HSA to a volume of 100 ml) were counted on a Packard Auto-Gamma Scintillation Spectrophotometer n. 5110 for a time designed to achieve a relative error of < 1% (10–20 min). The counts in the plasma samples were plotted against time and the line of best fit extrapolated to the time of injection and the plasma volume determined using the Formula

$$\text{Plasma Volume} = \frac{\text{no. counts in standard}}{\text{no. counts at } T_o} \times \frac{100}{1}$$

The method of least squares was used to determine the regression lines. Analysis of variance was used to assess the significance of the regressions. The four regression lines for the control fetuses were all significant at $P < 0.01$ and they were not significantly different from each other. The function describing the common regression was

blood volume (ml) = $-618.5 + 7.331$ (gestation in days)

This regression was significant at $P < 0.001$. The 95% confidence limits on the slope are 6.55 and 8.11.

The birthweight was known for 3 of the 4 control anmals. The final blood volume measurement ranged between 13.4% and 16.9% of the birthweight.

In all 12 water deprivation experiments the second blood volume measurement performed on the day of maximal maternal dehydration was greater than the control measurement. Thus the rate of increase in fetal blood volume was positive in all cases. In 5 of the 12 experiments the rate of increase in fetal blood volume was greater than controls (range 7.7–15.3 ml/day) and in 7 studies the rate of increase was less than controls (range 3.0–6.0 ml/day). Almost all the slopes lay outside the 95% confidence limits of the slope of the common regression line of the controls. The 7 slopes lying below the 95% confidence limit occurred in fetuses with hypotonic urine on the day of maximal maternal dehydration. Three of the 4 slopes lying above the 95% confidence limits occurred in fetuses with markedly hypertonic urine on the day of maximal maternal dehydration.

It has been established that the use of ^{125}I-labelled human serum albumin to measure plasma volume gives an over-estimation of blood volume when compared with a double-label method, by about 10% (6). However, as we were interested in the rate of change in blood volume in this study rather than absolute volume we were satisfied with this degree of over-estimation. The percentage of bodyweight made up by blood volume in the control animals in this study was very similar to that reported by another group (6) using the single-label method. Only 2 previous studies have evaluated the relationship between fetal blood volume and gestational age in chronically cannulated fetal sheep (7,8) and one of these studies (7) was limited by only one or two measurements being made in most fetuses near the end of gestation. The results of our control measurements which showed a highly significant association between gestational age and blood volume were consistent with the findings of the group (8) which also performed repeated measurements over the last third of pregnancy.

The results of the water deprivation studies have confirmed that maternal dehydration does not cause fetal hypovolaemia. An increase in fetal blood volume occurred during each maternal dehydration experiment (consistent with the fetus growing during the experiment) and there was no consistent effect of maternal water deprivation on the rate of increase in fetal blood volume. The greater variability in the rates of increase in blood volume during experiments compared with control data is probably because slopes determined during dehydration studies were based on 2 points and the slope of the control regression was based on many points.

The association between the relative expansion of blood volume (rate of increase above the 95% confidence limits of the slope of controls) during maternal dehydration and the presence of hypertonic urine in the fetus suggests that ADH may be involved in the regulation of fetal blood volume by acting to conserve water at the fetal kidney and also possibly at the placenta.

This study has confirmed that ADH release by the ovine fetus during maternal water deprivation is in response to the osmotic stimulus and not fetal hypovolaemia.

References

1. Bell, R. J., Congiu, M., Hardy, K. J. and Wintour, E. M. (1984). *Q. J. Exp. Physiol.* **69**, 187–195.
2. Robillard, J. E., Weitzman, R. E., Fisher, D. A. and Smith, F. G. (1979). *Pediat. Res.* **13**, 606–610.
3. Lingwood, B., Hardy, K. J., Horacek, I., McPhee, M. L., Scoggins, B. A. and Wintour, E. M. (1978). *Q. J. Exp. Physiol.* **63**, 315–330.
4. Wintour, E. M., Congiu, M., Hardy, K. J. and Hennessy, D. P. (1982). *Q. J. Exp. Physiol.* **67**, 427–435.
5. Coghlan, J. P., Fan, J. S. K., Scoggins, B. A. and Shulkes, A. A. (1977). *Aust. J. Biol. Sci.* **30**, 71–84.
6. Creasy, R. K., Drost, M., Green, M. V. and Morris, J. A. (1970). *Circulat. Res.* **27**(4), 487–494.
7. Stankewytsch-Janusch, B., Scroop, G. C., Marker, J. D. and Seamark, R. R. (1981). *J. Develop. Physiol.* **3**, 245–254.
8. Caton, D., Wilcox, C. J., Abrams, R. and Barron, D. H. (1975). *Q. J. Exp. Physiol.* **60**, 45–54.

Hydration in Normal, Growth Retarded and Premature Infants

D. B. Cheek, J. Wishart, A. H. MacLennan and R. R. Haslam*

Department of Obstetrics and Gynaecology, The University of Adelaide, South Australia and *Department of Neonatology, The Queen Victoria Hospital Inc., South Australia

The literature concerning total body water (TBW), extracellular volume (ECV) and intracellular water (ICW) in the neonate, has been confused. For example, it has been stated that weight loss is due to cell water loss (1), that caesarean section babies have a 20% increase in ICW (2), that loss of water from the cellular phase is dramatic (150 ml/kg) in the first 24 h (3) and that hyponatraemia occurs in small premature babies below 1.3 kg without any shift of water into the cells (4).

By contrast, in very early studies years ago, the corrected bromide space (ECV) *per se* in infants over the first week of life decreased progressively which accounted for, in the main, the weight loss of normal infants in early postnatal life (5). However, with the passage of time we have learned that criteria for assessing normal, premature and growth retarded or low weight for gestational age (LWGA) infants are strict—that so called normally grown infants have a narrow range of weight and that premature infants are either normally grown for gestational age or growth retarded (6). Earlier studies had no such adequate guidelines.

The present study involved 107 infants. Three groups of infants were selected for study:

37 Mature normally growth (38–41 weeks), birth weights 3.0–4.8 kg.

25 Premature infants, appropriate weights for gestational age (30–35 weeks), birth weights 1.4–2.6 kg.

45 Mature LWGA infants (37–40 weeks), birth weights 1.4–2.6 kg.

Gestational age was assessed by:

Accurate menstrual history, correlating with uterine size.

Ultrasonic examination before the 20th week.

Dubowitz assessment confirming within 2 weeks the calculated time.

The Physiological Development of the Fetus and Newborn
ISBN 0 12 389080 2

Copyright © 1985 by Academic Press, London.
All rights of reproduction in any form reserved.

Normal or retarded growth was assessed by:

Appropriate weight for gestation charts adjusted for maternal height and weight and infant's sex and birth rank.

Subscapular and triceps fat thickness.

Neonatal appearance, behaviour and weight gain.

Biochemical methods were improved such that TBW was determined with deuterium oxide, $^2HO_2$, given by stomach tube from a weighed syringe and determined by infrared spectrophotometry with the cell containing $^2HO_2$ corrected for temperature, thus improving sensitivity and precision (7). Urine of the neonate being very dilute is suitable for $^2HO_2$ determination (8).

Extracellular volume was determined as the corrected bromide space since Cl and Br distribute commensurately and the distribution of Cl in the body is known and accountable (9). Bromide was determined on plasma obtained by "heel stick" with the micro method of Goodwin (10) or by proton-induced X-ray emission (7,11).

Results

In this cross-sectional study, the weight changes of normal infants decreases over the first week as expected. The weight of premature infants remained at an approximately constant level over the first 2 weeks while an increase of some 200 g occurred in the LWGA group at 7 days.

The total body water of premature and LWGA age infants was over 800 g/kg due to lack of fat in adipose tissue, as has been known for years (12). The normal infant has a constant value of 750–760 g/kg. There was a progressive fall in ECV over the period of study in all 3 groups, indeed, the loss of ECV in the premature infants accounted for the loss of TBW.

Normally grown infants showed a progressive rise in ICW (TBW-ECV) after the second day and by 7 days the increase was significant by comparison with day 1. Premature infants were found to have no increase in ICW during the period of study (1–28 days). By contrast, LWGA infants showed a progressive increase in ICW which reached significance on days 7 and 14. At no time was hyponatraemia found to be present. The lowest values were in 3 premature infants at 7 days (133 mmol/l), when there was some suggestion of an increase in cell hydration.

Hydration of Normal Mature Infants born Vaginally or by Caesarean Section

Using similar techniques and protocols 65 infants were studied, 48 of whom were born vaginally and 17 by caesarean section. ECV during the first 24 hours of postnatal life in the vaginally born and caesarean section groups varied only from 343 ± 27 ml and 374 ± 31 ml at 6 hours to 358 ± 21 ml and 354 ± 29 ml at 24 hours respectively. Contrary to previous opinion neither TBW nor cell hydration differed in infants born by caesarean section compared with those born vaginally.

Discussion

It would appear that the fall in ECV in the newborn period is valid and significant (330-360 ml/kg in normal infants during the first week).

Clearly, weight loss is not due to cell water loss in the early days of postnatal life but rather there is a redistribution of water and ECW enters the cells. Loss of body weight after birth is related to a relative starvation not dehydration.

Infants of LWGA had a progressive gain in ICW which we believe is not related to water intoxication but rather to growth. The cell water : cell protein ratio is a constant in mammalian tissue. If cell protein increases, so does cell water (13). Sinclair and Silverman (14) showed in 1966 that the metabolic rate of the LWGA infant is higher than normal postnatally and our own studies have shown that water metabolism as measured by neonatal water turnover is much increases in these babies (15). It is important to point out that the earlier studies (1,2,3,4) that reported conflicting results to this paper all employed the use of antipyrine as a measure of TBW. This agent tags to protein, is metabolized in the liver and has not been proven to follow body water in the neonate or in pregnancy (16).

The fact that the premature is liable to hyponatraemia particularly where there is also a degree of growth retardation and exaggerated cell hydration as demonstrated in this study, emphasizes the risk of giving hypotonic fluid loads (180-200 ml/kg) (17,18).

References

1. MacLaurin, J. C. (1966). *Arch. Dis. Child.* **41**, 217, 286-291.
2. Cassady, G. (1971). *N. Engl. J. Med.* **284**, 16, 887-891.
3. Cassady, G. and Milstead, R. R. (1971). *Pediat. Res.* **5**, 673-682.
4. Roy, R. N., Chance, G. W., Radde, I. C., Hill, D. E., Willis, D. M. and Sheepers, J. (1976). *Pediat. Res.* **10**, 526-531.
5. Cheek, D. B., Maddison, T. G., Malinek, M. and Coldbeck, J. H. (1961). *Pediat.* **28**, 861-869.
6. Altman, D. G. and Coles, E. C. (1980). *Br. J. Obstet. Gynaec.* **87**, 2, 81-86.
7. Byers, F. M. (1979). *Ann. Biochem.* **98**, 208-213.
8. Cheek, D. B., Wishart, J., MacLennan, A. H., Haslam, R. R. and Fitzgerald, A. (1982). *Early Hum. Dev.* **7**, 323-330.
9. Cheek, D. B., West, C. D. and Golden, C. C. (1957). *J. Clin. Invest.* **36**, 2, 240-351.
10. Goodwin, J. F. (1971). *Clin. Chem.* **17**, 554-548.
11. Cheek, D. B., Hay, H. J. and Newton, C. S. (1979). *Aust. Phys. Sci. Med.* **2**, 85-93.
12. Clapp, W. M., Butterfield, J. and O'Brien, D. (1962). *Pediat.* **29**, 883-889.
13. Cheek, D. B., Habicht, J. P., Berall, J. and Holt, A. B. (1977). *Am. J. Clin. Nutr.* **30**, 851-860.
14. Sinclair, J. C. and Silverman, W. A. (1966). *Pediat.* **38**, 48-62.
15. MacLennan, A. H., Hocking, A., Seamark, R. F., Godfrey, B. and Haslam, R. R. (1983). *Early Human Dev.* **8**, 21-31.
16. Seitchik, J. and Alper, C. (1954). *Am. J. Obstet. Gynaecol.* **68**, 1540-1550.
17. Aperia, A. and Zetterstrom, R. (1982). *Clin. Perinatol.* **9**, 3, 523-533.
18. Oh, W. (1982). *Clin. Perinatol.* **9**, 3, 537-643.

Fetal Thoracic Duct Lymph Flow in the Chronically Catheterized Sheep

Robert A. Brace

Division of Perinatal Biology, Department of Physiology, School of Medicine,
Loma Linda University, Loma Linda, California, USA

Introduction

Recent studies in the fetal sheep (1,2) suggest that both the rate and extent of fluid and protein movement across the capillary wall may be significantly greater in the fetus than in the adult. Many previous studies have explored whole body lymph flow rates in the adult using flow from the left thoracic duct (3,4). Thus the purpose of this study was to catheterize left thoracic duct lymph flow rates in the sheep fetus under normal conditions.

Methods

Animal preparation

Pregnant Rambouillet-Columbia ewes with a single fetus underwent catheter implantation in the descending aorta, inferior vena cava through hindlimb vessels, and in the left carotid artery and jugular vein at 125–130 days. The fetal left thoracic duct was catheterized at its junction with the jugular and subclavian veins at the base of the neck. The lymphatic catheter was connected to the jugular catheter except during the lymph collection periods. Animals were maintained on daily antibiotics (2 ml of Combiotic intramuscularly to the ewe and 500 mg Ampicillin into the amniotic fluid).

For the first 7 postsurgical days, mean fetal thoracic duct lymph flow rate, vascular pressures, heart rate, and amniotic fluid pressure were measured over a 1 h period at 1 min intervals. On the 7th day, after measurement of control lymph flow, other experiments were performed.

Fetal arterial and venous pressures were recorded using amniotic fluid pressure as the zero pressure reference by subtracting the intra-uterine pressure from the

The Physiological Development of the Fetus and Newborn
ISBN 0 12 389080 2

Copyright © 1985 by Academic Press, London.
All rights of reproduction in any form reserved.

fetal vascular catheter pressures with the on-line computer. Lymph flow rate was determined by collecting the lymph in a continuously weighed sterile vial. The height of the outflow catheter was adjusted so that the pressure at its tip averaged -5 to -15 mmHg with respect to amniotic fluid pressure. The lymph was periodically returned to the fetus through a vascular catheter.

In addition to the 1 h observations, the effects of lymphatic catheter outflow pressure and outflow resistance were explored. At 20 min intervals, the height of the outflow catheter was changed randomly and lymph flow was recorded as a function of the hydrostatic pressure gradient between the lymphatic vessel at the point of catheterization and the amniotic fluid. Only data from the last 10 min of each 20 min period was accepted in order to avoid flows which may have been recorded during capacitative changes of the lymphatic system.

Data analysis

A two-way analysis of variance was used to determine whether the daily average lymph flow rates changed during the first 7 postsurgical days and tested for statistical significance using the Duncan's multiple range test. Differences at the P 0.05 level were taken as statistically significant.

Results

Fetal thoracic duct lymph flow rate was variable. The coefficient of variation for the first 7 postsurgical days in 5 fetuses averaged $29 \pm 6\%$ for the hourly average and was independent of the day. The hourly average lymph flow rates increased during the first few postsurgical days as shown in Table 1. Lymph flow varied with outflow pressure. As illustrated in Fig. 1, lymph flow rate was independent of outflow pressure whenever outflow pressure was less than zero. Lymph flow rate decreased at higher pressures and completely ceased at outflow pressures of 10–20 mmHg (mean 14 mmHg).

Approximately 60% of the hourly lymph flow averages were normally distributed about the mean (Fig. 2). A large majority of the non-normal distributions were associated with an exaggerated mode. Correlation and linear regression analyses showed that lymph flow rate was not dependent upon spontaneous changes in arterial, venous, or amniotic fluid pressures or fetal heart

Table 1. Average hourly thoracic duct lymph flow rates and average standard deviations in 5 chronically catheterized sheep fetuses for the first 7 postsurgical days

	Lymph flow rate (ml/min)						
	Postsurgical day						
	1	2	3	4	5	6	7
Mean	0.57	0.45	0.59	0.81	0.83	0.93	0.89
Average SD	0.10	0.09	0.19	0.18	0.27	0.16	0.15

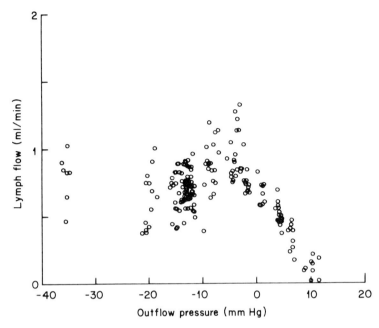

Figure 1. Illustration of the relationship between fetal thoracic duct lymph flow rate and lymphatic outflow pressure. Lymphatic outflow pressure is expressed relative to amniotic fluid pressure after correction for flow resistance in the lymphatic catheter.

rate. There were two exceptions to this finding. First, when lymph flow was low due to an elevated outflow pressure, flow rose during spontaneous increases in intra-uterine pressure. Obviously, this flow increase occurred because the net outflow pressure was significantly reduced by the elevation in intra-uterine pressure. Second, in some fetuses, lymph flow rate increases during spontaneous decreases in fetal heart rate. The cause for this is unknown but the changes in heart rate suggest that the increases in lymph flow may be associated with fetal movement.

Discussion

A large majority of the lymph which flows in the body is carried by the thoracic duct (4). Humphreys *et al.* (5) measured flow in anaesthetized, acutely catheterized fetal sheep and found average values of 0.04 ml/min/kg in fetuses of 120–130 days gestation and 0.09 ml/min/kg in fetuses of 138–147 days gestation, compared with 0.05 ml/min/kg in the adult. Smeaton *et al.* (6) reported that the thoracic duct of the fetal sheep could be chronically catheterized for up to 5 days and that lymph flow averaged 0.05–0.10 ml/min/kg. On a weight basis, fetal thoracic duct lymph flow rate averaged approximately 0.25–0.30 ml/min/kg in the present study, or 3–4 times the previously reported values. The cause of this difference

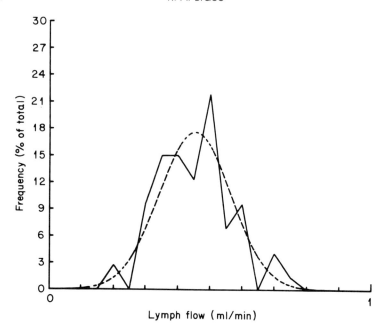

Figure 2. Histogram of fetal lymph flow rates illustrating that the observed distribution (solid line) is not significantly different from the normal distribution (dashed line) calculated from the mean and standard deviation. The interval width for this plot was 0.05 ml/min.

may be the pentobarbital anaesthesia, which was used by Humphreys *et al.* (5), and is known to reduce thoracic duct lymph flow by about 50% (3). In the study by Smeaton *et al.* (6) the thoracic duct was catheterized low in the chest instead of in the neck as in the present study, thereby excluding some of the thoracic sources on lymph.

One final factor which was not discussed in the previous studies is the effects of outflow pressure on fetal lymph flow. As illustrated in Fig. 1, at outflow pressures approximately equal to or less than fetal venous pressure, fetal lymph flow was not affected by outflow pressure. However, elevating the tip of the outflow catheter by only a few inches above the zero pressure for the amniotic fluid caused a dramatic decrease in lymph flow. In the present study, pressure at the inner tip of the lymphatic catheter averaged -5 to -15 mmHg during flow measurements for the 7 day observation period so the observed flows most likely represent the normal *in vivo* thoracic duct lymph flow rates in the sheep fetus.

In the sheep, adult left thoracic duct lymph flow ranges from 0.05 to 0.08 ml/min/kg (3). Thus the fetal thoracic duct lymph flows found in the present study are approximately 5 times adult sheep flow rates. The majority of the information regarding fetal lymph flows is derived from studies of fetal lung lymph flow as it relates to the clearance of fluid from the lungs at birth (5,7,8). This could indicate fetal sheep pulmonary lymph flow rates of 3–6 time adult values. Indeed Smeaton *et al.* (6) found that lymph flow from the lumbar trunk in the fetus averaged about 4 times adult levels.

It has long been established that lymph flow in the newborn is higher than in the adult (9). Thus, collectively the literature along with the present study suggest that whole body lymph flow rates in the fetus may be in the order of 5 times adult levels.

Acknowledgement

The author sincerely appreciates the technical assistance of Debra Brittingham and Kirk Turner. This study was funded in part by NIH grant HD17312.

References

1. Brace, R. A. (1983). *Circulat. Res.* **52**, 730–734.
2. Brace, R. A. (1983). *Am. J. Obstet. Gynecol.* **147**, 777–781.
3. Yoffey, J. M. and Courtice, F. C. (1970). "Lymphatics, Lymph and the Lymphomyeloid Complex". Academic Press, New York and London.
4. Brace, R. A. and Power, G. G. (1981). *Am. J. Physiol.* **240**, R282–R288.
5. Humphreys, P. W., Normand, I. C. S., Reynolds, E. O. R. and Strang, L. B. (1967). *J. Physiol.* **193**, 1–29.
6. Smeaton, T. C., Cole, G. J., Simpson-Morgan, M. W. and Morris, B. (1972). *Aust. J. Exp. Biol. Med. Sci.* **47**, 565–572.
7. Boston, R. W., Humphreys, P. W., Reynolds, E. O. R. and Strang, L. B. (1965). *Lancet* **2**, 473–474.
8. Bland, R. D., Bressack, M. A. and Haberkern, C. M. (1980). *Fed. Proc.* **39**, 280.
9. Holman, R. (1937). *Am. J. Physiol.* **118**, 354–358.

Prolactin Secretion Following Intracerebroventricular Infusion of Hypertonic Artificial Cerebrospinal Fluid in the Fetal Sheep at 115–130 Days Gestation

J. P. Figueroa, T. McDonald, T. Reimers,
P. D. Gluckman and P. W. Nathanielsz

Reproductive Studies, State University of New York,
College of Veterinary Medicine, Cornell University, Ithaca, New York, USA
and University of Auckland, School of Medicine, Department of Paediatrics,
Auckland, New Zealand

Introduction

Radioimmunoassayable prolactin (PRL) has been detected in fetal sheep plasma as early as 87 days gestation (12). Since PRL does not cross the ovine placenta, fetal PRL is most probably of fetal origin. However, human chorion-decidual tissue will synthesize PRL (4). PRL has been implicated in the control of water and salt balance in both the adult (5) and fetal (6) mammal. However, the evidence for a physiological significant role for fetal PRL in the regulation of fluid volume or composition in the fetus remains controversial.

Previous studies on the control of PRL secretion in the fetus have demonstrated that exogenously administered thyrotropin releasing hormone (TRH) (10) will stimulate fetal PRL release and bromoergocryptine (CB154), a dopamine agonist will inhibit the release of PRL (9).

The aim of the present studies was to investigate the response of the fetus to intracerebroventricular administration of hypertonic artificial cerebrospinal fluid (ACSF) on the secretion of PRL. Two different forms of hypertonic ACSF, 4.5% sodium chloride (NaCl, w/v) and urea 10% were used.

The Physiological Development of the Fetus and Newborn
ISBN 0 12 389080 2

Copyright © 1985 by Academic Press, London.
All rights of reproduction in any form reserved.

Materials and Methods

Four pregnant Rambouillet-Columbia ewes with a single mating date were studied. At 110 days gestation fetal jugular vein and carotid artery catheters were implanted as previously described (13). A lateral ventricular catheter was placed in the fetus under stereotactic guidance (3). At least 5 days were allowed to elapse postsurgery before any experiment was performed and at least 1 day elapsed between any 2 experiments on the same animal.

Intracerebroventricular Administration
of Different Solutions

Isotonic artificial CSF was prepared according to (8). The hypertonic solutions were made by adding either 4.5% NaCl w/v (hypertonic sodium chloride ACSF) or 10% urea w/v (hypertonic urea ACSF). Following a single fetal resting blood sample, a 4 h infusion of artificial ACSF (35 μl/min) either isotonic or hypertonic was commenced into the lateral ventricle. Fetal blood samples were taken at 15, 30, 60, 120 and 180 min. At 180 min, 5 μg thyrotropin releasing hormone (TRH Relefact, Organon) in saline was administered to the fetal jugular. Further blood samples were taken at 15 min (195 min from the commencement of the infusion), 30 and 60 min after the TRH challenge.

Radioimmunoassay for Fetal Plasma Prolactin (PRL)

PRL measurement was performed in 100 μl heparinized plasma as described by (1) using a prolactin antiserum (DJB-7-0330) kindly supplied by Dr D. J. Bolt (2). Ovine prolactin (LER-860-2), donated by Dr L. E. Reichert, Jr, Albany, NY, was radioiodinated using the chloramine-T procedure (6). Sensitivity of the assay was 2.5 ng/ml of NIAMMD-oPRL-I1, the reference preparation. Estimates of inter-assay and intra-assay precision have been reported (14).

Statistical Analysis

Data was analysed by one way analysis of variance (ANOVA) and Student's t test with the Bonferroni modification for multiple comparisons. To analyse potential changes in acid-base balance we have used [H+] rather than pH since pH data are distorted by log transformation.

Results

Outcome of preparations of blood gas responses
to the experimental procedure

Fetal blood gases and pH were within the normal range at the start of the intracerebroventricular infusions (13). During the infusion and the following 24 h fetal carotid PO_2 was unchanged (25.7 $\pm$ 2.8 Torr at the start of the infusion and

22.7±1.7 Torr 24 h after the beginning of the experiment). Fetal carotid pH was unchanged during the isotonic ACSF infusion but fell late in the experiments with hypertonic sodium chloride and urea ACSF infusions (Fig. 1). The fall observed in pH before the TRH administration in the hypertonic sodium chloride ACSF infusion was due to a fall in only one fetus (7.34 at 120 and 7.015 at 180). In both experimental protocols fetal carotid $[H+]$ rose after the TRH administration but was statistically significant only for the hypertonic urea infusion $(P < 0.01)$. All fetuses were alive and well with normal fetal pH and blood gases at least 3 days later when they were either examined for histology or used to test the response of the hypothalamus to exogenous CRF.

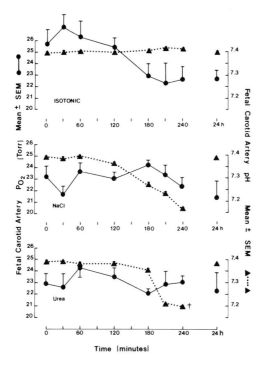

Figure 1. Fetal carotid pH (▲) and PO₂ (●) (mean ± SD) following the administration of 8.4 ml artificial CSF to the lateral cerebroventricular space over 4 h. Resting sample was taken at time 0.

Changes in fetal plasma PRL

Figure 2 shows the comparison of the administration of hypertonic sodium chloride ACSF and isotonic ACSF. Within 60 min of the commencement of the hypertonic ACSF to the lateral ventricle, fetal PRL had risen to 193% of the control levels $(P < 0.05)$; using the paired t test.

Figure 3 shows a similar comparison of the administration of hypertonic urea ACSF and isotonic ACSF. Within 60 min of the commencement of the hypertonic

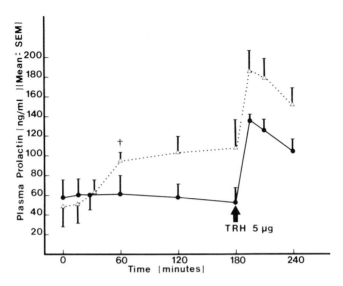

Figure 2. Fetal plasma prolactin concentration following the administration of 8.4 ml of either isotonic ACSF (●——●) or hypertonic sodium chloride ACSF (4.5%) (△ ······ △) to the lateral cerebroventricular space over 4 h *n*: 4 mean ± SEM for each group the resting sample was taken at 0 time immediately before the infusion.

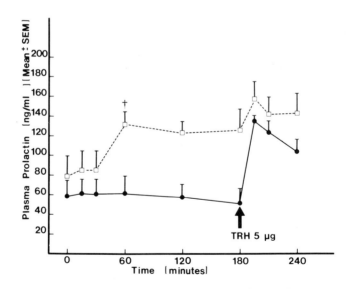

Figure 3. Fetal plasma prolactin concentration following the administration of 8.4 ml of either isotonic ACSF (●——●) or hypertonic urea (□ ----- □) to the lateral cerebroventricular space over 4 h *n*: 4 mean ± SEM for each group the resting sample was taken at 0 time immediately before the infusion.

saline to the lateral ventricle, fetal PRL had risen to 165% of the control levels ($P<0.05$ paired t test). With both hypertonic solutions, the effect of the TRH administration was additive.

Discussion

In vitro studies in which ovine PRL was added to the fetal side of human amniotic membrane have demonstrated that ovine PRL decreased the rate of passage of water from fetal to maternal sides of the amnion (7) other workers have observed an increase in water transport from fetus to mother (11). Whilst further work is required to reconcile these conflicting observations, the release of PRL that we have demonstrated in response to hypertonic solutions perfusing the cerebroventricular space suggests that central monitoring of the tonicity of fetal body fluids may constitute part of a homeostatic feedback control system regulating fetal water balance.

Acknowledgement

This work was supported by a grant from the NIH HD 12274. We would like to thank Karen Rasche for her assistance with this manuscript.

References

1. Davis, S. L., Reichert, Jr., L. E. and Niswender, G. D. (1971). *Biol. Reprod.* **4**, 145–153.
2. Echternkamp, S. E., Bolt, D. J. and Hawk, H. W. (1976). *J. Anim. Sci.* **42**, 893–900.
3. Gluckman, P. D. and Parsons, Y. (1984). *In:* "Animal Models in Fetal Medicine", Vol. III, (Nathanielsz, P. W., ed.) pp. 69–107. Perinatology Press, New York.
4. Golander, A., Hurley, T., Barrett, J., Hizi, A. and Handwerger, S. (1978). *Science* **202**, 311–313.
5. Horrobin, D. F., Lloyd, I. J., Lipton, A., Burstyn, P. G., Durkin, N. and Muiruri, K. L. (1971). *Lancet*, 332–354.
6. Hunter, W. M. and Greenwood, F. C. (1963). *Nature* **194**, 495–496.
7. Leontic, E. A. and Tyson, J. E. (1976). *Am. J. Physiol.* **232**(3), R124–R127.
8. Levine, J. E. and Ramirez, V. D. (1980). *Endocrinology* **107**, 1782.
9. Lowe, K. C., Beck, N. F. G., McNaughton, D. C., Gluckman, P. D., Kaplan, S. L., Grumbach, M. M. and Nathanielsz, P. W. (1979). *Am. J. Obstet. Gynecol.* **135**, 773–777.
10. Lowe, K. C., Magyar, D. M., Eisner, C. W., Buster, J. E. and Nathanielsz, P. W. (1980). *Society Gynecol. Inv.* Abstract No. 304.
11. Manku, M. S., Mrabji, J. P. and Horrobin, D. F. (1975). *Nature* **258**, 78–80.
12. Mueller, P. L., Gluckman, P. D., Kaplan, S. L., Rudolph, A. M. and Grumbach, M. M. (1979). *Endocrinology* **105**, 129–134.
13. Nathanielsz, P. W., Abel, M. H., Bass, F. G., Krane, E. J., Thomas, A. L. and Liggins, G. C. (1978). *Q. J. Exp. Physiol.* **63**, 211–219.
14. Reimers, T. J., McCann, J. P. and Cowan, R. G. (1983). *J. Anim. Sci.* **57**, 683–691.

Maternal Factors Related to the Role of the Fetal Kidney in the Prevention of Hypertension in Fetal Lambs

J. C. Mott, I. M. Fore, A. Dutton and L. M. Valdes Cruz

The Nuffield Institute for Medical Research,
University of Oxford, Oxford, UK

Binder *et al.* (1) found on average no significant difference between mean arterial pressures of bilaterally nephrectomized fetal lambs (41.5 ± 3.0 SEM mmHg) and those of intact lambs (4.59 ± 1.4 SEM mmHg). This contrasts with high pressures (77 ± 4 SEM mmHg) previously reported in nephrectomized fetal lambs (2). Nevertheless, the ranges of pressures recorded (26–73 (1)) and (26–83 (2)) are not dissimilar. Binder *et al.* (1) rejected observations on lambs with pH values below 7.30 but we have not found nephrectomized lambs to be more acidaemic than intact ones. The main difference between the investigations of the Oregon workers and ourselves is that their ewes received alfalfa and oats whereas ours were fed on grain based concentrate with $>40\%$ available carbohydrate (*vs* 1.5% for grass) and containing supplementary sodium chloride. However, bilateral nephrectomy occasionally fails to induce hypertension in lambs of ewes consuming concentrate.

Further measurements have now been made in nephrectomized and intact lambs of ewes given concentrate without added sodium chloride and also in those of ewes given hay or grass.

Methods

Food was withheld for 24 h before operation at 117–125 days gestation when ewes and lambs were catheterized under general anaesthesia and the kidneys removed from some lambs. Appetite built up gradually during the first few postoperative days and the weight of food eaten each day was noted. Water was always available and its consumption measured. Fetal mean arterial and venous

The Physiological Development of the Fetus and Newborn
ISBN 0 12 389080 2

Copyright © 1985 by Academic Press, London.
All rights of reproduction in any form reserved.

pressures (corrected for amniotic pressure) and heart rate were recorded continuously and blood gases measured daily.

Sodium

Table 1 shows that reduction of the (normal) sodium content of concentrate from 200 to the endogenous level of 26 mmol/kg did not prevent development of hypertension in nephrectomized fetal lambs. However the arbitrary pressure threshold of 60 mmHg was reached on average about 12 h later in a lesser proportion (57% *vs* 75%) of lambs when no sodium chloride was added to the concentrate.

Table 1. Incidence of raised arterial pressure (normal ~44 mmHg) following bilateral nephrectomy in fetal lambs

Ewes fed concentrate	Na^+	26	200
containing mmol/kg	K^+	215	217
no. lambs		7	12
no. with bp >60 mmHg		4	9
days from nephrectomy	mean	4.5	3.9
	range	(3–6)	(2–6)
Maternal urinary excretion	Na^+ mmol/day	9 ± 1.6	78 ± 13.5

Hay and Grass

The sodium content of hay and grass used lay between that of the concentrate with and without a sodium supplement (Table 2). The arterial pressures found in the first 6 nephrectomized lambs of ewes given either hay or grass were all lower ($P < 0.001$) than predicted from previous measurements of fetal plasma Na^+, K^+ and PCV (3 and unpublished). Within the group of hay/grass fed animals hypertension was significantly associated with restricted maternal energy

Table 2. Composition* of ewes' food

		Hay	Compressed grass		Concentrate no added	+ Na^+
			82/83	83/84	Na^+	
Dry matter	%	89	90	90	89	90
Crude protein	% DM	9.6	20.8	22.5	15.8	
Metabolizable energy (estimated)	MJ/kg	9.0	9.0	10.2	13.45	
Available carbohydrate	% DM			1.5	45.5	
Na^+	mmol/kg	73.9	30.4	78.3	26.1	200
K^+	mmol/kg	558	248	382	215	217

*Analyses carried out by the Nutrition Chemistry Department MAFF, Coley Park, Reading, UK

intake ($P<0.02$). At comprable energy intakes pressures were higher in the concentrate fed group. However for the combined groups arterial pressure was inversely related ($P<0.02$) to the crude protein intake of the ewes. The values for each animal were averaged over the 5th and 8th postoperative day. For the combined group of 9 lambs of ewes eating hay or grass and 7 lambs whose mothers were fed on concentrate yielded the relationship

arterial pressure (mmHg) = 67.8 − 6.5x g crude protein/kg/ewe/day   (1)

Conclusion

While increased Na$^+$ intake by concentrate fed ewes somewhat exacerbates the hypertension developed by their nephrectomized lambs (Table 1) it is not the main cause of this phenomenon.

Equation (1) implies that fetal arterial pressure in nephrectomized lambs should be supranormal when protein consumption is <3.7 g/kg/ewe/day and subnormal at higher protein intake. It appears that, subject to sufficient appetite in the ewe,

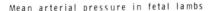

Mean arterial pressure in fetal lambs

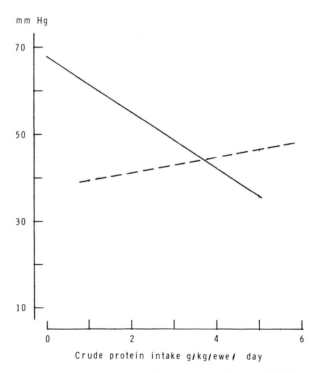

Figure 1. Average arterial pressure of (− − −) 6 intact ($r=0.707$, $n=6$ NS) and (———) fetal ($r=-0.590$, $n=17$, $P<0.02$) lambs in relation to the calculated intake of crude protein (g/kg/ewe/day) by their mothers.

arterial pressure can be controlled in nephrectomized fetal lambs by appropriate adjustment of maternal food. The significant factor may be protein or some component occurring in comparable proportions.

The original purpose of fetal bilateral nephrectomy was to demonstrate a fall of fetal arterial pressure due to the absence of circulating angiotensin II. The present observations suggest that this will only be achieved in lambs carried by ewes receiving adequate protein (Fig. 1). This may have happened in 11 of 19 lambs reported in (1).

The range of plasma glucose levels in nephrectomized lambs with supranormal arterial pressures is similar to that of intact lambs (Bassett and Mott unpublished). Thus the raised catecholamine levels found in these lambs (see (2)) are not directly attributable to hypoglycaemia.

It is tentatively concluded that in the intact fetus an unidentified renal mechanism prevents development of hypertension under conditions of maternal food restriction. Alternatively or in addition food restriction may affect some aspect of placental function.

References

1. Binder, N. D., Anderson, D. F., Potter, D. M., Thornburg, K. L. and Faber, J. J. (1982). *Biol. Neonate* **42**, 50–58.
2. Mott, J. C. (1981). *Adv. Physiol. Sci.* **8**, 299–307.
3. Mott, J. C. and Dutton, A. (1985). *Int. J. Pediat. Nephrol.* (in press).

The Probable Role of Antidiuretic Hormone in the Pathophysiology of Fetal Secondary Growth Defect

A. Merialdi and M. Fatone

Department of Obstetrics and Gynaecology, University of Parma, Italy

Introduction

Arginine-Vasopressin (AVP) acts on the kidney by binding the receptors in collecting duct cell membranes and activating adenylate cyclase. This results in cyclic AMP production which increases permeability of the luminal membrane to water and facilitates reabsorption of free water from the collecting duct (12). AVP secretion is mainly determined by changes in plasma osmolality, as detected by osmosensitive cells in the anterior hypothalamus. It is also affected by changes in blood pressure and extracellular volume (12) via the α- and β-adrenergic receptors found in the carotid sinus, along the aortic arch, and in the left atrium. In addition AVP is released in several stressful situations, such as hypoxia, even without a change in blood volume (10).

There is much experimental evidence suggesting that AVP is secreted by the neurohypophysis of the fetus and is active in prenatal life (10). In the fetus AVP may possibly be involved in following situations: responses to hypoxia, haemorrhage, control of fetal body fluids. All involve reflex secretion of several hormones as well and cardiovascular changes (10). Less is known of the role of AVP in human fetus especially in abnormal conditions.

The objective of the present study was to define the role of AVP secretion in the pathophysiology of secondary growth defect in human.

Material and Methods

Five fetuses with secondary growth defect born to mothers affected by pregnancy-induced hypertension and 5 normal fetuses born to mothers without any apparent pregnancy complication were investigated.

The Physiological Development of the Fetus and Newborn
ISBN 0 12 389080 2

Copyright © 1985 by Academic Press, London.
All rights of reproduction in any form reserved.

Poor intra-uterine growth had been assessed by echographic (biparietal and antero-posterior abdominal diameter) and clinical methods (Symphysis-fundus uterine distance and birth weight centile according to Parma chart (1)).

Both groups of fetuses were delivered by elective caesarean section. Amniotic fluid was aspirated by a syringe before uterine incision. The cord was clamped before the first breathing and venous and arterial cord blood immediately collected. Gas analysis of venous and arterial cord blood was carried out by Automatic Gas System, 940, Comesa. The placental weight was assessed after removing infarcted areas.

For AVP determinations 3 ml of plasma or amniotic fluid were collected into chilled tubes containing EDTA (1 mg/ml) and Trasylol (100 IU/ml) and were extracted for AVP using DEAE Sephadex A 25 column (1×7 cm) eluted with 0.02 M ammonium acetate buffer pH 5.5 and 1 ml was collected and lyophilized. Each fraction was solubilized in 0.2 ml of ammonium hydrogen carbonate buffer. The AVP (Ferring-Sweden) was iodinated by the chloramine T method (7) and purified on Sephadex A 25 column (1×7 cm) equilibrated with 0.02 M ammonium acetate buffer pH 5.5. Antiserum to AVP (Ferring) was prepared according to the method (11) and previously tested for cross-reactivity (5). The limit of detection of the assay was 0.5 pg/tube.

Recovery of added AVP from amniotic fluid and plasma by using DEAE Sephadex A 25 was 70%. The mean intra-assay coefficient of variation was 11.2% and the mean inter-assay coefficient of variation was 12.8%. The samples (0.2 ml) and antiserum (0.1 ml) were incubated for 48 h at 4°C, after the addition of 0.1 ml labelled hormone (about 10 000 count/180 s), the reaction was continued for a further 96 h at 4°C. Bound hormone was precipitated adding to each tube normal rabbit serum (0.1 ml) and goat anti-rabbit gammaglobulin (0.1 ml), incubation at 4°C for 48 h.

The data were analysed statistically using Student's impaired t test.

Results and Discussion

The levels of AVP found in arterial cord blood and in amniotic fluid of affected fetuses were higher than those found in normal fetuses (see Table 1). As for the significant of these results neither haemorrhage nor hypoxia should be responsible since both groups of fetuses were delivered by caesarean section and did not show any significant difference as regards pH and gas tension (see Table 1). On the basis of the fact that the weight of cotyledonary mass was lower in the group of fetuses affected by reduced growth (Table 1) we suggest that the following mechanism may be involved. In the fetuses with reduced growth owing to the low placental weight, an increase in umbilical resistance and systemic arterial pressure could be anticipated to occur, on the basis of researches in animal (2). The high arterial pressure could lead to an increase in renal blood flow and consequently to an increase in Glomerular Filtration Rate (GFR). Because the tubules of perinatal kidney have low active reabsorptive capacity largely due to their small size, an excessive amount of water and electrolytes would be lost as a consequence of the increased GFR, unless some compensatory mechanism take

Table 1. Arginine-vasopressin in cord blood and in amniotic fluid

	5 fetuses affected by secondary reduced fetal growth, born to mothers with pregnancy induced hypertension (caes. sect.)	5 normal fetuses born to mothers without any apparent pregnancy complication (caes. sect.)	
AVP (pg/ml)	M ± SD	M ± SD	t test
Umb. vein	25.7 ± 2.5	18.7 ± 2.1	P < 0.025
Umb. art.	60.6 ± 7.9	42.8 ± 7.1	P < 0.01
Amn. fluid	64.1 ± 4.3	39.4 ± 1.4	P < 0.0005
Umb. vein			
pH	7.18 ± 0.12	7.26 ± 0.09	NS
pO$_2$	22.67 ± 12.50	22.00 ± 7.07	NS
Umb. art.			
pH	7.16 ± 0.10	7.23 ± 0.04	NS
pO$_2$	12.67 ± 7.51	15.50 ± 3.87	NS
Placental weight	403.33 ± 112.40	502.50 ± 88.08	NS
Viscosity			
Umb. blood	5.78 ± 0.84	5.26 ± 0.51	NS

place (6). This compensatory mechanism could just be the augmented secretion of antidiuretic hormone that would maintain normal rheologic conditions in fetal blood in spite of the presence of profound circulatory changes. When we measured the blood viscosity (4,13) in another group of fetuses with growth defect we did not find any significant difference when compared with normal fetuses (Table 1).

References

1. Bevilacqua, G. and Moretti, M. (1975). *In:* "Therapy of Feto Placental Insufficiency", (Salvadori, B. ed.) Springer Verlag.
2. Dawes, G. S. (1978). "Foetal and Neonatal Physiology", Year Book Medical Publish Inc., Chicago.
3. De Vane, G. W. and Porter, J. C. (1980). *J. Clin. Endocrin. Metab.* **51**, 1412.
4. Fatone, M. and Merialdi, A. (1983). *In:* "Dilemmas in Gestosis", (Janisch, H. and Reinold, E., eds) G. T. Verlag, Stuttgart and New York.
5. Fyhrquist, M., Wallenius, M. and Hollemans, H. J. (1976). *Scand. J. Clin. Lab. Invest.* **36**, 841.
6. Kleinman, L. I. (1978). *In:* "Perinatal Physiology", (Stave, U. ed.) Plenum Medical Book Company, New York and London.
7. Legros, J. J. and Franchimont, P. (1971). "Radioimmunoassay Methods" (Kirkham, K. E. and Hunter, W. M., eds) p. 40, Churchill-Livingstone, Edinburgh.
8. Merialdi, A., Chiodera, P. and Fatone, M. (1982). *In:* "Fetal and Postnatal outcome in EPH Gestosis", (Salvadori, B., Merialdi, A. and Rippmann, E. T., eds) Excerpta Medica, Amsterdam.

9. Merialdi, A. and Fatone, M. (1983). *In:* "Dilemmas in Gestosis", (Janisch, H. and Reinold, E., eds) G. T. Verlag, Stuttgart and New York.
10. Nathanielsz, P. W. (1976). "Fetal Endocrinology: An Experimental Approach". North Holland Publishing Company, Amsterdam.
11. Skowsky, W. R., Rosenbloom, A. A. and Fisher, D. A. (1974). *J. Clin. Endocrin. Metab.* **38**, 276.
12. Tulchinsky, D. and Ryan, K. J. (1980). "Maternal-Fetal Endocrinology". W. B. Saunders, Philadelphia.
13. Wright, D. J. and Jenkins, D. E. (1970). *Blood* **36**, 516.

The Contribution of Research on Vision to the Understanding of the Organization of the Brain during Development

D. Whitteride

Department of Experimental Psychology,
Oxford University, Oxford, UK

For the last 25 years, the visual area of the cerebral cortex has been studied intensively. This has established 3 main points.

1. There is a map of the visual hemifield on each striate area (V1). This was deduced from war wounds and the visual defects they produced for man by Holmes (1), and a detailed map of V1 in the monkey was constructed by neurophysiological methods by Daniel and myself (2). It can reasonably be called point-to-point, but is distorted by the great magnification of the foveal region, and correspondingly small representation of the extreme periphery.

2. This map is complicated by the need to represent both the retinal areas which are excited by one and the same visual hemifield. This is achieved by dividing the representation of each eye into strips about 0.4 mm wide in the receptive layer 4C (3). These strips appear side-by-side alternatively with receptive fields each of which overlaps those of its neighbour by half its width. These ocular dominance columns in the monkey have the same width throughout the cortex, but they can fuse and break up, giving zebra like patterns. The existance of these strips or rather columns has been established by making lesions in one layer of the lateral geniculate (LGN), and following the terminal degeneration in the cortex, which in the binocular parts of the field is discontinuous. Injections of radioactive proline into one eye gives autoradiographic marking of the appropriate layers in the LGN,

The Physiological Development of the Fetus and Newborn
ISBN 0 12 389080 2

Copyright © 1985 by Academic Press, London.
All rights of reproduction in any form reserved.

and the marker crosses the synapses of the LGN and is carried to the cortex, where it marks the ocular dominance columns (4).

3. The first striking discovery made by Hubel and Wiesel was that at least 90% of cortical cells, unlike their predecessors in the visual pathway in the retina and the LGN, are most easily driven by bars and illuminated slits, and the orientation of these stimuli is a constant property of the cell. Further, cells from layer 2 to layer 6 of the cortex with the same orientation are arranged in vertical columns radial to the surface. A set of orientation columns covering all possible orientations occupies about as much space as a pair of ocular dominance columns, and it is convenient to think of orientation columns as roughly orthogonal to ocular dominance columns (3).

When they had established these points, Hubel and Wiesel looked at the visual cortex in the newborn kitten, and to their surprise found little difference qualitatively between the properties of the cells of the kitten without any visual experience and those of the adult cat. Unfortunately the kitten's visual system is very difficult to work on as the eyes are not open for 9–10 days, the media are cloudy and recording is difficult. Nevertheless, after some initial controversy, the salient facts as stated by Hubel and Wiesel (5) have been confirmed. They went on to work on the newborn monkey and Ramachandran *et al.* and Kennedy *et al.* (6,7) have worked on the newborn lamb. In both animals it is possible to record on the day of birth before any visual experience. The map of the visual field on the cortex is no different from that in the adult. In the lamb only about 80% of cells in the visual striate area (V1) have orientation preferences, as compared with 95% in the adult (7).

Sequences of orientation columns are present in the lamb, but orientation tuning is a little wider, fewer cells are directionally selective, and fewer prefer as stimuli short rather than long bars (called end-stopping). Binocular cells which can be driven by receptive fields in each eye are found but there is much less facilitatory effect of one field on the other than is seen in the adult. Obligate binocular cells, which can only be driven by simultaneous excitation of both receptive fields, are almost completely absent in the newborn, and appear only after 1–2 months of visual experience. In general, the main cell group are present at birth, but they are less sharply tuned and less exacting in their requirements. In the cat the conduction rate of the fibres in the optic radiations is much less than that in the adult, which is not surprising since myelinization of the optic radiations is not completed until after birth (8).

The acuity of cortical cells in the monkey at birth is 5cyc/deg. and rises to the adult figure of 50 cyc/deg. in the first 3 months of life (9).

The two main morphological differences to be seen in the newborn are the incomplete differentiation of the ocular dominance columns and of the band of callosally connecting fibres at the V1/V2 border which is seen in the adult. Although ocular dominance columns are recognizable functionally at birth, layer 4 at this stage can be filled almost uniformly by autoradiographically marked fibres from either eye. According to Rakic (10) slight differences in density at 0.8 mm intervals can only be detected by counting grains. This beginning of segregation of fibres from the two eyes begins in the monkey in the last 2-3 weeks of fetal life. However the process does not need visual experience, and if both eyes are closed at birth, the process will continue until segregation is complete at about 6 weeks. Fibres apparently withdraw from cells, so that layer 4 comes to consist of cells driven exclusively by one or the other eye.

In the adult monkey, fibres which have come from the opposite hemisphere via the corpus callosum project to a narrow band about 1-2 mm wide at the V1/V2 border. These fibres have visual fields limited to the region of the vertical meridian as Choudhury *et al.* (11) showed some 20 years ago, and arise from roughly corresponding points in the opposite hemisphere.

This border zone was called OBy by von Economo and is quite uniform in appearance and width from the fovea to the extreme periphery. In the cat this zone is a little wider and contains the terminations of the callosal but their cells of origin extend a little outside it.

In the newborn kitten, callosal fibres are distributed over the whole of V1 and V2 as are their cell bodies, and gradually disappear from everywhere except the V1/V2 border during the next 4-6 weeks of life. By double retrograde staining of the cell bodies Innocenti (12) has shown that some at least of the callosal axons die off, leaving their cell bodies with connections to their own hemisphere only. It is possible that cell death accounts for the disappearance of other axons.

The other unexpected and very important phenomenon discovered by Hubel and Wiesel (5) was the effect of closure of one eye on development of the visual pathway and on vision in that eye. If an eye is closed in the kitten for more than 3-4 days any time from the 9th day of life to the 6-8th week, when that eye is reopened the kitten behaves as though that eye is blind. If both eyes are left open, little or no recovery occurs for a month, and it remains permanently impaired. If eye closure is delayed until 3 months of age, there is very little effect. Similar critical periods have been seen in the monkey and the sheep, but in both it lasts longer—perhaps up to 6 months.

Critical periods have been described previously, for example the effect seen by McCance and Widdowson of a low level of nutrition at stages which require a considerable amount of protein, producing a permanent dwarfing of the animal. The amblyopia and the morphological changes to be described can be reversed if the eye is opened before the end of the critical period and the animal is forced to use it by closing the good eye. This is termed "reverse suture".

In human babies severe amblyopias have been seen after the accidental closure of an eye for a month during the first 6 months of life, and these amblyopias are permanent if untreated in very early life. The length of the critical period in man is not known with certainty, but it probably does not exceed 2 years.

Hubel and Wiesel (13) have followed the effect of closing one eye on the segregation of the ocular dominance columns using autoradiography and find that this process is severely disturbed. There seems to be competition for the cells of layer 4 between fibres from the two eyes, and where that competition does not occur the pathway from the closed eye is unimpaired. This can be seen in the area of monocular representation of the peripheral field, opposite the blind spot, or opposite an experimental destruction of the retina of the open eye (14).

Elsewhere, the number of layer 4 cells driven by the closed eye is much reduced, and the corresponding cells of the LGN cease to grow.

Simple reopening of the closed eye has little effect as long as the good eye is also open, but various substances which increase cell excitability such as 4HT, will increase the effectiveness of the previously deprived eye, provided deprivation has not lasted for more than 4 days. Vigorous stimulation using revolving disks of black and white sections or gratings is also effective in speeding recovery provided again that the eye has not been closed for more than 4 days (15).

In the experiments of Blakemore on monkeys (16), reverse suture produces a remarkable degree of recovery after only 5 days, and he has autoradiographic evidence of an increase in the number of fibres making contact with cells of layer 4 even in that short time.

Any interference with sharply focussed images falling on corresponding points in the two eyes during the critical period disrupts binocular vision and usually abolishes stereopsis. This is seen clearly in artificial squints produced in cats or monkeys by severing the lateral rectus muscle. This produces a very large decrease in dominance group 4 cells, that is in cells which are driven equally by the two eyes, and the near disappearance of obligate binocular cells. Closing one eye, or 'penalizing' one eye by instilling enough atropine to abolish accommodation both greatly reduce the number of binocular cells. Artificial squint and closure of one eye also leads to the persistence in the adult of cells well away from the V1/V2 border.

If both the eyes are closed for 3–4 weeks during the critical perod, both eyes continue to drive their own cortical cells in layer 4 monocularly, but there is a slow decrease in the binocularly driven cells, which seem to need experience of binocular vision.

Although the salient features of the development of cortical visual systems are now known, we can at present only speculate about the cellular mechanism responsible. There are two good examples of axon distributions which are widespread at first and become more sharply localized during development, namely the formation of ocular dominance columns and the narrowing down of the callosal projections. In the first case the cell normally ceases to accept synapses from one eye. Presumably the initial bias to one eye is determined genetically and impulses from the favoured eye seem to inhibit and finally "destabilize" synapses from the other eye. We know equally little about the stabilization and the destabilization of synapses, but Changeux (17) has some interesting suggestions on how such a process could occur at the nerve-muscle junction, a process involving the production of diffusible substances following successful excitation of the junction. Swindale (18) has produced in a model in which zebra-like stripes appear if cells can excite others within 200μ and inhibit those over 600μ. However it still seems unlikely that one and the same cell can excite its near neighbours and inhibit its more distant neighbours.

The binocularly driven and the callosally driven cells have the different requirement that synapse from two different sources should persist on their dendrites and perikarya, and to do so, these must be driven roughly simultaneously. Clearly such synapses could facilitate each other, and the problem of making such changes permanent is familiar to us in the problem of learning, where it is equally unsolved. The difference is that in the synapses of the visual cortex the synapses are "stabilized" by the end of the critical period, whereas elsewhere in the cortex synapses concerned with learning remain more or less plastic for the whole of life.

It is very likely that the need for visual experience for the proper functioning of binocular mechanisms, a need seen from the frog to man, is connected with the maintenance of proper alignment of the eyes.

In the case of ocular dominance, the competition between the two eyes merely reinforces genetic mechanisms which can perfectly well produce negation of ocular dominance columns on their own.

References

1. Holmes, G. (1945). *Proc. Roy. Soc.* B**132**, 348–361.
2. Daniel, P. M. and Whitteridge, D. (1961). *J. Physiol.* **159**, 203–221.
3. Hubel, D. H. and Wiesel, T. N. (1978). *J. Comp. Neurol.* **146**, 421–450.
4. Hubel, D. H. and Wiesel, T. N. (1977). *Proc. R. Soc.* B**198**, 1–59.
5. Hubel, D. H. and Wiesel, T. N. (1965). *J. Neurophysiol.* **28**, 1029–1040.
6. Ramachandran, V. S., Clarke, P. G. H. and Whitteridge, D. (1977). *Nature* **268**, 333–335.
7. Kennedy, H., Martin, K. A. C. and Whitteridge, D. (1983). *Neuroscience* **10**, 295–300.
8. Friedlander, M. J. and Martin, K. A. C. (1982). *J. Physiol.* **325**, 79.
9. Blakemore, C. and Vital-Durand, F. (1983). *J. Physiol.* **345**, 40.
10. Rakic, P. (1977). *Phil. Trans. R. Soc. Lond.* **278**, 245–260.
11. Choudhury, B. P., Whitteridge, D. and Wilson, M. E. (1965). *Q. J. Exp. Physiol.* **50**, 214–219.
12. Innocenti, G. M. (1979). *Nature,* **280**, 231–234.
13. Hubel, D. H. and Wiesel, T. N. (1977). *Phil. Trans. R. Soc. Lond.* **278**, 377–409.
14. Guillery, R. W. (1972). *J. Comp. Neurol.* **144**, 117–130.
15. Kennedy, H., Martin, K. A. C. and Whitteridge, D. (1982). *Exp. Brain Res.* **47**, 313–316.
16. Swindale, N. V., Vital-Durand, F. and Blakemore, C. (1981). *Proc. R. Soc. Lond.* B**213**, 435–450.
17. Changeux, J.-P. (1983). *In:* "Molecular and Cellular Interactions Underlying Higher Brain Functions". (J.-P. Changeux, ed.) pp. 465–478. Elsevier, Amsterdam and New York.
18. Swindale, N. V. (1980). *Proc. R. Soc. Lond.* B**208**, 243–264.

Cardiovascular Development in Normal Infants and Infants at Risk

Ronald M. Harper

Brain Research Institute, Department of Anatomy, School of Medicine, University of California (Los Angeles), Los Angeles, California, USA

Introduction

Trends in heart rate and heart rate variability rapidly change over the first 6 months of life, and provide useful markers for development during that period. There are a large number of factors which affect heart rate and variability during early postnatal life, however, and it is the purpose of this paper to discuss the influence of several of these factors. Cardiac activity is a prime example of an aspect of physiology that is heavily dependent on the interaction of a great many variables. Both heart rate and variability measures, as well as cardiac waveform (1) are greatly affected by sleep–waking state, as well as ultradian (< 24 h) and circadian (approximately 24 h) rhythms. These circadian rhythms are altered with age (2). Any description of heart rate and variability must also consider respiratory influences on the cardiac cycle, since these influences are major. Moreover, respiratory patterns rapidly change over the first few weeks of life, and the subsequent interaction between respiration and cardiac activity will thus markedly change with development. Finally, respiratory patterning is markedly state dependent, thus, state-dependent cardiac activity changes often result from state-related alterations in respiratory patterns.

Because cardiac rate and variability are sensitive to developmental influences, respiratory effort, and circadian and ultradian effects, any developmental modification in these influences, or any modification by illness, will alter cardiac rate and variability values. Thus, assessment of cardiac rate and variability, while controlling for developmental aspects of these various influences, can provide a useful tool for evaluating dysfunction. This paper will describe normal development of cardiac rate and variability, and some of the influences acting on these physiological parameters, together with some of the deviations

The Physiological Development of the Fetus and Newborn
ISBN 0 12 389080 2

Copyright © 1985 by Academic Press, London.
All rights of reproduction in any form reserved.

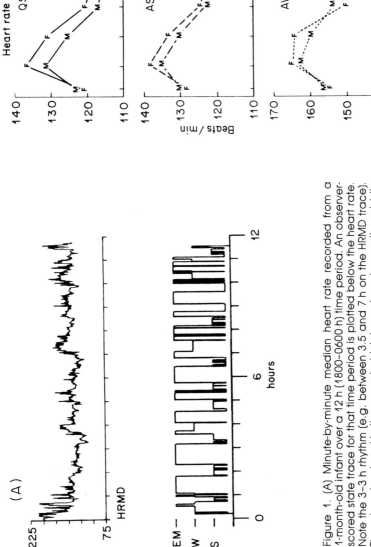

Figure 1. (A) Minute-by-minute median heart rate recorded from a 1-month-old infant over a 12 h (1800–0600 h) time period. An observer-scored state trace for that time period is plotted below the heart rate. Note the 3–3 h rhythm (e.g. between 3.5 and 7 h on the HRMD trace). There is a slow trend in the record which has a trough near the middle of the night; this probably represents one-half of the circadian rhythm. (B) Median heart rate is plotted for 9 females and 16 males over the first 6 months of life; measures were taken from 12 h night-time recordings. Note the large increase in rate from the newborn period to the first month of age, and the decline in rate thereafter. Note that the Y axes have different scales, and that state has a very large effect on rate.

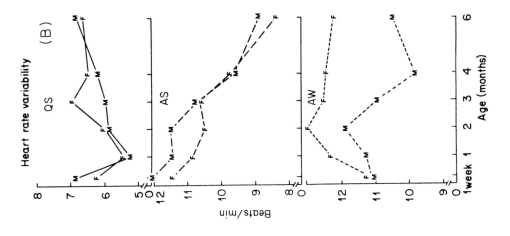

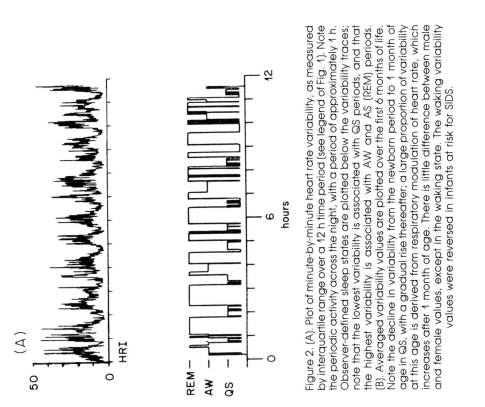

Figure 2. (A), Plot of minute-by-minute heart rate variability, as measured by interquartile range over a 12 h time period (see legend of Fig. 1). Note the periodic activity across the night, with a period of approximately 1 h. Observer-defined sleep states are plotted below the variability traces; note that the lowest variability is associated with QS periods, and that the highest variability is associated with AW and AS (REM) periods. (B), Averaged variability values are plotted over the first 6 months of life. Note the decline in variability from the newborn period to 1 month of age in QS, with a gradual rise thereafter; a large proportion of variability at this age is derived from respiratory modulation of heart rate, which increases after 1 month of age. There is little difference between male and female values, except in the waking state. The waking variability values were reversed in infants at risk for SIDS.

observed in infants who are ill or who are at risk for certain pathological syndromes.

Normal Development of Heart Rate and Variability

It is now apparent that assessment of heart rate and variability without reference to state is meaningless, since state effects are so pervasive on both rate and variability parameters. Figure 1 illustrates the validity of this statement; in this figure minute-by-minute median heart rate values are plotted across an entire night for a 1-month-old infant, together with an observer-defined state coding. Figures 1A and 2A illustrate that rate and variability are extremely dependent on state. Figure 1B illustrates the generality of that principle; in this figure, averaged median values for quiet sleep (QS), rapid eye movement or active sleep (REM or AS), and waking (AW) are plotted over the first 6 months of life for a group of 25 normal infants (9 female, 16 male) recorded over 12-h night-time periods at 6 different ages. The very different values in each state at each age are apparent from this grouped data.

The time-of-day characterization of the data is important since there is a strong circadian influence operating on heart rate. In Fig. 1A, a very shallow "trough", centred about 6–7 h into the night, represents one portion of the 24 h cycle that cannot be completely observed in this 12 h record, but illustrates the substantial influence of a circadian oscillator on rate.

Figure 1B illustrates little influence contributed by gender on heart rate development. There is a minor gender difference in heart rate variability (see Fig. 2B), but only in the awake state at one age (see below). There is no other systematic difference in developmental cardiac activity contributed by gender after state parameters are controlled (3).

Cardiac output is very high in the newborn compared to the adult (4). The principal mechanism in the infant for increasing cardiac output is by increasing heart rate; and rate increases over the first month of life.

Variability of heart rate from all sources is also greatly dependent on state, as is seen in Fig. 2A. This figure illustrates minute-by-minute values of the interquartile range (an assessment of variability which is less sensitive to outliers than a measure such as the standard deviation) plotted over a 12 h night-time recording period. A plot of minute-by-minute state classification is drawn below the variability values, and illustrates the state-dependency of variability values.

The generality of the state-dependency of variability values is shown in Fig. 2B, which illustrates the developmental trends for 25 normal infants over the first 6 months of life. This figure illustrates that the developmental trends for variability vary greatly with state; this state effect is largely manifested by different contributions to heart rate variability in each state, rather than an enhanced degree of a particular kind of variability. Gender is responsible for only a portion of the variability, with females having lower heart rate variability during the awake state at 3 months.

Variability: Contribution of Respiration

Some of the contributions to variability can be observed in Fig. 3A. This figure is a plot of cardiac R-R intervals, and illustrates the instantaneous changes in rate that occur in normal infants during each state. The plots indicate that heart rate values during waking are high and relatively fixed compared to the instantaneous changes during QS; this reduction in variation is inversely related to rate (5) with respect to short-term variation. The primary contribution to variation in heart rate during QS is that caused by respiration, i.e., the increase in rate with inspiration and the decrease with expiration. Variability from this source is reflected as a near-sinusoidal modulation of heart rate at the respiratory frequency (Fig. 3A). This respiratory, or sinus, arrhythmia forms the principal contribution to variation during QS; only an occasional bradycardia-tachycardia sequence is observed in that state, perhaps in response to a sigh or other sustained respiratory effort. The contribution of respiratory modulation of heart rate variation to the entire observed variability can be partitioned using time series analysis procedures. Specifically, spectral estimates of heart rate variation in the respiratory frequency can be determined, and developmental trends for this source of variation can be established (6,7). Trends for normal infants over the first 6 months of life for each state have been described elsewhere (8); the amplitude of respiratory arrhythmia falls over the first month of life, and then rises. This trend of respiratory modulation of heart rate variation in QS closely parallels that for overall variability in that state (Fig. 2B), since the major contribution of variation during that state is from respiration.

In addition to the heart rate variation contributed by the normal respiratory cycle, there are slower rhythms present on the QS traces, as can be seen in plots of R-R intervals during that state (Fig. 3). The portion of the QS record represented by the underline is one such slower rhythm. It appears that a portion of the slower variation on cardiac R-R intervals is contributed by an oscillatory process with a frequency similar to that found for periodic breathing (9).

REM or AS in the infant is accompanied by a large number of tachycardia-bradycardia sequences intermixed with respiratory modulation of heart rate. These episodic sequences are usually associated with transient arousals or phasic events of REM sleep. Because of the episodic nature of these sequences, it is frequently more difficult to quantify their presence with time series procedures that demand stationarity as a requirement for assessment.

One can further assess the contribution of respiration to heart rate variability by measuring the degree of coherence, or coupling, of respiratory to heart rate variability. A plot of coherence values across a 12 h recording is shown in Fig. 3B. Coherence is very much enhanced during QS; these results address the question of sleep state contributions to heart rate variability. These measures have an incidental advantage of greatly assisting machine classification of sleep state.

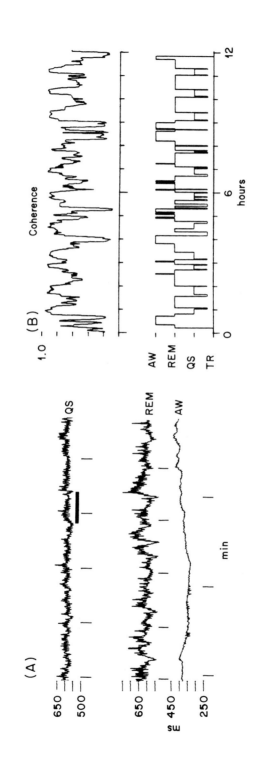

Figure 3. (A). Plot of successive cardiac R-R intervals during 3 states for a 3-month-old infant. Successive minutes are represented by short vertical lines. Note the near-sinusoidal modulation of intervals during QS at the respiratory frequency (approximately 28/min), the near absence of activity at that frequency during AW, and a mixture of respiratory activity together with episodes of tachycardia and bradycardia during REM. Note also the presence of slower variation on the QS record (an underline represents one cycle). The variability during AW can be large, but is derived from nonrespiratory sources. (B). Plot of coupling between variation of heart rate at the respiratory frequency (coherence) and respiration across a 12 h recording from a 3-month-old infant. Note the enhanced coherence during QS, intermediate values in REM, and lowest values during AW and transition periods (TR).

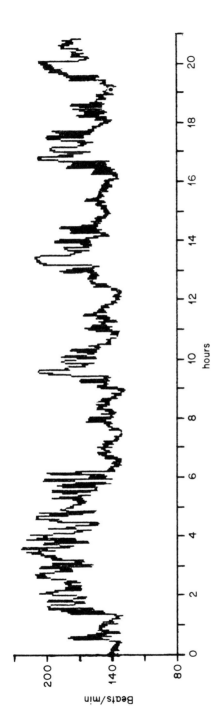

Figure 4. Plot of median heart rate across an entire day from a 1-month-old infant, with the recording beginning in the daytime. Note the higher rates during daytime, and the 3–4 h modulation of rate at night.

Rate and Variability: Circadian
and Ultradian Contributions

The importance of the contribution of circadian and shorter ultradian rhythms to heart rate and variability values cannot be overemphasized. As can be seen from Fig. 4, heart rate measured during quiet periods of daytime hours may greatly exceed active night-time periods. Thus, values for heart rate occurring during sleeping states on a peak of the 24 h cycle may approach values normally found during waking near the trough of the circadian cycle. Similarly, a prominent 3–4 h rhythm is superimposed on the circadian and hourly sleep rhythms. This 3–4 h rhythm has long been known (10), and it has been suggested that the cycle represents a feeding rhythm. In young infants, heart rate is higher in QS and REM following feeding periods than during waking periods in which there are no feedings (11); however, this was not the case with older infants. Thus, food intake may alter the overall level of "arousal", and contribute to overall heart rate variation, particularly in young infants.

From Fig. 4, it is apparent that assessment of heart rate and variability obtained by examining only a small amount of time ignores major aspects of cardiac control, and may provide an overly simplified assessment of cardiovascular integrity. These data argue for very long-term monitoring to ascertain an appropriate assessment of cardiovascular development.

Rate and Variability in Infants at Risk

Changes in heart rate or variability in rate have long been known to be associated with certain severe dysfunctions in infants (12,13,14). The ability to partition sources that contribute to heart rate variation over the first 6 months of life allow the potential to unmask subtle differences between groups at risk for syndromes which exhibit few obvious signs of distress. Partitioning heart rate by state, for example, reveals that, during QS, heart rate is higher in a group of 25 siblings of victims of the Sudden Infant Death Syndrome (SIDS) than in a group of control infants. An important characteristic of this syndrome is that few obvious signs of dysfunction are present; typically SIDS victims have been described as otherwise healthy. It is significant to note that we found no differences in heart rate of variability *unless* the effect of state were partitioned; the reasons for that result are immediately obvious by examining the extraordinary contribution to variability by state, as exemplified in Figs 1 and 2. Similarly a heart rate difference can be found between preterm and full-term infants if the state effect is partitioned (15). These results question the value of attempting to find rate differences between risk groups on the basis of long-term monitoring *without* adequate indication of state.

Heart rate variability is reduced in the first week of life in siblings of SIDS infants. That reduction, however, is observed only in QS, again illustrating the need for a partitioning of state in assessing differences between groups. The principal contribution of variation to heart rate during QS is respiration, and it is that source of variation which is diminished in the newborn period in siblings of SIDS victims.

The assessment of ultradian organization of cardiac rate can be useful in separating at-risk infants from control infants. In particular, the coherence of minute-by-minute cardiac rate values with respiratory rate at a 4 min periodicity, together with measures of coherence of respiratory rate and other parameters, provides a powerful discriminator for separating siblings of SIDs victims from control infants (16), who are at a 5-fold risk for the syndrome (17).

Conclusion

Development of heart rate and variability over the first 6 months of life provides dramatic insights into ongoing maturational processes which, when disturbed, provide useful indexes of risk. The assessment of cardiac parameters, however, must be taken in the context of sleep state, time of day, relationship to ongoing circadian and ultradian rhythms, and relationship to respiratory activity. A primary working concept is that of interaction; assessment of any one aspect of cardiac activity must also control for contributions from other sources. This partitioning can often be accomplished mathematically by means of digital filtering techniques. For example, the contribution of circadian and the shorter 3–4 h ultradian rhythms can be separated by selective digital filtering to attain the "pure" contribution by state. In this fashion, particular aspects of cardiac rate and variability can be assessed. Utilizing such partitioning allows for subtle discrimination of infants at risk. The assessment of interactions of variables at particular biological oscillatory frequencies may also be usful in this determination. These interactions may exist at very short time intervals (e.g. respiratory modulation of heart variation) or between heart rate and respiration at longer oscillatory periods (approximately 12 min). These determinations assume that healthy development is associated with the simultaneous interactions among several physiological systems.

Acknowledgements

A large number of investigators made contributions to these studies, including Drs T. Hoppenbrouwers and J. Hodgman, Los Angeles County-USC Women's Hospital, Drs M. B. Sterman of the Sepulveda Veterans' Administration Medical Center, and Drs R. C. Frysinger and B. Leake of UCLA. E. Hoffmann, S. Geidel, J. Marks, and D. Taube provided valuable technical assistance. This research was supported by NIH-NICHD HD-1-4608-04. Data collection efforts were previously supported by HD-4-2810 and HD-2-2777.

References

1. Haddad, G. G., Krongrad, E., Epstein, R. A., Epstein, M. A. F., Law, H. S., Katz, J. B., Mazza, N. M. and Mellins, R. B. (1979). *Pediat. Res.* **13**, 139–141.
2. Hoppenbrouwers, T., Jensen, D. K., Hodgman, J. E., Harper, R. M. and Sterman, M. B. (1980). *Pediat. Res.* **14**, 345–351.

3. Harper, R. M., Leake, B., Hodgman, J. E. and Hoppenbrouwers, T. (1982). *Sleep* **5**, 28–38.
4. Dawes, G. S. (1968). *Am. J. Cardiol.* **22**, 469–478.
5. Mazza, N. M., Epstein, M. A. F., Haddad, G. G., Law, H. S., Mellins, R. B. and Epstein, R. A. (1980). *Pediat. Res.* **14**, 232–235.
6. Sayers, B. McA. (1973). *Ergonomics* **16**, 17–32.
7. Harper, R. M., Sclabassi, R. J. and Estrin, T. E. (1974). *IEEE Trans Autom. Cntl.* **6**, 932–943.
8. Harper, R. M., Walter, D. O., Leake, B., Hoffman, H. J., Sieck, G. C., Sterman, M. B., Hoppenbrouwers, T. and Hodgman, J. (1978). *Sleep* **1**, 33–48.
9. Finley, J. P. and Nugent, S. T. (1983). *Can. J. Pharmacol.* **61**, 329–335.
10. Kleitman, M. (1967). *Res. Nerv. Ment. Dis.* **45**, 30–38.
11. Harper, R. M., Hoppenbrouwers, T., Bannett, D., Hodgman, J., Sterman, M. B. and McGinty, D. J. (1977). *Develop. Psychobiol.* **10**, 507–517.
12. Watanabe, K., Iwase, K. and Hara, K. (1973). *Biol. Neonate* **22**, 87–98.
13. Valimaki, I., Rautaharju, P. M., Roy, S. B. and Scott, K. E. (1974). *Eur. J. Cardiol.* **1**, 411–419.
14. Rudolph, A. J., Valbona, C. and Desmond, M. M. (1965). *Pediat.* **36**, 551–559.
15. Katona, P. G. and Egbert, J. R. (1978). *Pediat.* **62**, 91–95.
16. Frostig, Z. and Harper, R. M. (1984). *Soc. Neurosci. Abs.* (in press).
17. Froggatt, P., Lynas, M. A. and MacKenzie, C. (1971). *Br. J. Prevent. Soc. Med.* **25**, 119–134.

The Normal Progression of Maturation: The Development of Systems, *pari passu*

Michael H. Chase

Brain Research Institute, and Departments of Physiology and Anatomy, School of Medicine, University of California (Los Angeles), Los Angeles, California, USA

Introduction

Not all reflexes are created equal, neither in the kitten nor in the adult cat. In the adult cat, two of the primary reflexive actions which control the jaw musculature react differently in a manner dependent on the behavioural state of the animal. The jaw-closing (masseteric) reflex is largest during wakefulness, smaller during quiet sleep and of minimal amplitude during active sleep. The jaw-opening (digastric) reflex is largest during quiet sleep and it exhibits a general equivalence of amplitude during the states of wakefulness and active sleep. An essential difference between these reflexes, in terms of their behavioural reactivity, is that the masseteric reflex is large during wakefulness and it increases in amplitude during arousal, while the digastric is small during wakefulness and it decreases in amplitude during arousal.

In other publications I have reviewed the actions of these reflexes and examined the physiological bases for their differential state-dependent patterns of activity (1,2,3,4). In this present forum I will first present an overview of the modulation of these jaw reflexes in developing kittens, and then describe some of the physiological processes that could account for their immature patterns of activity. In the final section I intend (a) to develop a foundation for the concept that there are key synaptic interactions that are forged according to strict time-dependent schedules and (b) to advance the hypothesis that the maintenance of these temporal schedules is a prerequisite for the normal progression of maturation.

The Physiological Development of the Fetus and Newborn
ISBN 0 12 389080 2

Copyright © 1985 by Academic Press, London.
All rights of reproduction in any form reserved.

Overview

The monosynaptic masseteric reflex was monitored electromyographically from the masseter muscle (Fig. 1A (1), oscilloscopic record) (2). The reflex consisted of a single monophasic wave and, when induced by electrical stimulation of the mesencephalic Vth nucleus, resulted in jaw closure. The disynaptic digastric reflex was recorded from the anterior belly of the digastric muscle (Fig. 1B (1), oscilloscopic record); behaviourally it was correlated with jaw opening (2).

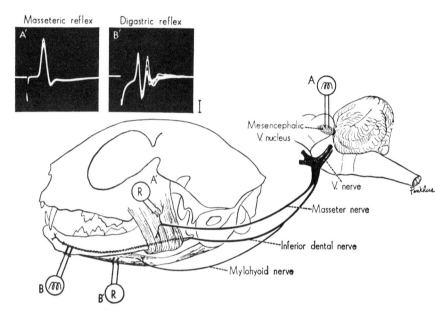

Figure 1. Stimulation and recording paradigm: The masseteric reflex was induced by stimulation of the sensory cell bodies within the mesencephalic nucleus of the 5th nerve (A), which innervate proprioceptors of the masseter muscle. Contraction of the masseter muscle followed which consisted of a single monophasic wave (A'). The digastric reflex was initiated by excitation of the inferior dental nerve via screw electrodes which were placed within the mandibular canal (B). A biphasic polysynaptic reflex was induced which resulted in contraction of the anterior belly of the digastric muscle (B'). Calibration: 200 μV; sweep speed, 5 ms (2).

The masseteric reflex, which was easily evoked in 2-week-old kittens, was of large amplitude (Fig. 1). Its waveform was similar to that reported in the adult (5). In contrast, the digastric reflex was of low amplitude in kittens 1 week of age and it could be induced only at levels of stimulation higher than those used in animals 2 weeks of age or older.

A similar pattern of reflex development during sleep and wakefulness was observed in each kitten. The only difference among animals appeared to reflect their relative degree of development. For example, a 2-week-old kitten, which was behaviourally more mature and weighed more than other kittens at this age, often exhibited a pattern of reflex modulation that was typical of a 3-week-old animal. Thus, the pattern of progression of maturational change was the same, although there were variations in the temporal degree of development.

As others have reported (6), I observed that kittens during early development exhibited rapid transitions from the awake state to that of active sleep, whereas in the adult there are prolonged intervening periods of quiet sleep (7). This immature pattern was accompanied by comparably abrupt, state-dependent changes in the amplitude of the masseteric and digastric reflexes. Additionally, in the neonate, periods of active sleep were often interrupted by short episodes of quiet sleep or wakefulness. Both reflexes exhibited specific, state-dependent changes in amplitude during these brief state transitions.

Masseteric Reflex Activity during Sleep and Wakefulness

In the adult cat the masseteric reflex, in a manner generally consistent with many other reflexes (3,4,8), decreases in amplitude as the animal progresses from the awake state to quiet sleep, and then again from quiet sleep to active sleep (9). A diametrically opposite pattern occurred in the young kitten, for the masseteric reflex increased in amplitude during comparable state transitions, in the following manner.

In kittens, from 7–14 days of age, the reflex was smallest during the awake state and of intermediate size during quiet sleep; it was largest during active sleep (Figs 2, 3). A reduction in reflex amplitude occurred whenever there were brief periods of arousal either during quiet sleep or ongoing episodes of awake behaviour (Figs 2, 4). Only occasionally was there a reduction in reflex amplitude during bursts of eye movement accompanying active sleep. However, toward the end of this early developmental period, there were more consistent episodes of phasic reflex suppression during active sleep which occurred in conjunction with rapid eye movements (Fig. 3).

The relative increase in response during the awake state equalled the decrease during active sleep immediately prior to the occurrence of the adult pattern (at about 3 weeks of age). Thus, for a day or so, and in some kittens for a period lasting only a few hours, *no* state-dependent changes in reflex amplitude were present (Figs 5, 6). Quiet sleep during this time-frame could be viewed as a fulcrum, with the forces responsible for the amplitude of the masseteric reflex during wakefulness being precisely balanced by those mediating its amplitude during active sleep, i.e., the amplitude of the masseteric reflex during the awake state was equal to that of active sleep, and both were equal to that of quiet sleep.

By 4 weeks of age, reflex modulation was comparable to that which we previously reported for the adult cat (Figs 3, 6) (5), as follows: (a) there was a decrease in amplitude during quiet sleep compared with wakefulness and during active sleep compared with quiet sleep; (b) facilitation (and occasionally suppression) occurred during arousal; and (c) phasic reductions in amplitude were present during active sleep in conjunction with bursts of rapid eye movements.

KITTEN (IO days old)

MASSETERIC REFLEX (Continuous Record)

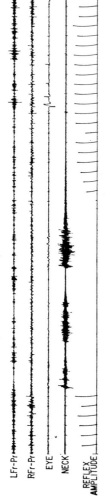
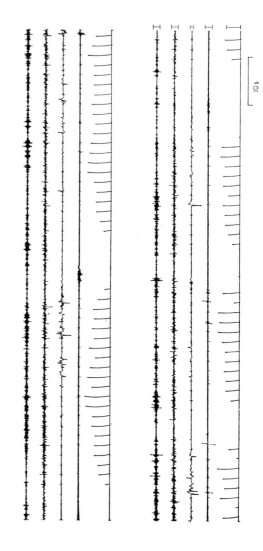

Figure 2. Correlation between rapid changes in state and the response of the masseteric reflex. Note the reduction in reflex amplitude during arousal and its increase during active sleep. This figure also illustrates the reduction in response during brief periods of quiet sleep (which occur in the 2nd and 3rd sets of traces) and the rapid increase in reflex amplitude coincident with the onset of active sleep. Stimulation parameters: Reflex −3 V. 0.75 ms, 0.5/s. Calibration: EEG, EOG, EMG, 50 μV; Reflex, 500 μV (2).

MASSETERIC REFLEX

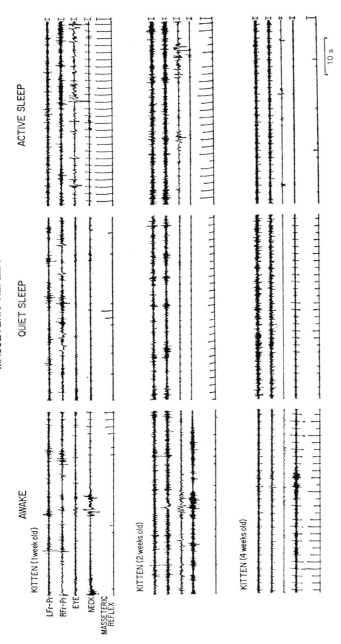

Figure 3. Masseteric reflex modulation in the 1-, 2- and 4-week-old kitten. This reflex was of greatest amplitude during active sleep in the 1- and 2-week-old kitten. By 4 weeks of age the mean amplitude of the reflex was largest during the awake state and smallest during active sleep. Note the lack of a clearly differentiable state-dependent EEG pattern in the 1-week-old kitten. Stimulation parameters: Masseteric reflex — 3 V, 0.5 ms, 0.5/s. Calibration: EEG, EOG, EMG, 50 μV; Reflex, 500 μV. For this and subsequent figures the following abbreviations for the cortical recording sites were employed: LFr-Pr, left frontal to left parietal; RFr-Pr, right frontal to right parietal; Trans-Fr, transfrontal (3).

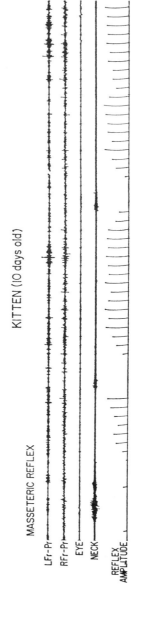

Figure 4. The masseteric reflex during arousal. This reflex exhibited a reduction in amplitude during periods of arousal in the 10-day-old kitten. In the adult, during comparable episodes, the masseteric reflex increases in mean amplitude above the background level. Stimulation parameters: Masseteric reflex — 2.5 V, 0.5 ms, 0.5/s. Calibration: EEG, EOG, EMG, 50 μV; Reflex, 500 μV (2).

KITTEN (3 weeks old)

MASSETERIC REFLEX (Continuous Record)

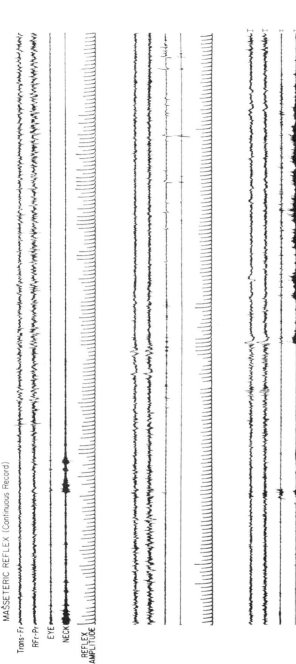

Trans-Fr

RFr-Pr

EYE

NECK

REFLEX
AMPLITUDE

20 s

Figure 5. At approximately 3 weeks of age the masseteric reflex exhibited only minor variations in amplitude as the animal changed state. Apparently at this point in development those factors which lead to progressively greater responses during the awake state are equal to those processes which tend to suppress activity during active sleep. This pattern is observed for only a very short time, usually less than a couple of days. Stimulation parameters: Masseteric Reflex—4 V, 0.5 ms, 1/s. Calibration: EEG, EOG, EMG, 50 μV; Reflex, 1 mV (2).

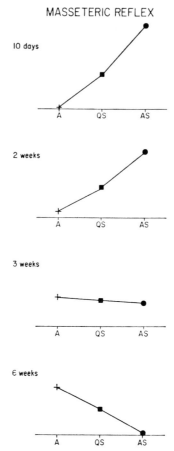

Figure 6. The mean amplitude of 100 consecutively induced reflex responses (evoked at the rate of 0.5/s) is plotted in this figure on an arbitrary but relative scale for each age group. The pattern of masseteric reflex activity during wakefulness and active sleep in the first 2 postnatal weeks was the opposite from that which occurred at 4 weeks of age, when the responses were similar to those reported in the mature cat (2).

The Digastric Reflex during Sleep and Wakefulness

In the developing kitten, the digastric reflex was smaller during arousal than during the quiet alert state; its amplitude increased during quiet sleep (Figs 7, 8). In the youngest population of kittens (7–10 days old), no obvious changes in reflex amplitude were evident when active sleep was compared with quiet sleep; a slight decrease occurred in 2-week-old kittens and depression similar to the adult pattern was observed in 4-week-old animals (Figs 7, 8).

Wakefulness, in kittens at 2 weeks of age, consisted predominantly of aroused or active behaviour which was correlated with depression of the digastric reflex

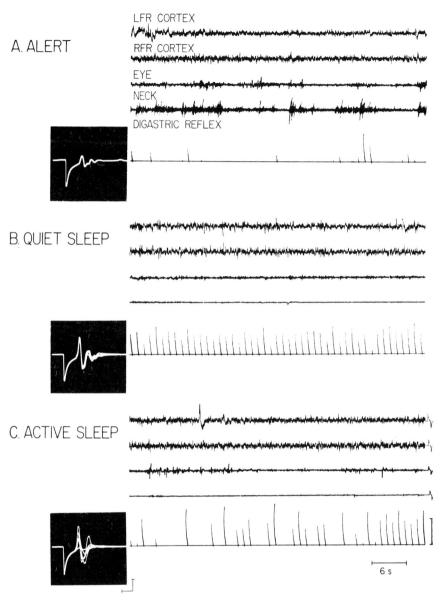

Figure 7. Digastric reflex during sleep and wakefulness in the kitten. Kitten (2 weeks old): On-line record of the EEG, EOG, EMG and of the reflex response. The polygraphic record of the digastric reflex represents the peak amplitude of its first component. This record was obtained at the same time as the oscilloscopic recordings (5 superimposed traces). Note in the oscilloscopic records that both components fluctuated in parallel during sleep and wakefulness. Inferior dental nerve: 1.2 V, 0.01 ms, 1/s. Calibration: 200 μV, 5 ms (oscilloscopic records); 50 μV (EEG, EOG, EMG), 500 μV (digastric reflex) (1).

590   M. H. Chase

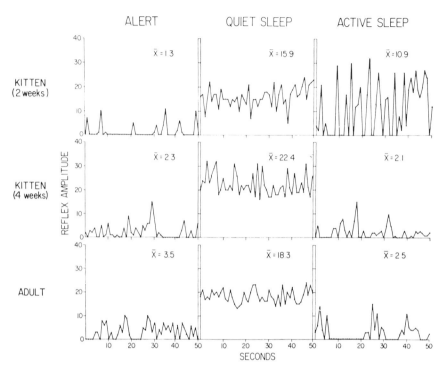

Figure 8. Digastric reflex fluctuations during sleep and wakefulness; comparison of results obtained in the 2-week-old and 4-week-old kitten and the adult cat. Reflex amplitudes were plotted for each animal on an arbitrary, but relative scale. For the kitten data, the amplitude fluctuations of the initial wave are presented. These records were obtained in each animal during consecutive alert, quiet, and active sleep states. Inferior dental nerve: 1.0 V, 0.1 ms (2-week-old kitten); 1.2 V, 0.05 ms (4-week-old kitten); 1.5 V, 0.1 ms (adult) (1).

(Fig. 7). The degree of sustained arousal appeared greater in the kitten than in the adult and, as the kitten became more aroused, the degree of reflex depression increased. During wakefulness there were brief period of 10–20 s when a reflex failed to occur, even when it was induced at levels which resulted in very large amplitude responses during quiet and active sleep (Figs 7, 8). In accord with previous observations, quiet wakefulness or the drowsy state were observed only as brief transitions from the alert to the quiet sleep state (7); these transitional states were accompanied by a relative increase in reflex amplitude.

An increase in reflex amplitude also occurred during quiet sleep, compared with the waking or drowsy states. In the youngest animals, the demarcation between quiet and active sleep was often difficult to assess from polygraphic records; it was also difficult to distinguish these states by an analysis of the digastric reflex response. There were, however, indications of reflex facilitation during active sleep, relative to quiet sleep, in the 1-week-old kitten. By 2 weeks of age, reflex depression occurred constantly throughout active sleep during rapid eye movement periods as well as in the nonrapid eye movement periods, i.e., those active sleep episodes lacking EOG or EMG activity (Figs 7C, 8). At this age, during active sleep, a few responses were equal to those obtained during quiet sleep; however, the majority were either suppressed or were greater than those which occurred during quiet sleep (Figs 7, 8).

Discussion

In the young kitten, spontaneous periods of sustained arousal are maintained for prolonged periods during wakefulness, but in the adult, in general, they occur only when specific initiating stimuli are present (personal observation). This behavioural trait of young kittens may, perhaps, be due to a paucity of tonic forebrain inhibitory influences acting upon the excitatory regions of the mesencephalic reticular formation, which could also account for the depression of the digastric reflex in the kitten during wakefulness and aroused behaviour. In this regard, the hypothesis that the reticular activating system is not inhibited by forebrain structures in the kitten is supported by the finding that in the adult cat, with an intact neuraxis, digastric reflex inhibition gradually decreases during prolonged mesencephalic reticular stimulation (10,11). In the diencephalic preparation, with the elimination of forebrain influences, reflex suppression is present as long as reticular stimulation is maintained (10,11). The cessation of sustained inhibition in the intact preparation is ascribed to corticofugal suppression of the reticular activating system (10,11). In the young kitten (2 weeks old), if corticofugal inhibitory projections are not active, reticular activation would be expected to induce prolonged periods of arousal and reflex depression. As with such concepts, this one is not all-encompassing, for it does not account for facilitation of the masseteric reflex during wakefulness that is present in the adult cat.

The increase in the amplitude of both the masseteric and digastric reflexes in the kitten during active sleep, above levels obtained during wakefulness or quiet sleep, may be a reflection of the "intensity" of active sleep in the young animal. Kittens in this age group spend a greater percentage of time in active sleep (7) and the frequency and extent of rapid eye movements and myoclonic jerks appear greater than in the adult cat (personal observation). Because mesencephalic reticular stimulation exerts a dual effect on digastric reflex activity (at very high levels of reticular stimulation, reflex facilitation (10,12) and not inhibition occurs), then it is possible that the increased digastric reflex response during active sleep may be due to a higher level of reticular activity in the kitten during this state. Masseteric reflex facilitation during active sleep in the kitten may also be due to delayed development of inhibitory systems, for in the adult cat reticular stimulation induces reflex facilitation during wakefulness and quiet sleep, and inhibition during active sleep (13). Thus, it is possible that the inhibitory active sleep-dependent forces of the adult central nervous system are not functional during this early developmental period.

There are other views, of course, that may be taken of the fact that these reflexes, in the kitten, are suppressed during wakefulness and facilitated during active sleep. But rather than exhaustively explore alternative hypotheses, we should at least challenge the notion that the terms "reflex suppression" and "reflex facilitation" are accurately employed, for their very nature leads one to make certain assumptions. It is possible that these reflexes, in the young kitten, are truly "suppressed" during wakefulness, but that they are not facilitated during active sleep, for the active sleep level may represent a true baseline of excitability, i.e., a level not influenced by either extrasegmentally driven facilitation or suppression. Of course, the same argument can be turned 180°, with the level of activity during wakefulness being viewed as a baseline, and active sleep the state when extrasegmental effects, in this case facilitation, become prominent. Finally, it is possible that most extrasegmental modulating influences are present from birth, but that the local segmental reflex circuitry has to mature in order to be sensitive, or receptive, to this in put. In support of this argument is the fact that EMG activity in the newborn kitten appears to be reduced during active sleep and is of greater magnitude during wakefulness, almost in defiance of the increase and decrease in reflex activity that occur during these respective states (Figs 2–4, 7).

The control of reflex activity in the developing kitten certainly seems to rest upon shifting sands, for reflex amplitude is not only temporally labile and but also state-dependent. Thus, at any given moment in the developmental schedule of these reflexes, and dependent on the point in time in the developmental schedule of the states of sleep and wakefulness, various state-dependent patterns of reflex responsivity occur. For example, we have observed an adult pattern of modulation for the masseteric reflex in the early morning, only to see it replaced by a previously documented immature pattern a few hours later, and then, the very next day, a permanent re-establishment of the adult pattern. It appeared as if a variety of factors were modulating reflex amplitude, and that some synaptic drives were only tentatively functional at first, or that they were unable to maintain control, at first, for more than a brief period of time.

Summary

Since first publishing these basic data a number of years ago, I have remained very impressed by the dynamic nature of the developmental forces that control motor activity and the fashion in which one set of synaptic drives is replaced or superceded by another during development. I believe that there are critical time-dependent synaptic windows which open briefly, and that it is at these moments that certain key neuronal contacts must be formed. All within the first 4 weeks of the kitten's postnatal life! And, if there are key synaptic links that must be forged within circumscribed time frames, as seems likely, then the accelerated or delayed development of either pre- or postsynaptic elements must represent factors of considerable risk. And if there are key interactions between key systems that must be formed at specific times to preserve the normal progression of maturation, then an accelerated or delayed schedule might put the entire organism at risk. I suggest that "timing is all", and that accelerated development can be as deleterious as delayed development. Therefore, one would hope to find, when assessing the normal progression of maturation, that all of the key elements within a system or those linking systems are proceeding, *pari passu*.

References

1. Chase, M. H. (1970). *Arch. Ital. Biol.* **108**, 403–422.
2. Chase, M. H. (1971). *Physiol. Behav.* **7**, 165–172.
3. Chase, M. H. (1972). *In:* "Maturation of Brain Mechanisms Related to Sheep Behavior", (Clemente, C. D., Purpura, D. P. and Meyer, F. E. eds) pp. 253–285, Academic Press, New York and London.
4. Chase, M. H. (1974). *In:* "Basic Sleep Mechanisms", (Petre-Quadens, O. and Schlag, J., eds) pp. 249–267, Academic Press, New York and London.
5. Chase, M. H. and McGinty, D. J. (1970). *Brain Res.* **19**, 127–136.
6. Jouvet-Mounier, D., Astic, L. and Lacote, D. (1970). *Develop. Psychobiol.* **2**, 216–239.
7. Chase, M. H. and Sterman, M. B. (1967). *Brain Res.* **5**, 319–329.
8. Pompeiano, O. (1967). *In:* "Sleep and Altered States of Consciousness" (Res. Publ. Assoc. Res. Nerv. Ment Dis., Vol. 45), pp. 351–423 (Kety, S. S., Evarts, E. V. and Williams, H. L. eds) William and Wilkins, Baltimore.
9. Chase, M. H., McGinty, D. J. and Sterman, M. B. (1968). *Experientia* **24**, 47–48.
10. Dumont, S. (1964). *Contribution a l'étude du controle reticulaire des integrations sensorimotrices au cours de la vigilance.* Faculté des Sciences de l'Université de Paris.
11. Hugelin, A. and Dumont, S. (1961). *Arch. Ital. Biol.* **99**, 244–269.
12. Hugelin, A. (1955). *C. R. Soc. Biol. (Paris)* **149**, 1893–1898.
13. Chase, M. H. (1983). *In:* "International Review of Neurobiology", Vol. 24, (Bradley, R. J. ed.) pp. 213–258, Academic Press, New York and London.

Studies of Carotid Baroreceptor Afferents in Fetal and Newborn Lambs

C. E. Blanco*, G. S. Dawes**,
M. A. Hanson and H. B. McCooke

Department of Physiology and Biochemistry, University of Reading,
Reading, UK, *Department of Paediatrics, University of Mastricht, Netherlands
and ** Nuffield Institute for Medical Research, Oxford University, Oxford, UK

Introduction

There is disagreement about the magnitude of the baroreflex in fetal lambs near term. Dawes *et al.* (3) reported that the reflex sensitivity, assessed from the change in heart rate produced by administering phenylephrine or methoxamine iv or by inflating a balloon in the descending aorta, is lower in the fetus aged 118–142 days than in the newborn lamb or adult. They suggested that the threshold for baroreceptor activity is above the normal range of arterial pressure in the fetus. On the other hand, on the basis of the effects of bilateral carotid sinus and aortic nerve section, Itskovitz *et al.* (6) concluded that the baroreflex is functional at basal blood pressure in the fetus, because they observed that the denervation increased heart rate variation. This denervation would remove both baroreceptor and chemoreceptor afferent inputs to the medulla, and since it has been shown that the carotid chemoreceptors are spontaneously active in fetal sheep from 90 days (1), the studies of Itskovitz *et al.* (6) are hard to interpret. As a first approach to resolving some of these problems, we have determined directly the stimulus-response curves of carotid baroreceptors in fetuses over two ranges of gestational ages and of 1-month-old lambs. This provides information about the afferent limb of the baroreflex over this period of development.

Methods

Mule-cross sheep between 88–113 or 131–144 days gestation were anaesthetized with halothane and a fetus exteriorized. Newborn lambs were anaesthetized with

The Physiological Development of the Fetus and Newborn
ISBN 0 12 389080 2

Copyright © 1985 by Academic Press, London.
All rights of reproduction in any form reserved.

halothane or pentobarbitone. The left carotid sinus nerve was exposed and cut near to its junction with the glossopharyngeal nerve, and activity of single or few-fibre afferents was recorded as described previously (1). Baroreceptor discharge was recorded during the transient rise in arterial blood pressure produced by occluding the abdominal aorta or by administration of 100–500 μg angiotensin II iv. Discharge was analysed on a beat-to-beat basis, taking only the rising limb of the response to avoid the problems of hysteresis (see ref. 2 for discussion). For each beat analysed mean baroreceptor discharge, expressed as impulses/s, was related to mean arterial pressure.

Results

In all animals regardless of age, carotid baroreceptors were phasically active in synchrony with the arterial pressure pulse (Fig. 1) and their discharge increased when arterial pressure was raised (e.g. Fig. 2). The results are compiled in Table 1. Basal mean arterial blood pressure increased with gestational age and then increased further after birth. There was, however, no significant increase with age in the basal discharge of the baroreceptors, expressed as a percentage of their individual maximum discharge. Thus their stimulus-response curves move

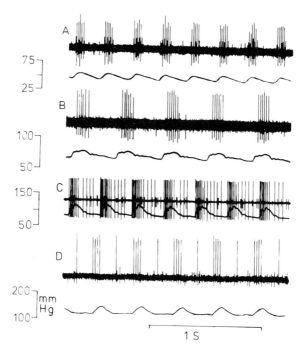

Figure 1. Examples of discharge of carotid baroreceptors at basal arterial pressure at various ages. A: fetus, 109 days gestation; B: fetus, 131 days gestation; C: lamb, day of birth; D: lamb, 28 days postnatal.

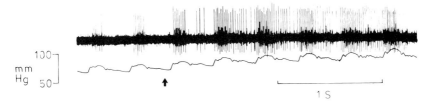

Figure 2. Response of baroreceptors to aortic compression performed at arrow.

Table 1. Mean basal arterial blood pressure, basal carotid baroreceptor activity (% of the maximum response) and slope of the steep portion of the response curve, before and after birth

Gestational age or postnatal age[†] (days)	Number of animals	Basal mean arterial blood pressure (mmHg) $\bar{x} \pm SEM$	Basal baroreceptor discharge (% of maximum) $\bar{x} \pm SEM$	Slope of the steep portion (%/mmHg) $\bar{x} \pm SEM$
88–113	6	49.1 ± 10.1	23.5 ± 5.1	7.89 ± 1.57
131–144	5	74.4 ± 1.7	36.2 ± 8.3	5.14 ± 1.06
30–40[†]	4	87.5 ± 10.2	36.01 ± 3.56	1.82 ± 0.37

to the right with age as basal arterial pressure increases. In addition, the slope of the steep portion of the curve was significantly reduced with age.

Discussion

Whilst reports differ about the magnitude of the baroreflex in unanaesthetized fetal sheep *in utero* (3,5,6,8,9), we have found that the carotid baroreceptors are active at basal arterial pressure from 88 days in the fetal lamb. Furthermore, the baroreceptors responded to increases in arterial pressure above basal, the slope of the response being significantly steeper in the fetus than the 1-month-old lamb. Our studies had of necessity to be conducted on anaesthetized, exteriorized fetuses, but there is no evidence that anaesthesia affects the sensitivity of the receptors, and the basal arterial pressures of the fetuses were in the range reported for the unanaesthetized fetus *in utero* (3). Thus it is clear that at least the afferent limb of the baroreflex is functional from 88 days in the fetal lamb. We observed this whether the arterial pressure was elevated by aortic compression or by angiotensin II administration, methods which have been reported to produce different reflex effects (5). We are not at present able to decide the extent to which central influences intervene to modify the reflex effects of changes in afferent baroreceptor traffic at different ages, or whether the suggestion (5) that angiotensin II has some central actions is correct.

Our results indicate that baroreceptor resetting occurs as mean arterial blood pressure increases during late gestation and in early postnatal life. This resetting has two aspects: first, a movement of the stimulus-responsive curve to the right; secondly, the slope of the steep portion of the curve is reduced, i.e. the sensitivity of the receptors is reduced. Similar conclusions may be inferred from the work of Downing (4, Fig. 10) on newborn rabbits. We do not know how rapidly these resetting processes occur, or whether they are akin to those occurring in the adults of other species during hypertension (7). The two aspects of the resetting may not occur at the same rate: in the adult dog Coleridge *et al.* (2) observed a parallel shift to the right in the stimulus-response curve of aortic baroreceptors after elevation of arterial pressure for only 20 min. We conclude that, surprisingly, the sensitivity of the baroreceptors is high in early fetal life when that of the baroreflex is low.

References

1. Blanco, C. E., Dawes, G. S., Hanson, M. A. and McCooke, H. B. (1984). *J. Physiol.* **351**, 25–37.
2. Coleridge, H. M., Coleridge, J. C. G., Poore, E. R., Roberts, A. M. and Schultz, H. D. (1984). *J. Physiol.* **350**, 309–326.
3. Dawes, G. S., Johnston, B. M. and Walker, D. W. (1980). *J. Physiol.* **309**, 405–417.
4. Downing, S. E. (1960). *J. Physiol.* **150**, 201–213.
5. Ismay, M. J. A., Lumbers, E. R. and Stevens, A. D. (1979). *J. Physiol.* **288**, 467–479.
6. Itskovitz, J., LaGamma, E. F. and Rudolph, A. M. (1983). *Circulat. Res.* **52**, 589–596.
7. Korner, P. I., West, M. J., Shaw, J. and Uther, J. B. (1974). *Clin. Exp. Pharmacol. Physiol.* **1**, 65–76.
8. Maloney, J. E., Cannata, J., Dowling, M. H., Else, W. and Ritchie, B. (1977). Baroreflex activity in conscious fetal and newborn lambs. *Biol. Neonate* **31**, 340–350.
9. Shinebourne, E. A., Vapaavuorri, E. K., Williams, R. L., Heymann, M. A. and Rudolph, A. M. (1972). *Circulat. Res.* **31**, 710–718.

Localization of Vasoactive Sites in the Thalamus of Newborn Swine

Phyllis M. Gootman, Barbara J. Buckley*,
Norman Gootman* and Maria-Eliana Salinas-Zeballos

Department of Physiology, State University of New York, Downstate Medical
Center, Brooklyn, New York, USA and *Division of Pediatric Cardiology,
Schneider Children's Hospital, Long Island Jewish-Hillside Medical Center,
New Hyde Park, New York, USA

Introduction

There have been a limited number of attempts to localize central neural vasoactive sites in the perinatal brain stem (1–9). Medulary vasoactive sites were located in piglets (1,7,8). Age-related aortic pressure and femoral flow responses have been obtained from a number of different brain stem sites in neonatal swine (2–5). Due to space limitations, the present paper describes cardiovascular responses to stimulation of vasoactive sites in the thalamus. While there have been some reports in the adult literature indicating the location of thalamic sites (10–12), there has been no such study in neonates, except for a preliminary report by Gootman *et al.* (13).

Methods

Experiments were performed on lighly anaesthetized piglets, ranging in age from birth to 14 days; see references (1,14–16) for general and (1–5,13) for central stimulation (STIM) methodology. Exploration of thalamic (THAL) sites was successfully carried out using bipolar electrodes for STIM (biphasic pulses: 0.01–1.0 ms, 1–100 Hz in 10 s trains, intervals between trains, 3–4 min) of grids of points along dorsoventral tracks at 0.5–1.0 mm intervals. Vasoactive sites were located by exploring a track with 0.8 mA stimuli at 50 Hz and were identified histologically (1,2). Aortic pressure (AoP), EKG and femoral (Fem), carotid (Car) and/or renal (Ren) arterial flow (F) responses to STIM of THAL sites were

The Physiological Development of the Fetus and Newborn
ISBN 0 12 389080 2

Copyright © 1985 by Academic Press, London.
All rights of reproduction in any form reserved.

recorded. Threshold for AoP response was found for all vasoactive sites. Then frequency was changed in random order while holding intensity constant and vice versa (2).

Results

All of the observed responses to THAL STIM had short latencies and were very well localized. STIM of a site ≥ 1.0 mm distant from an active locus usually resulted in loss of response.

Eight vasoactive sites were located within the THAL (Fig. 1) (17). Decreases in AoP were elicited by STIM of anterior medialis (AM), centralis lateralis (CL), ventralis lateralis (VL) (Fig. 2) and from a site located between nucleus lateralis

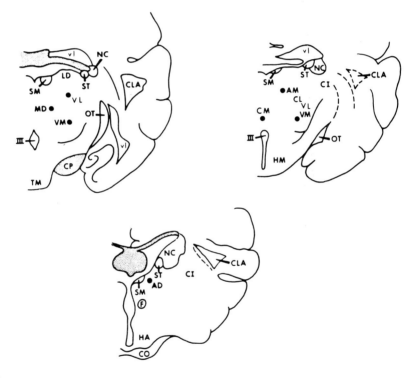

Figure 1. Diagrams of coronal sections drawn from histological material indicating the vasoactive (●) sites located in the thalamus. Abbreviations (17); AD, nucleus anterior dorsalis thalami; AM, nucleus anterior medialis thalami; CI, internal capsule; CL, nucleus centralis lateralis thalami; CLA, claustrum; CM, nucleus centromedialis thalami; CO, chiasma opticum; CP, cerebral peduncle; F, fornix; HA, anterior hypothalamus; HM, medial hypothalamus; LD, nucleus lateralis dorsalis thalami; MD, nucleus medialis dorsalis thalami; OT, optic tract; SM, stria medullaris; ST, stria terminalis; TM, tuberculum mamillaris; VL, nucleus ventralis lateralis thalami; vl, lateral ventricle; VM, nucleus ventromedialis thalami; III, third ventricle.

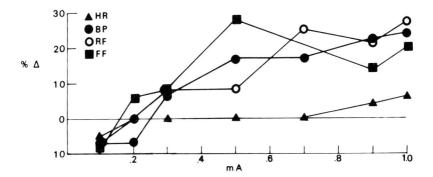

Figure 2. Intensity-response curves of cardiovascular responses elicited by stimulation (0.1 ms, 50 Hz) of nucleus ventralis lateralis thalami in a 14-day-old piglet. Abbreviations: BP, mean aortic pressure; HR, heart rate; RF, mean renal arterial blood flow; FF, mean femoral arterial blood flow.

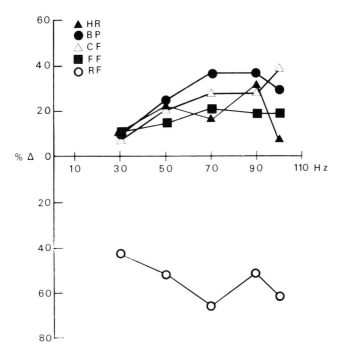

Figure 3. Frequency-response curves of cardiovascular responses to stimulation (0.5 ms, 0.8 mA) of nucleus medialis dorsalis thalami in a 7-day-old piglet. Abbreviations: CF, mean carotid arterial blood flow; see Fig. 2 for explanation of other abbreviations.

P. M. Gootman *et al.*

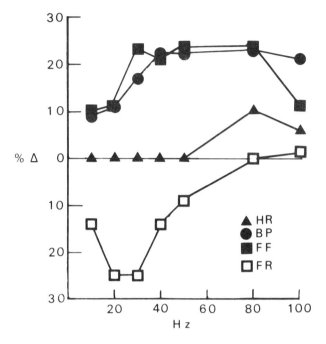

Figure 4. Frequency-response curves of cardiovascular responses obtained to stimulation (0.1 ms, 2.0 mA) of nucleus ventralis lateralis thalami in a 1-day-old piglet. Note the marked femoral vasoconstriction. Abbreviations: FR, femoral vascular resistance; see Fig. 2 for explanation of other abbreviations.

dorsalis and VL. Increases in AoP were elicited with STIM of nucleus centromedialis (CM), nucleus medialis dorsalis (MD) (Fig. 3), VL (Figs 2 and 4) and nucleus anterior dorsalis (AD). HR increased to STIM of MD (Fig. 3) and ventromedialis (VM), decreased with STIM of CL and CM, did not change significantly to VL (Figs 2 and 4) and varied with STIM of other THAL sites. Low frequency or intensity STIM of VL (Figs 2 and 4) elicited decreases in AoP, Ren F and Fem F without an accompanying change in HR. High frequency or intensity STIM of VL increased AoP, Ren F and HR (Figs 2 and 4). Responses to THAL STIM were lost in the presence of hypercapnia.

Discussion

The results of this study are part of a detailed investigation concerned with the localization of central nervous system vasoactive sites in developing swine (1–5). This paper reports that sites within the THAL can elicit blood pressure, heart rate and regional blood flow responses. These cardiovascular responses were quite similar to those observed in adult mammals (10–12). The loss of responses in neonatal swine observed to THAL STIM during stress has also been reported with STIM of other sites in the diencephalon (2–5). In addition, hypoxia has been reported to inhibit responses to posterior hypothalamic STIM in puppies (6). Such an effect of stress was not seen with STIM of medullary vasomotor sites in piglets (4,5). Thus our results indicate that STIM of sites within the CNS, similar to those reported in adults of other species, can produce changes in cardiovascular function in the neonatal pig. CNS vasomotor sites undergo postnatal maturation; their immaturity is indicated by the age-related differences in magnitude of responses to STIM under normal experimental conditions (2–5) and by the loss of responses in the presence of stress.

Acknowledgements

This work was supported by USPHS grant HL-20864 from the HLBI of NIH awarded to PMG and an American Heart Association Grant, Nassau Chapter awarded to NG.

References

1. Gootman, N., Gootman, P. M., Cohen, M. I., Levine, M. I. and Spielberg, R. (1972). *Am. J. Physiol.* **222**, 994–999.
2. Gootman, P. M., Buckley, N. M. and Gootman, N. (1978). *In:* "Fetal and Newborn Cardiovascular Function, vol. 1. Developmental Aspects", (L. D. Longo and D. D. Reneau, eds.) pp. 93–152, Garland STPM Press, New York.
3. Gootman, P. M., Buckley, N. M. and Gootman, N. (1979). *In:* "Reviews in Perinatal Medicine, vol. 3", (E. M. Scarpelli and E. V. Cosmi, eds.) pp. 1–72, Raven Press, New York.
4. Gootman, P. M., Gootman, N. and Buckley, B. J. (1983). *Federation Proc.* **42**, 1648–1655.
5. Gootman, P. M., Gootman, N., Turlapaty, P., Yao, A. C., Buckley, B. J. and Altura, B. M. (1981). *In:* "Ciba Foundation Symposium No. 83; Development of the Autonomic Nervous System" (Burnstock, G., ed.) pp. 70–93, Pitman Medical Ltd., UK.
6. Broadie, T. A., Devedas, M., Rysavy, J., Delaney, J. P. and Leonard, A. S. (1973). *J. Pediat. Surg.* **8**, 747–756.
7. Marshall, A. E. and Breazile, J. E. (1974). *Am. J. Vet. Res.* **35**, 223–229.
8. Marshall, A. E. and Breazile, J. E. (1974). *Am. J. Vet. Res.* **35**, 2341–2346.
9. Williams, R. L., Hof, R. P., Heymann, M. A. and Rudolph, A. M. (1976). *Pediat. Res.* **10**, 40–45.
10. Gootman, P. M., Baez, S. and Feldman, S. M. (1973). *Am. J. Physiol.* **225**, 1375–1383.
11. Evans, M. H. (1980). *Brain Res.* **183**, 329–340.
12. Jurf, A. N. and Blake, W. D. (1972). *Circulat. Res.* **30**, 322–331.
13. Gootman, P. M., Gootman, N., Buckley, B. J. and Salinas-Zeballos, M.-E. (1983). *Fed. Proc.* **42**, 1120.
14. Gootman, N., Buckley, B. J., Gootman, P. M. and Nagelberg, J. S. (1982). *Develop. Pharmacol. Ther.* **4**, 139–150.

15. Gootman, N., Buckley, B. J., Gootman, P. M., Griswold, P. G., Mele, J. D. and Nudel, D. B. (1983). *Develop. Pharmacol. Ther.* **6**, 9–22.
16. Buckley, B. J., Gootman, N., Nagelberg, J. S., Griswold, P. G. and Gootman, P. M. (1984). *Am. J. Physiol.* **247**, R626–R633.
17. Salinas-Zeballos, M.-E., Zabellos, G. A. and Gootman, P. M. (1985). *J. Comp. Neurol.* (submitted).

Changes in Organ Blood Flow between High and Low Voltage Electrocortical Activity and during Isocapnic Hypoxia in Intact and Brain Stem Transected Fetal Lambs

A. Jensen, O. S. Bamford, G. S. Dawes,
G. J. Hofmeyr and M. J. Parkes

The Nuffield Institute for Medical Research, University of Oxford, Oxford, UK

Introduction

The electrocortical activity of unanaesthetized fetal lambs is differentiated into episodes of high and low voltage activity at about 125 days gestation (term is at 147 days). During the former, most of the breathing movements are inhibited (5) and active movements of the limbs and neck are clustered together (11). Low voltage activity is the more active state, caused by cortical desynchronization in which the reticular formation of the brain stem is involved (8). In adults of other species in acute experiments under general anaesthesia, low voltage electrocortical activity is accompanied by increased cerebral oxygen consumption (7).

Isocapnic hypoxia causes arrest of breathing in the near-term fetus (1) and body movements are reduced (11). There is circulatory centralization as a result of hypoxia or asphyxia with blood supply being favoured to the brain, heart and adrenals (2,4,9,10) at the expense of almost every other organ.

Transection of the fetal brain stem, at the level of the inferior colliculi or upper pons, dissociated breathing from electrocortical activity and conversed the normal response during hypoxia from arrest of breathing to hyperpnoea (6). It was suggested that this may be due to a failure of increase in blood flow to the medulla and to the central chemoreceptors during hypoxia, causing local acidosis which in turn stimulates breathing.

The Physiological Development of the Fetus and Newborn
ISBN 0 12 389080 2

Copyright © 1985 by Academic Press, London.
All rights of reproduction in any form reserved.

In the present study we have avoided uterine contractions and have investigated the effects of high and low voltage activity on the distribution of blood flow within the brain, spinal cord and systemically.

Methods

Organ blood flow distribution in high and low voltage electrocortical activity as compared with changes after 30 min isocapnic hypoxia was measured in 5 unanaesthetized chronically prepared fetal lambs at a mean gestational age of 126 ± 1.1 days, by the microsphere reference sample technique (13). Four injections were made in high (H) and low (L) voltage alternately (i.e. H L L H or L H H L), followed by a 5th injection during hypoxia. The effects of brain stem transection on the blood flow distribution in normoxia was determined in 6 fetal lambs and compared with 5 animals at a mean gestational age of 127 ± 1.2 and 129 ± 1.6 days, respectively. Two injections were made in high and in low voltage electrocortical activity, the average being taken for comparison between animals: 5 and 4 of these animals, respectively, were subjected to isocapnic hypoxia with blood flow measurements made after 15 min.

After anaesthetizing the ewe with halothane, fetal catheters were inserted into a carotid and brachial artery, tarsal vein and femoral artery, trachea and amniotic cavity. Pairs of stainless steel wire electrodes were placed bi-parietally on the dura (3) to record the electrocortical activity. Wire electrodes were also used to record the electrocardiogramme for heart rate measurements, and to record the diaphragm and uterine electromyographic activity. Maternal catheters were implanted in a carotid artery and jugular vein. The fetal brain stem was sectioned at the inferior colliculi/upper pontine level after removal of the cerebellum by suction (M. J. Parkes) which results in enhancement rather than arrest of breathing during hypoxia.

Blood flow measurements were made with 5 batches of radioactively labelled microspheres (^{141}Ce, ^{113}Sn, ^{103}Ru, ^{95}Nb and ^{46}Sc, 15 μ diameter). An Autogamma Spectrometer (Packard 5320 Modumatic II) was used, connected to a multichannel (1024) pulse height analyser (Nuclear Data Inc., ND 62), interfaced on line to a programmable computer (Nascom 2, Warwick, UK). Microspheres ($2.5 \pm 0.3 \times 10^6$) were injected into the caudal vena cava and reference samples were withdrawn from a femoral and carotid or brachial artery, this volume (5 ml/min altogether) being simultaneously replaced by dextran. After formalin infusion, fetal tissues were dissected and counted. The number of microspheres in the samples exceeded 500, except for the ductus arteriosus in which about 200 spheres were counted. The adrenal medulla was separated from the cortex by punching (12).

Physiological variables, as described elsewhere (6), were recorded continuously on a Schwarzer polygraph from 24 h after the operation. The animals were allowed to recover for at least 5 days before they were studied. Blood samples were drawn from the carotid artery. Isocapnic hypoxia was produced by giving the ewe a gas mixture to breathe containing 8.5% O_2 with 2.5% CO_2 in N_2 for 30 min.

For statistical evaluation paired t tests and Wilcoxon Rank Tests were used. The results are given as means $\pm$ SEM.

Results

Electrocortical activity and blood flow

The blood gases, pH (Table 1) and the packed cell volume ($29 \pm 1.2\%$ and $28 \pm 1.6\%$, respectively) were within the normal range for chronic unanaesthetized preparations *in utero* and were not significantly different ($P > 0.05$) during high or low voltage electrocortical activity. But there was a fall in blood pressure ($P < 0.02$), a decrease in heart rate ($P = 0.06$) and a small increase in the arterial carotid PO_2 ($P < 0.1$) during low voltage states. Changes in the electrocortical activity were associated with blood flow changes in a number of organs. Although the arterial blood pressure decreased, there was an increase in flow during low voltage as compared with high voltage activity to the brain stem between 15 and 25% including the diencephalon ($P = 0.01$), midbrain ($P = 0.02$ and medulla (total, $P = 0.07$), and to the stomach ($+ 26\%$, $P = 0.03$), small ($+ 27\%$, $P = 0.03$), small ($+ 27\%$, $P = 0.01$) and large gut ($+ 31\%$, $P = 0.02$), pancreas ($+ 36\%$, $P = 0.03$), liver ($+ 32\%$, $P = 0.06$), and spleen ($+ 25\%$, $P = 0.07$). A decrease in blood flow during low voltage activity was measured in the wall of the ductus arteriosus ($- 35\%$, $P = 0.07$). A decrease in blood flow during low voltage activity was measured in the wall of the ductus arteriosus ($- 35\%$, $P = 0.07$), possibly suggesting constriction in this state of activity, and in the cardiac atria ($- 14\%$, $P = 0.06$). The detailed analysis of blood flow changes in the brain (Fig. 1) showed that the regions in which flow increased during low voltage approximate closely to the arborization of the reticular formation.

Table 1. Changes with high or low voltage electrocortical activity in normoxia ($n = 5$) and in isocapnic hypoxia ($n = 4$) in unanaesthetized fetal lambs at a mean gestational age of 126 ± 1.1 days

		Normoxia		30 min Hypoxia
ECOG	(voltage)	20 ± 1.4	21 ± 1.5	$11.8 \pm 0.4^{\star}$
PCO_2	(mmHg)	47.6 ± 1.3	45.7 ± 0.8	26.2 ± 2.9
pH		7.32 ± 0.01	7.33 ± 0.01	$7.27 \pm 0.03^{\star}$
BP	(mmHg)	45 ± 3.0	$42 \pm 3.0^{\star}$	$49.5 \pm 4.8^{\star}$
FHR	(bpm)	216 ± 15	197 ± 14	$178 \pm 25^{\star}$

$^{\star}P < 0.05$.

The blood flow measurements during hypoxia were compared with control values in a similar electrocortical state. The flow changes during hypoxia were quantitatively different in the brain and qualitatively different in the peripheral organs as compared with changes observed during low voltage. There was a significant increase in blood flow to the brain stem (97 to 123%), cerebrum ($+ 54\%$), cerebellum ($+ 78\%$), upper ($+ 136\%$) and lower ($+ 53\%$) spinal enlargements, hypophysis ($+ 116\%$), diaphragm ($+ 46\%$) and placenta ($+ 15\%$). There was also an increase in blood flow to the adrenal glands ($+ 145\%$, $P = 0.03$) that was not significantly different in the cortex or in the medulla, though the

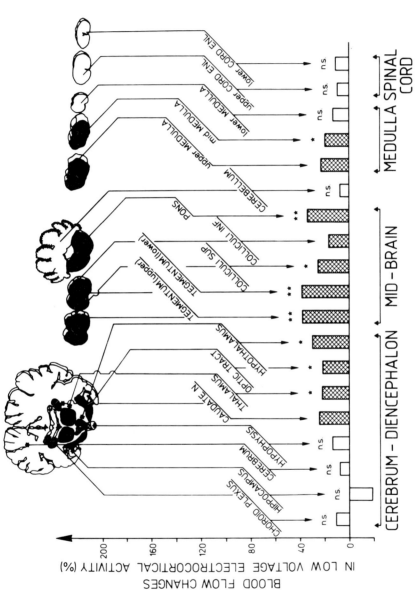

Figure 1. Blood flow changes in various parts of the brain and spinal cord in normoxia during low voltage electrocortical activity as % of the blood flow during high voltage in 5 unanaesthetized fetal lambs at a mean gestational age of 126 ± 1.1 days. Note: the regions in which there is a significant increase in blood flow during low voltage activity (hatched bars ($P<0.1$) corresponding to the black areas in the diagram) approximate closely to the arborization of the reticular formation in the brain stem. $^*P<0.5$; $^{**}P<0.01$.

absolute values (248 ± 71 and 511 ± 155 ml/100/min, respectively) at control differed considerably. Blood flow was reduced to the stomach (-40%, $P=0.005$), small gut (-24%, $P=0.08$), lung (-40%, $P=0.05$), brown adipose tissue (-70%, $P=0.09$) and skin (-23%, $P=0.05$). Thus, the changes of organ blood flow distribution from high to low voltage activity and those observed during isocapnic hypoxia were different.

Brain stem transection and blood flow

In the control period the arterial blood gases (PO_2 19.3 ± 1.4 mmHg, PCO_2 45.0 ± 1 mmHg), pH (7.33 ± 0.01), blood pressure (46.9 ± 1.9 mmHg) and the heart rate (178 ± 4 bpm) in the brain stem transected fetal lambs were no different as compared with intact animals. But the blood flow distribution in normoxia was different in brain stem transected animals. There was an increase in flow to the spleen ($+95\%$, $P=0.005$), small gut ($+20\%$, $P=0.05$), large gut ($+51\%$, $P=0.02$), thyroid gland ($+64\%$, $P=0.05$), brown adipose tissue ($+35\%$, $P=0.07$), bone ($+73\%$, $P=0.07$) and diaphragm ($+195\%$, $P=0.003$). But there was no significant change in blood flow to the principal organs such as brain, heart, lungs, adrenals and kidneys.

Isocapnic hypoxia caused hyperventilation in all brain stem transected lambs, while breathing was arrested in the intact animals. After 15 min there were no differences in the blood gas values between intact and brain stem transected animals, but, unlike in the intact animals, the arterial blood pressure failed to increase and the heart rate had already recovered in the latter group. Blood flow values of most of the organs measured were no different during hypoxia in transected or intact animals, including the flows to the medulla, diencephalon, cerebrum, heart, lungs, kidneys, stomach, small gut, muscle and skin. The redistribution of blood flow to the vital organs at the expense of the peripheral organs was maintained. Although the blood pressure had not risen in the brain stem transected animals during hypoxia there was a significant increase in blood flow to the medulla ($+63\%$, $P<0.001$), diencephalon ($+33\%$, $P<0.001$), cerebrum ($+15\%$, $P=0.01$), heart ($+97\%$, $P<0.001$), adrenals ($P=0.001$), brown adipose tissue ($P=0.06$), thyroid gland ($P=0.01$) and to the wall of the ductus arteriosus ($+33\%$, $P=0.008$), whereas the blood flow was reduced to the lungs ($P=0.005$), small and large gut ($P<0.05$), spleen ($P=0.02$), muscle ($P=0.01$) and choroid plexus ($P=0.05$). The % increase in medullary blood flow during hypoxia was not significantly different in brain stem transected fetuses compared with intact animals.

Conclusions

It is concluded first, that low voltage electrocortical activity is not only associated with an increase in blood flow to the brain stem areas, that approximate closely to the arborization of the reticular formation, but also with increased flows to the gastro-intestinal tract and the pancreas. These flow changes are different from those observed after 30 min isocapnic hypoxia. It is suggested that the inferred constriction of the ductus arteriosus during low voltage activity may represent a mechanism causing preferential streaming of oxygenated blood to the heart and brain, but more direct evidence is needed.

Secondly, brain stem transection alters the flow distribution in normoxia, but the circulatory centralization in favour of the vital organs during 15 min, isocapnic hypoxia is maintained. Since the medullary flow rose as in intact animals it is very unlikely, that the enhancement of breathing during hypoxia in brain stem transected fetuses is due to a failure of increase in blood flow to the medulla and the central chemoreceptors.

Acknowledgements

A. Jensen supported by the MRC and DFG Je 108/2-2. We are grateful for support from the Medical Research Council. We thank E. Stanley, F. Knight, C. Hanson, R. Belcher, G. Payne and S. Arkinstall for technical assistance.

References

1. Boddy, K., Dawes, G. S. and Robinson, J. (1974). *In:* "Modern Perinatal Medicine", (Gluck, L., ed.) pp. 381–389, Yearbook Medical Publishers, Chicago.
2. Campbell, A. G. M., Dawes, G. S., Fishman, A. P. and Hyman, A. I. (1967). *Circulat. Res.* **21**, 229–236.
3. Clewlow, F., Dawes, G. S., Johnston, B. M. and Walker, D. W. (1983). *J. Physiol.* **341**, 463–476.
4. Cohn, E. H., Sacks, E. J., Heymann, M. A. and Rudolph, A. M. (1974). *Am. J. Obstet. Gynecol.* **120**, 817–824.
5. Dawes, G. S., Fox, H. E., Leduc, B. M., Liggins, G. C. and Richards, R. T. (1970). *J. Physiol.* **210**, 47–48.
6. Dawes, G. S., Gardner, W. N., Johnston, B. M. and Walker, D. W. (1983). *J. Physiol.* **335**, 535–553.
7. Gleichmann, U., Ingvar, D. H., Lassen, J. A., Lübbers, D. W., Siesjö, B. K. and Thews, G. (1962). *Acta Physiol. Scand.* **55**, 82–94.
8. Ingvar, D. H. and Söderberg, U. (1958). *Acta Physiol. Scand.* **42**, 130–143.
9. Jensen, A., Künzel, W. and Hohmann, M. (1982). *Pflügers Arch. Europ. J. Physiol.* **394** (suppl.), 20.
10. Jensen, A., Künzel, W. and Hohmann, M. (1985). *In:* "The Physiological Development of the Fetus and Newborn", (Jones, C. T. and Nathanielsz, P. W., eds) pp. 405–410. Academic Press, London and Orlando.
11. Natale, R., Clewlow, F. and Dawes, G. S. (1981). *Am. J. Obstet. Gynecol.* **140**, 545–551.
12. Palkovits, M. (1973). *Brain Res.* **64**, 146–147.
13. Rudolph, A. M. and Heymann, M. A. (1967). *Circulat. Res.* **21**, 163–184.

Caffeine Effects: Mouse Neonate Sciatic Nerve

K. S. Amankwah, R. C. Kaufmann and A. Weberg

Division of Maternal/Fetal Medicine, Department of Obstetrics and Gynecology, Southern Illinois University School of Medicine, Springfield, Illinois, USA

Introduction

Caffeine is one of the most common drugs ingested in beverages. It is also extensively used as a therapeutic agent, e.g., in the treatment of apnoea in premature infants. Yet, little is known concerning its fate in the body, its effects upon fetus and newborn, or the metabolism of the drug by fetus and newborn. Khanna *et al.* (1) were the first to demonstrate that the fetus can convert caffeine to theophylline and vice versa. Warszwaski *et al.* (2) in their premature human autopsy and drug studies concluded that in cases of maternal caffeine ingestion there is a greater caffeine concentration in newborn than in adult tissues. In both adults and infants, caffeine is known to easily diffuse through the blood–brain barrier (2,3). At the brain level, caffeine and theophylline have been shown empirically to depress myelin-protein synthesis in the newborn (4). Accordingly, this preliminary animal study was designed to test the hypothesis that myelin synthesis in the fetal sciatic nerve is depressed by caffeine.

Methods and Materials

Animals

All mice in this investigation were of the C57BL/KsJ strain acquired from Jackson Laboratory, Bar Harbor, Maine. Male and female, 2- to 3-month-old mice were housed in cages in a room at 25°C with a 12 h light/12 h dark cycle. The control animals (Group I) were fed dry food and tap water. The study group (II) was given dry chow also but was additionally fed coffee with sugar. The sugar had to be added to induce the mice to drink the coffee. A third group (III) was fed

The Physiological Development of the Fetus and Newborn
ISBN 0 12 389080 2

Copyright © 1985 by Academic Press, London.
All rights of reproduction in any form reserved.

the same dry chow and tap water concentrated with the amount of sugar fed the study group. The total intake of food and fluids was measured for each group.

The coffee was commercially available canned coffee (Folgers Automatic Drip) purchased in 3 lb cans. To prepare a pot of coffee, 7 heaped teaspoonfuls were measured into the filter, and one pot of tap water was poured into the coffee maker. The brewed coffee was cooled to room temperature and poured into graduated bottles. For each 8 fl. oz of coffee, 3/4 teaspoons of D-glucose anhydrous (granular, analytical grade, Mallinckrodt) was added and the bottle swirled.

Virgin mice were examined daily for a vaginal plug, and the day a plug was found was designated Day Zero of gestation. The pregnant mice were then removed to a separate cage with free access to food and the liquid appropriate to the group to which they belonged. These mice were followed until delivery at which time, 6 pups from each of the 3 groups were chosen for study.

Tissue preparation

Upon spontaneous vaginal birth, each pup was sacrificed by neck fracture whereupon the entire animal was immediately immersed in a solution of 3% glutaraldehyde in 0.1 M cacodylate buffer at pH 7.3 for dissection. While under this solution, the neonatal sciatic nerve was promptly dissected from the body and then sliced into pieces. Following this, specimens were fixed overnight in a fresh solution of the 3% glutaraldehyde solution. Next day, specimens were rinsed in 0.1 M cacodylate buffer and post-fixed in 1:1 ratio of 2% aqueous osmium tetroxide and 3% potassium ferrocyanide for 2 h, rinsed in cacodylate buffer, dehydrated in a graded series of ethyl alcohol, and embedded in Spurr medium. Thick sections were stained with toluidine blue and examined by light microscope. Thin sections were cut with a diamond knife on a Reichert OM U-3 ultramicrotome, mounted on copper grids, and stained with uranyl acetate and lead citrate. Sections were then examined in a JEOL 100B electron microscope for ultrastructural changes.

Results

The C57BL/KsJ mice were divided into 3 groups for this experiment. The mean weights of the pups from Groups I, II, and III were 1.3620 ± 0.0040, 1.217 ± 0.0517, and 1.354 ± 0.0753 g respectively. The pups from Group II whose mothers had been on coffee were the smallest, and the difference in weights was significant at $P < 0.5$. Fluid and food intake was the same in each group. All pups were delivered between gestational Days 19–21 as was expected of this strain.

Group I. The females in this group were given tap water, and all pups from these mothers demonstrated some myelinated nerve fibres in sciatic nerve tissue. A total of 12 sciatic nerves from 6 pups were examined, and Fig. 1 shows a representative section.

Group II. The females in this category received coffee with sugar. Only 1 out of 10 offspring revealed any myelination in sciatic nerve tissue. Figure 2 shows typical sciatic nerve micrographs from this group. Note the complete absence of myelination.

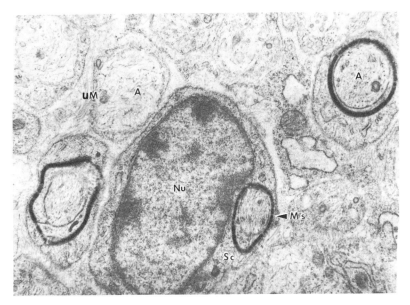

Figure 1. Cross-section of sural nerve from a neonatal mouse born to a mother on tap water throughout gestation, showing several myelinated nerves (Ms) and unmyelinated fibres (UM). A: axons, Sc: Schwann cell, Nu: nucleus ($\times$ 11 368).

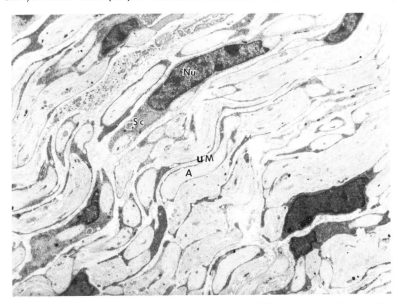

Figure 2. Section through the sural nerve from neonatal mouse born to a mother on brewed coffee mixed with dextrose throughout gestation, showing only unmyelinated fibres (uM). Sc: Schwann cell, Nu: nucleus ($\times$ 3185).

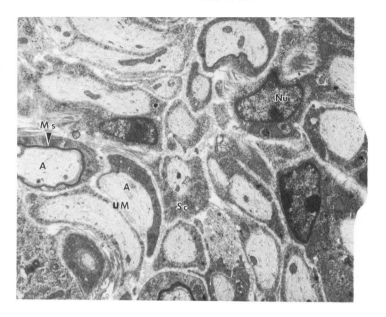

Figure 3. Section through the sural nerve from a neonatal mouse born to a mother on tap water mixed with dextrose throughout gestation, showing myelinated (Ms) and unmyelinated fibres (UM). A: axon, Sc: Schwann cell, Nu: nucleus (×5645).

Group III. These females were fed tap water with sugar, and all tissue samples from offspring of this group of mothers showed myelination of the sciatic nerves. Fig. 3 reveals both myelinated and nonmyelinated nerve fibres present in a total of 6 specimens from the neonates in this group.

Discussion

It was not the purpose of this experiment to determine fetal metabolism of caffeine but rather to investigate whether maternal coffee ingestion did, in fact, affect myelination of fetal peripheral nerves as exemplified by the neonatal sciatic nerve. The results obtained demonstrate that brewed coffee fed to a pregnant mouse over a prolonged period of time can, indeed, affect myelination of fetal sciatic nerves.

These findings are not really surprising since Fuller and Wiggins (4) previously demonstrated possible caffeine and/or other methylxanthine effects on postnatal myelination in the rat brain. These caffeine effects may be similar to the caffeine effects on cholesterol and sulfatide which were notably reduced in culture studies of dissociated neonatal brain tissue (5). Instances of such hypomyelination have also been found in cases of nutritional insufficiency (6). The hypomyelination in fetal brain tissue was considered the result of a failure of oligodendroglia to mature and to initiate myelin formation (6).

Another finding of note in this investigation was that coffee-fed mice demonstrate lower than normal maternal and fetal weights even though they apparently eat and drink as much or more than control animals. These low weights have not yet been explained, and one wonders whether the ability to absorb and/or to utilize nutrients has been impaired in some way. Similar findings were noted by Fuller and Wiggins (4). Another question concerns whether the obvious lack of myelination in Group II pups is due to the caffeine alone or whether it is indicative of the results of caffeine in combination with another as yet undiscovered factor relating to fetal *in utero* nutrition.

References

1. Bada, H. S., Khanna, N. N., Somani, S. M. and Tin, A. A. (1979). *J. Pediat.* **94**, 993–995.
2. Warszawski, D. and Gorodischer, R. (1981). *Pediat. Pharmacol.* **1**, 341–346.
3. Somani, S. M., Khanna, N. N. and Bada, H. S. (1980). *J. Pediat.* **96**, 1091–1093.
4. Fuller, A. N. and Wiggins, R. C. (1981). *Brain Res.* **213**, 476–480.
5. Siegrist, H. P., Burkart, T., Hoffmann, K., Wiesmann, V. and Herschkowitz, N. (1980). *Pediat. Res.* **14**, 1226–1229.
6. Wiggins, R. C. (1982). *Brain Res. Rev.* **4**, 151–175.

Towards an Ultrasonic Characterization of Fetal Brain Development

Jason C. Birnholz and Elaine E. Farrell

Departments of Radiology and Obstetrics, Rush Medical College and the
Division of Neonatology, Department of Pediatrics, Northwestern University,
Chicago, Illinois, USA

Fetal brain development has been inferred, for some time, from ultrasonic measurements of external cranial dimensions. Progressive improvement in ultrasonic technology has led to antenatal detection of a range of intracranial (and spinal) malformations and to possibilities for functional and behavioural evaluations of the central nervous system through subjective, 2-dimensional, observation of movement patterns (1–3), statistical analysis of individual movement frequency and periodicity (4), and attempts to recognize distinct behavioural states (5). This work introduces new capabilities for anatomic study of the fetal brain with recently developed magnification ultrasonic imaging.

Magnification or "super-resolution" instrumentation utilizes effective transducer apertures about 4 times longer than conventional devices (Acuson 128, Mountain View, CA: 80 mm at 3.5 mHz centre frequency, 58 mm at 5.0 mHz). Multi-element array transducer design and simultaneous computer control of each data channel permits operator adjustment of focal depth in receive and transmit modes. Acoustic data is processed digitally and displayed from a matrix (1024 pixels by 480 TV lines), which is itself allocated dynamically, depending upon field of view and imaging rate. The end result is a uniform beam focal pattern for the entire field of view. Lateral resolution spreading is eliminated, and parenchymal grey scale gradients are enhanced. The entire array and display can be concentrated on an arbitrary region of interest with further improvement in image resolution. Acoustic sampling and display rate are, typically, around 30 Hz. The larger aperture also lessens the degrading effects of skull bones (and maternal adipose thickness) on ultrasonic image quality, which is germane to fetal brain visualization.

The Physiological Development of the Fetus and Newborn
ISBN 0 12 389080 2

Copyright © 1985 by Academic Press, London.
All rights of reproduction in any form reserved.

Anatomic Observations

Brain parenchyma is portrayed as a uniform, low level backscatter region from the 3rd to 4th months of pregnancy, with sharp delineation of the cerebral and cerebellar boundaries externally and the ventricular margins internally. Cerebral echodensity remains uniform throughout pregnancy. The cerebellar hemispheres begin to show selective increase in reflectivity of the peripheral cortex to the lateral lobes in the mid-third trimester.

The major arteries are identified by their movement patterns throughout the 2nd and 3rd trimesters. These are the carotids and basilar arteries and the circle of Willis branches in base plane views. The peripheral middle cerebral arteries are also seen in this view, but can be compared in the Sylvian fissure regions on coronal views. Sagittal views reveal the pericallosal artery and other anterior cerebral branches, and selective magnification views of the posterior fossa demonstrate both superior and inferior cerebellar arteries. Arterial pulsations can also be monitored within the spinal canal along the dorsal surface of the cord.

The lateral ventricles have the relatively small, "newborn" appearance from the 4th month, with failure to distinguish brain parenchyma (with its water content in excess of 90%) from ventricle with early equipment presumed to account for the misconception that relative ventriculomegaly persists past the middle of the second trimester. Ventricular dilatation at 16–17 weeks is pathological, representing delayed cerebral development (as in Down's syndrome) or the onset of hydrocephalus.

We have been interested particularly in sulcation and have attempted to reproduce neuropathologic observations on surface markings (6–7) *in utero*. We strive for a midline sagittal view depicting the full length of the corpus callosum, which appears to be formed fully by 20-weeks gestational age (Fig. 1). This view is optimal for documenting the appearance of a cingulate sulcus (25 weeks) and the callosal marginal sulcus (26.5 weeks). Sulci are graded subjectively by tortuosity and branch pattern, which increase progressively between 28 and 32 weeks and after 36 weeks. Midline sagittal views cannot be obtained well when the cranial vertex presents below the symphysis. Transverse base plane views, however, can nearly always be recorded for study of temporal sulci. We have concentrated upon the length and tortuosity of the insular boundary and the depth of the lateral temporal sulci in the 3rd trimester. Because of a meniscus lens effect of the fetal skull, markings on the far side of the brain are more readily seen than those ipsilateral to the probe. We have not studied, specifically, laterality in development, although this is present.

We have also studied eye development in the 2nd and 3rd trimesters with measurement of average globe diameter and calculation of vitreous volume. These parameters do not increase linearly with gestation but rather show surges between 16 and 20 weeks, 28–32 weeks, and after 37 weeks with mild-plateaus between 20 and 24 and 32 and 36 weeks. This pattern is in concert with volume and surface area increase of the cerebral hemispheres. It is possible that this technically simple measurement may provide an index of cerebral development. Conversely, relative degrees of microphthalmia and mental retardation are associated strongly (8).

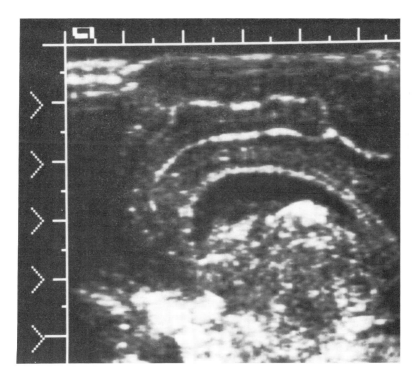

Figure 1. Magnification of midline sagittal image showing the callosomarginal and cingulate sulci at 27.1 weeks gestational age. The corpus callosum overlies the echo-free cavum septi pellucidi.

Summary

Magnification ultrasonic imaging provides new capabilities for studying anatomic brain development antenatally. Observable anatomic features are gross by a neuropathologic standard. Severe deformations are evident, and more subtle derangements may be inferred from delayed appearance or retarded maturation of the gyral pattern or, perhaps, from developmental delay in other features such as corpus callosal length, cerebellar foliation or vitreous volume of the eye.

We also suggest that anatomic studies be pursued in close conjunction with equally detailed observations of functional development, including directed stimulus–response patterns (9).

References

1. Birnholz, J. C., Stephens, J. D. and Faria, M. (1978). *Am. J. Roentgenol.* **130**, 537–540.
2. Birnholz, J. C. (1981). *Science* **213**, 679–681.

3. deVries, J. I. P., Visser, G. H. A. and Prechtl, H. F. R. (1982). *Early Hum. Dev.* **7**, 301–322.
4. Campbell, K., MacNeill, I. and Patrick, J. (1980). *J. Biomed. Eng.* **2**, 108–112.
5. Prechtl, H. F. R. (1974). *Brain Res.* **76**, 185–203.
6. Dorovini-Zis, K. and Dolman, C. L. (1977). *Arch. Path. Lab. Med.* **101**, 192–195.
7. Chi, J. G., Dooling, E. C., Gilles, F. H. (1977). *Ann. Neurol.* **1**, 86–93.
8. Warburg, M. (1971). *Birth Defects: Orig. Art. Ser.* **7**, 136–154.
9. Birnholz, J. C. and Benacerraf, B. R. (1983). *Science* **222**, 516–518.

The Effects of Mid-brain Lesions on Breathing in Fetal Lambs

Barbara M. Johnston, P. D. Gluckman
and Yvonne Parsons

Developmental Physiology Laboratory, Department of Paediatrics,
University of Auckland, Auckland, New Zealand

Introduction

In late gestation fetal lambs, experimental hypoxia causes a large reduction or complete abolition of breathing movements (1). Recent experiments in which the brain stem was transected at the level of the rostral pons or inferior colliculus have resulted in fetal lambs in which breathing movements are no longer inhibited by hypoxia and are sometimes stimulated (2,3). In addition, the incidence of breathing gradually increases so that by 10 days postsurgery it is almost continuous and quite dissociated from electrocortical activity. However transections at levels rostral to the posterior hypothalamus do not affect the inhibition of breathing during hypoxia, nor its episodic nature (3). This suggests that there are neural networks in or above the rostral pons but below the posterior hypothalamus which are involved not only in the inhibition of breathing during hypoxia but also in the generation of apnoea associated with high voltage electrocortical activity. We have therefore performed additional brain stem transections, plus a series of multiple mid-brain electrolytic lesions in order to try to locate these areas more precisely.

Methods

Operations were carried out on 16 pregnant sheep of 119–121 days gestation. Under halothane anaesthesia and using sterile techniques, catheters were implanted into the fetal carotid artery, jugular vein, trachea and amniotic sac. Electrodes made from stainles steel wire (Cooner Wire Co. Calif.) were implanted to record the electrocorticogram (ECOG) and the electromyogram (EMG) of the

The Physiological Development of the Fetus and Newborn
ISBN 0 12 389080 2
Copyright © 1985 by Academic Press, London.
All rights of reproduction in any form reserved.

nuchal and diaphragm muscles. Using the coordinates of the atlas of Gluckman and Parsons (4) a transection of the brain was made in each of 3 fetuses at AP + 20 mm, AP + 19 mm and AP + 17.5 mm with a wire knife angled at 44° backwards from the vertical plane. In a further 14 fetuses bilateral electrolytic lesions were made in the mid-brain using a monopolar needle electrode insulated except at the tip and positioned stereotaxically. A constant current of 5–10 mAmp was passed for 20–30 s. Initially multiple lesions were made in the same coronal plane and depending on the response to hypoxia progressively smaller areas were lesioned in subsequent fetuses. After surgery the ewes were housed in metabolic cages at constant temperature (20°C) and humidity (50%), and given free access to water and food. Continuous polygraphic recordings were made for 8–12 days of ECOG, integrated nuchal and diaphragm EMGs plus tracheal pressure, arterial pressure and heart rate. From the 4th or 5th postoperative days the response to hypoxia was tested on several occasions by allowing the ewe to breathe from a large plastic bag flushed with 9% O_2 in N_2 to which 3% CO_2 was added to maintain isocapnia. The duration of the hypoxia was usually 15 min. The ewe and fetus were sacrificed electively at 8–12 days postsurgery and the fetal head perfused with 10% buffered formalin in preparation for subsequent histological examination.

Results

Transection experiments

Of the 3 brain stem transected fetuses, the 2 with the rostral cuts (at AP + 19 and AP + 20) showed largely episodic breathing which was abolished by hypoxia. Electrocortical activity was not differentiated into any organized pattern and for 3–4 days after surgery an almost continuous series of small convulsive episodes was seen. The histological examination showed extensive damage throughout the thalamus and hypothalamus but with most of the midbrain, pons and medulla unaffected.

The fetus with the caudal cut (at AP + 17.5 mm) showed breathing which occurred for long periods and which was stimulated by hypoxia. The electrocortical activity was not differentiated and histological examination showed extensive damage in the mid-brain and pons.

A diagrammatic representation of the location of the transections is shown in Fig. 1 and taken together these results suggest that the likely area(s) involved in the hypoxic depression of breathing lies within the upper pons or mid-brain.

Midbrain lesions

In a total of 13 fetuses to date, multiple lesions were made in the vertical plane of the atlas at a level of + 16 mm in the anterior-posterior plane as shown in Fig. 1. Multple lesions which effectively transected the dorsal half of the brain stem did not abolish the hypoxic depression of breathing whereas multiple lesions in the ventral half caused a stimulation of breathing by hypoxia. Subsequent lesions at the same level but confined to the central areas of the brain stem also had

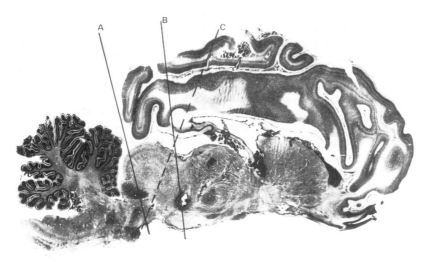

Figure 1. A sagittal section cut 2 mm from the midline from a 120 day gestation fetal lamb. Lines A and B are superimposed to show the approximate level and plane of section of the transections at 17.5 mm (A) and 20 mm (B). The dotted line (C) shows the level and plane of the electrode when making lesions at AP 16 mm.

no effect on the hypoxic depression of breathing. However hypoxia augmented breathing in a total of 5 fetuses with lesions encompassing the lateral mid-brain reticular formation, the lateral lemniscus and lateral parts of the pons. Figure 2 shows the smallest lesion to date which has resulted in a stimulation of breathing during hypoxia. In one fetus in which there was bilateral destruction of the pons but very little damage extending rostrally into the midbrain, breathing was inhibited by hypoxia.

None of the lesions caused breathing to become continuous although the normal episodic pattern seen in intact fetuses was disturbed in many cases, particularly in those fetuses in which the lesion encompassed the lateral mid-brain. When the proportion of time spent breathing was analysed over a continuous 48 h period, 4–6 days after surgery, those fetuses with lesions which induced breathing during hypoxia spent $55\pm6\%$ ($n=4$) of the time breathing compared with $47\pm5\%$ ($n=7$) in those fetuses with lesions which did not affect the response to hypoxia.

The effects on electrocortical activity were variable and it was frequently difficult to discern clear periods of low and high voltage activity. When they could be seen the ratio of low:high voltage activity ranged from 1.3–2.5 except in one with a lesion in the central part of the brain stem dorsal to the cerebral aquaduct, which had a ratio of only 0.8:1.

Breathing was dissociated from ECOG in all fetuses with damage to the lateral parts of the mid-brain whereas in those fetuses in which the lesions were confined to the dorsal or central areas breathing eventually came to be associated with low voltage ECOG for much of the time.

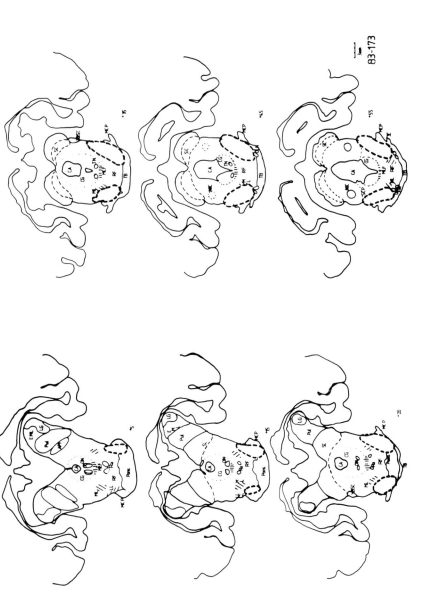

83-173

Figure 2. Diagrams drawn from serial coronal sections to show the extent of the smallest lesion to date which abolishes the hypoxic depression of breathing. APt, anterior prefectal nucleus; BSC, brachium superior colliculus; CA, cerebral aquaduct; CG, central grey; MCP, middle cerebellar peduncle; ML, medial lemniscus; MLF, medial longitudinal fasciculus; LL, lateral lemniscus; NIC, nucleus inferior colliculus; ON, occulomotor nerve nuclei; Pul, pulvinar; Ra, raphe nuclei; RF, reticular formation; SC, superior colliculus; TB, trapezoid body.

Discussion

Our present results agree with the conclusions of Dawes *et al.* (2,3) that there is an area above the pons which is involved in the inhibition of breathing during hypoxia in late gestation fetal lambs. We still cannot be sure whether this area is in itself chemosensitive (to O_2 lack) or even whether it is a discrete enough area to deserve the term "centre". However from the present results it seems unlikely that a diffuse neural network extending throughout the mid-brain or thalamus is involved, but rather it is a smaller more localized area in the region of the pontine/mid-brain junction. While we have not yet done the appropriate experiments to distinguish damage to cell bodies from that of fibres of passage, the available transection data would suggest that the cell bodies of the inhibitory neurones of interest must lie at approximately the level of these electrolytic lesions.

It appears that it is the lateroventral parts of the brain stem in the region of the upper pons/mid-brain border that are involved in the response since neither small nor extensive lesions in the central or dorsal brain stem at this level affect the normal depression of breathing during hypoxia. Although the lesions we have made are relatively small compared with the damage caused by the cruder technique of brain stem section, to date the smallest lesion which we have found to abolish the hypoxic depression of breathing is nevertheless in the order of $2 \times 3 \times 5$ mm. Experiments are in progress in which we are making smaller lesions in an attempt to delineate the area more precisely.

Acknowledgements

This work was supported by grants from the Cot Death Division of the National Children's Health Research Foundation and the Medical Research Council of New Zealand.

References

1. Boddy, K., Dawes, G. S., Fisher, R., Pinter, S. and Robinson, J. S. (1974). *J. Physiol.* **243**, 599–618.
2. Dawes, G. S., Gardner, W. N., Johnston, B. M. and Walker, D. W. (1980). *J. Physiol.* **307**, 47–48.
3. Dawes, G. S., Gardner, W. N., Johnston, B. M. and Walker, D. W. (1983). *J. Physiol.* **335**, 535–553.
4. Gluckman, P. D. and Parsons, Y. (1984). *In:* "Animal Models in Fetal Medicine" (Nathanielsz, P. W., ed.) Perinatology Press, New York.

Prenatal Influences on the Brain Stem Development of Preterm Infants

David J. Henderson-Smart, Alan G. Pettigrew
and Deborah A. Edwards

Department of Perinatal Medicine, King George V Memorial Hospital,
Camperdown, New South Wales, Australia and Department of Physiology,
University of Sydney, New South Wales, Australia

Introduction

Preterm small for gestational age (SGA) infants are reported to be at increased risk of neurological handicap in later life, particularly where growth retardation commences before 34 weeks gestation (9,14). Some authors have attributed this to intrapartum and neonatal complications such as asphyxia (2,16). The possibility that brain development may be altered prenatally is suggested from the clinical observations by Gould *et al.* (7) and Amiel-Tison (1) of infants exposed to chronic intra-uterine "stress". The accelerated neurological maturation observed by these authors is supported recently by similar findings of altered gyral patterns in the cerebral hemisphere of SGA infants (8).

This study examined the effect of some prenatal factors on the neurophysiological maturation of the brain stem in preterm infants using auditory evoked responses. Preliminary results (5) indicated that SGA infants have shorter brain stem conduction times and show a slower postnatal development of the response. Over half of the SGA infants were born to hypertensive mothers, the majority of whom were treated with either alpha methyl dopa or clonidine HCl, drugs known to alter brain stem neurotransmitter levels. This study indicated that altered brain stem development is related to intra-uterine growth retardation rather than to maternal hypertension or the drugs used to treat it.

Methods

All of the 109 preterm infants in this study were delivered at King George V Memorial Hospital before 35 weeks gestation. Each was studied at various

The Physiological Development of the Fetus and Newborn
ISBN 0 12 389080 2

Copyright © 1985 by Academic Press, London.
All rights of reproduction in any form reserved.

postmenstrual ages up to term equivalent age, using brain stem evoked response. Clinical details were obtained from the hospital records. Gestational age was based on the maternal menstrual history or an ultrasound assessment prior to 20 weeks. If neither were available, a neonatal clinical assessment of gestational age, as described by Dubowitz *et al.* (4), was used. Infants excluded from this study included those with clinical or ultrasonic evidence of periventricular haemorrhage; birth asphyxia based on an umbilical cord arterial pH < 7.02 (−2SD) or clinical signs of asphyxia in the neonatal period; maternal narcotic abuse; fetal alcohol syndrome or profound hearing loss that precluded latency measurements. No infant had evidence of congenital abnormality of the central nervous system or intra-uterine infection.

Details of the 3 groups of infants are shown in Table 1. The control group consisted of 68 infants whose growth was appropriate for gestational age (AGA) and whose mothers were normotensive. The 2nd group was made up of 19 AGA infants whose mothers were hypertensive during pregnancy. Hypertension was defined as a blood pressure of more than 140/90 or a rise of more than 15 mmHg during pregnancy. The 3rd group of 22 infants consisted of those who were small for gestational age (SGA, weight < 10th percentile (11)) and whose mothers were hypertensive during pregnancy.

Table 1. Details of the 3 groups of infants studied

		AGA no HDP	HDP AGA	HDP SGA
Number		68	19	22
Gestational age	Mean ± SD	30.8 ± 2.2	29.9 ± 2.5	32 ± 1.8
(weeks)	Range	26–34	27–34	27–34
Male:Female		41:27	7:12	11:11
Antihypertensive	Nil	68	2	3
drugs*	Clonidine HCl	—	13	13
	Alpha methyl dopa	—	3	7
	Hydralazine HCL	—	10	10
	Diazoxide	—	9	8
Duration of drug	Mean	—	38	23
treatment (days)	Range	—	1–200	1–134

*Some infants received multiple drugs

The brain stem auditory evoked response was recorded in all infants using the same Amplaid Mk4 signal processor. Details of the recording techniques have been published previously (10). The latencies measured in this study were those of peaks generated by neural activity in the cochlea and auditory nerve (Wave I and the large negative wave immediately following this, IIn), and near the inferior collicus (Wave V). The time difference between Wave I and Wave V and between IIn and V were used as 2 measures of the brain stem conduction time (BCT).

Statistical comparisons of means was assessed using the students *t* test with Yates correction. Linear regression and analysis of covariance was used to study and compare whole groups.

Results

The brain stem conduction time (BCT) of the auditory evoked response in the 68 control preterm infants who were of appropriate weight for gestational age (AGA) decreased with advancing postmenstrual age (Fig. 1). This was true for both the I-V and IIn-V intervals and was substantiated by regression analysis of all data points against age ($P < 0.001$). Overall the BCTs of the 19 AGA infants born to hypertensive mothers followed the same time course of shortening with postmenstrual age (Fig. 1). At 30–31 weeks the difference in their mean BCT was just significantly shorter ($P < 0.05$).

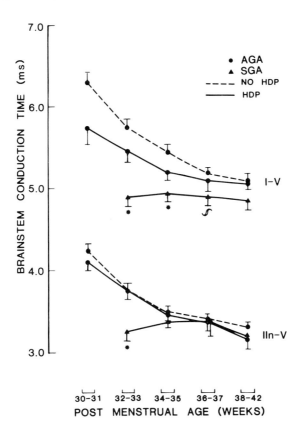

Figure 1. Means ($\pm$SEM) of brain stem conduction times (I-V and IIn-V intervals) for 68 control infants whose growth was appropriate for gestational age (AGA no HDP), 19 AGA infants born to hypertensive mothers (HDP AGA) and 22 small for gestational age infants whose mothers were hypertensive (HDP SGA). Statistically significant differences between HDP SGA and AGA no HDP are indicated (*$P < 0.001$, §$P < 0.02$). Differences also exist between HDP SGA and HDP AGA at 32–33 weeks ($P < 0.002$) and between HDP AGA and AGA no HDP at 30–31 weeks ($P < 0.05$).

The small for gestational age (SGA) infants born to hypertensive mothers had shorter BCTs than AGA control infants (Fig. 1). At 32–33 weeks the mean BCT of SGA infants was also significantly shorter than AGA infants born to hypertensive mothers. No significant change in the BCT occurred during postnatal development to term equivalent age in these SGA infants.

Discussion

The data concerning the development of BCT in AGA preterm infants agrees well with a number of other studies of "normal" preterm infants (3,6,13), especially when SGA infants were deliberately excluded from the test population (6).

The major finding of our preliminary study (5) was that the group mean BCT of nonasphyxiated SGA infants born at less than 35 weeks gestation was significantly shorter than that for age-matched AGA infants during the early preterm period. This suggests that the altered brain stem function is of prenatal origin. The present results indicate that it is intra-uterine growth retardation, rather than hypertensive disease in the mother of the drugs used to treat it, that is the main marker of altered neural development. Our data are consistent with the clinical findings of Gould *et al.* (7) and Amiel-Tison (1) which showed that prenatal stress can enhance the level of neural performance seen in the first weeks of life. Recent anatomical studies of cerebral gyral patterns also suggest accelerated maturation of the central nervous system (8). Furthermore, infants with short BCTs for their gestational ages have more mature respiratory control, as judged by the incidence of recurrent apnoea (10).

The shorter mean BCT of the SGA infants could be due to faster nerve conduction or to changes in synaptic function. Studies of peripheral nerve conduction velocity have shown no difference between preterm SGA infants and AGA infants (15) and a poor correlation between this measure and the BCT (12). In the present study 5 of the SGA infants with short BCTs had peripheral nerve conduction velocities which were in the normal range for postmenstrual age (Kesson *et al.*, unpublished data). It is also unlikely that the faster conduction time in the SGA infants is due simply to the reduced dimensions of the head since there was a poor correlation between the BCT and head circumference.

Infants with early symmetrical intra-uterine growth retardation tend to show persistence of somatic growth failure postnatally (9,14). It has been suggested that this may be due to a reduction of total cell number which is the result of an early switch in fetal development from a phase of cell hyperplasia to one of cellular maturation (17). The present data showing acceleration of brain stem "maturation" supports this concept. It has yet to be determined whether the early alteration of brain stem development in preterm SGA infants is correlated with later neural handicap.

Acknowledgements

This research was supported by grants from the National Health and Medical Research Council of Australia, Ramaciotti Foundations and Postgraduate Medical

Foundation of the University of Sydney. Thanks go to Bruce Storey and the nursing staff who assisted with clinical data collection and to Gwen Cox for typing the manuscript.

References

1. Amiel-Tison, C. (1980). *J. Obstet. Gynaecol.* **138**, 303–306.
2. Coomey, J. O. O. and Fitzhardinge, P. M. (1979). *J. Pediat.* **94**, 779–786.
3. Despland, P. A. and Galambos, R. (1980). *Neuropediat.* **11**, 99–107.
4. Dubowitz, L. N. S., Dubowitz, V. and Goldberg, C. (1980). *J. Pediat.* **77**, 1–10.
5. Edwards, D., Pettigrew, A. G. and Henderson-Smart, D. J. (1983). *Exerpta Medica, Asian Pacific Cong. Ser.* **18**, 59.
6. Goldstein, P. J., Krumholz, A., Felix, J. K., Shannon, D. and Carr, R. F. (1979). *Am. J. Obstet. Gynecol.* **135**, 622–628.
7. Gould, J. B., Gluck, L. and Kulovich, M. V. (1977). *Am. J. Obstet. Gynecol.* **127**, 181–186.
8. Hadi, H. A. (1984). *Obstet. Gynecol.* **63**, 214–219.
9. Harvey, D., Prince, J., Bunton, J., Parkinson, C. and Campbell, S. (1982). *Pediat.* **69**, 296–300.
10. Henderson-Smart, D. J., Pettigrew, A. G. and Campbell, D. J. (1983). *N. Engl. J. Med.* **308**, 353–357.
11. Kitchen, W. H., Robinson, H. P. and Dickinson, A. J. (1983). *Aust. Pediat. J.* **19**, 157–160.
12. Miller, G., Skouteli, H., Dubowitz, L. M. S. and Lary, S. (1984). *Neuropaediat.* **15** (1), 25.
13. Starr, A., Amlie, R. N., Martin, W. H. and Sanders, S. (1977). *Pediat.* **60**, 831–839.
14. Stave, U. and Ruvalo, C. (1980). *Early Hum. Dev.* **4**, 229–241.
15. Thibeault, D. W., Laul, V. and Gulak, H. (1975). *Pediat. Res.* **9**, 107–110.
16. Tudehope, D. I., Burns, Y., O'Callaghan, M., Mohay, H. and Silcock, A. (1983). *Aust. Paediat. J.* **19**, 3–8.
17. Winick, M. and Rosso, P. (1969). *Pediat. Res.* **3**, 181–184.

Morphine-induced Depression and Stimulation of Breathing Movements in the Fetal Lamb

George D. Olsen and G. S. Dawes

Department of Pharmacology, School of Medicine, Oregon Health Sciences University, Portland, Oregon, USA and the Nuffield Institute for Medical Research, University of Oxford, Oxford, UK

Infusion of morphine into 4 fetal lambs in the last 5th of gestation had a dual effect; the depth of breathing was first increased early in the infusion and then breathing was suppressed, even during long episodes of low voltage electrocortical activity. Breathing returned after the infusion was stopped. Section of the brain rostral to the pons did not prevent these responses.

Introduction

Exposure to opioid drugs during fetal development has undesirable effects upon neonatal health. Breathing control is altered (1), sleep is disturbed (2), and the incidence of sudden infant death is increased (3). After 120 days gestation (term is 147 days) breathing movements in the normal fetal lamb are intermittent and episodic, and cycle in phase with changes in electrocortical activity (4). Morphine was administered to fetal lambs to study its action upon breathing movements (FBM) and the relationship of breathing to electrocortical activity.

Methods

In 4 ewes at 117–120 days gestation under halothane anaesthesia, electrodes were sewn into the diaphragm, around one eye to record the electro-oculogram (EOG), and were placed on the parietal dura to record the electrocorticogram (ECoG; (5)). Catheters were placed into the trachea, amniotic cavity, a carotid artery and a jugular vein. One fetus underwent midcollicular brain stem section (6). The

The Physiological Development of the Fetus and Newborn
ISBN 0 12 389080 2

Copyright © 1985 by Academic Press, London.
All rights of reproduction in any form reserved.

diaphragm electromyogram (EMG) was filtered and integrated (I Dia; (7)). Amniotic pressure was subtracted electronically from tracheal pressure and arterial blood pressure. Heart rate was obtained from the pressure pulse.

Fourteen experiments were done, 4 in the transected lamb, 4 each in 2 intact lambs and 2 in the third. Experiments were spaced an average of 4 days apart between 121 and 139 days gestation. Morphine was infused into either a fetal carotid artery or jugular vein; the route did not influence the results. The infusion rate was 14–30 μg/min/kg estimated fetal weight (2.0–3.2 kg) for 5 h in all but one lamb (3.5 h).

The electrocorticogram was differentiated into high and low voltage in all but the first 2 of 4 experiments in one intact lamb. These are included in the analysis; the breathing response was the same as in other experiments. Data was analysed each minute for breathing and electrocortical activity and every 10 min for heart rate and blood pressure. The presence of breathing was defined as 4 or more breaths/min. The data was analysed for 18 h divided into 3 consecutive 6 h sections, the first immediately preceding the infusion. The second, infusion period, was started with the infusion. The last, postinfusion period, was the final 6 h. The two-tailed, unpaired t test was used: 18 h records from the day before morphine infusion were available for 6 experiments in the 4 fetuses. The mean data did not change from one 6 h period to another, nor from the pretreatment period on the day of the experiment.

Results

Fetal arterial blood pH (7.364±0.007), PO_2 (21.9±0.5), PCO_2 (44.4±0.8) and haematocrit (31±1) were not changed by morphine infusion, nor were the heart rate or arterial blood pressure (Table 1). Morphine had a dual effect on breathing in the transected and intact fetal lamb (Fig. 1). The depth was increased in

Table 1. Fetal measurements before, during and after infusion of morphine (mean±SEM)

	Preinfusion	Infusion	Postinfusion
Heart rate (beats/min)	154±7	151±6	152±6
Mean blood pressure (mmHg)	59±2	57±2	54±2
Maximum tracheal amplitude (mmHg)[†]	3.0±0.4	7.6±1.0***	4.9±0.6*
Maximum breathing episode (min)	30±3	82±25*	76±19*
Maximum apnoeic episode (min)	34±7	92±12***	28±4
LV ECoG (% time)[‡‡]	62±2	82±4***	78±2***
Maximum LV ECoG episode (min)	33±1	214±49**	63±15
Incidence of FBM during LV ECoG (% time)	79±3	54±5***	76±5

*$P<0.05$ **$P<0.005$ ***$P<0.001$ (compared to the pretreatment period).
[†]Average amplitude during hour with greatest average depth of breathing.
[‡‡]% time = $\dfrac{min}{360\ min}$ × 100.

one-half of the experiments, usually beginning during the first 2 h of infusion (Fig. 1B, Table 1). During the 4th or 5th hour, and for the 1st h after the infusion was stopped, breathing was suppressed in 13 of 14 experiments (Fig. 1C, Table 1). One intact lamb did not respond to infusion of 17 μg/min/kg morphine for 5 h at 131 days gestation, but responded with depression 3 days later at 30 μg/min/kg. Increased breathing activity returned in 8 experiments, usually by 2 h after the infusion was stopped (Table 1).

The incidence of low voltage (LV) ECoG activity increased significantly in the treatment and posttreatment periods compared to the pretreatment control; the duration of the longest episode of low voltage activity increased with morphine treatment (Table 1). Breathing was often suppressed during long episodes of low voltage activity. The overall decrease in the incidence of breathing during low voltage was one-third during the infusion period (Table 1). The effects disappeared within 7 h after the end of the infusion.

Discussion

There is ample evidence of multiple opioid receptors, as proposed by Martin *et al.* (8) and Lord *et al.* (9), although there are no studies in sheep. Stimulation of breathing by morphine in fetal sheep has been reported by several investigators (10–12), but the dual effect has only been reported by us in a preliminary communication (13). Our results suggest that there may be at least 2 receptors for opioid drugs in the fetal lamb and that the affinity may differ for each receptor. At the beginning of the infusion, when blood and brain drug concentrations are low, breathing is stimulated. After several hours when drug concentration has reached a plateau (unpublished observations), breathing is depressed. When the infusion is stopped and blood levels of drug are declining the stimulated breathing returns.

The location of these opioid receptors may be in the medulla or the spinal cord. It is unlikely that they are rostral to the pons since the fetus with a mid-collicular brain stem section experienced both stimulation and depression of breathing. Millhorn has studied the effect of morphine on the intercostal-phrenic nerve reflex in C_1 spinalized cats. Small doses of morphine excited this reflex, a 10-fold increase in dose had little or no effect upon it, and a 100-fold increase in morphine caused a large inhibition.

The effects of brief morphine treatment in our study reversed. The fetal effects of chronic treatment during a critical period of development may not be reversible. A permanent change in the neurological control of breathing after fetal opioid exposure might explain some cases of sudden infant death (3), whereas a permanent or prolonged alteration of normal electrocortical cycling may be related to the sheep disturbances reported in the neonate after chronic opioid exposure (2).

Acknowledgements

This work was supported by the NIH Fogarty Senior International, NATO Senior Scientist and Tartar Research Fellowships, by the Wellcome Trust and the

A

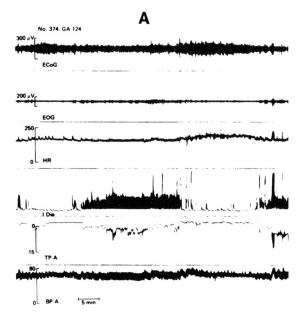

No. 374. GA 124

300 μV — ECoG

200 μV — EOG

250 / 0 — HR

.I Dia

0 / 15 — TP-A

80 / 0 — BP-A

5 min

B

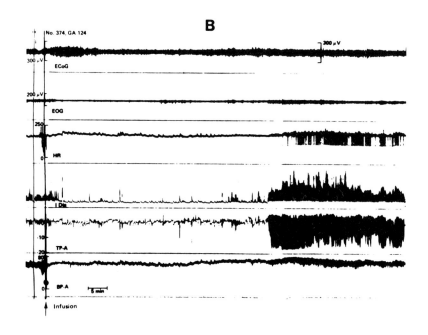

No. 374, GA 124

300 μV

300 μV — ECoG

200 μV — EOG

250 / 0 — HR

I Dia

-10 / -20 — TP-A

80 / 0 — BP-A

5 min

↑ Infusion

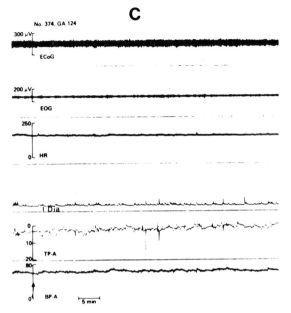

Figure 1. Recordings in an intact fetal lamb at 124 days gestation before (A) and during a 5 h morphine infusion (22 μg/min/kg). (B) Morphine-induced stimulation of breathing during the 1st 90 min of infusion. (C) Morphine-induced depression of breathing beginning in the 4th hour of the infusion; from above downwards electrocortical activity (ECoG), eye movements (EOG), heart rate (bpm), diaphragm activity (arbitrary units), tracheal and arterial pressures (mmHg).

Medical Research Council. We thank Dr Brian J. Koos and Frank Clewlow for their assistance at the beginning of these studies.

References

1. Olsen, G. D. and Lees, M. H. (1980). *J. Pediat.* **96**, 983–989.
2. Dinges, D. F., Davis, M. M. and Glass, P. (1980). *Science* **209**, 619–621.
3. Chavez, C. J., Ostrea, E. M. Jr., Stryker, J. C. and Smialek, Z. (1979). *J. Pediat.* **95**, 407–409.
4. Dawes, G. S., Fox, H. E., Leduc, B. M., Liggins, G. C. and Richards, R. T. (1972). *J. Physiol.* **220**, 119–143.
5. Clewlow, F., Dawes, G. S., Johnston, B. M. and Walker, D. W. (1983). *J. Physiol.* **341**, 463–476.
6. Dawes, G. S., Gardner, W. N., Johnston, B. M. and Walker, D. W. (1983). *J. Physiol.* **335**, 535–553.
7. Dawes, G. S., Gardner, W. N., Johnston, B. M. and Walker, D. W. (1982). *J. Physiol.* **326**, 461–474.

8. Martin, W. R., Eades, C. G., Thompson, J. A., Huppler, R. E. and Gilbert, P. E. (1976). *J. Pharmacol. Exp. Ther.* **197**, 517–532.
9. Lord, J. A. H., Waterfield, A. A., Hughes, J. and Kosterlitz, H. W. (1977). *Nature* **267**, 495–499.
10. Olsen, G. D., Hohimer, A. R. and Mathis, M. D. (1983). *Life Sci.* **33** (Suppl. I), 751–754.
11. Umans, J. G. and Szeto, H. H. (1983). *Life Sci.* **33** (Suppl. I), 639–642.
12. Toubas, P. L. and Sheldon, R. E. (1983). *Pediat. Res.* **17**, 143A.
13. Olsen, G. D. and Dawes, G. S. (1983). *Fed. Proc.* **42**, 1251.
14. Millhorn, D. E. (1983). Personal Communication.

Studies *in utero* of the Mechanism of Chemoreceptor Resetting

C. E. Blanco*, M. A. Hanson and H. B. McCooke

Department of Physiology and Biochemistry, University of Reading, Reading, UK and *Department of Pediatrics, St Annadal Hospital, Maastricht, Netherlands

Introduction

We recently reported (1) that in fetal lambs carotid chemoreceptor activity is greatly reduced at birth when arterial PO_2 rises. The range of chemoreceptor sensitivity is shifted to its adult position in early postnatal life. This raises the question of whether the chemoreceptor resetting is itself initiated by, and is dependent on, the rise in PO_2 or whether it is produced by some other event at birth, for example the sudden removal of a maternal humoral agent. In order to study this we have performed mechanical ventilation of unanaesthesized term fetuses *in utero* (2) so that arterial PO_2 was maintained above 70 mmHg and arterial PCO_2 was held in the normal range for 24–26 h.

Methods

Mule-cross sheep at 140–145 days gestation were anaesthetized with halothane and the fetal head and neck were exteriorized. A carotid artery was cannulated. The trachea was cannulated with a tube of interior diameter 5 mm. This was connected to a Y-piece so that the fetus could be ventilated with low deadspace via 2 tubes led out through the flank of the ewe and connected to a constant flow, time cycled respirator. The inspiratory gas used to ventilate the fetus was warmed, humidified and passed through a bacterial filter. The fetus was returned to the uterus and anaesthesia was discontinued. Ventilation was continued for 24–26 h, arterial PO_2, PCO_2 and pH being sampled at hourly intervals. At the end of this time the ewe was anaesthetized again and the fetus was delivered by caesarean section, ventilation being continued throughout. After the umbilicus had been ligated, 1–2% halothane was added to the gas used to ventilate the fetus.

The Physiological Development of the Fetus and Newborn
ISBN 0 12 389080 2

Copyright © 1985 by Academic Press, London.
All rights of reproduction in any form reserved.

Body temperature was kept at 39°C. The left carotid sinus nerve was identified and activity of chemoreceptor afferent fibres was recorded as described previously (1). The response of chemoreceptors to isocapnic hypoxia was studied by manipulating the gas delivered to the ventilator, keeping total flow constant.

The hypoxic responses of chemoreceptors from 2 term fetuses subjected to 24–26 h of hyperoxia *in utero* were compared to those of 2 term fetuses which were exteriorized acutely and where the cord was tied and ventilation was started only when chemoreceptor discharge was being recorded.

Results

The hypoxic responses of the carotid chemoreceptors of the fetuses ventilated for 24–26 h were similar to those of the fetuses without prior hyperoxic ventilation. The responses lay within the range described for fetal arterial chemoreceptors (1). However, in 1 fetus ventilated for 26 h the hypoxic response curve of the chemoreceptors was to the far right of the fetal range (Fig. 1). Whether this represents the beginning of resetting in this animal we do not know.

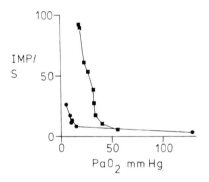

Figure 1. Isocapnic responses of carotid chemoreceptors. Squares: response determined at arterial PCO_2 of 53.9 ± 1.8 mmHg for term fetus ventilated *in utero* for 26 h to keep arterial PO_2 at 139 ± 25 mmHg and arterial PCO_2 at 42.8 ± 2.0 mmHg. Circles: response determined at arterial PCO_2 of 51.7 ± 3.0 mmHg for term fetus not ventilated before determination of the response curve.

Discussion

Our results confirm and extend those of our previous study (1), that carotid chemoreceptor sensitivity has not been reset to the adult range 24 h after the rise in PO_2 occurring at birth. But in the present experiments the umbilical circulation was maintained, and the fetus remained *in utero*, for its 1st 24 h of hyperoxia. Of itself this result suggests that some factor other than the rise in PO_2 may produce chemoreceptor resetting. However, in one of the fetuses ventilated for 26 h, the hypoxic response curve of the chemoreceptors was to the right of the fetal range. This might represent the beginning of resetting, in which case it suggests that the process is slow in onset after the rise in arterial PO_2.

References

1. Blanco, C. E., Dawes, G. S., Hanson, M. A. and McCooke, H. B. (1984). *J. Physiol.* (in press).
2. Blanco, C. E., Martin, C. B., Hanson, M. A. and McCooke, H. B. (1984). *Proc. Soc. Study Fetal Physiol. (Oxford)* July.

The Effect of Morphine on Breathing and Behaviour in Fetal Sheep

Henrique Rigatto, David Lee, Rebecca Caces,
Susan Albersheim and Michael Moore

Department of Pediatrics, University of Manitoba, Winnipeg, Canada

Introduction

Drugs like indomethacin, 5 hydroxytryptophan, and pilocarpine have been shown to induce continuous breathing in fetal sheep (1,3,4). Recently, Sheldon *et al.* showed that administration of morphine also induced fetal breathing (8). This finding was provocative as morphine is expected to depress breathing in the newborn. However, in this preliminary observation, measurements of breathing pattern or fetal behaviour were not made.

We designed the present study therefore to examine the changes in respiratory pattern and fetal behaviour associated with the administration of morphine to the fetal sheep.

Experimental

Ten chronically instrumented fetal sheep were studied on 13 occasions. Surgery was done at 120–128 days of gestation and studies were performed at 130–146 days. Each study consisted of a) monitoring one low voltage period of electrocortical activity (ECoG, *resting conditions*), b) infusing 1 ml/kg of saline solution in the jugular vein during the subsequent low voltage ECoG period (*control*), and c) injecting 1 mg/kg of morphine sulphate, by push, in the jugular vein during the following low voltage ECoG period (*morphine treatment*). During each of these steps, the fetus was observed and videotaped (Panasonic Model NV-8310) in order to assess fetal behaviour (5,6,7). Fetal behaviour was assessed by measuring fetal breathing, eye movements, jerky or slow movements of the head, sucking or swallowing and licking. Fetal wakefulness was defined by opened eyes and purposeful movements of the head.

The Physiological Development of the Fetus and Newborn
ISBN 0 12 389080 2

Copyright © 1985 by Academic Press, London.
All rights of reproduction in any form reserved.

Instrumentation of the fetus according to conventional methods (2,7) permitted measurements of electrocortical activity (ECoG), eye movements (EOG), electromyography of the diaphragm (EMG_{Di}), electromyography of the neck muscles (EMG_{neck}), tracheal pressure (TP), carotid pressure (CP), and amniotic pressure (AP) (Fig. 1). A catheter was inserted in the external jugular vein for administration of saline solution or morphine. Respiratory pattern was evaluated by measuring inspiratory time (Ti), total duration of the respiratory cycle (T_{tot}), mean inspiratory increase in tracheal pressure (TP/Ti), mean inspiratory rise in integrated diaphragmatic activity ($\int EMG_{Di}/Ti$) and "duty cycle" (Ti/T_{tot}). Ti was measured from the beginning to the peak of the TP deflection and also from the duration of diaphragmatic activity. Statistical significance of the differences between control and treatment periods were assessed by using the two-tailed pair *t* test.

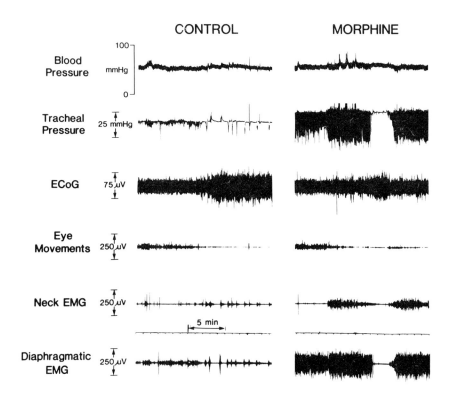

Figure 1. Representative tracing showing that the administration of morphine induces an increase in fetal breathing. Note the increase in TP and in EMG_{Di} after morphine.

Results

Fetal breathing

The administration of a saline solution produced no breathing response. We therefore compared values after morphine administration with those during saline infusion only. With morphine there was an initial apnoea followed by an increase in fetal breathing activity, TP and $\int EMG_{Di}$. Frequency increased from 57 ± 6 breaths/min to 83 ± 12. The delay time measured from end of morphine injection to beginning of apnoea was 0.76 ± 0.44 (SEM) min. The length of apnoea was 8.4 ± 2.3 min. The length of hyperpnoea was 121.9 ± 19.9 min. The changes observed are illustrated in Table 1. The hyperpnoea phase was also associated with significant increases in TP/Ti from 14.0 ± 2.3 mmHg to 58.6 ± 8.3 ($P=0.0003$) and in $\int EMG_{Di}$/Ti from 23.8 ± 7.9 mmHg to 60.9 ± 9.2 ($P=0.0002$). Large breaths of the type "pressure on the top of a pressure" also appeared during morphine administration in a frequency of 2.72 ± 0.46 breaths/min. The changes in the shape of the breath in response to morphine are illustrated in Fig. 2. PO_2

Table 1. Physiologic measurements during control and after the administration of morphine in fetal sheep

	TP (mmHg)	$\int EMG_{Di}$ (arbitrary units)	Ti_{TP} (s)	Ti_{Di} (s)	T_{tot} (s)	TP/Ti (mmHg/s)	$\int EMG_{Di/Ti}$ (arbitrary units/s)	$^{Ti}Di/T_{tot}$
Control	5.0 ±0.8	8.4 ±2.1	0.43 ±0.06	0.42 ±0.04	1.21 ±0.10	14.0 ±2.3	23.8 ±7.9	0.366 ±0.023
Morphine	17.2* ±2.9	18.8* ±2.9	0.25* ±0.02	0.31* ±0.03	0.88* ±0.10	58.6* ±8.3	60.9* ±9.2	0.393 ±0.028
Morphine (large breaths)	32.3* ±2.7	23.5* ±3.3	0.33 ±0.03	0.43 ±0.05	1.32 ±0.21	105.7* ±14.5	65.3* ±11.4	0.367 ±0.048

*$P<0.05$ in relation to control values using the two-tailed paired t test.

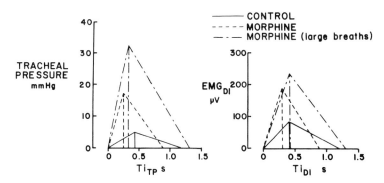

Figure 2. The size of a breath increases with morphine. Note the increase in TP/Ti and $\int EMG_{Di}$/Ti after administration of morphine.

decreased from 19 ± 0.8 mmHg during control to 15 ± 0.5 after morphine administration. PCO_2 and pH did not change. Heart rate increased from 151 ± 6 beats/min during control to 188 ± 15 during morphine ($P=0.04$). Systolic arterial blood pressure increased from 56.4 ± 2.2 mmHg to 64.9 ± 4.1 ($P=0.02$) with no significant change in diastolic blood pressure.

Fetal behaviour

During resting conditions and during saline administration the fetus alternated between periods of activity (REM sleep) and inactivity (quiet sleep). During REM sleep (low voltage ECog) breathing, eye movements, jerky ante- and retro-flexion movements of the head or slow rotation of the head, sucking or swallowing and licking were present. At the end of REM sleep, a general and powerful tonic muscle discharge preceded the transition from low to high voltage ECoG. During high voltage ECoG the fetus was inactive except for general periodic tonic muscular discharge. After morphine administration, the general behavioural pattern seen during the control period remained, but the proportion of time spent in low voltage increased from $31\pm2\%$ to 68 ± 10 ($P=0.01$). Breathing was observed, at times, during high voltage ECoG. Fetal wakefulness was not observed.

Discussion

We found that the administration of morphine induced a change in breathing in fetal sheep which was biphasic in nature. Shortly after injection there was a brief apnoea which was followed by pronounced hyperpnoea. The response was associated with an increase in the duration of low voltage electrocortical activity. There was no evidence of fetal wakefulness. We suggest that the opioid receptors responsible for apnoea are different from those responsible for hyperpnoea.

Previous investigators have shown that administration of morphine given to fetal sheep induced hyperpnoea, but they failed to demonstrate an initial apnoea (8). This omission may have been related to the lack of sleep and behaviour analysis in their study. Unless morphine is given during low voltage electrocortical activity while the fetus is breathing it may be difficult to detect the initial apnoea.

Analysis of breathing pattern showed that the response to morphine produced an increase in tracheal pressure, integrated diaphragmatic activity and in frequency. This increase in breathing was associated with an increase in the rate of rise in inspiratory activity as reflected by increase in TP/Ti and $\int EMG_{Di}/Ti$. Morphine, therefore, induced a breathing pattern which was not different from that induced by other agents capable of stimulating breathing, such as CO_2, indomethacin and pilocarpine. Morphine caused the appearance of large breaths which had a pressure on the top of a pressure pattern. These large breaths had an average rate of rise during inspiration similar to that of smaller breathing during morphine. This similarity related to an increase in TP and $\int EMG_{Di}$ with a proportional increase in T_{tot}. The mechanism for appearance of these large breaths remains unknown.

The behavioural assessment showed that during resting conditions the fetus behaved as reported previously (5,6,7). During REM sleep (low voltage ECoG) the fetus was active. Breathing, body and eye movements, sucking or swallowing and licking were present. During quiet sleep (high voltage ECoG) the fetus was inactive, except for periodic general tonic muscular discharges. During administration of morphine, there was a prolongation of REM sleep. Breathing usually stopped during high voltage ECoG but in some occasions it did not. Except for this occasional presence of breathing activity during quiet sleep and a prolongation of REM sleep the behavioural activity of the fetus after morphine did not change from control periods. Wakefulness defined by opened eyes and purposeful movements of the head was not seen during control or treatment periods.

Arterial PaO_2 decreased significantly during hyperpnoea as compared to control. It is likely that this decrease was related to an increased O_2 consumption during the powerful breathing induced by morphine. The increase in pulse pressure and in heart rate with morphine may reflect the central stimulant effects of morphine during hyperpnoea.

In summary, we found that administration of morphine to fetal sheep produces a "biphasic" change in fetal breathing, with initial "apnoea" followed by "hyperpnoea". These changes were associated with an increase in REM sleep but fetal wakefulness was not observed. During hyperpnoea there was an increase in respiratory output as defined by increased in TP and $\int EMG_{Di}$. Frequency also increased. We suggest that morphine releases the inhibition to breathe in the fetal sheep. This is *not* mediated through fetal arousal. It is likely that apnoea and hyperpnoea are reflections of morphine actions on different opioid receptors.

References

1. Brown, E. R., Lawson, E. E., Tauesch, H. W. and Chernick, V. (1978). *Pediat. Res.* **12**, 402.
2. Dawes, G. S., Fox, H. E., Leduc, B. M. and Liggins, G. C. (1972). *J. Physiol.* **220**, 119.
3. Kitterman, J. A., Liggins, G. C., Clements, J. A. and Tooley, W. H. (1979). *J. Develop. Physiol.* **1**, 453–466.
4. Quilligan, E. J., Clewlow, F., Johnston, B. M. and Walker, D. W. (1981). *Am. J. Obstet. Gynecol.* **141**, 271–275.
5. Rigatto, H., Moore, M., Horvath, L., Winter, A., Luz, J. and Cates, D. (1983). *Pediat. Res.* **17**, 332A.
6. Rigatto, H., Moore, M. and Cates, D. (1984). *Pediat. Res.* **18**, 112A.
7. Rigatto, H. (1984). *In:* "Animal Models in Fetal Medicine", Vol. III. (Nathanielsz, P. W., ed.) Perinatology Press, New York.
8. Sheldon, R. E. and Toubas, P. L. (1985). *J. Appl. Physiol.* (in press).

The Effects of a Stable Adenosine Analogue on Fetal Behavioural, Respiratory and Cardiovascular Functions

Hazel H. Szeto and Jason G. Umans

Department of Pharmacology, Cornell University Medical College, New York, USA

Introduction

Purinergic agonists have been shown to cause a receptor-mediated depression in cardiovascular and respiratory function, and an increase in slow-wave sleep at the expense of wakefulness in adult laboratory animals (1,2). More recently, adenosine analogues have been shown to depress respiratory function in neonatal (3) and preterm (4) rabbits. However, the effects of purinergic agonists on cardiovascular and neurobehavioural function in the immature animal have not been examined. Using the metabolically stable adenosine analogue, 1-phenylisopropyl-adenosine (PIA), we sought to determine the functional dependence of these same effects on purinergic stimulation in the 3rd trimester ovine fetus.

Methods

Eight unanaesthetized, unrestrained pregnant ewes between 123 and 138 days of gestation (term being 145 days) were studied 8–34 days following the surgical implantation of cannulae and electrodes to monitor fetal blood pressure, heart rate, tracheal pressure, diaphragmatic EMG, electrocortical activity, eye movements and EMg of the dorsal neck muscle and hindlimb muscle. Details of the surgical and recording procedures were as described previously (5,6).

PIA (10–500 μg) was administered iv directly to the fetus. All physiologic

The Physiological Development of the Fetus and Newborn
ISBN 0 12 389080 2
Copyright © 1985 by Academic Press, London.
All rights of reproduction in any form reserved.

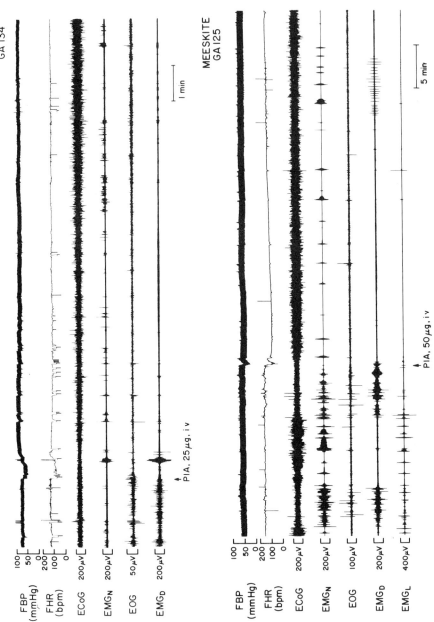

Figures 1 and 2. Polygraphic traces showing effects of PIA on the fetus. Abbr: FBP, fetal blood pressure; FHR, fetal heart rate; ECoG, electrocorticogram; EOG, electrooculogram; EMG$_D$, diaphragmatic EMG; EMG$_N$, nuchal EMG; EMG$_L$, hindlimb EMG; bpm, beats/min.

parameters were monitored continuously for at least 2 h before and after the administration of PIA.

The polygraphic recordings were scored in 1 min epochs by visual analysis. The criteria for behavioural state scoring have been previously described (5,6). The % incidence of fetal breathing movements (FBMs) was calculated as [(min containing FBMs/total time) × 100%]. The peak cardiovascular effects were reported as changes from the predrug control values.

Results

PIA resulted in immediate bradycardia and hypotension in all fetuses (see Figs 1,2). The magnitude and duration of the bradycardia was dose-related, as demonstrated in Table 1. Higher doses (> 250 μg) resulted in cardiac standstill.

Table 1. PIA-Induced changes in cardiovascular parameters

Dose	n	HR (beats/min)	Systolic BP (mmHg)	Diastolic BP (mmHg)
10	4	-41 ± 8.9*	-12.5 ± 3.1	-13.5 ± 2.4
25	3	-49 ± 5.5	-13.0 ± 4.2	-16.0 ± 5.1
50	4	-59 ± 6.6	-16.0 ± 4.5	-17.0 ± 4.8
100	1	-110	-25.0	-28.0

*mean $\pm$ SEM

At doses greater than 10 μg, PIA also resulted in synchronization of the ECoG with total suppression of FBMs. The effects of PIA on the incidence of FBMs and the incidence of synchronized electrocortical activity are summarized in Table 2. The duration of synchronized ECoG was directly dose-related, ranging from 24 min following 25 μg to 120 min following 100 μg. The duration of apnoea generally exceeded that of the synchronized ECoG.

Table 2. Respiratory and neurobehavioural effects of PIA

Dose	n	Incidence of FBMs		Incidence of synch ECoG	
		predrug	postdrug	predrug	postdrug
10	4	41.2 ± 3.7	34.4 ± 6.4	46.0 ± 5.0	44.0 ± 5.5
25	3	41.2 ± 4.3	26.0 ± 7.3	45.3 ± 4.3	59.3 ± 7.8
50	4	44.5 ± 1.8	10.9 ± 2.8	44.1 ± 4.3	77.7 ± 1.6
100	1	47.3	3.8	47.3	96.2

Associated with the synchronized ECoG, there was also a reduction in muscular activity and the absence of rapid eye movements, consistent with the state of quiet sleep (5,6). Both arousal and rapid eye movement sleep were decreased in a dose-related fashion.

Discussion

The metabolically stable adenosine analogue, PIA, resulted in a depression of cardiovascular, respiratory and neurobehavioural function in the fetal lamb. The effects were consistent with those observed in neonatal and adult animals (1-4,7).

At doses less than 25 µg, PIA resulted in a significant bradycardia without significant changes in blood pressure, breathing movements or behavioural activity. This suggests that the cardiac depressant effect may be due to direct stimulation of myocardial adenosine (A_1) receptors (8).

At doses greater than 25 µg, PIA resulted in prolonged quiet sleep at the expense of both rapid eye movement sleep and arousal. These results differ from those found in adult rats. Radulovacki *et al.* (7) reported that adenosine analogues increased slow-wave sleep but did not decrease rapid eye movement sleep except at very high doses.

The suppression of FBMs may in part be due to the increase in quiet sleep since FBMs are generally absent during quiet sleep. However, FBMs were still absent upon recovery of rapid eye movement sleep and arousal, suggesting that PIA may directly inhibit respiration in the fetal lamb.

Acknowledgement

Supported by NIDA-02475-04 and BRSG-2-SO7-RR05396-22. H. H. Szeto is the recipient of a Research Scientist Development Award from NIDA (KO2-00100-01), and J. G. Umans is the recipient of a Research Fellowship from the Charles H. Revson Foundation.

References

1. Hedner, T., Hedner, J., Wessberg, P. and Jonason, J. (1982). *Neurosci. Lett.* **33**, 147-151.
2. Radulovacki, M., Miletich, R. S. and Green, R. D. (1982). *Brain Res.* **246**, 178-180.
3. Lagercrantz, H., Yamamoto, Y., Fredholm, B. B., Prabhakar, N. R. and von Euler, C. (1984). *Pediat. Res.* **18**, 387-390.
4. Hedner, T., Hedner, J., Jonason, J. and Wessberg, P. (1984). *Eur. J. Resp. Dis.* **65**, 153-156.
5. Szeto, H. H. (1983). *Am. J. Obstet. Gynecol.* **146**, 211-218.
6. Umans, J. G. and Szeto, H. H. (1983). *Life Sci.* **33** (Supp. 1), 639-642.
7. Radulovacki, M., Virus, R. M., Djuricic-Nedelson, M. and Green, R. D. (1984). *J. Pharmacol. Exp. Ther.* **228**, 268-274.
8. Leung, E., Johnston, C. I. and Woodcock, E. A. (1983). *Biochem. Biophys. Res. Comm.* **110**, 208-215.

Methionine-enkephalin and the Arrest of Fetal breathing

G. J. Hofmeyr*, O. S. Bamford,
T. Howlett** and M. J. Parkes

Nuffield Institute for Medical Research, University of Oxford, Oxford, UK,
*Witwatersrand University Council Overseas Research Fellow, **Department
of Chemical Endocrinology, St Bartholomew's Hospital Medical College,
London, UK

Introduction

Isocapnic hypoxia, which stimulates breathing in the adult and neonate, causes arrest of breathing in fetal lambs (1). A possible explanation for this difference is that the arrest of breathing in the fetus is dependent upon one or more placental products. One site of production of methionine enkephalin (met-enkephalin) is the placenta (2). When infused into fetal lambs met-enkephalin causes arrest of breathing (3). We have investigated the hypothesis that met-enkephalin is a factor in the arrest of breathing during hypoxia.

Materials and Methods

Fetal lambs were operated under general anaesthesia (1). Cortical, diaphragmatic and precordial electrodes, and aortic and inferior vena caval catheters were inserted. In 4 fetuses the cerebellum was removed by suction and the brain stem was transected at the level of the inferior colliculus under direct vision. A minimum of 4 days recovery (7 days after transection) was allowed before experimentation at 123–133 days gestation.

Met-enkephalin (Peninsula Laboratories) was diluted in acidified normal saline (pH 3) and stored at $-20\,^{\circ}\mathrm{C}$ until use. Control injections were made with equal volumes of acidified or normal saline. Isocapnic hypoxia was induced in all fetuses. Room air was administered to the ewe through a box over her head at 40 l/min for 30 min, followed by oxygen 8.5% with carbon dioxide 1.2% in N_2 for 1 h.

The Physiological Development of the Fetus and Newborn
ISBN 0 12 389080 2
Copyright © 1985 by Academic Press, London.
All rights of reproduction in any form reserved.

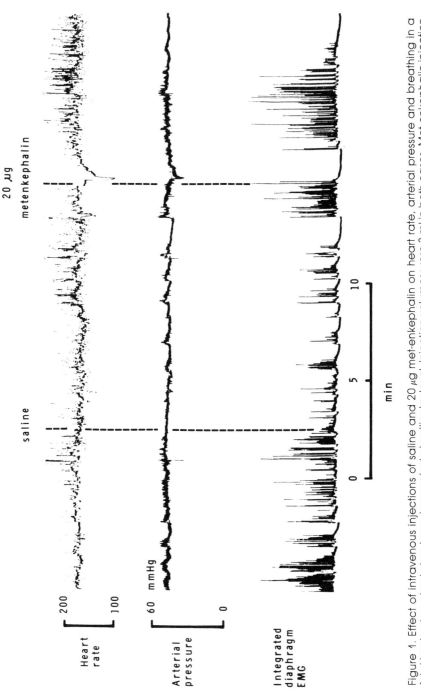

Figure 1. Effect of intravenous injections of saline and 20 μg met-enkephalin on heart rate, arterial pressure and breathing in a fetal lamb whose brain has been transected at collicular level. Injection volumes were 3 ml in both cases. Met-enkephalin injection was followed by an arrest of breathing, bradycardia and a fall in arterial pressure.

For met-enkephalin assay blood samples of 10 ml were added to lithium heparin tubes containing aprotinin (Trasylol Bayer) 10 000 KI units, centrifuged at 4°C and the plasma was acidified with 750 μl glycine/HCl (1.6% w/v glycine in 1M HCl) per 5 ml of plasma and frozen at -20°C. Met-enkephalin was measured by a specific extracted radioimmunoassay (4).

Results

The 8 intact fetal lambs showed the normal arrest of breathing during isocapnic hypoxia (PO_2 reduced from 20 ± 1 to 11.3 ± 6 mmHg, mean$\pm$SEM), whereas the 4 with brain stem transection responded to isocapnic hypoxia (PO_2 reduced from 19 ± 1 to 11 ± 0.8 mmHg) with enhanced breathing. Injection of met-enkephalin (20 μg into the IVC) caused a consistent abrupt arrest of breathing lasting 30–180 s, accompanied by a fall in heart rate and blood pressure in intact lambs as reported by others (3). The response of the transected fetuses to met-enkephalin injection (Figs 1 and 2) was indistinguishable from that of the normal fetuses.

Continuous intravenous infusion of naloxone (0.8 mg, followed by 1.6 mg/h in 6 intact fetuses) failed to modify the effect of isocapnic hypoxia on fetal breathing. Rapid injection of naloxone (2.8 mg) during apnoea induced by hypoxia

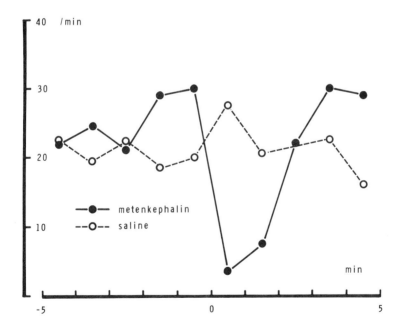

Figure 2. Effect of intravenous injections at time 0 of met-enkephalin and saline on breathing rate in consecutive 1 min periods. The values shown are the means of 2 experiments on each of 2 fetuses with brain stem transection and were measured by computerized analysis of diaphragm electromyogram and tracheal pressure recordings.

also failed to induce breathing. During the control period, naloxone did not prevent the arrest of breathing during high-voltage electrocortical activity.

After 20–30 min hypoxia the fetal arterial plasma met-enkephalin concentration was *reduced* from a control value of 45 ± 6 (mean $\pm$ SEM) to 37 ± 6 ng/l ($P < 0.02$, Wilcoxon sign ranked test). Maternal values were 33 and 23 ng/l respectively. In 1 lamb the umbilical vein (sampled from the placental surface) met-enkephalin concentration was 94 ± 6 and that in the umbilical artery was 76 ± 14 ng/ml (mean of 4 sets of samples).

Discussion

Upper pontine transection reversed the effect of hypoxia upon fetal breathing, but had no effect upon the arrest of breathing by met-enkephalin. The mechanisms whereby hypoxia and met-enkephalin cause arrest of breathing are therefore different. Whereas the arrest of fetal breathing caused by hypoxia (and by barbiturates (5)) is dependent upon a suprapontine mechanism, that caused by met-enkephalin, as by ethanol (6), is not. The opioid peptide may act by a direct effect upon the medulla or spinal cord.

Naloxone was described as enhancing the ventilatory response to carbon dioxide in partly exteriorized fetal lambs (7). However infusion or injection of naloxone failed to inhibit the arrest of breathing during hypoxia in unanaesthetized lambs *in utero*, in agreement with Adamson and Patrick (8).

Thus while opioid peptides may modify fetal breathing in certain circumstances, the evidence using naloxone does not support their implication in the arrest of breathing during hypoxia.

The number of met-enkephalin measurements in the umbilical artery and vein was too small to be conclusive. However, the mean increase across the placenta is in agreement with the findings of others (2).

The small decrease in plasma met-enkephalin after 20–30 min hypoxia is quite different from the response of β-endorphin and β-lipoprotein, which increase 3–4 fold after 15 and 30 min hypoxia (9). It is possible that met-enkephalin may increase after more prolonged hypoxia or during recovery. However the early decrease is inconsistent with the hypothesis that met-enkephalin is responsible for the arrest of breathing early in hypoxia.

We conclude that met-enkephalin is not responsible for the arrest of fetal breathing by hypoxia.

Acknowledgements

We thank the MRC for a grant to Professor G. S. Dawes; C. T. Jones for a supply of met-enkephalin; and S. Tomlin, H. Elvidge and C. Hanson for technical assistance.

References

1. Boddy, K., Dawes, G. S., Fisher, R., Pinter, S. and Robinson, J. S. (1974). *J. Physiol.* **243**, 599–618.

2. Jones, C. T. Personal communication.
3. La Gamma, E. F., Itskovitz, J. and Rudolph, A. M. (1983). *Pediat. Res.* **17**(2), 162–167.
4. Clement-Jones, V., Lowry, P. J., Rees, L. H. and Besser, G. M. (1980). *J. Endocrinol.* **86**, 231–243.
5. Dawes, G. S., Gardner, W. N., Johnston, B. M. and Walker, D. W. (1983). *J. Physiol.* **335**, 535–553.
6. Bamford, O. S., Dawes, G. S., Hofmeyr, G. J., Parkes, M. J. and Quail, A. W. Effects of maternally administered ethanol on fetal sheep. (in prep.).
7. Moss, I. R. and Scarpelli, E. M. (1979). *J. Appl. Physiol.* **47**, 527–531.
8. Adamson, L. and Patrick, J. (1983). *Proc. 30th Meeting, Soc. Gynaecol. Invest.* March.
9. Wardlaw, G. L., Stark, R. I., Daniel, S. and Frantz, A. G. (1981). *Endocrinology* **108**, 1710–1715.

When does Sexual Differentiation of the Human Brain Occur?

D. R. Abramovich, I. A. Davidson,
A. Longstaff and C. K. Pearson

Departments of Obstetrics and Gynaecology and Biochemistry,
University of Aberdeen, Aberdeen, Scotland

Testosterone (T) secreted by the testes during a "critical" period influences certain aspects of brain development leading to masculinization of behaviour and neuroendocrine function (1). In all species so far studied CNS sexual differentiation either follows or overlaps differentiation of the reproductive tract and occurs at a time when plasma T concentrations are higher in males than females. For many mammals (rat, mouse, hamster, ferret and dog) this is a perinatal event; for others (guinea-pig, sheep and rhesus monkey) it is prenatal (1).

The exact timing of human brain sexual differentiation is unknown but it has been suggested on morphological (2) and psychological evidence (3) to be between the 4th and 7th month of fetal life. A sex difference in plasma T concentration occurs in the human fetus between 12–18 weeks (4). In view of the involvement of estrogen and androgen receptors in brain sexual differentiation reported in rodents, we examined human fetal brain cytosol between 14 and 20 weeks gestation for these receptors.

Receptor Assays

Ligands used

Estrogen. (11B-methoxy-^{3}H) Moxestrol (R2858), New England Nuclear. This was used because it does not bind to contaminating plasma proteins and unlike the natural estrogens it was not sulphated by fetal tissues (5).

Androgen. (17α-methyl-^{3}H) methyltrienolone (R1881), New England Nuclear. It is neither aromatized nor metabolized and does not bind to SHBG (6).

The Physiological Development of the Fetus and Newborn
ISBN 0 12 389080 2

Copyright © 1985 by Academic Press, London.
All rights of reproduction in any form reserved.

Tissue

Fetuses (14–20 weeks gestation) were obtained following prostaglandin induced abortion or by hysterotomy. Cytosols were prepared from either whole brain or from the following regions: hypothalamus, frontal lobe, temporal lobe, hind brain, occipital lobe and cortex. Human endometrium and neonatal rat brain were used as control tissues for estrogen receptors. similarly rat prostate was used as the control for androgen receptors.

Methodology

We attempted to tackle the question of *in utero* sexual differentiation of the human brain by examining this tissue for the presence of estrogen and androgen receptors. Tissue cytosols were incubated with either R2858 or R1881 in the presence and absence of a 100 times molar excess unlabelled ligand. Bound and free steroid were separated using the following techniques: Sephadex LH-20 chromatography, dextran-coated charcoal and sucrose density gradient centrifugation.

Endogenous steroids which may be saturating receptor binding sites were removed by passing cytosol through a Sephadex LH-20 column prior to incubation.

Results

No estrogen or androgen receptors were detected in any area of human fetal brain between 14 and 20 weeks after exhaustive investigation. However, receptors could routinely be detected in control tissues with the above methodology. The removal of the endogenous steroids from the human brain cytosol preparations made no difference to binding. Also mixing human brain cytosol with rat brain cytosol did not destroy rat receptor activity, suggesting that there is nothing interfering with receptor binding in human cytosol.

Androgen levels

Cord bloods were obtained from 26–36 week infants and from term deliveries. Bloods were collected from infants from day 0 up to 7 months of age. T and DHT were measured by radioimmunoassay.

Results

Plasma T and DHT levels are shown in Tables 1 and 2 respectively.

Discussion

Work with rodents has shown that steroids acting on the brain during a "critical" period of development can influence its sexual differentiation (7). Although no biochemical proof is available it is firmly believed by most workers that sexual differentiation of the human brain is a prenatal event (1,2,3,8).

Table 1. Plasma T

| Age | Testosterone (nmol) Mean ± SEM (n) | | t test |
	Male	Female	
Fetal 26–36 weeks	5.49 ± 0.57 (13)	5.01 ± 0.55 (9)	P < 0.3
Birth	6.65 ± 0.52 (19)	6.46 ± 0.69 (16)	P < 0.4
0–24 h	12.30 ± 1.19 (15)	7.40 ± 0.96 (8)	P < 0.01
1–5 days	7.8 ± 1.2 (28)	5.40 ± 0.85 (12)	P < 0.1
5–10 days	4.8 ± 0.61 (5)	6.1 ± 1.23 (5)	P < 0.2
> 10 days	7.0 ± 0.87 (36)	4.5 ± 1.10 (22)	P < 0.1

Table 2. Plasma DHT

| Age | Testosterone (nmol) Mean ± SEM (n) | | t test |
	Male	Female	
Fetal 26–36 weeks	3.76 ± 0.33 (14)	3.10 ± 0.32 (8)	P < 0.15
Birth	7.59 ± 0.48 (19)	7.27 ± 0.32 (16)	P < 0.3
0–24 h	5.47 ± 0.67 (17)	2.53 ± 0.30 (5)	P < 0.0125
1–5 days	2.60 ± 0.23 (42)	1.64 ± 0.21 (20)	P < 0.005
5–10 days	2.3 ± 0.32 (15)	1.3 ± 0.24 (5)	P < 0.4
> 10 days	2.4 ± 0.32	1.3 ± 0.18 (10)	P < 0.025

The absence of estrogen and androgen receptors suggests that no differentiation occurs in the human brain between 14–20 weeks *in utero*, despite the presence of a plasma androgen sex difference in fetuses of this age. The above plasma results show that the only other time when there is an androgen sex-difference is in the neonatal period. It is feasible that this could be the period where sexual differentiation of the human brain could occur. The implications of this hypothesis are of interest.

Acknowledgements

This work was supported by the Medical Research Council, Grampian Health Board, and Masson Medical Research Foundation.

References

1. McEwen, B. S. (1983). *Int. Rev. Physiol.* **27**, 99–145.
2. Dorner, G. and Staudt, J. (1972). *Endokrinologie* **89**, 152–155.
3. Ehrhardt, A. A. (1977). *In:* "Handbook of Sexology", (Money, J. and Musaph, H., eds) pp. 258–287. Excerpta Medica, Amsterdam.
4. Abramovich, D. R. and Rowe, P. (1973). *J. Endocrinol.* **56**, 621–622.

5. Davidson, I. A., Stott, J. E., Longstaff, A., Abramovich, D. R. and Pearson, C. K. (1983). *J. Ster. Biochem.* **18**, 525–529.
6. Fichman, K. R., Nyburg, L. M., Bujnovsky, P., Brown, T. R. and Walsh, P. C. (1981). *J. Clin. Endocrinol. Metab.* **52**, 919–923.
7. Baum, M. J. (1979). *Neurosci. Biobehav. Rev.* **3**, 265–284.
8. Rubin, R. T., Reinisch, J. M. and Hawkett, R. F. (1981). *Science* **211**, 1318–1324.

Blockade of Endogenous Opiates in the Ventral Medulla induces Wakefulness and Continuous Fetal Breathing in Exteriorized Fetal Sheep

S. Ioffe, A. H. Jansen and V. Chernick

Perinatal Physiology Laboratory, Department of Pediatrics,
University of Manitoba, Winnipeg, Canada

Introduction

Fetal asphyxia or low O_2 breathing in neonates is associated with apnoea and ventilatory depression (1,2). In neonates, these can be markedly reduced by naloxone (2,3). These effects are not seen in the adult, perhaps because of fewer opiate receptors in the medulla at the time of birth (4). Paradoxically, iv administration of morphine has been shown to cause continuous fetal breathing in sheep (5). The present study was undertaken to explore the site of action of morphine and naloxone on the fetal medulla.

Methods

Twelve pregnant ewes were operated under pentobarbitone anaesthesia at 130–133 days gestation. Catheters were placed in the fetal femoral artery and jugular vein. Electrodes were placed in the fetal diaphragm, lateral rectus muscle and on the fetal cortical dura for ECoG recording (6). A portion (15 mm diameter) of the occipital bone and the cerebellum were removed to allow access to the 4th ventricle. The fetus was replaced in the uterus and catheters exteriorized through the flank of the ewe. After 3 days recovery *in utero* the fetus was exteriorized into a saline bath (39.5–40°C) under maternal spinal anaesthesia. Morphine (0.5 mg, in 1 ml), naloxone (0.5–2 mg, in 1 ml) or saline (1 ml) were injected into the subarachnoid space of the ventral medulla via direct injection or a catheter inserted laterally around the dorsal medulla ($n = 27$).

The Physiological Development of the Fetus and Newborn
ISBN 0 12 389080 2
Copyright © 1985 by Academic Press, London.
All rights of reproduction in any form reserved.

Following each injection, sleep state and diaphragmatic EMG activity were monitored for at least 1 h. In addition, the effects of iv morphine (2 mg), naloxone (9 mg) or saline on fetal breathing and sleep state were studied ($n = 20$) and compared to those of direct medullary injections.

Results

Ventral medullary injection

Naloxone caused arousal within 5–15 min associated with a large increase in diaphragmatic EMG amplitude and frequency (Fig. 1B). When the fetus

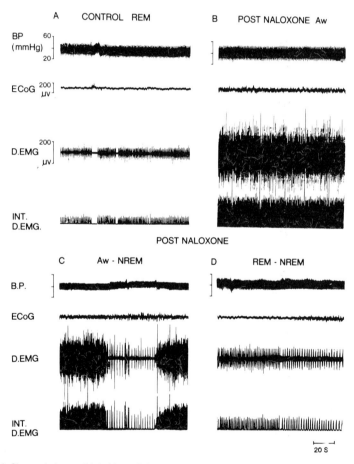

Figure 1. Sleep state and fetal breathing activity in 1 fetus at 137 days gestation before (A) and after (B,C,D) injection of 1.5 mg naloxone in the area of the ventral medulla. BP, blood pressure; D EMG, diaphragmatic EMG; Int D EMG, integrated diaphragmatic EMG.

spontaneously went from the awake state to NREM sleep the amplitude and frequency of diaphragmatic EMG activity decreased (Fig. 1C). A decrease in diaphragmatic EMG activity also occurred when REM changed to NREM sleep (Fig. 1D). Following stimulation of breathing activity by naloxone the injection of 0.25 ml 2% xylocaine in the same area was associated with an immediate decrease in the amplitude of breathing activity and blood pressure (Fig. 2, top). Similarly, pentobarbitone sodium injected intravenously (10–20 mg) following stimulation of breathing activity by naloxone caused a rapid decrease in fetal breathing but had no effect on blood pressure (Fig. 2, bottom). A much smaller dose of pentobarbitone (1–2 mg iv) injected directly into the fetus during REM sleep abolished fetal breathing in the nonstimulated fetus (Jansen *et al.*, unpublished observations).

Injection of an equal volume of 0.9% NaCl solution did not produce measurable

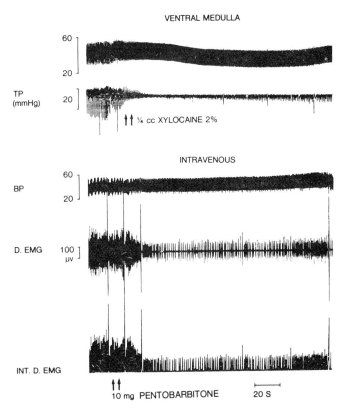

Figure 2. (Top) Injection of xylocaine into the region of the ventral medulla following stimulation of fetal breathing by injection of naloxone at the same site. Time of injection between the arrows. TP, tracheal pressure. (Bottom) Injection of 10 mg pentobarbitone IV in a fetus in whom naloxone had been previously administered to the area of the ventral medulla. Time of injection between the arrows.

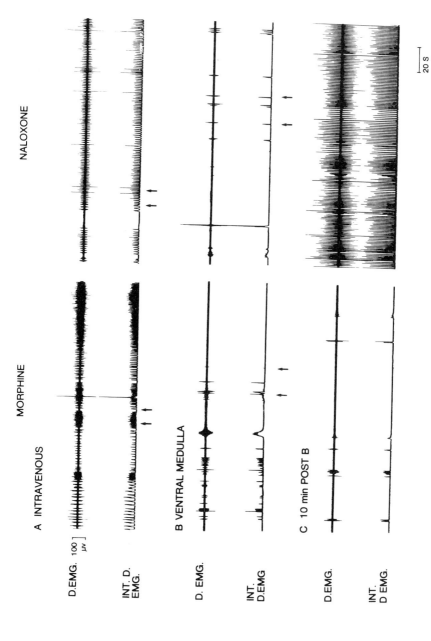

Figure 3. (Left) Comparison of the effects on fetal breathing activity of intravenous and ventral medullary injection of morphine. (Right) Similar comparison of naloxone injections.

changes in sleep state or breathing activity. Similarly, morphine injected into the same area had no effect on sleep state or breathing activity (Fig. 3B, 3C, left).

Intravenous injections

Fetal breathing was increased in amplitude when naloxone injection was associated with arousal. There was no dramatic change in diaphragmatic EMG activity when naloxone was injected during REM sleep and no arousal occurred (Fig. 3A, right). Saline injection had no effect. Intravenous morphine during REM sleep caused an immediate increase in fetal breathing (Fig. 3A, left) with no change in ECoG activity. When morphine was injected during NREM sleep, no response was seen until the fetus switched to REM sleep at which time there again was an increase in breathing activity.

Discussion

This study clearly demonstrates a complex mechanism of action of drugs on fetal breathing dependent on the site of injection. The findings are:

1. The action of centrally applied naloxone is not mediated by arousal or central chemoreceptors.

2. Arousal caused initiation of fetal breathing during iv naloxone.

3. Morphine does not act directly on fetal respiratory neurones but possibly stimulates breathing activity via the reticular formation.

References

1. Bystrzycka, E., Nail, B. S. and Purves, M. J. (1975). *Resp. Physiol.* **25**, 199–215.
2. Grunstein, M. M., Hazinski, T. A. and Schlueter, M. A. (1981). *J. Appl. Physiol. Resp. Env. Ex. Physiol.* **51**, 122–130.
3. Chernick, V. and Craig, R. J. (1982). *Science* **216**, 1252–1253.
4. Villiger, J. W., Taylor, K. M. and Gluckman, P. D. (1982). *Pediat. Pharmacol.* **2**, 349–356.
5. Olsen, G. D., Hohimer, A. R. and Mathis, M. D. (1983). *Life Sci.* **33**, 751–754.
6. Ioffe, S., Jansen, A. H. and Chernick, V. (1985). *J. Appl. Physiol. Resp. Env. Ex. Physiol.* (in press).

Clinical Significance of Fetal Breathing and Other Movements

John Patrick and Bryan Richardson

MRC Group in Reproductive Biology, Departments of Obstetrics and
Gynecology and of Physiology, University of Western Ontario, London,
Ontario, Canada

Clinical Significance of Fetal Breathing and Other Movements

Until recent years, obstetricians considered that attention to the health of pregnant women consulted in acceptable fetal outcome. By the mid-1960s maternal mortality had been reduced to very low levels and obstetricians and paediatricians turned their attention to the health of fetuses and sick newborns.

The radical concepts of Liley and others in dealing with Rh-sensitized pregnancies led to three new lines of obstetrical thought:

1. use of an invasive test to directly measure fetal health,
2. accurate tests of fetal health to permit delivery of sick fetuses who would do better in the nursery than in the uterus,
3. invasive testing may permit treatment of fetuses *in utero* before birth.

However, underlying these new concepts is the fact that an understanding of the physiology and pathophysiology of health and disease can lead to effective management and, in the case of Rh immune globulin, effective, safe preventive measures which eventually eliminate the need to expensive tests and treatment.

Pregnant women and persons interested in their care have long recognized the significance of fetal movements as a sign of fetal life and health. However, until the development of newer noninvasive technology, it was impossible to study comprehensively fetal activity in humans. In the 1970s, with the development of chronic fetal lamb preparations by physiologists, cardiologists, obstetricians and paediatricians, it became possible to study, in controlled circumstances, the physiology of fetal activity.

The Physiological Development of the Fetus and Newborn
ISBN 0 12 389080 2

Copyright © 1985 by Academic Press, London.
All rights of reproduction in any form reserved.

Fetal Breathing Movements

Initial studies examined fetal breathing movements by recording negative tracheal pressure, tracheal flow or diaphragmatic electromyogram in fetal animals. Led by Geoffrey Dawes' group in Oxford, it was reported that during the last third of pregnancy in sheep, fetuses normally made breathing movements 30–40% of the time (1). Breathing movements, which were episodic, were reported to occur only during low voltage electrocortical activity with rapid eye movements (1). There was a circadian rhythm in fetal breathing movements in healthy fetuses (2). Infusions of glucose led to an increase in the incidence of fetal breathing movements. Administration of an isocapnic hypoxia mixture to the ewe resulted in complete suppression of fetal breathing movements, yet hypercapnia caused an increase in the incidence of fetal breathing movements (3). Hyperoxia had no influence on fetal breathing movements but hypercapnia resulted in diminished fetal breathing activity. Fetal asphyxia resulted in suppression of normal fetal breathing movements and development of abnormal gasping patterns (4). During the last 2–3 days before spontaneous labour, fetal breathing movements were diminished (5).

The observation that fetal breathing movements disappeared during times of fetal hypoxaemia and that gasping movements preceded death and occurred with fetal asphyxia was received enthusiastically by clinicians who hoped to use the measurement of fetal breathing movements as a sign of fetal health or sickness in humans. Initially, technology was a problem and the first ultrasonic methods developed by Boddy and Robinson (6) were found to be difficult and undependable when used in the clinic. However, the real-time ultrasonic scanner permitted obstetricians to observe directly for the first time echoes of the human fetus in real time. Clinicians used two strategies in the examination of fetal breathing movements. Some moved directly to the clinic and the others to clinical laboratories to study natural patterns and influences on fetal breathing movements.

Studies of Human Fetal Breathing Movements in Clinical Laboratories

Clinical investigators using healthy pregnant volunteers made observations of human fetal breathing movements under controlled conditions. It was possible, during the last 10 weeks of pregnancy, to observe fetal breathing movements. Real-time ultrasound transducers were placed on the maternal abdominal wall and a longitudinal cross-section of fetal chest and abdominal wall echoes was selected. During each fetal breath, anterior chest wall echoes moved inward 2–5 mm and anterior abdominal wall echoes moved outward in the opposite direction about 3–8 mm. Following each inspiratory movement chest wall and abdominal wall echoes returned to a resting state. Investigators identified individual breaths and coded them on chart paper using event markers.

During the last 10 weeks of pregnancy, human fetal breathing movements are episodic and occur about 30% of the time (7,8). As a result, the incidence of fetal breathing movements can be altered substantially by the length of recording

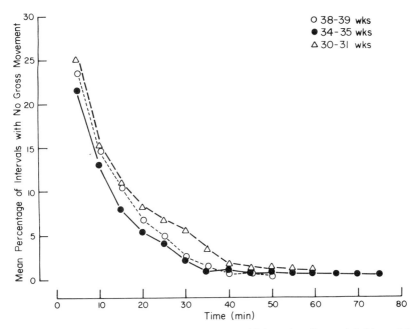

Figure 1. Composite plot of the percentage of intervals with no fetal breathing movements in 9 fetuses at 30–31 weeks, 11 at 34–35 weeks and 11 at 38–39 weeks demonstrating a similar distribution at the different gestational ages. The longest apnoeic interval was 65 min at 30–31 weeks, 105 min at 34–35 weeks and 120 min at 38–39 weeks in fetuses observed continuously over 24 h observation intervals (from Ref. 9).

intervals. Because fetal breathing movements occur in episodes and are separated by periods of apnoea, it was necessary to record for at least 2 h to be certain the recording interval did not entirely consist of a normal period of fetal apnoea (Fig. 1) (9).

Although episodic fetal breathing movements occur about 30% of the time, the hourly incidence over 24 h observation intervals can vary according to time of day and maternal meals. During the last 10 weeks of pregnancy the incidence of fetal breathing movements is significantly increased at 1–3 h after maternal meals and overnight while mothers are asleep (7,8). The increase in fetal breathing movements following maternal meals can be reproduced by giving fasted women a glucose drink or injection and no similar increase occurred if women were not fed or given glucose during the day (10). The increase in fetal breathing movements between 0200–0700 h while mothers sleep seems to reflect a circadian rhythm in fetal breathing movements. In women receiving exogenous glucocorticoid and in whom the circadian rhythm in cortisol was depressed or absent, no similar increase in fetal breathing movement occurs overnight (11).

There is evidence of maturation in control of patterns of fetal breathing movements during pregnancy. Recent reports of studies of human fetuses under

20 weeks gestational age have suggested that breathing movements occur either as isolated breaths or groups of breaths which last a few seconds. Trudinger and Knight studied 8 patients serially from 20 weeks' gestational age and reported that at 20 and 24 weeks fetal breathing movements occurred in rapid isolated births of 4–10 breaths (12). By 28–30 weeks, fetal breathing movements began to occur in episodes. Furthermore, the rate of fetal breathing movements decreased during the last 10 weeks of pregnancy from 58 breaths/min at 30–31 weeks to 47 breaths/min at 38–39 weeks and the distribution of breath intervals was broader at 30–31 than at 38–39 weeks (9). Therefore, fetal breathing movements, when present, are more regular in older fetuses.

Carbon Dioxide and Oxygen

Few studies on the influence of increased concentrations of CO_2 in fetal breathing movements have been conducted during human pregnancy. Ritchie and Lakhani (13) administered 5% CO_2 in air to pregnant women for 15 min and measured a threefold increase in the incidence of fetal breathing movements in uncomplicated pregnancies. Similar observations were made by Van Weering et al. (14) who used a 10% mixture of CO_2 for 5 min intervals and noted that the incidence of fetal breathing movements usually increased. They reported that, in some fetuses which were small for gestational age, no similar response was observed to this stimulus. Richardson et al. (15) studied the effect of administering 4% CO_2 in air to healthy pregnant women over 15 min observation intervals at 30, 34 and 38 weeks' gestational age. They reported a significant increase in the incidence of fetal breathing movements at all 3 gestational ages after administration of CO_2 but the increase was significantly greater in fetuses at 34 and 38 weeks compared to the same fetuses at 30 weeks. They concluded that a maturational change in the sensitivity of the fetal respiratory centre to CO_2 may occur during the last 10 weeks of pregnancy.

Marsal et al. (16) demonstrated that maternal hyperventilation during human pregnancy sufficient to reduce maternal arterial P_{CO_2}, results in a reduction in the incidence of fetal breathing movements.

Investigators found no change in the incidence of fetal breathing movements in healthy fetuses whose mothers were given 50% O_2 by mask (17,18). Ritchie and Lakhani (17) reported that, in mothers with small for gestational age fetuses, the incidence of fetal breathing movements was not significantly different from normal but increased dramatically during maternal oxygen administration.

No controlled human studies can be ethically conducted to examine the effects of hypoxia. However, Manning and Platt (19) reported that fetal breathing movements were observed in a woman suffering from homozygous haemoglobin S disease and in whom two episodes of sickle cell crises occurred. They observed fetal breathing movements 23–80% of the time when maternal PO_2 was greater than 60 mmHg, but during the two episodes of crises when maternal PO_2 fell to 40 mmHg, no fetal breathing movements were observed. This experiment of nature suggested that acute hypoxia during human pregnancy results in absence of fetal breathing movements which had been reported in experimentally induced hypoxia in sheep (3).

In fetal lambs, asphyxia results in the appearance of abnormal gasping patterns. Anecdotal reports suggest that human fetuses make gasping movements prior to death *in utero*. Clinically, one characteristic of the asphyxiated human fetus is the presence of meconium which has been inhaled deeply into the air way before death. Manning *et al.* (20) reported that when real-time ultrasonic observations were made on dying fetal rhesus monkeys, gasping activity could not be differentiated from normal breathing movements despite repeated detailed video analysis. Direct recordings with newer ultrasonic tracking devices may provide an opportunity for examining the structure of fetal gasping movements in the dying human fetus. However, no comprehensive investigation of these phenomena can be expected from clinical investigators.

Cigarette Smoking and Drugs

It has been demonstrated that cigarette smoking results in a decreased incidence of fetal breathing movements for about 1 h (21). Recent studies have demonstrated that fetal breathing movements are virtually abolished for up to 3.5 h after maternal ingestion of ethanol (0.25 g/kg) (22).

Preliminary reports on small numbers of patients have appeared concerning the effects of meperidine, diazepam, amylobarbital, salbutamol, terbutaline, methyldopa and caffeine on human fetal breathing movements and were reviewed by Lewis and Boylan (23).

Richardson *et al.* (24) reported that fetuses of mothers taking methadone had a diminished response to CO_2 both before or after maternal methadone ingestion. The incidence of fetal breathing movements, in women taking methadone, was decreased in relationship to maternal end tidal PCO_2 when compared to normal controls.

Parturition and Prostaglandins

During human (Fig. 2) (25) and sheep pregnancy (5), the incidence of fetal breathing movements decreases during the last 3 days before spontaneous parturition at term. In both species there is strong evidence that fetal breathing movements are virtually abolished during active labour at term (Fig. 3) (26).

It has been demonstrated, in sheep, that infusions of prostaglandin synthetase inhibitors into the fetal lamb results in a dramatic increase in fetal breathing activity during the first 12 h following infusion (27). Conversely, Kitterman *et al.* (28) reported a significant decrease in the incidence of fetal breathing movements following infusion of prostaglandin E_2 intravenously into healthy fetal lambs. They reported that similar intravenous infusions of prostaglandin $F_{2\alpha}$ caused slightly diminished fetal breathing activity and that no change in fetal breathing activity occurred following infusions of endoperoxides. It has been suggested that the decrease in fetal breathing activity normally observed just before and during active labour in sheep, rhesus monkeys and humans may be due to

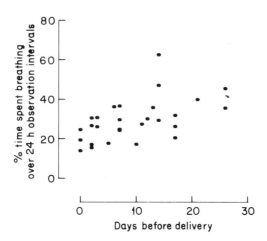

Figure 2. Incidence of human fetal breathing movements over 24 h observation intervals was plotted in relationship to days before delivery at term and demonstrated a decrease in breathing activity during the last few days before parturition (from Ref. 25).

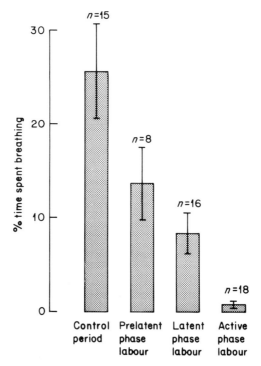

Figure 3. Mean percentage time spent breathing (±SEM) during a control period, prelatent-phase labour, latent-phase labour and active-phase labour in women being electively induced at term (from Ref. 26).

an increase in fetal prostaglandin E_2 concentrations. It has been demonstrated that prostaglandin E concentrations increase in amniotic fluid during active labour in humans (29). In sheep, a model for preterm parturition was developed using fetal intravenous injections of adrenocorticotrophic hormone (ACTH) over 100 h starting at day 127 (term = 147 days in sheep) (30). In this study, fetal carotid arterial prostaglandin E_2 concentrations rose to a peak during the last 8 h before the onset of labour. The incidence of fetal breathing movements was not influenced by ACTH infusions but fell during the last 12 h before the onset of labour from 33 to 15%. The incidence of fetal breathing movements was inverse to fetal arterial prostaglandin E_2 concentrations which further suggested a role for prostaglandin E_2 in the control of fetal breathing activity.

Preterm Labour

In humans, Castle and Turnbull (31) recently measured fetal breathing movements over short observation intervals in women in preterm labour. Unfortunately some of the patients received tocolytic drugs, some both tocolytic and glucocorticoid drugs and others no treatment. It appeared that the absence of fetal breathing movements predicted fetuses that would actually deliver when women presented in preterm labour, whereas the presence of fetal breathing movements in women with similar symptoms was a predictor that fetuses would not deliver within 48 h of testing. If this observation is valid, it will be possible to select out those patients that would actually benefit from tocolytic and steroid medications from those who would not deliver in any case and therefore not require exposure to potentially harmful drugs. However, fetal breathing movements occur episodically about 30% of the time in human fetuses and do not completely arrest until active labour (25,26,30) when treatment would not be effective or appropriate. We recently observed fetal breathing movements in 7 women presenting with signs of preterm labour and measured breathing activity 15% of the time over 2 h observation intervals in 3 women who delivered within 12 h of study. These data suggest that, although the incidence of fetal breathing movements is decreased prior to spontaneous labour at term in women, the movements do persist. As a result, some caution needs to be raised regarding the prediction of preterm delivery when clinical observations are made over short intervals.

Clinical Use of Fetal Breathing Movements

In experiments on sheep, isocapnic hypoxia resulted in arrest of fetal breathing movements (3) and asphyxia resulted in appearance of abnormal gasping movements (4). Clinicians hoped these observations might prove useful in assessment of human fetal health. Preliminary reports by Boddy (32), in a study of 800 pregnancies, suggested the incidence of fetal breathing movements was decreased in growth-retarded fetuses and fetuses that developed distress in labour. However, Marsal (33) examined fetal breathing movements in 100 consecutive pregnancies and, while he did measure a decreased incidence of fetal breathing movements in complicated pregnancies, he reported no correlation between the incidence of fetal breathing movements and the subsequent course and outcome of pregnancies. Other investigators reported similar observations. It was soon apparent that clinical measurement of fetal breathing movements for assessing health was disappointing. The presence of fetal breathing movements was reassuring at the time of the test but did not predict outcome in labour or at delivery. Furthermore, the absence of fetal breathing movements over short (usually 30 min) observation intervals was usually a poor predictor of fetal outcome, because few of these fetuses showed any signs of hypoxia at birth.

In retrospect it is not difficult to understand the problem clinicians faced in attempting to use fetal breathing movements as a sign of health in high risk pregnancies. Fetal breathing movements are episodic and normally influenced by many variables. Even in chronic fetal lamb preparations, it is not possible to assess health over short observation intervals. In normal human fetuses, apnoea for up to 120 min is not unusual and as a result observation intervals of less than 2 h would occasionally result in a diagnosis of fetal apnoea which is a part of the normal periodicity of breathing activity and not a reflection of fetal ill health (Fig. 1).

Fetal breathing movements are significantly reduced during hypoxaemia in sheep and should be a good indicator of fetal hypoxia in humans. Unfortunately, it is often not clinically practical to make observations of 2–4 h to be sure fetuses are in fact apnoeic due to hypoxaemia and not to a physiologic period of apnoea. Furthermore, little is known regarding events leading up to death or asphyxial damage during human pregnancy. It is not clear that human fetuses experience prolonged periods of hypoxia before death. One exception is the intra-uterine growth-retarded fetus which may experience prolonged hypoxaemia prior to death. Indeed, Trudinger et al. (34) reported that in growth-retarded fetuses the incidence of fetal breathing movements was usually less than in normal fetuses. However, there was a significant overlap between the incidence of fetal breathing movements in growth-retarded and in normal fetuses. Using a fetal sheep model of growth retardation, Worthington et al. (35) demonstrated that the incidence of fetal breathing movements over 24 h intervals was about one-half that of normal controls. However, it is impractical to make such prolonged observations in the clinical setting.

A review of clinical reports suggest that the presence of fetal breathing movements is an indicator of health at the time of the test but use of the absence of fetal breathing movements has been disappointing as an indicator of fetal ill health. Further, some fetuses with normal patterns of breathing movements may subsequently have poor outcomes despite testing. It will be important for clinicians to examine the natural patterns of breathing movements leading up to death or damage in pregnancies. At the present time little is known about patterns of breathing activity preceding human fetal death in utero.

Human Fetal Body Movements

Fetal body movements were first comprehensively studied in humans using the real-time scanner or strain gauges placed on the maternal abdominal wall. Initially, investigators studying fetal breathing movements were annoyed by gross fetal body movements as they interrupted the observation of breathing movements and caused repositioning of ultrasound transducers. However, it soon became apparent that body movements were different from breathing movements in pattern and distribution.

Gross fetal body movements occur about 10% of the time during the last third of pregnancy, when measured with real-time scanners (36). Fetuses make 20–50 gross fetal body movements/h. Body movements are episodic and may be absent for up to 75 min in healthy fetuses during the last 10 weeks of pregnancy (Fig. 4). Gross fetal body movements are not influenced by maternal plasma glucose concentrations or maternal meals. Recent studies demonstrated that gross fetal body movements, unlike fetal breathing movements, do not diminish during the last 3 days prior to spontaneous labour at term (25). Furthermore, Richardson

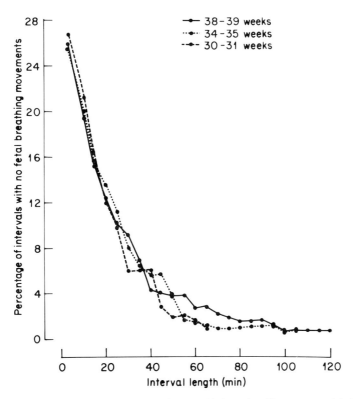

Figure 4. Composite plot of the percentage of intervals with no gross fetal body movements in 9 fetuses at 30–31 weeks, 11 at 34–35 weeks and 11 at 38–39 weeks, demonstrating a similar distribution at the different gestational ages. The longest period of fetal rest was 60 min at 30–31 weeks, 75 min at 34–35 weeks and 50 min at 38–39 weeks in fetuses observed continuously over 24 h observation intervals (from Ref. 36).

et al. (26) demonstrated that gross fetal body movements diminish only slightly during electively induced labour at term.

It is clear that accelerations, which appear in the fetal heart rate during the last 10 weeks of pregnancy, coincide with gross fetal body movements. Timor-Tritsch *et al.* (37) reported that when fetuses, near term, move for 3 s or more, accelerations are always present in the fetal heart rate recording.

Studies of Fetal Body Movements in Sheep

There are few studies of fetal body movements using chronic fetal lamb preparations. Movements of the fetal head and limbs occur during both quiet and active sleep in chronic fetal lamb preparations and complex fetal movements such as combined movements of the neck, limb and trunk occur 300–600 times/day (38). This type of activity appears to occur in episodes especially during quiet sleep. Natale *et al.* (39) measured fetal forelimb movements in chronic fetal lambs before or after isocapnic hypoxia and reported that these movements are almost completely abolished during fetal hypoxaemia. Recent reports have indicated that fetal body movements in lambs usually coincide with heart rate accelerations.

Clinical Use of Fetal Body Movements

Human fetal body movements have been suggested as a method of evaluating fetal well-being (40,41). It has been suggested that, if women report less than 4–10 fetal movements in a 12 h period, fetuses may be in jeopardy. These findings need further confirmation, as all reports are not in agreement (42). Maternal reports of fetal body movements are a noninvasive method of measuring fetal activity but women may not be aware of all fetal activity. When maternal subjective awareness is compared with ultrasonic real-time scanning at 32–34 weeks it was reported that one-third of women did not perceive movements observed by ultrasound (43). Some women report movements that are actually Braxton-Hicks contractions and some sense movements that are due to maternal aortic pulsation and respiration. Indeed, Hertogs *et al.* (43) reported that 1 woman, with an intra-uterine fetal death, reported fetal activity. It appears that most women can sense gross fetal body movements and report them consistently, but some are inconsistent in their reports and may even be unaware of most fetal activity.

Measurement of fetal body movements is also complicated by the fact that fetuses may spend prolonged periods of time at rest. Under normal conditions, newborns sleep approximately 90% of the time. Two states of sleep in newborns have been described using direct measurements. Quiet sleep is characterized by low frequency, high voltage electro-encephalogram (EEG), tonic activity of muscles, absence of gross movements, lack of variability in heart rate and respiratory rate patterns. Active sleep (rapid eye movement sleep) is characterized by high frequency, low voltage EEG, gross movements of one limb or generalized body movements as well as irregular heart rate and respiratory rate patterns. Active sleep in newborns occurs roughly 20–60 min out of every 90 min. It is tempting to speculate that human fetuses may have similar patterns of sleep prior to birth.

During human labour, Rosen *et al.* (14) recorded EEG patterns in fetuses that resemble patterns seen during quiet sleep, active sleep and awake state in newborns.

We measured fetal body movements with a real-time scanner continuously over 24 h observation intervals and, after observing periods of rest and activity in these measurements, attempted to develop mathematical models which might be used to predict patterns of movement and rest in healthy fetuses. We used the Box-Jenkins modelling system and reported that gross body movements were pseudoperiodic in occurrence and best represented by a first-order auto-regression with an iterative moving average system with a formula which represented most of the variability in the measurement (45). The mathematical model scientifically expressed the variability of movement patterns in human fetuses but did not help the clinician because it cannot predict when the next movement episode would be.

It has been suggested that stimuli such as sound, light and physical stimulation be used to alter periods of fetal rest during human pregnancy. However, there is no evidence that any external stimulus can alter prolonged periods of fetal rest. Controlled experiments in sheep demonstrated that fetuses do not move when hypoxaemic (39) but healthy human fetuses may remain at rest for periods of up to 75 min (36).

An easier way to describe patterns of fetal activity during the last 10 weeks of pregnancy is illustrated in Fig. 4. These data represent 744 h of recording time in 31 fetuses (36). The plots represent 5 min intervals and multiples of 5 min intervals during which time no gross fetal body movements occurred. It can be seen that about 75% of the time fetuses move in any 5 min interval but some healthy fetuses were at rest for long periods up to 75 min.

The clinical dilemma is how to separate human fetuses who are normal, but at rest, from fetuses that are not moving because of hypoxaemia and/or asphyxia. As was mentioned above, little is known regarding events leading up to death or asphyxial damage during human pregnancy. Absence of gross body movements over a 2 h interval, as indicated by absence of accelerations in fetal heart rate tracings, has been reported as a good sign of fetal ill health (46). However, absence of gross fetal body movements over short observation intervals could be expected to be a poor indicator of fetal outcome as it would be impossible to determine whether the fetus was not moving because it was hypoxaemic or because it was experiencing a normal period of fetal rest.

Combination of Fetal Breathing and Body Movements as a Sign of Health

Manning *et al.* (47) suggested that a combination of tests of fetal activity might be superior to single tests of fetal breathing, body movements or heart rate. Fetal breathing, gross fetal body movements, tone, fetal heart rate and qualitative amniotic fluid volume were measured as an index of fetal health in 216 high risk pregnancies. Fetal outcome was assessed by a 5 min apgar score, fetal distress in labour and perinatal mortality. They reported that, for any single measurement, the positive predictive value was low. However, the combination of all 5 tests, using a scoring system, resulted in high positive and negative predictive values for fetal outcome. Manning *et al.* (48) subsequently reported a prospective study of outcome in 1184 high-risk patients, using the 5 measurements, which suggested that a significant reduction in perinatal mortality coincided with the use of the test. However, while these preliminary results are impressive, the test requires expensive equipment and skilled operators. Further, it is not yet clear what contribution is made to fetal outcome by exposure of high-risk patients to careful reassessment by a skilled team of clinicians and nurses, despite fetal testing. Manning *et al.* (48) also noted that ultrasound screening of high-risk patients resulted in *antepartum* recognition of most major fetal anomalies which is clinically important in the management of women during labour.

Clinical Dilemmas

Periodicity of fetal movements is a characteristic of health. The presence of movements is reassuring but absence of fetal breathing for up to 2 h and body movements for up to 80 min is not unusual in healthy fetuses. Fetal animal studies and clinical observations in humans demonstrate that hypoxaemia is associated with absence of fetal breathing and body movements. The clinical dilemma is how to separate human fetuses that are normal, but at rest, from fetuses that are not moving because of hypoxaemia and/or asphyxia. It is now clear that, during the last third of human pregnancy, clinical studies need to account for the normal periods of fetal apnoea and rest by using flexible testing intervals. Fetal breathing and gross body movements cannot be considered absent unless tests have been conducted continuously for at least 2 h. Conversely, if clinicians are reassured by the presence of these activities, most tests would be complete within 10 min. Published data demonstrate that few normal fetuses would be apnoeic or inactive for a full 2 h. The false positive rate for diagnosis of fetal hypoxia would be greatly reduced if recording intervals of human tests were made more flexible. The fact remains that, even in high risk pregnancies, there are very few hypoxic fetuses.

A second dilemma is that tests of fetal breathing, gross fetal body movements and heart rate are reflections of health at the time of the test. There is no evidence that normal fetal activity can predict subsequent health or outcome. Practising clinicians are often unaware of this fact and may be falsely reassured by a normal test. Clinical investigators should make it clear, to practising physicians, that tests of fetal activity are not a replacement for good clinical judgment.

The most serious clinical dilemma is that, at present, there is no good evidence that human fetuses are hypoxaemic for prolonged periods of time before death. In most clinical studies, the interval between oxygen delivery sufficient to sustain both normal fetal breathing and body movements and severe hypoxaemia or death may be very short. Indeed, "true positive" tests of fetal activity in the literature are usually reported in severely growth-retarded fetuses, extreme postmaturity or prolonged rupture of membranes. Finally, our experience with tests of fetal activity in assessment of health (46) suggests there may be no significant interval of transition between the presence of normal fetal activity and the absence of activity. If there is a grey area, it must be very short. There is a real need for longitudinal documentation of activity in fetuses at risk of hypoxia in pregnancy complications which predispose to intra-uterine asphyxia or death. It is surprising such data are not available, given the widespread use of fetal testing.

The last 10 years were a time of rapid development of noninvasive technology. It is unfortunate that much of the technology has been immediately used in clinical management. Indeed, in some countries, it is difficult to obtain ethical permission to conduct controlled studies of the human physiology of new high tech measurements. Frequently, the only human data available are from measurements made of experiments of nature in uncontrolled settings. In future, parallel studies using noninvasive measurements of controlled human observations and invasive measurements in fetal animals should be encouraged. Clinical strategies could be suggested from these studies but application of new technology should await evaluation by controlled clinical trials.

Acknowledgements

We wish to thank Misses Lesley Carmichael and Carol Probert for their interest in this work and Mrs T. Clarke for her excellent secretarial assistance.

This work was supported by the Canadian Medical Research Council. B.R. is a Canadian MRC Scholar.

References

1. Dawes, G. S., Fox, H. E., Leduc, B. M., Liggins, G. C. and Richards, R. T. (1972). *J. Physiol.* **220**, 119–143.
2. Boddy, K., Dawes, G. S. and Robinson, J. S. (1973). *In:* "Foetal and Neonatal Physiology, Sir J. Barcroft Centenary Symposium", (Comline, R. S., Cross, K. W., Dawes, G. S. and Nathanielsz, P. W., eds) pp. 63–66. Cambridge University Press, Cambridge.
3. Boddy, K., Dawes, G. S., Fisher, R. L., Pinter, S. and Robinson, J. S. (1974). *J. Physiol.* **243**, 599–618.
4. Patrick, J. E., Dalton, K. J. and Dawes, G. S. (1976). *Am. J. Obstet. Gynecol.* **125**, 73–78.
5. Boddy, K. and Dawes, G. S. (1975). *Br. Med. Bull.* **31**, 3–7.
6. Boddy, K. and Robinson, J. S. (1971). *Lancet* **ii**, 1231–1233.
7. Patrick, J., Natale, R. and Richardson, B. (1978). *Am. J. Obstet. Gynecol.* **132**, 507–513.
8. Patrick, J., Campbell, K., Carmichael, L., Natale, R. and Richardson, B. (1980). *Obstet. Gynecol.* **56**, 24–30.
9. Patrick, J., Campbell, K., Carmichael, L., Natale, R. and Richardson, B. (1980). *Am. J. Obstet. Gynecol.* **136**, 471–477.
10. Natale, R., Patrick, J. and Richardson, B. (1978). *Am. J. Obstet. Gynecol.* **132**, 36–41.
11. Patrick, J., Challis, J., Campbell, K., Carmichael, L., Richardson, B. and Tevaarwerk, G. (1981). *Am. J. Obstet. Gynecol.* **139**, 324–328.
12. Trudinger, B. J. and Knight, P. C. (1980). *Am. J. Obstet. Gynecol.* **137**, 724–728.
13. Ritchie, J. W. K. and Lakhani, K. (1980). *Am. J. Obstet. Gynecol.* **136**, 386–388.
14. Van Weering, H. K., Wladimiroff, J. W., Roodenburg, P. J. (1978). *In:* "Proceedings of the Fifth Conference on Fetal Breathing", (Eskes, T. J. B. and DeHaan, J., eds) p. 62. University of Nijmegen, Nijmegen.

15. Richardson, B. S., O'Grady, J. P. and Johnson, K. (1982). Society of Gynecological Investigation, Dallas, Abstract 11.
16. Marsal, K., Gennser, G. and Lofgren, O. (1979). *Acta Obstet. Gynecol. Scand.* **58**, 335-342.
17. Ritchie, J. W. K. and Lakhani, K. (1980). *Br. J. Obstet. Gynaec.* **87**, 1084-1086.
18. Devoe, L. D., Abduljabbar, H., Carmichael, L., Probert, C. and Patrick, J. (1984). *Am. J. Obstet. Gynecol.* **148**, 790-794.
19. Manning, F. A. and Platt, L. D. (1979). *Obstet. Gynecol.* **53**, 758-760.
20. Manning, F. A., Martin, C. B., Murata, Y., Miyaki, K. and Danzler, G. (1979). *Am. J. Obstet. Gynecol.* **135**, 71-76.
21. Manning, F. A., Wyn Pugh, E. and Boddy, K. (1975). *Br. Med. J.* **1**, 552-553.
22. McLeod, W., Brien, J., Loomis, C., Carmichael, L., Probert, C. and Patrick, J. (1983). *Am. J. Obstet. Gynecol.* **145**, 251-257.
23. Lewis, P. and Bovlan, P. (1979). *Am. J. Obstet. Gynecol.* **134**, 587-598.
24. Richardson, B. S., O'Grady, J. P. and Olsen, G. D. (1984). *Am. J. Obstet. Gynecol.* **150**, 400-405.
25. Carmichael, L., Campbell, K. and Patrick, J. (1984). *Am. J. Obstet. Gynecol.* **148**, 675-679.
26. Richardson, B., Natale, R. and Patrick, J. (1979). *Am. J. Obstet. Gynecol.* **133**, 247-255.
27. Kitterman, J. A., Liggins, G. C., Clements, J. A. and Tooley, W. H. (1979). *J. Develop. Physiol.* **1**, 453-466.
28. Kitterman, J. A., Liggins, G. C., Fewell, J. E. and Tooley, W. H. (1983). *J. Appl. Physiol.* **54**, 687-692.
29. Keirse, M. J. N. C. and Turnbull, A. C. (1973). *J. Obstet. Gynaecol. Brit. Commonwealth* **80**, 970-973.
30. Patrick, J., Challis, J., Olson, D. and Lye, S. (1985). In preparation.
31. Castle, B. M. and Turnbull, A. C. (1983). *Lancet* **2**(1), 471-472.
32. Boddy, K. (1976). *In:* "Fetal Physiology and Medicine", (Beard, R. W. and Nathanielsz, P. W., eds) pp. 302-328. W. B. Saunders, London.
33. Marsal, K. (1978). *Obstet. Gynecol.* **52**, 394-401.
34. Trudinger, B. J., Lewis, P. J. and Pettit, B. (1979). *Br. J. Obstet. Gynaec.* **86**, 432-436.
35. Worthington, D., Piercy, W. N. and Smith, B. T. (1981). *Obstet. Gynecol.* **58**, 215-221.
36. Patrick, J., Campbell, K., Carmichael, L., Natale, R. and Richardson, B. (1982). *Am. J. Obstet. Gynecol.* **142**, 363-371.
37. Timor-Tritsch, I. E., Dierker, L. J., Zador, I., Hertz, R. H. and Rosen, M. G. (1978). *Am. J. Obstet. Gynecol.* **131**, 276-280.
38. Ruckebusch, Y., Gaujoux, M. and Eghbali, B. (1977). *Electroencephalogr. Clin. Neurophysiol.* **42**, 226-237.
39. Natale, R., Clewlow, F. and Dawes, G. S. (1981). *Am. J. Obstet. Gynecol.* **140**, 545-551.
40. Pearson, J. F. and Weaver, J. B. (1976). *Br. Med. J.* **1**, 1305-1307.
41. Sadovsky, E. and Polishuk, W. Z. (1977). *Obstet. Gynecol.* **50**, 49-55.
42. Mathews, D. D. (1978). *Obstet. Gynecol.* **51**, 281-283.
43. Hertogs, K., Roberts, A. B., Cooper, D. and Campbell, S. (1979). *Br. Med. J.* **2**, 1183-1185.
44. Rosen, M. G., Scibetta, J. J., Chik, L. and Borgstedt, A. D. (1973). *Am. J. Obstet. Gynecol.* **115**, 37-47.
45. Campbell, K., MacNeill, I. and Patrick, J. (1981). *Ultrasonic Imaging* **3**, 330-341.
46. Brown, R. and Patrick, J. (1981). *Am. J. Obstet. Gynecol.* **141**, 646-651.
47. Manning, F. A., Platt, L. D. and Sipos, L. (1980). *Am. J. Obstet. Gynecol.* **136**, 787-795.
48. Manning, F. A., Baskett, T. F., Morrison, I. and Lange, I. (1981). *Am. J. Obstet. Gynecol.* **140**, 289-294.

Ultrasound and the Analysis of Fetal Growth

J. S. Robinson

Faculty of Medicine, University of Newcastle,
New South Wales, Australia

Ultrasound has been used in obstetrics for more than 25 years (15). The range of measurements that can now be made has increased considerably in parallel with the improvement of the instruments available. The measurements of size have been correlated with fetal age, and in women in whom there is doubt about the duration of pregnancy, estimation of age has been a standard procedure in many institutions for more than a decade. Initially, the biparietal diameter was utilized (5) but more recently it has been suggested that other variables such as femur length may be more accurate (59). The biparietal diameter, together with abdominal circumference, has also been utilized to provide a reasonable estimate of fetal weight (57). These estimates of fetal weight, particularly before 34 weeks, now assist in the decision of when, where and how to deliver the at-risk fetus.

The rapid changes in the ability of ultrasonographers to identify abnormal growth of the fetus has posed new dilemmas in obstetrics. Identification of problems such as urinary tract abnormalities (28) or hydrocephalus (2) has led these authors to attempt fetal surgical procedures but others have taken a more cautious view of these interventions (42).

The purpose of this brief review is to describe the growth of the fetus and its analysis by ultrasound. Since improvement in ultrasound techniques allows prenatal identification of problems previously more in the realm of paediatrics, attention will be given to some of these "new" problems.

Early Pregnancy

In early pregnancy the growth of the conceptus was first assessed by measurement of the gestational sac. Various measurements (diameters, circumference and calculated volume) have been related to gestational age but the main value of

The Physiological Development of the Fetus and Newborn
ISBN 0 12 389080 2

Copyright © 1985 by Academic Press, London.
All rights of reproduction in any form reserved.

these measurements lies in the assessment of viability of the conceptus (40). The yolk sac has also been identified (41) and reaches a maximum diameter of 7 mm (11). The latter report suggested that abnormalities of yolk sac development might provide an early indicator of subsequent fetal death.

Crown–rump length is used to assess fetal size in the first trimester in order to determine fetal age. The mean crown–rump length at 6.5 weeks was 5 mm, increasing to 18 mm at 18.5 weeks (50). A curvilinear of parabolic relationship between crown–rump length and gestational age has been described (16,51). Although using this, Robinson (50) was able to calculate gestational age with considerable accuracy, Nelson (45) found that a significant proportion of measurements are outside the 95% confidence limits derived by Robinson and Fleming (51). The prediction of the date of delivery using crown–rump length is similar to that using biparietal diameter in the second trimester of pregnancy (39).

Cephalometry

The most widely used measurement to assess fetal growth is cephalometry. Measurement of the biparietal diameter was chosen, since this can be recognized easily and the relationship between the biparietal diameter and fetal age has been the subject of numerous investigations (see 14,52). Separate curves have been established for males and females and the curve for males was consistently above that for females from the 20th week of pregnancy (48). These separate curves should now be used antenatally when fetal sex has been determined ultrasonically or by other means. Sabbagha et al. (54) observed that the majority (90%) of fetuses maintain the same biparietal diameter percentile rank from midpregnancy onwards. Thus, the growth potential for a particular fetus can be determined and if the biparietal diameter falls from above 80th to the 30th centile then the risk of intra-uterine growth retardation increases sixfold to 20% (53). Persson et al. (49) suggested that heavy infants exhibit a continuously fast growth rate, whereas the deviation of the curve for the light infants occurred later in pregnancy and that this can be accounted for by increasing effects of environmental influences. For example, they found that increase of the biparietal diameter with age was significantly delayed in fetuses of smoking mothers, both light (1–10 cigarettes/day) and heavy smokers (>10 cigarettes/day) (49).

The growth rate of the biparietal diameter of the second twin lags behind that of the first twin (the twin presenting to the pelvis) and after 32 weeks the growth of both twins is retarded compared to singletons (25). Discrepancy and divergence of the biparietal diameters is associated with a high incidence of growth retardation of one or both twins.

Campbell (4) defined two patterns of abnormal fetal growth, late flattening and low profile. Follow-up studies of children, divided into groups according to the time of onset of growth retardation, have been provided (17,29). Growth failure before 26 weeks of gestation was associated with a lower general cognitive index on McCarthy scales, principally due to perceptual-performance and motor deficits.

The occipito–frontal diameter has been the subject of fewer studies than the biparietal diameter. Perhaps the most interesting suggesting was that the ratio of the occipito–frontal to biparietal diameter would identify fetuses with Down's syndrome (3). Later studies have failed to confirm this but it would be of interest to know what proportion of children with brachycephaly have Down's syndrome and how this compares with the incidence of this syndrome with increasing maternal age.

Intracranial anatomy can be defined using ultrasound and growth curves for ventricular size have been published which include identity of different parts of the lateral ventricles (12,33). The accuracy of the diagnosis of fetal hydrocephalus has been assessed by Chervenak *et al.* (8) who described 30 fetuses with hydrocephalus. While it was possible to determine the severity of the hydrocephalus by assessment of the ratio of the width of the lateral ventricle to the width of the hemisphere in the majority, identification of other anomalies was not as successful. Isolated hydrocephalus without other anomalies was only present in 4 of the 30 cases. One false negative evaluation occurred in a patient with a family history of X-linked aqueductal stenosis who was examined at 20 and 24 weeks of gestation. Similar false negative assessments have been made at 24 and 30 weeks in a woman with a history of X-linked hydrocephalus yet significant hydrocephalus was present by 34 weeks (J. S. Robinson, unpublished observation).

The high incidence of associated anomalies suggests that fetal surgery either by cephalocentesis (2) or by insertion of a ventriculo-amniotic shunt (9) will only be worthwhile in carefully selected cases, e.g. early onset of sex-linked hydrocephalus.

Estimation of Fetal Weight

Although measurements of the biparietal diameter accurately describe the growth of the fetal head, the correlation of these measurements with birthweight is not sufficiently close to allow prediction of birthweight accurate enough for clinical purposes. Estimation of fetal weight from abdominal circumference alone or with the biparietal diameter provides a more accurate prediction (6,27,30). Warsof and his colleagues (57) tested a number of empirically derived equations and demonstrated that birthweight (BW) was predicted most accurately using a logarithmic function of abdominal circumference (AC) and biparietal diameter (BPD)

$$(\log_{10}(BW) = -1.599 + 0.144(BPD) + 0.032(AC) - 0.111(BPD^2 \times AC)/1000).$$

The standard deviation of this regression was 106 g/kg fetal weight. The accuracy of the equation for fetal weight production was found to be greater for preterm infants whose birthweights were between 500 and 1500 g. The mean error of the estimated fetal weight was -15.1 ± 71.5 g, $n = 50$ and the absolute error was 52.3 ± 48.5 g with a correlation coefficient for the regression line of estimated weight on birthweight of 0.98 (37). These authors suggested that this technique is one that can be used by obstetricians with basic real-time ultrasound skills. Results of other evaluations have supported these conclusions (13,18).

Warsof *et al.* (57) provided reference tables to avoid the need for calculation of weight.

Intra-uterine growth retardation has proved difficult to diagnose accurately by clinical methods such as abdominal palpation but may be identified more accurately by measurement of symphysial–fundal height (55). Two stage ultrasound has proved even more accurate, the initial ultrasound examination early in the mid-trimester being used to confirm the gestational age and to exclude anomalies. The second examination was conducted early in the third trimester. Measurement of biparietal diameter and abdominal circumference or trunk area plus or minus estimation of crown–rump length have enabled up to 94% of growth-retarded fetuses to be detected. The false-positive rate of 12% must not be ignored since it may lead to inappropriate intervention (44). Additional assessment of oligohydramnios, determined ultrasonically by absence of pockets of amniotic fluid of more than 1 cm in broadest diameter, will help to detect the fetuses most at risk (31). This two-stage procedure ensures that the majority of multiple pregnancies are detected early in pregnancy (25).

Renal Function

Growth of the kidneys has been followed ultrasonically by measurement of the anteroposterior dimension and the length of the kidney (1,32). Unlike the increase in the biparietal diameter, the kidney dimensions increase in a curvilinear fashion but without slowing of growth late in gestation. Production of urine by the fetus has been estimated by measuring the fetal bladder in three planes. First, the largest outline of the bladder was measured, then the two measurements of the largest transverse diameters. Volume of the bladder was then determined from the formula

$$\frac{4}{3}\pi \times \frac{\text{diameter}}{2} \times \frac{\text{diameter t1}}{2} \times \frac{\text{diameter t2}}{2}.$$

Campbell *et al.* (7) validated this method by scanning the bladder of a stillborn infant in the tank of water. Changes in the fetal bladder volume were used to calculate the hourly fetal urine production rate. Urine production increased from 12.2 ml/h at 32 weeks to 28.2 ml/h at 40 weeks. We have measured hourly fetal urine production rates from 19–32 weeks. The volume produced increased from 1.6 to 16.2 ml/h at 33 weeks (43). Reduced urine production was found in complicated pregnancies and there was a highly significant increase in the number of growth-retarded infants in this group of fetuses with low urine output (58). Polyhydramnios associated with poorly controlled maternal diabetes was associated with normal or reduced urine flow (56).

In contrast, significant renal anomalies are more likely to be detected by changes in bladder size. Enlargement of the bladder is associated with urethral valves, urethral atresia, meatal stenosis and the prune belly syndrome. When the bladder is not visualized, despite prolonged and repeated observation, then renal agenesis or dysplasia needs to be excluded. Enlargement of the kidneys, unilaterally or bilaterally is associated with multicystic kidneys and vesico-ureteric reflux. On a few occasions, Beckwith syndrome with enlarged kidneys, or renal tumours, have been detected ultrasonically (20,42). Severe oligohydramnios with dysplastic kidneys was not associated with surviving fetuses, with death usually occurring from respiratory failure due to pulmonary hypoplasia. Confusion can result if absence of renal function due to urethral obstruction occurs in association with oesophageal atresia when oligohydramnios is not severe, as we observed in the VATER syndrome (Robinson, unpublished observation).

Reduction in renal function may be unilateral or bilateral and, in the former, no case can be made for intervention (26). In the latter, intervention has been undertaken. Harrison *et al.* (28) performed bilateral ureterostomy at 21 weeks. Although distension of the urinary tract was reduced and pregnancy continued until 35 weeks, the infant died from pulmonary hypoplasia. Catheter drainage to the exterior for 13 days was undertaken by McFayden *et al.* (42). An epidural catheter was inserted into the right renal pelvis and urine drained freely for 9 days but then the catheter blocked. It was cleared by flushing, but, despite continued drainage, the right hydronephrosis worsened. The child was found after delivery to have posterior urethral valves which were resected endoscopically. In a second case, the distended fetal bladder was emptied but the catheter was removed later when micturition was observed. This child subsequently died from respiratory distress at 35 weeks. McFayden and his colleagues (42) concluded that too interventionist an approach is restricted by frequent failure, to demonstrate that drainage has improved renal function and that obstruction appearing before 20 weeks is associated with irreversible lung hypoplasia and these fetuses will not survive.

Femur Length

As mentioned previously, the length of the fetal femur has been measured from 12 weeks of pregnancy. O'Brien and Queenan (46) found that the growth of the femur can be described by an asymptotic curve similar to that for the biparietal diameter with comparable limits of 2 SD. They suggested that it could be used to assess gestational age up to 24 weeks of pregnancy. In contrast, Yeh *et al.* (59) suggested that the increase of the length of the femur can be described accurately by a simple regression equation. Furthermore, they suggested that measurement of the length of the femur would provide a more precise index of gestational age than the biparietal diameter. Further studies are required to confirm this suggestion.

Detailed examination of the fetal limbs as a routine will result in detection of short-limbed dwarfs from time to time. Thanatophoric dwarfism, achondrogenesis, asphyxiating thoracic dystrophy or Ellis-Van-Creeld have all been detected by ultrasound in time for some pregnancies to be terminated (10,22,34,60). For each of these cases it is important to ensure that careful autopsy or examination of the newborn is made so that genetic counselling can be provided.

Placenta

No discussion on the growth of the fetus would be complete without mention of the placenta, since this organ plays a pivotal role in transport between the mother and the fetus. A series of changes in the appearance of the placenta have been found with increasing gestational age when it is examined by ultrasound (19). After 10 weeks the placenta takes on a finely granular appearance. Later the membranes becomes visible and echo-free spaces develop within the placenta and probably correspond with blood spaces. Calcification and intercotyledonary septa become visible in the succeeding weeks. These changes were comparable to those seen when the placenta was cut after delivery or when X-ray photographs were taken. A grading system from 0 to III has been devised for these changes by Grannum *et al.* (24). Fisher *et al.* (19) noted that the appearance of the placenta matured earlier when intra-uterine growth retardation was present. Early placental maturation (grade III before 34 weeks) identified a group of fetuses with a fourfold increase in growth retardation to 16% (47), whereas others found the incidence as high as 59% (36). Grade III placentas were found to be a reliable predictor of lung maturation (23), though others found this to hold only at term but not in preterm complicated pregnancies (35).

Conclusions

During the last 25 years, our knowledge of the growth of the human fetus has increased considerably. Initially, ultrasound was used to assist in the assessment of gestational age. Later, with improvement in equipment, more and more disturbances of fetal growth have been recognized. Many major anomalies can be detected in time to offer termination of pregnancy and for others fetal surgery may have a role.

Although static determinations of growth have been presented here, functional correlates of growth are beginning to play a role in the management of the at-risk fetus. The most obvious of these are heart rate and fetal activity. Micturition was mentioned earlier but, as yet, we know little about the factors controlling urine flow in the human fetus. Even less is known about placental blood flow, and after the beginnings described by Gill *et al.* (21), we can expect assessment of changes in umbilical blood flow in complicated pregnancies. Increased umbilical blood flow is associated with fetal anaemia (38). Changes in umbilical blood flow with oxygenation and nutrition are awaited with interest and the relationship of all these to placental grading may provide further and more accurate assessment of fetal growth.

Finally, it can be seen that the use of ultrasound to study fetal growth has expanded rapidly in the 25 years in which it has been used in clinical practice. New equipment and computer-assisted enhancement of images is likely to ensure that finer details of fetal anatomy will be available for scrutiny.

References

1. Bertagnoli, L., Lalalta, F., Gallicchio, R., Fantuzzi, M., Rusca, M., Zorzoli, A. and Deter, R. L. (1983). *J. Clin. Ultrasound* **11**, 349–356.
2. Birnholz, J. C. and Frigoletto, F. D. (1980). *N. Engl. J. Med.* **303**, 1021–1023.

3. Buttery, B. W. (1979). *Med. J. Aust.* **2**, 662-664.
4. Campbell, S. (1974). *In:* "Size at Birth", Ciba Foundation Symposium No. 27, pp. 275-303. Elsevier Exerpta Medica, Amsterdam.
5. Campbell, S. and Newman, G. B. (1971). *J. Obstet. Gynaecol. Brit. Commonwealth* **78**, 513-519.
6. Campbell, S. and Wilkin, D. (1975). *Br. J. Obstet. Gynaec.* **82**, 689-697.
7. Campbell, S., Wladimiroff, J. W. and Dewhurst, C. J. (1973). *J. Obstet. Gynaecol. Brit. Commonwealth* **80**, 680-686.
8. Chervenak, F. A., Berkowitz, R. L., Romero, R., Tortora, M., Mayden, K., Duncan, C., Mahoney, M. J. and Hobbins, J. C. (1983). *Am. J. Obstet. Gynecol.* **147**, 703-716.
9. Clewell, W. H., Johnson, M. L., Meier, P. R., Newkirk, J. B., Zide, S. L., Hendee, R. W., Bowes, W. A., Hecht, F., O'Keeffe, D., Henry, G. P. and Shikes, R. H. (1982). *N. Engl. J. Med.* **306**, 1320-1325.
10. Cremin, B. J. and Shaff, M. I. (1977). *Radiology* **124**, 479-480.
11. Crooij, M. J., Westhuis, M., Shoemaker, J. and Exalto, N. (1982). *Br. J. Obstet. Gynaec.* **89**, 931-934.
12. Denkhaus, H. and Winsberg, F. (1979). *Radiology* **131**, 781-787.
13. Deter, R. L., Hadlock, F. P., Harrist, R. B. and Carpenter, R. J. (1981). *J. Clin. Ultrasound* **9**, 421-425.
14. Deter, R. L., Harrist, R. B., Hadlock, F. P. and Carpenter, R. J. (1981). *J. Clin. Ultrasound* **9**, 481-493.
15. Donald, I., MacVicar, J. and Brown, T. G. (1958). *Lancet* **i**, 1188-1195.
16. Drumm, J. E., Clinch, J. and MacKenzie, G. (1976). *Br. J. Obstet. Gynaec.* **83**, 417-421.
17. Fancourt, R., Campbell, S., Harvey, D. and Norman, A. P. (1976). *Br. Med. J.* **1**, 1435-1437.
18. Finikiotis, G., MacLennan, A. H., Verco, P. W. and Ogden, S. E. (1980). *Aust. N.Z. J. Obstet. Gynecol.* **20**, 135-138.
19. Fisher, C. C., Garrett, W. and Kossoff, M. E. (1976). *Am. J. Obstet. Gynecol.* **124**, 483-488.
20. Ford, W. D. A., Ahmed, S., Verco, P. W. and Jureidini, K. F. (1984). *Aust. Paediat.* **20**, 67-72.
21. Gill, R. W., Trudinger, B. J., Garrett, W. J., Kossof, G. and Warren, P. S. (1981). *Am. J. Obstet. Gynecol.* **139**, 720-725.
22. Graham, D., Tracey, J., Winn, K., Corson, V. and Sanders, R. C. (1983). *J. Clin. Ultrasound* **11**, 336-338.
23. Grannum, P. (1979). *Clin. Diagnost. Ultrasound* **3**, 41-55.
24. Grannum, P., Berkowitz, R. and Hobbins, J. C. (1979). *Am. J. Obstet. Gynecol.* **133**, 915-922.
25. Grennert, L., Persson, P. H. and Gennser, G. (1978). *Acta Obstet. Gynecol. Scand. Suppl.* **78**, 1-5.
26. Gruenewald, S. M., Crocker, E. F., Walker, A. G. and Trudinger, B. J. (1983). *Am. J. Obstet. Gynecol.* **148**, 278-283.
27. Hansmann, M. (1974). *Gynakologe* **7**, 26-35.
28. Harrison, M. R., Golbus, M. S., Filly, R. A., Callen, P. W., Katz, M. and de Lorimer, A. A. (1982). *N. Engl. J. Med.* **306**, 591-593.
29. Harvey, D., Prince, J., Bunton, P., Parkinson, C. and Campbell, S. (1982). *Pediat.* **69**, 296-300.
30. Higginbottom, J., Slater, J., Porter, G. and Whitfield, C. R. (1975). *Br. J. Obstet. Gynaec.* **82**, 698-701.

31. Hill, L. M., Breckle, R., Wolfgram, K. R. and O'Brien, P. C. (1983). *Am. J. Obstet. Gynecol.* **147**, 407–410.
32. Jeanty, P., Dramaix-Wilmet, M., Elkhazen, N., Hubinont, C. and van Regemorter, N. (1982). *Radiology* **144**, 159–162.
33. Johnson, M. L., Dunne, M. G. and Mack, L. A. (1980). *J. Clin. Ultrasound* **8**, 311–315.
34. Jorgensen, C., Ingemarsson, I. and Svenningsen, N. W. (1983). *Br. J. Obstet. Gynaec.* **90**, 162–166.
35. Kazzi, G. M., Gross, T. L., Rosen, M. and Jaatoul-Kazzi, N. Y. (1984). *Am. J. Obstet. Gynecol.* **148**, 54–58.
36. Kazzi, G. M., Gross, T. L., Sokol, R. J. and Kazzi, N. J. (1983). *Am. J. Obstet. Gynecol.* **145**, 733–737.
37. Key, T. C., Dattel, B. J. and Resnik, R. (1983). *Am. J. Obstet. Gynecol.* **145**, 574–578.
38. Kirkinen, P., Jouppila, P. and Eik-Nes, S. (1983). *Br. J. Obstet. Gynaec.* **90**, 640–643.
39. Kopta, M. M., May, R. R. and Crane, J. P. (1983). *Am. J. Obstet. Gynecol.* **145**, 562–565.
40. Levi, S. (1976). *In:* "Present and Future of Diagnostic Ultrasound", (Donald, I. and Levi, S., eds) pp. 76–95. Wiley, New York.
41. Mantoni, M. and Pedersen, J. F. (1979). *J. Clin. Ultrasound* **7**, 459–461.
42. McFayden, I. R., Wigglesworth, J. S. and Dillon, M. J. (1983). *Br. J. Obstet. Gynaec.* **90**, 342–349.
43. Moore, K. H. and Robinson, J. S. (1984). *Aust. N.Z. J. Obstet. Gynecol.* (submitted).
44. Neilson, J. P., Whitfield, C. R. and Aitchison, T. C. (1980). *Br. Med. J.* **1**, 1203–1206.
45. Nelson, L. H. (1981). *J. Clin. Ultrasound* **9**, 67–70.
46. O'Brien, G. D. and Queenan, J. T. (1981). *Am. J. Obstet. Gynecol.* **141**, 833–837.
47. Patterson, R. M., Hayashi, R. H., Cavazos, D. (1983). *Am. J. Obstet. Gynecol.* **147**, 773–777.
48. Persson, P. H., Grennert, L. and Gennser, G. (1978). *Acta Obst. Gynecol. Scand. Suppl.* **78**, 21–27.
49. Persson, P. H., Grennert, L., Gennser, G. and Kullander, S. (1978). *Acta Obst. Gynecol. Scand. Suppl.* **78**, 33–39.
50. Robinson, H. P. (1973). *Br. Med. J.* **4**, 28–32.
51. Robinson, H. P. and Fleming, J. E. E. (1975). *Br. J. Obstet. Gynaec.* **82**, 702–710.
52. Robinson, J. S. (1979). *Br. Med. Bull.* **35**, 137–144.
53. Sabbagha, R. E. (1978). *Obstet. Gynecol.* **52**, 252–256.
54. Sabbagha, R. E., Barton, B. A., Barton, F. B., Kingas, E., Orgill, J. and Turner, H. J. (1976). *Am. J. Obstet. Gynecol.* **126**, 485–490.
55. Taylor, P., Coulthard, A. C. and Robinson, J. S. (1985). *Aust. N.Z. J. Obstet. Gynecol.* (in press).
56. van Otterlo, L. C., Wladimiroff, J. W. and Wallenburg, H. S. C. (1977). *Br. J. Obstet. Gynaec.* **84**, 205–209.
57. Warsof, S. L., Gohari, P., Berkowitz, R. L. and Hobbins, J. C. (1977). *Am. J. Obstet. Gynecol.* **128**, 881–892.
58. Wladimiroff, J. W. and Campbell, S. (1974). *Lancet* **i**, 151–154.
59. Yeh, M. N., Bracero, L., Reilly, K. B., Murtha, L., Aboulafia, M. and Barron, B. A. (1982). *Am. J. Obstet. Gynecol.* **144**, 519–522.
60. Zimmer, E. Z., Weinraub, Z., Raijman, A., Pery, M. and Peretz, B. A. (1984). *J. Clin. Ultrasound* **12**, 112–114.

The Assessment of Placental Function

R. J. Norman and T. Chard

Departments of Obstetrics, Gynaecology and Reproductive Physiology,
St Bartholomew's Hospital Medical College and the London Hospital Medical
College, London, UK

The main physiological function of the placenta is to exchange gas, nutrients
and waste products between maternal and fetal compartments. Impairment of
this process is responsible for much of the risk to the fetus in the latter half of
pregnancy. Therefore, modern antenatal care has emphasized the importance of
detection of fetoplacental dysfunction to reduce perinatal mortality and morbidity.
At the present time there are no useful direct tests of placental gas and nutrient
exchange. Instead, a group of techniques has been developed over the past

Table 1. Placental products which have been advocated for clinical use
in the 3rd trimester of pregnancy

	Group 1	Group 2
Examples	Steroids (e.g. estriol)	Placental proteins 5 and 12
	Enzymes (e.g. heat-stable alkaline phosphatase, cystine amino peptidase)	PAPP-A
	Placental protein hormones (e.g. hPL, hCG)	
	Placental proteins (e.g. SP1)	
Postulated functions	Hormonal	Local (immune and coagulation)
Pathological implications	Fetal pathology including growth retardation and fetal distress	Placental pathology including placental abruption, preterm labour and pre-eclampsia

Abbreviations: hPL, human placental lactogen; SP1, Schwangerschaftsprotein 1; PAPP-A, pregnancy-associated placental protein A.

The Physiological Development of the Fetus and Newborn
ISBN 0 12 389080 2

Copyright © 1985 by Academic Press, London.
All rights of reproduction in any form reserved.

2 decades to measure the export into the maternal compartment of a number of products which can loosely be described as "specific" to the placenta. These compounds may be conveniently subdivided into 2 groups largely based upon their probable site of action and function (Table 1).

Group 1 Products

These have received the greatest attention in the past and include human placental lactogen (hPL) and estriol, the most widely applied tests in clinical obstetrics. Despite the recent popularity of biophysical assessment of placental function, biochemical measurements of placental function (hPL and possibly estriol) still have an important role in several clinical situations (1,2). Much of the literature on this subject is difficult to interpret because of inadequate analysis and reporting of results. The last few years have seen a more uniform use of terms such as sensitivity, specificity and predictive value and the use of these statistical techniques should serve to clarify the rela role of these tests. One example of such an approach is that of Grudzinskas *et al.* (3), who demonstrated that values of hPL below the 10th percentile, observed during routine screening, were more effective than many other factors widely considered to be of great value in antenatal diagnosis. The sensitivity of a low hPL in this study was 17% and its predictive value 25%. Furthermore, a high hPL value was predictive of a favourable outcome of pregnancy. It is doubtful that biophysical monitoring techniques could improve on such results on an unselected population.

A more recently identified member of the Group 1 products is SP1 (Schwangerschaftspecifiches protein 1; pregnancy-specific β-1 glycoprotein), a glycoprotein of molecular weight 90 000. SP1 concentrations are elevated in early pregnancy immediately before or at the same time as human chorionic gonadotrophin and rise to a plateau at about 37 weeks. The concentration of SP1 in maternal blood closely reflects the weight of the placenta throughout gestation as emphasized by the positive relationship between low birthweight and low serum SP1 levels (4,5). In these characteristics SP1 is very similar to hPL although the former is found in concentrations 20 times higher and has a much longer half-life. Various clinical studies have shown SP1 measurements to be similar but probably not superior to those of hPL in routine screening for fetoplacental dysfunction.

All Group 1 products tend to be reduced in growth retardation, pre-eclampsia, prolonged gestation and fetal distress. Given the heterogeneous nature of these conditions, it is not surprising that the predictive value of these measurements is not especially high (20–25%). However, with judicious use there is still an undoubted role for measurement of at least one Group 1 product in patients at increased fetal risk of impaired growth or hypoxia.

Group 2 Products

Recently, much interest has been focussed on several newer placental proteins such as PAPP-A (pregnancy-associated plasma protein A) and PP5 (placental

Table 2. Comparison of the characteristics of Group 1 placental products (hPL/SP1 etc.) with Group 2 products (PP5/PAPP-A)

	hPL/SP1	PP5/PAPP-A
Complex with heparin	−	+
Plateau at term	+	−/+
Serum protease inhibition	−	+
Correlation with fetal weight	+	+/−
Prediction of growth retardation	+	+/−
Blood levels in pre-eclampsia	↓	↑
Blood levels in abruptio	↓	↑
Prediction of preterm labour	−	+

protein 5) (1,6). This interest has arisen from the observation that the postulated functions and characteristics of this group may differ significantly from those of Group 1 (Table 2).

PAPP-A is a glycoprotein with a high molecular weight (800 000 daltons), α-2 electrophoretic mobility and an ability to complex with heparin. It is probably produced by several other tissues in addition to the trophoblast (e.g. decidua, endometrium). Concentration rises rapidly in pregnancy and probably continues to rise until the end of gestation without reaching a plateau. PP5 is another glycoprotein of lower molecular weight (36 000 daltons) found in the placenta, seminal plasma and ovarian follicle. Maternal levels show a continuing rise during pregnancy but, unlike PAPP-A, seem to reach a plateau near term. Of particular interest has been the observation that both PAPP-A and PP5 levels are *increased* in pre-eclampsia and abruptio placentae (1,6). This has led to the hypothesis that these products may have a local action within the placenta with respect to blood coagulation and immune mechanisms. For example, Salem *et al.* (7) have suggested that PP5 may be the placental equivalent of antithrombin III. In contrast to Group 1 products, Group 2 compounds actually may be *increased* during episodes of placental damage and may prove to have predictive value in these conditions.

Conclusions

The past decade has seen a radical transformation of attitudes to antenatal screening for fetoplacental function. With the increasing enthusiasm for biophysical tests of fetal well-being, such as antenatal cardiotocography, advocates of biochemical assessment have had to review critically their approach and investigation of fetoplacental dysfunction in the third trimester. Undoubtedly, traditional indices such as hPL and estriol still have a role in antenatal care but measurement of the Group 2 products may ultimately prove more valuable in certain clinical situations. The practice of antenatal cardiotocography has been accepted by many with far less critical evaluation than that of biochemical testing and there is considerable evidence that a comparison of the two approaches will not necessarily favour the former.

References

1. Chard, T. and Klopper, A. (1982). "Placental Function Tests". Springer-Verlag, New York.
2. Tulchinsky, D. (1983). *Clin. Perinatol.* **10**, 763–776.
3. Grudzinskas, J. G., Gordon, Y. B., Wadsworth, J., Menabawey, M. and Chard, T. (1981). *Aust. N.Z. J. Obstet. Gynecol.* **21**, 103.
4. Gordon, Y. B., Grudzinskas, J. G., Jeffrey, D., Chard, T., Letchworth, A. T. (1977). *Lancet* **i**, 331–333.
5. Chapman, M. G. and Jones, W. R. (1978). *Aust. N.Z. J. Obstet. Gynecol.* **18**, 172.
6. Bischof, P. and Klopper, A. (1983). *In:* "Progress in Obstetrics and Gynaecology" (Studd, J. ed.) Vol. 3, pp. 57–72. Churchill Livingstone, Edinburgh.
7. Salem, H. T., Seppala, M. and Chard, T. (1981). *Placenta* **2**, 205–208.

Fetal Heart Rate Monitoring

G. S. Dawes

The Nuffield Institute for Medical Research, University of Oxford, Oxford, UK

Fetal heart rate monitoring was introduced nearly a quarter of a century ago (1). Flattening of the trace antenatally, with loss of fetal movements and the appearance of decelerations, is still the best index of incipient death. Indeed, introduction of antenatal monitoring in 1976 was associated with halving of the stillbirth rate in Oxford. So it seemed useful to determine whether a more sophisticated computerized analysis would uncover more information.

We knew from observations in pregnant sheep that the fetal heart rate pattern was dependent on gestational age, on the presence or absence of respiratory movements and on episodic changes in electrocortical activity, that it had a diurnal variation and that there were multiple rhythms of different frequencies, some very low, so that the duration of a record of itself altered the measured variation (2). In the fetal lamb, isocapnic hypoxaemia induced a large rise in heart rate variation, prolonged over many hours in the absence of acidaemia (2). In addition, recent evidence shows that cardiac accelerations are associated with but not due to fetal movement, since they are not abolished by neuromuscular blockade.

Many of these principles have been shown to apply to the human fetus. There is a diurnal variation in the fetal heart rate and its pattern (3), a prominent effect of gestational age on heart rate variation (with a 3-fold rise in the number of accelerations/hour during the last 12 weeks) and, over the same period, an episodic change develops analogous to that associated with electrocortical states or sleep cycles postnatally (4,5). The basic pattern is modulated in association with breathing and other movements as shown by several authors (6–8). However, the modulation by human fetal breathing is of high frequency, and breathing episodes do not always coincide with other signals indicative of changing electrocortical state.

Another important feature of computerized human studies has been the evidence of high signal loss (20–50%) commonly experienced with commercial Doppler ultrasound instruments (9), without range-gating (10) or autocorrelation (11).

The Physiological Development of the Fetus and Newborn
ISBN 0 12 389080 2

Copyright © 1985 by Academic Press, London.
All rights of reproduction in any form reserved.

Signal loss is greater earlier in gestation and, even with modern instruments, can rise briefly to unacceptable limits during vigorous movements or hiccoughs (12). It is still essential to identify signal loss. While experienced practitioners have well based confidence in visual analysis of heart rate records, they do not usually comment on this high signal loss. In addition, observer variability has been high (13,14). Computerized analysis at the bedside also permits detection of errors as they occur, when it is often possible for the nurse to rectify them.

It has been suggested that human fetuses can be "aroused" *in utero*, by sensory stimuli (tactile or auditory) to develop accelerations in a hitherto flat fetal heart rate trace. Well controlled trials have only been executed on tactile stimuli (shaking the fetus vigorously) which proved ineffective, either generally (15) or in episodes of low heart rate variation (16). It is indeed common knowledge that newborn infants are difficult to arouse from quiet sleep. Auditory stimuli have been said to evoke fetal responses for nearly half a century (17), and in 1984 these are advocated in Europe (18) and America (19) as a useful index of health, preferable on logistic and medical grounds to an induced uterine contraction test. However, further critical trials of the fetal response to auditory stimuli are required to take account both of the state of the fetus in episodes of low heart rate variation and of the normal pattern of accelerations at a modal frequency of 2/min near term (8) in episodes of high variation. In the absence of such evidence, the repeated statements that the fetus responds to sound remain controversial.

Turning now to some practical issues, let us consider flattening of the fetal heart rate pattern. This occurs in growth-retarded infants before the development of acidaemia (20), possibly with a fall of fetal PaO_2 (21). It is less easy to be certain of the significance of changes in PaO_2 than in pH on Caesarean delivery of such infants as compared with a control group. In sheep the maintenance of normal fetal heart rate variation depends on the integrity of the autonomic nervous system, and on sensory input from the systemic baro- and chemoreceptors. If all these receptors are denervated, heart rate variation is *increased* (22). The cause of flattening of the fetal heart rate in human growth retardation is uncertain. It could be a sign of coma, comparable to loss of the medullary centres (23), or to suppression of their activity by opiates. Yet the effects of morphine, the type substance, are complex, causing stimulation before depression in fetal lambs, as in some adult species. And the origin, sites of action and effects of natural opiates are still uncertain; the clinical phenomenon has not yet been reproduced experimentally.

We need to take into account adaptation of the sensory receptors as a factor in what is likely to be a complex pathophysiological process. The baroreceptors accommodate rapidly in adult animals; in fetal hypertension developing a few days after bilateral nephrectomy, the heart rate is somewhat increased (24). The chemoreceptors reset within 3 days of birth (25); in fetal lambs which become hypoxaemic in growth retardation the heart rate is also close to normal (26,27).

Finally, there is evidence of an unexpectedly wide frequency distribution of human fetal heart rate variation, shown by the presence of low variation ($< $5th centile, comparable with that in growth retardation) at 32 weeks gestation, with normal delivery at term (28). This pattern persists in an individual until after delivery (29). So we may need to redirect our attention to the question of whether the trace commonly considered as flat is outside the range of normality. It has always been obvious that fetal heart rate monitoring, however sophisticated, provides only one of the many pieces of information on which fetal health must be assessed. The measurement of heart rate forms a small part of the evidence of health postnatally. A full neurological prognosis is often not possible before a year from birth. And antenatally the health of the mother may be of predominant importance.

Acknowledgements

It is a pleasure to acknowledge this generous support of the Medical Research Council, and of my many clinical colleagues, especially Dr C. W. G. Redman.

References

1. Hon, E. H. (1960). *Clin. Obstet. Gynecol.* **3**, 860.
2. Dalton, K. J., Dawes, G. S. and Patrick, J. E. (1977). *Am. J. Obstet. Gynecol.* **127**, 414–424.
3. Visser, G. H. A., Goodman, J. D. S., Levine, D. H. and Dawes, G. S. (1982). *Am. J. Obstet. Gynecol.* **142**, 535–544.
4. Visser, G. H. A., Dawes, G. S. and Redman, C. W. G. (1981). *Br. J. Obstet. Gynaec.* **88**, 792–802.
5. Dawes, G. S., Houghton, C. R. S., Redman, C. W. G. and Visser, G. H. A. (1982). *Br. J. Obstet. Gynaec.* **89**, 276–284.
6. Timor-Tritsch, I. E., Dierker, L. J., Zador, I., Hertz, R. H. and Rosen, M. G. (1978). *Am. J. Obstet. Gynecol.* **131**, 276–280.
7. Wheeler, T., Gennser, G., Lindvall, R. and Murrills, R. J. (1980). *Br. J. Obstet. Gynaec.* **87**, 1068–1079.
8. Dawes, G. S., Visser, G. H. A., Goodman, J. D. S. and Levine, D. H. (1981). *Am. J. Obstet. Gynecol.* **140**, 535–544.
9. Dawes, G. S., Visser, G. H. A., Goodman, J. D. S. and Redman, C. W. G. (1981). *Am. J. Obstet. Gynecol.* **141**, 43–52.
10. Lawson, G., Dawes, G. S. and Redman, C. W. G. (1982). *Am. J. Obstet. Gynecol.* **143**, 840–842.
11. Lawson, G. W., Belcher, R., Dawes, G. S. and Redman, C. W. G. (1983). *Am. J. Obstet. Gynecol.* **147**, 721–722.
12. Dawes, G. S., Redman, C. W. G. and Smith, J. (1985). *Br. J. Obstet. Gynaec.* (in press).
13. Trimbos, J. B. and Keirse, M. J. N. C. (1978). *Br. J. Obstet. Gynaec.* **85**, 900–906.
14. Lotgering, F. K., Wallenberg, H. C. S. and Schouten, H. J. A. (1982). *Am. J. Obstet. Gynecol.* **144**, 701–705.
15. Richardson, B., Campbell, K., Carmichael, L. and Patrick, J. (1981). *Am. J. Obstet. Gynecol.* **139**, 344–352.
16. Visser, G. H. A., Zeelenberg, H. J., de Vries, J. I. P. and Dawes, G. S. (1983). *Am. J. Obstet. Gynecol.* **145**, 579–584.
17. Grimwade, J. C., Walker, D. W., Bartlett, M., Gordon, S. and Wood, C. (1971). *Am. J. Obstet. Gynecol.* **109**, 86–93.

18. Jensen, O. H. (1984). *Acta Obstet. Gynecol. Scand.* **63**, 97–101.
19. Serafini, P., Lindsay, M. B. J., Nagey, D. A., Pipkin, M. J., Tseng, P. and Crenshaw, C. (1984). *Am. J. Obstet. Gynecol.* **148**, 41–45.
20. Henson, G., Dawes, G. S. and Redman, C. W. G. (1983). *Br. J. Obstet. Gynaec.* **90**, 516–521.
21. Bekedam, D. J. and Visser, G. H. A. (1984). *Proc. Soc. Fetal Physiol.* **C11**.
22. Itskovitz, J., La Gamma, E. F. and Rudolph, A. M. (1983). *Circ. Res.* **52**, 589–596.
23. Dawes, G. S., Gardner, W. N., Johnston, B. M. and Walker, D. W. (1983). *J. Physiol.* **335**, 535–553.
24. Mott, J. C. (1980). *Adv. Physiol. Sci., 28th Int. Congress, Budapest* **8**, 299–307.
25. Blanco, C. E., Dawes, G. S., Hanson, M. A. and McCooke, H. B. (1984). *J. Physiol.* **351**, 25–37.
26. Robinson, J. S., Jones, C. T. and Kingston, E. J. (1983). *J. Develop. Physiol.* **5**, 89–100.
27. Walker, A. M., Berger, P. J., Cannata, J., Horne, R. and Maloney, J. E. (1984). *Proc. Soc. Fetal Physiol.* **C6**.
28. Lawson, G. W., Dawes, G. S. and Redman, C. W. G. (1984). *Br. J. Obstet. Gynaec.* **91**, 542–551.
29. Smith, J., Dawes, G. S. and Redman, C. W. G. (1984). *Proc. Soc. Fetal Physiol.* **P21**.

Hypertension in Pregnancy— Physiology or Pathology?

Fiona Broughton Pipkin

Department of Obstetrics and Gynaecology, University Hospital, Queen's Medical Centre, Nottingham, UK

In the search for the cause of pregnancy-induced or associated hypertension (PIH), it has always been assumed that it is a pathological response. However, with the advent of sophisticated data retrieval systems it emerges that, in Western Europe and North America, hypertension arising late in pregnancy, and not accompanied by proteinuria is neither associated with any increase in perinatal mortality or morbidity nor with a decreased birthweight (1–3). In the rarer, severe form of the disease, usually arising late in the second trimester and usually accompanied by significant proteinuria, there is an increased perinatal mortality and morbidity with decreased fetal birthweight. It must also be remembered that pregnancy induced or associated hypertension is the single most frequently cited cause of maternal mortality in places as diverse as Washington State in the USA (4) and Mozambique (5).

It is generally agreed that even in the most highly developed nations, with almost universal health care, approximately 1 woman in 10 will become hypertensive (systemic arterial pressure in excess of 140/90 mmHg) during the course of her first pregnancy. This figure rises sharply with worsening poverty and delivery of health care. Yet childbearing is, biologically speaking, the most important part of a woman's life. It seems improbable that a totally harmful process should be present at such high incidence in the population. Arguing teleologically, it seems far more likely that it is in some way an adaptive phenomenon, of intrinsic survival value, which in some women breaks down, converting a physiological process into one of pathology.

True PIH is a self-limiting disease, resolving rapidly after delivery. There is some evidence to suggest that a tendency to the form of the disease which gives rise to its most dangerous manifestation, eclampsia (convulsions) can be genetically determined (6), possibly by simple Mendelian recessive inheritance. This is not

The Physiological Development of the Fetus and Newborn
ISBN 0 12 389080 2

Copyright © 1985 by Academic Press, London.
All rights of reproduction in any form reserved.

so for the mild and moderate forms of the disease. Since eclampsia can occur at relatively low diastolic pressures, and since it can also occur *postpartum*, the relevance of observations made in eclamptic patients to the very large majority of hypertensive primigravidae may be questioned.

However, few people now would question the hypothesis that some factor or factors occurring in very early pregnancy is the ultimate cause of the disease, the secondary effects being manifested finally as hypertension. In normal pregnancy, there is a secondary trophoblast invasion of the maternal spiral arteries reaching beyond the deciduo-myometrial junction, and resulting in the almost total erosion of the musculo-elastic tissues of the vessel wall (7). The arteries thus become unresponsive to neural or hormonal stimuli, and are functionally reduced to wide-bore conduits. Changes in the Doppler-derived blood velocity waveforms in the arcuate artery observed serially from 14 to 20 weeks gestation have shown a marked increase in velocity at this time, temporally coincident with the structural changes in the spiral arteries (8). However, in hypertensive pregnancy, the secondary trophoblastic invasion is halted at the deciduo-myometrial junction, so that a reactive segment of spiral artery remains (7). A broadly similar picture of failed erosion has also been demonstrated in severe intra-uterine growth retardation (IUGR) (9), although not all the changes seen in the spiral arteries in PIH are duplicated in IUGR (10). A good correlation has been demonstrated at delivery between changes in the placental bed characteristic of pregnancy hypertension and abnormal flow velocity waveforms indicating increased resistance and decreased flow (11). Such decreased uteroplacental blood flow (UPBF) in PIH was first shown 30 years ago (12), since when various authors using different techniques have confirmed the findings.

It is not simply in the spiral arteries that changes in vascular reactivity may be observed in pregnancy. The loss of reactivity in the spiral arteries has an anatomical basis; a similar loss of reactivity occurs in the systemic vasculature, but its cause is less well understood. Abdul-Karim and Assali (13) were the first to record a reduced pressor sensitivity to angiotensin II (AII) in pregnant as opposed to nonpregnant women, an observation since repeatedly confirmed. A similar diminution in pressor responsiveness may occur in relation to vasopressin, but this has not been as extensively studied (14). The alteration in response appears to be confined to the small polypeptides; both systemic pressor (15) and hand vascular reactivity (16) to noradrenaline are unchanged in normal pregnancy. It was initially felt that the alteration in response to AII was related to the high circulating concentrations of AII found in most normal pregnant women. However, experiments in both pregnant sheep (17) and humans (18) have shown that acute volume expansion, with a demonstrated fall in plasma renin activity is not associated with any change in vascular reactivity to AII. Alterations in plasma sodium concentration are associated with changes in vasoconstrictor responsiveness to AII (18–20). However, these changes do not affect responsiveness to AII alone, at least in nonpregnant subjects (20), and are more likely to reflect the nonspecific effect of structural changes in the vessel wall as the intracellular sodium concentration changes.

At present, the most likely factor specifically modifying the pressor response to AII in pregnancy seems to be the family of vasodilator prostanoids. These hormones are usually synthesized at or near their sites of action and can markedly alter vascular responsiveness to other vasoactive substances (see 21). There appears to be a functional renin–angiotensin system within at least some major arteries capable of local production of AII (22), which is also a circulating hormone. Thus, a balance between the 2 hormons systems has been proposed as regulating the moment by moment blood flow in such tissue beds as the kidney (23,24). The infusion of prostaglandin E_2 (PGE_2) has been shown to blunt the pressor response to AII in pregnant rabbits, while the administration of indomethacin enhances it (25). Similar effects obtain in human pregnancy. Thus the administration of cyclo-oxygenase inhibitors is associated with enhanced pressor responsiveness to AII (18,26) while the infusion of PGE_2 or PGE_1 is associated with a blunting of response (27,28).

Prostaglandins (PGs) also appear to inhibit the neuronal release of noradrenaline (NOR) (21). The normal pregnant uterus can synthesize high concentrations of PGs and it is possible that the functional denervation of the normal pregnant human uterus (29,30) with minimal tissue NOR present reflects this.

Factors which control the blood pressure (BP) in normal pregnancy are not well understood. The initial fall in diastolic BP, reaching a nadir at around 16–20 weeks gestation is assumed to be due to a fall in total peripheral resistance (TPR), since cardiac output is increased from early in pregnancy. The fall in TPR is presumably caused by a progressive withdrawal of sympathetic tone, since the vascular reactivity to NOR *per se* is unchanged in pregnancy (see above). Some alteration in sympathetic nervous control is also suggested by the inappropriate vasodilation in response to a cold pressor test seen in some pregnant women in the second trimester (31).

The BP begins to rise again after mid-pregnancy, usually coming close to nonpregnant levels by term. Maximum cardiac output is attained by mid-pregnancy, so we may postulate increasing vasoconstrictor influence. The work of Assali and his colleagues (32), which showed an increasing hypotensive effect of ganglion blockade as pregnancy progressed, suggests that the autonomic nervous system is implicated. However, vascular reactivity to angiotensin II also increases in late pregnancy (33). Experiments with chronically cannulated pregnant sheep have shown that blockade of the renin–angiotensin system, whether with angiotensin-converting enzyme inhibitor (34) or with the receptor blocker [Sar^1] [Ala^8] angiotensin II (35,36) lowers maternal BP. It thus seems possible that the renin–angiotensin system may also have a role in maintaining BP in late pregnancy.

In hypertensive pregnancies, the rise in BP is accelerated. Autonomic control seems to be of markedly lesser importance, since ganglion blockade in these patients resulted in only a small fall in BP (32). However, Gant *et al.* (33) showed that, in primigravidae who subsequently became hypertensive, the pressor response to AII increased sharply from mid-pregnancy, reaching or exceeding nonpregnant levels. This enhanced response to AII in PIH was noted 20 years ago by Chesley (14) and is now very well documented. Its implications in PIH are discussed below.

Deteriorating renal function and proteinuria accompany severe PIH but the time course of their onset suggests that they are secondary to the intense vasoconstriction of the condition, and are not primary events (37). Again, many, but not all cases of severe PIH are accompanied by low plasma volume in the second trimester in association with IUGR (38). This has been interpreted as an early, inadequate, maternal response to pregnancy, but the overlap of ranges is large. Related may be the haemoconcentration and increased plasma viscosity noted in this condition which are apparent from the beginning of the 3rd trimester (39). Dintenfass (40) has postulated that there is a certain critical arteriolar diameter, below which there is a dramatic increase in resistance, consequent upon the rigidity/deformability of the red blood cells. Erythrocyte deformability is reduced in PIH (39). There is also good evidence for widespread disseminated intravascular coagulation in the severe disease but, again, the time course of its development suggests it to be an epiphenomenon (37).

It thus appears that many of the symptoms associated with PIH postdate the onset of the clinically defined hypertension, which in turn occurs after the failure of secondary trophoblast invasion and the start of the return to nonpregnant values of pressor response to AII, which occur roughly synchronously. If the autonomic nervous system is not implicated, then we must look for other vasoactive substances which show "inappropriate" activity in PIH. However, it must be remembered that the measurement of plasma concentrations of any hormone may not be a useful guide to its biological effect. Thus, during sodium restriction, when plasma AII concentrations rise, adrenal glomerulosa cells become more, and the vasculature less, sensitive to AII (19).

Considering the catecholamines first, assessment of their concentration in plasma has been hindered by the lack of sensitivity and specificity of the assays used. Clarification should have been achieved with the advent of radio-enzymatic assays, but of 5 recent studies using this technique, one has reported raised NOR concentrations (41), 3 report unchanged NOR and adrenaline (AD) levels (42,43, Professor D. A. Davey, pers. comm.), while 1 reports reduced NOR concentrations (44). The method of blood sampling and handling is critical for catecholamine determinations and has not been standardized.

The measurement of plasma NOR, which does not differ in normotensive women pre- and postpartum (42,43) illustrates well the importance of considering tissue content as well as plasma concentration. O'Shaughnessy et al. (30) showed that in normal pregnancy uterine NOR content fell to ~ 2% of nonpregnant levels, levels in the placental bed itself being even lower. Tissue levels of dopamine and AD were only slightly lower than in the nonpregnant uterus. Interestingly, tissues from hypertensive patients, while still having substantially lower NOR contents than nonpregnant women, nevertheless showed several-fold higher tissue NOR than normotensive controls.

Antidiuretic hormone (ADH; vasopressin) would be an interesting hormone to study in PIH in view of the contracted plasma volume and later deterioration in renal function. However, its measurement is also technically difficult, and the single comparative study to date showed that although plasma ADH concentration was increased in both normo- and hypertensive pregnancies, by comparison by nonpregnant women, the 2 pregnant groups did not differ from each other (45). Isolated reports in the 1930s and 1940s (see 46) suggested an enhanced pressor response to ADH in some hypertensive pregnant women, but the response was inconsistent and nonspecific and investigations were abandoned after the occurrence of oliguria apparently related to the administration of ADH.

The 2 hormone systems most studied, both in isolation from each other and in terms of their joint action, are the renin–angiotensin system (RAS) and the prostanoids. Activity of the RAS is increased at around the time of ovulation and, should conception occur, levels of renin, AII and aldosterone (ALD) continue to rise, falling again only in late pregnancy (47–49). Similarly, fetal plasma renin concentration (PRC) and activity (PRA) are markedly raised by 16 weeks gestation (50), falling off in the 3rd trimester to values approximating maternal following delivery by caesarean section (51,52). Studies in the chronically cannulated fetal lamb have shown that, although PRA is raised by comparison with maternal levels, plasma AII concentrations are very similar (53); both are considerably in excess of nonpregnant values.

It is felt that the primary cause of activation of the maternal RAS is the necessity to conserve sodium in the face of high concentrations of circulating progesterone concentrations, which antagonize the action of aldosterone at the distal tubule. The demonstrated dissociation between vascular and adrenal cortical receptor number in the face of changing sodium concentration (19) may partially explain the lack of a pressor effect consequent upon the high AII concentrations of normal pregnancy. The lowered BP of the second trimester may also act as a stimulus to AII production.

Animal studies have shown that the high circulating AII concentrations may have a role in the maintenance of maternal BP in late pregnancy (34–36). At low doses, AII administration is associated with an increased uterine blood flow (54,55) but at higher doses uterine blood flow decreases. AII may normally assist in maintaining ovine uterine blood flow, since blockade of the RAS decreases uterine blood flow. Since BP also falls under these conditions, this may be a response to diminished perfusion pressure, although the fall seems disproportionately large (36,56).

On the fetal side of the circulation, a marked sensitivity to AII has been shown in the resistance vessels of the human placenta (57,58). Animal experiments show a variable response of both fetal blood pressure and umbilical blood flow following the administration of [Sar^1] [Ala^8] AII, the overall effect being a diminution in both, the size of which may depend on fetal maturity (35,36,59).

The placental capacity to produce prostanoids is very large, and is established early in pregnancy. Amnion, chorion, decidua and placental tissue both contain and can synthesize large amounts of E and F series prostaglandins (PGEs, PGFs) prostacyclin (PGI_2) and thromboxane (TxA_2) (60–62). Interestingly, while the decidua tends to the production of the primarily vasoconstrictor PGF and TxA_2, the fetal membranes and blood vessels mainly produce the primarily vasodilator PGEs and PGI_2. Human umbilical arteries and placental veins synthesize almost entirely PGI_2, and in much higher amounts than do adult blood vessels (63). Uterine arteries can also synthesize PGI_2 (64).

PGE$_1$ and PGI$_2$ have a biphasic effect on human umbilical and chorionic plate vasculature, eliciting relaxation at low doses and contraction at higher (65–67). However, TxA$_2$, PGE$_2$ and PGF$_2$ all constrict both umbilical and placental vasculature (65,68). Indomethacin evokes vasoconstriction in both the cotyledonary (placental) and extracotyledonary vasculature in the pregnant ewe, which suggests an overall vasodilator effect of the prostanoids in these sites (69,70).

The acute administration of PGI$_2$ increases uterine blood flow in the ewe (71) as does PGE$_1$ (72). Interestingly, a direct association has been shown between umbilical arterial PGI$_2$ production and umbilical blood flow in human fetuses (73). Conversely, the administration of indomethacin reduces uterine blood flow in rabbits and dogs (74,75).

Thus it appears that in both the fetal and maternal circulations in normal pregnancy, the RAS and the prostanoids play important roles in the regulation of blood flow and hence of oxygen and nutrient supply. What happens in PIH? It appears that in the mild forms of the disease maternal plasma AII concentrations are unchanged (76) or raised (77) and an association can be demonstrated between plasma AII concentration and diastolic BP (77). Plasma AII concentrations are also raised in the fetuses of such mothers (52) and there is indirect evidence that the placenta may actually be contributing to the higher levels (78). However, in early-onset PIH, activity of the RAS is suppressed (79,80). At the same time, the vascular responsiveness to AII is enhanced (see above). The balance between these 2 phenomena, in terms of net effect on BP, has yet to be determined.

One factor which may be permitting enhanced responsiveness to AII in severe PIH is that, in these same patients, both maternal and fetal tissues have a much diminished content and capacity for the production of vasodilator prostanoids (61,63,81–83). It has been reported that placental tissues from patients with PIH have a diminished capacity to metabolize PGE$_1$ (84). Since PGE$_1$ is vasodilator at low concentrations but vasoconstrictor at higher (see above), this may also be of relevance in terms of vasoconstriction. Recent measurements of plasma concentrations of PGI$_2$ and TxA$_2$ metabolites have shown a decrease in the former and an increase in the latter in severe PIH (85,86). Both metabolites are present in higher concentration in uterine venous than peripheral venous blood, suggesting a uteroplacental contribution to circulating concentrations.

How may we synthesize a coherent hypothesis as to the pathogenesis of PIH from this observational data, and such animal data as we have concerning secondary effects?

The biological imperative of reproductive has allowed massive manipulation of maternal physiology to permit a successful outcome to pregnancy. Among these adaptations may be supposed to be those relating to the threat of inadequate nutrient supply consequential on impaired uteroplacental blood flow. To consider an analogy: if renal perfusion pressure drops outside physiological limits, the RAS is stimulated resulting in the increased production of AII which acts on the systemic circulation to increase systemic BP and thus perfusion pressure. It also acts on the adrenal cortex to promote aldosterone (ALD) release with consequent antinatriuretic and antidiuretic effects at the distal tubule. At the same time, the renal release of vasodilator prostanoids is also markedly increased (87).

There is a complex mutual stimulation of intrarenal synthesis and release between these 2 hormone families (88). The balance between vasoconstrictor and vasodilator hormones then determines to which part of the kidney flow is preferentially directed. If PG synthesis is inhibited, AII exerts an unopposed renal vasoconstrictor effect (89).

It has been shown that acute uterine ischaemia in bitches is associated with a 4-fold rise in uterine venous AII-like concentration in uterine venous blood (90). This arterio-venous difference is similar in magnitude to that reported across the canine kidney during acute renal ischaemia. The administration of low-dose AII is associated not only with increased uterine blood flow (see above) but also with the release of PGEs into the venous effluent (75,91). When PG synthesis is inhibited, uteroplacental blood flow falls (74) and the increase in uterine blood flow in response to AII is prevented (92). Conversely, the administration of an angiotensin-converting enzyme inhibitor was associated with a fall in both uterine blood flow and in uterine venous PGE concentration (56).

Thus we can postulate that in late-onset PIH, the inadequate uteroplacental blood flow arising as a mechanical consequence of the failure of erosion of the deep spiral arteries is compensated for by mechanisms analogous with those in the kidney. The uteroplacental–fetal complex is, in fact, second only to the kidney in its content of and synthetic capacity for both components of the RAS and the vasodilator prostanoids. The increasing AII concentrations both increase systemic, and thus uteroplacental perfusion, pressure and also stimulate sufficient local vasodilator activity to overcome their intrinsic vasoconstrictor effect and permit an increased blood flow to the uterus and its contents. Fetoplacental needs are thus met at a cost to the mother of a degree of systemic hypertension.

However, when the capacity to synthesize the vasodilator prostanoids is lost, as in severe PIH, this physiological balance will tip to the pathological. Instead of the potential uterine vasoconstrictor effects of AII being offset by PG production, they will exert an unopposed vasoconstrictor effect. Lack of PG production in the systemic vasculature allows an enhanced pressor response to such AII concentrations as are present. The renal medullary failure to produce PGEs in this condition (42,93) also permits the uninterrupted intrarenal effects of AII. In the nonpregnant state, the infusion of AII has been shown to reduce urate clearance, primarily through a decrease in renal blood flow (94); a rise in serum uric acid concentration accompanies the development of severe PIH. The proteinuria which also accompanies the condition is characteristic of "vasoactive" proteinuria. It has been known since 1940 that the experimental administration of renin or AII is associated with the development of proteinuria, apparently by an alteration in glomerular basement membrane permeability, as well as by their haemodynamic effects (95). Thus it is possible to consider several of the secondary symptoms of PIH in terms of the unopposed actions of AII secondary to failure of production of the vasodilator prostanoids.

The disturbance in platelet vascular homeostasis in severe PIH could well be a consequence of imbalance between PGI_2 and TxA_2 production, with *in vivo* platelet activation and consumption and widespread disseminated intravascular coagulation.

In conclusion, we have to admit that the primary cause of PIH eludes us. It is, however, the hypertension *per se* which gives rise to clinical concern, not the failure of trophoblast migration. The data here outlined, and the hypothesis arising from them, suggest that the mild form of the disease may be of positive physiological benefit and its high incidence thus not surprising. The severe form of the disease would then be a breakdown of a normal safety mechanism, with consequent harmful effects not only to the fetus but also to the mother.

References

1. Page, E. W. and Christianson, R. (1976). *Am. J. Obstet. Gynecol.* **126**, 821–829.
2. Clinch, J. (1980). *J. Irish Med. Assoc.* **73**, 348–349.
3. Chamberlain, G. (1981). *Br. J. Hosp. Med.* **26**, 127–133.
4. Benedetti, T. J., Starzyk, P. and Frost, F. (in press). *Clin. Exp. Hypertension B.*
5. Liljestrand, J., Axemo, P. and Bergström, S. (in press). *Clin. Exp. Hypertension B.*
6. Chesley, L. C. (1978). "Hypertensive Disorders in Pregnancy". Appleton Century Crofts, New York.
7. Robertson, W. B., Brosens, I. and Dixon, H. G. (1967). *J. Path. Bact.* **93**, 581–592.
8. Cohen-Overbeek, T., Hernandez, C., Meisner, I., Pearce, M. and Campbell, S. (in press). *Clin. Exp. Hypertension B.*
9. Sheppard, B. L. and Bonnar, J. (1980). *Placenta* **1**, 145–156.
10. Fox, H. (1982). *In:* "Pregnancy Hypertension", (Sammour, M. B., Symonds, E. M., Zuspan, F. P. and El-Tomi, N., eds) pp. 249–253. Ain Shams University Press, Cairo.
11. Khong, T. Y., Pearce, J. M. F., Robertson, W. B. and Campbell, S. (in press). *Clin. Exp. Hypertension B.*
12. Browne, J. C. M. and Veall, M. (1953). *J. Obstet. Gynaecol. Brit. Empire* **60**, 141–147.
13. Abdul-Karim, R. and Assali, N. S. (1961). *Am. J. Obstet. Gynecol.* **82**, 246–251.
14. Chesley, L. C. (1966). *Clin. Obstet. Gynecol.* **9**, 871–880.
15. Chesley, L. C., Talledo, E., Bohler, C. S. and Zuspan, F. P. (1965). *Am. J. Obstet. Gynecol.* **91**, 837–842.
16. Lumbers, E. R. (1970). *Aust. J. Exp. Biol. Med. Sci.* **48**, 493–500.
17. Matsuura, S., Naden, R. P., Gant, N. F., Parker, C. R. and Rosenfeld, C. R. (1981). *Am. J. Physiol.* **240**, H908–H913.
18. Everett, R. B., Worley, R. J., MacDonald, P. C., Chand, S. and Gant, N. F. (1978). *Semin. Perinatol.* **2**, 3–13.
19. Aguilera, G. and Catt, K. (1981). *Circulat. Res.* **49**, 751–758.
20. Heistad, D. D., Abboud, F. M. and Ballard, D. R. (1971). *J. Clin. Invest.* **50**, 2022–2032.
21. McGiff, J. C., Malik, K. U. and Terragno, N. A. (1976). *Fed. Proc.* **35**, 2382–2387.
22. Loudon, M., Bing, R. F., Swales, J. D. and Thurston, H. (1982). *Clin. Exp. Hypertension A* **4**, 2049–2061.
23. Messina, E. J., Weiner, R. and Kaley, G. (1976). *Fed. Proc.* **35**, 2367–2375.
24. Horton, R., Zipser, R. and Fichman, M. (1981). *Med. Clin. North Am.* **65**, 891–914.
25. O'Brien, P. M. S., Filshie, G. M. and Broughton Pipkin, F. (1977). *Prostaglandins* **13**, 171–181.
26. Jaspers, W. J. M., De Jong, P. A. and Mulder, A. W. (1981). *Europ. J. Obstet. Gynec. Reprod. Biol.* **11**, 379–384.
27. Broughton Pipkin, F., Hunter, J. C., Turner, S. R. and O'Brien, P. M. S. (1982). *Am. J. Obstet. Gynecol.* **142**, 168–176.

28. Broughton Pipkin, F., O'Brien, P. M. S. and Sant-Cassia, L. J. (1982). *Clin. Exp. Hypertension B* **1**, 493–504.
29. Thorbert, G., Alm, P., Björklund, A. B., Owman, C. and Sjöberg, N.-O. (1979). *Am. J. Obstet. Gynecol.* **135**, 223–226.
30. O'Shaughnessy, R. W., O'Toole, R., Tuttle, S. and Zuspan, F. P. (1983). *Clin. Exp. Hypertension B* **2**, 447–457.
31. Macpherson, M., Cowley, A., Morrison, R., Stanmuir, K. and Broughton Pipkin, F. (in press). *Clin. Exp. Hypertension B.*
32. Assali, N. S., Vergon, J. M., Tada, Y. and Garber, S. T. (1952). *Am. J. Obstet. Gynecol.* **63**, 978–988.
33. Gant, N. F., Daley, G. L., Chand, S., Whalley, P. J. and MacDonald, P. C. (1973). *J. Clin. Invest.* **52**, 2682–2689.
34. Broughton Pipkin, F., Symonds, E. M. and Turner, S. R. (1982). *J. Physiol.* **323**, 415–422.
35. Broughton Pipkin, F. and O'Brien, P. M. S. (1978). *Am. J. Obstet. Gynecol.* **132**, 7-15.
36. McLaughlin, M. K. and Chez, R. A. (1980). *Clin. Exp. Hyp.* **2**, 851–863.
37. Dunlop, W., Hill, L. M., Landon, M. J., Oxley, A. and Jones, P. (1978). *Lancet* **ii**, 346–349.
38. Gerretsen, G., Huisjes, H. J. and Elema, J. D. (1981). *Br. J. Obstet. Gynaec.* **88**, 876–881.
39. Thorburn, J., Drummond, M. M., Wigham, K. A., Lowe, C. D. O., Forbes, C. D., Prentice, C. R. M. and Whitfield, C. R. (1982). *Br. J. Obstet. Gynaec.* **89**, 117–122.
40. Dintenfass, L. (1982). *Clin. Hemorheol.* **2**, 175–188.
41. Coevoet, B., Fievet, P., Comoy, E., Legrand, F., Makdassi, R., Verhoest, P., Boulanger, J. C. and Fournier, A. (1982). *Clin. Exp. Hypertension* **1**, 479–491.
42. Pedersen, E. B., Christensen, N. J., Christensen, P., Johannesen, P., Kornerup, H. J., Kristensen, S., Lauritsen, J. G., Leyssac, P. P., Rasmussen, A. and Wohlert, M. (1983). *Hypertension* **5**, 105–111.
43. Rubin, P. C., Butters, L. and Reid, J. L. (1983). *Clin. Exp. Hypertension B* **2**, 421–428.
44. Tunbridge, R. D. G. and Donnai, P. (1981). *Br. J. Obstet. Gynaec.* **88**, 105–108.
45. Weir, R. J., Doig, A., Fraser, R., Morton, J. J., Parboosingh, J., Robertson, J. I. S. and Wilson, A. (1976). *In:* "Hypertension in Pregnancy", (Lindheimer, M. D., Katz, A. I. and Zuspan, F. P., eds) pp. 251–261. John Wiley, New York.
46. MacGillivray, I. (1984). "Pre-eclampsia. The Hypertensive Disease of Pregnancy". W. B. Saunders, London.
47. Sundsfjord, J. A. and Aakvaag, A. (1973). *Acta Endocrinol.* **73**, 499–508.
48. Weir, R. J., Brown, J. J., Fraser, R., Lever, A. F., Logan, R. W., McIlwaine, G. M., Morton, J. J., Robertson, J. I. S. and Tree, M. (1975). *J. Clin. Endocrin. Metab.* **40**, 108–115.
49. Oats, J. N., Broughton Pipkin, F., Symonds, E. M. and Craven, D. J. (1981). *Br. J. Obstet. Gynaec.* **88**, 1204–1210.
50. Franks, R. C. and Hayashi, R. H. (1979). *Am. J. Obstet. Gynecol.* **134**, 20–22.
51. Richer, C., Hornych, H., Amiel-Tison, C., Relier, J.-P. and Giudicelli, J.-F. (1977). *Biol. Neonate* **31**, 301–304.
52. Broughton Pipkin, F. and Symonds, E. M. (1977). *Clin. Sci. Mol. Med.* **52**, 449–456.
53. Broughton Pipkin, F., Lumbers, E. R. and Mott, J. C. (1974). *J. Physiol.* **243**, 619–636.
54. Bruce, S. L., Morishima, H. O., Petrie, R. H., Sakuma, K., Daniel, S. S. and Yeh, S.-Y. (1981). *Am. J. Obstet. Gynecol.* **141**, 495–498.
55. Naden, R. P. and Rosenfeld, C. R. (1981). *J. Clin. Invest.* **68**, 468–474.
56. Ferris, T. F. and Weir, E. K. (1983). *J. Clin. Invest.* **71**, 809–815.
57. Tulenko, T. N. (1979). *Am. J. Obstet. Gynecol.* **135**, 629–636.

58. Abramovich, D. R., Page, K. R. and Wright, F. (1983). *Br. J. Pharmacol.* **79**, 53–56.
59. Iwamoto, H. S. and Rudolph, A. M. (1979). *J. Develop. Physiol.* **1**, 283–293.
60. Myatt, L. and Elder, M. G. (1977). *Nature* **268**, 159–160.
61. Robinson, J. S., Redman, C. W. G., Clover, L. and Mitchell, M. D. (1979). *Prostaglan. Med.* **3**, 223–234.
62. Mitchell, M. D. (1981). *In:* "Clinical Pharmacology of Prostacyclin", (Lewis, P. J. and O'Grady, J., eds) pp. 121–129. Raven Press, New York.
63. Remuzzi, G., Misiani, R., Muratore, D., Marchesi, D., Livio, M., Schieppati, A., Mecca, G., de Gaetano, G. and Donati, M. B. (1979). *Prostaglandins* **18**, 341–348.
64. Kawano, M. and Mori, N. (1983). *Prostaglandins* **26**, 645–662.
65. Tuvemo, T. (1980). *Semin. Perinatol.* **4**, 91–95.
66. Pomerantz, K., Sintetos, A. and Ramwell, P. (1978). *Prostaglandins* **15**, 1035–1044.
67. Kitson, G. E. and Broughton Pipkin, F. (1981). *Am. J. Obstet. Gynecol.* **140**, 683–688.
68. Mak, K. K.-W., Gude, N. M., Walters, W. A. W. and Boura, A. L. A. (1984). *Br. J. Obstet. Gynaeco.* **91**, 99–106.
69. McLaughlin, M. K., Brennan, S. C. and Chez, R. A. (1978). *Am. J. Obstet. Gynecol.* **132**, 430–435.
70. Rankin, J. H. G., Berssenbrugge, A., Anderson, D. and Phernetton, T. (1979). *Am. J. Physiol.* **236**, H61–H64.
71. Clark, K. E., Austin, J. E. and Seeds, A. E. (1982). *Am. J. Obstet. Gynecol.* **142**, 261–268.
72. Resnik, R. and Brink, G. W. (1978). *Am. J. Physiol.* **234**, H557–H561.
73. Mäkilä, U.-M., Jouppila, P., Kirkinen, P., Viinikka, L. and Ylikorkala, O. (1983). *Lancet* **i**, 728–729.
74. Venuto, R. C., O'Dorisio, T., Stein, J. H. and Ferris, T. F. (1975). *J. Clin. Invest.* **55**, 193–197.
75. Terragno, N. A., Terragno, D. A., Pacholczyk, D. and McGiff, J. C. (1974). *Nature* **249**, 57–58.
76. Gordon, R. D., Symonds, E. M., Wilmshurst, E. G. and Pawsey, C. G. T. (1973). *Clin. Sci. Mol. Med.* **45**, 115–127.
77. Symonds, E. M., Broughton Pipkin, F. and Craven, D. J. (1975). *Br. J. Obstet. Gynaec.* **82**, 643–650.
78. Broughton Pipkin, F. and Symonds, E. M. (1976). *J. Physiol.* **256**, 121–122P.
79. Helmer, O. M. and Judson, W. E. (1967). *Am. J. Obstet. Gynecol.* **99**, 9–17.
80. Weir, R. J., Fraser, R., Lever, A. F., Morton, J. J., Brown, J. J., Kraszewski, A., McIlwaine, G. M., Robertson, J. I. S. and Tree, M. (1973). *Lancet* **i**, 291–294.
81. Downing, I., Shepherd, G. L. and Lewis, P. J. (1980). *Lancet* **ii**, 1374.
82. Carreras, L. O., Defreyn, G., van Houtte, E., Vermylen, J. and van Assche, A. (1981). *Lancet* **i**, 442.
83. Stuart, M. J., Sunderji, S. G., Yambo, T., Clark, D. A., Allen, J. B., Elrad, H. and Slott, J. H. (1981). *Lancet* **i**, 1126–1128.
84. Alam, N. A., Clary, P. and Russell, P. L. (1973). *Prostaglandins* **4**, 363–370.
85. Lewis, P. J., Shepherd, G. L., Ritter, J., Chan, S. M. T., Bolton, P. J., Jogee, M., Myatt, L. and Elder, M. G. (1981). *Lancet* **i**, 559.
86. Märtensson, L. and Wallenburg, H. C. S. (1984). *Proc. Soc. Gynecol. Invest.* San Francisco, Abstract 410, p. 243.
87. Ånggård, E., Larsson, C. and Weber, P. (1976). *Adv. Prostaglandin Thromboxane Res.* **2**, 587–594.
88. Vane, J. R., Bunting, S. and Moncada, S. (1982). *Int. Rev. Exp. Path.* **23**, 161–207.

89. Aiken, J. W. and Vane, J. R. (1973). *J. Pharmacol. Exp. Ther.* **184**, 678–687.
90. Bell, C. (1973). *Am. J. Obstet. Gynecol.* **117**, 1088–1092.
91. Franklin, G. O., Dowd, A. J., Caldwell, B. V. and Speroff, L. (1974). *Prostaglandins* **6**, 271–280.
92. Speroff, L., Haning, R. V. and Levin, R. M. (1977). *Obstet. Gynecol.* **50**, 611–614.
93. Moutquin, J. M. and Leblanc, N. (1982). *Clin. Exp. Hypertension B* **1**, 539–552.
94. Ferris, T. F. and Gorden, P. (1968). *Am. J. Med.* **44**, 359–365.
95. Bohrer, M. P., Deen, W. M., Robertson, C. R. and Brenner, B. M. (1977). *Am. J. Physiol.* **233**, F13–F21.

Maternal Exercise and Fetal Development

James Metcalfe, A. Roger Hohimer and Mark J. Morton

Department of Physiology, School of Medicine,
Oregon Health Sciences University, Portland, Oregon, USA

Introduction

Dynamic exercise is associated with a major increase in blood flow to working muscles. The increase in perfusion is due to a local metabolic vasodilatation in the active muscles and also to the maintenance of (or actual increase in) arterial blood pressure that is possible because of both an increase in cardiac output and vasoconstriction in nonworking tissues. The augmentation of cardiac output requires adequate venous return in order to maintain cardiac filling. During exercise, there is a decrease in plasma volume as fluid is translocated from the vascular space into the extracellular space of the working muscles. This loss of vascular volume appears to be compensated for by shifts in blood volume out of visceral and somatic venous pools. Hyperthermia, whether due to an elevated environmental temperature or humidity, or merely to the body's own heat production, and the upright posture further complicate the haemodynamic challenge of exercise for the human (1).

Haemodynamic Changes During Exercise

Cardiac output

Cardiac output is the product of heart rate and stroke volume. Because the variability of rate is much greater than that of stroke volume, changes in heart rate are quantitatively more important than changes in stroke volume in altering cardiac output when venous return is increased: the normal ejection fraction approximates 65% under resting conditions so there is not much room for improvement with exercise. Heart rate is kept proportional to oxygen uptake during exercise by decreasing vagal tone and increasing sympathetic activity.

The Physiological Development of the Fetus and Newborn
ISBN 0 12 389080 2

Copyright © 1985 by Academic Press, London.
All rights of reproduction in any form reserved.

Stroke volume is the other component of cardiac output. The Starling mechanism links stroke volume to end-diastolic volume so that ejection fraction remains relatively constant: this is the predominant intrinsic mechanism controlling stroke volume. Because of the shape of the pressure–volume curve of the ventricle, end-diastolic pressure rises sharply when end-diastolic volume is significantly increased in supine subjects. Careful measurements have shown that only minor increases in filling pressure occur in normal humans during supine exercise. In the upright position, however, resting end-diastolic volume is reduced, so that the ventricles are operating on the steep portion of their Starling curves; in consequence, small increases in end-diastolic pressure will increase stroke volume. More important is the concept that, regardless of posture, any *decrease* in venous return will cause a fall in end-diastolic volume and substantially diminish stroke volume.

Extrinsically, the rate and extent of cardiac muscle shortening during systole are inversely related to afterload, which is best approximated in the beating heart by average ventricular wall stress. This is determined by the instantaneous intraventricular pressure and by geometric factors that are approximated by the ratio of ventricular radius to the thickness of the ventricular wall. The relationship beween intraventricular pressure and the mechanics of ventricular ejection are influenced by aortic impedance. For example, when systemic vascular resistance is lowered, or aortic capacitance increased, aortic pressure will be lower at any given amount of left ventricular ejection. As a result, ventricular wall stress will be reduced and the rate and extent of ventricular shortening will be increased. During exercise, peripheral vascular resistance falls, allowing the left ventricle to eject a larger stroke volume at a faster rate against a smaller afterload.

The other short-term determinant of stroke volume is ventricular contractility. During exercise, catecholamines released at nerve endings within the myocardium, as well as those brought to the heart by circulating blood, cause contractility to increase. As is the case with the extrinsic regulation of heart rate, contractility during exercise is correlated with the activity of the exercising muscles.

Catecholamines also increase the rate of ventricular muscle relaxation (2). This is important as the heart rate increases; there must be time in the cardiac cycle for the relatively passive process of ventricular filling during diastole.

Distribution of blood flow

As already noted, muscular exercise is accompanied by increased activity of the sympathetic nervous system. The increased neural outflow is manifested by a marked redistribution of cardiac output; blood flow is diverted away from inactive regions, including the splanchnic, renal and cutaneous vascular beds, and from nonworking muscles toward working muscles. The amount of the reduction in visceral blood flow is proportional to the intensity of the exercise: during extreme exertion visceral blood flow falls to only about 20% of its resting level (1). During upright exercise, if venous return increases adequately, cardiac output can be increased to provide a 4-fold increase in oxygen delivery. The 80% reduction in splanchnic and renal blood flow that occurs during maximal exercise would make approximately 2 l/min of blood available to working muscles. Assuming a similar vasoconstriction for skin and nonworking muscle (and assuming that 50% of the total muscle mass is not working), a total of 3 l/min of blood could be redirected to active muscle during extreme exertion (1). Thus, in a healthy individual, redistribution of blood flow is quantitatively much less important than augmentation of cardiac output in supplying exercising muscles with additional blood. In a patient with heart disease who is unable to increase cardiac output, redistribution of blood would allow a doubling of oxygen uptake (1). So, the relative importance of redistribution depends upon the ability of the subject to generate an increased cardiac output.

Venous capacitance and effective blood volume

As we have already emphasized, changes in venous return are of fundamental importance for the maintenance of cardiac output during exercise, especially in upright subjects. Of course, the "muscle pump" acts to return blood from the veins of working muscles back to the central circulation. Splanchnic veins are known to have adrenergic receptors and nervous innervation, but the importance of active venoconstriction during exercise has been difficult to determine (3). It is possible that the fall in distending pressure that results from precapillary vasoconstriction combined with a fall in intrathoracic pressure due to hyperpnoea cause the veins of inactive tissues to empty passively during muscular exercise. However, redistribution of blood *volume* probably plays a larger role in the haemodynamic response to exercise than does the redistribution of blood *flow* that is the more obvious result of sympathetic vasoconstriction.

Exercise causes a decrease in circulating blood volume (4,5). This phenomenon is associated with a rise in haematocrit and occurs soon after the onset of muscular exercise, so most of its is due to increased transudation of fluid into the extravascular spaces. Although the resultant haemoconcentration acts to maintain oxygen delivery to the tissues, the decrement in blood volume compounds the problem of maintaining venous return.

Hyperthermia during exercise

When exercise is conducted in a hot environment or maintained for more than a few minutes, the problem of heat dissipation affects the cardiovascular system. In humans, skin blood flow has been shown to rise from normothermic resting levels approximating 200 ml/min to levels approaching 3 l/min. Hyperthermia also affects venous return. Two mechanisms are involved: first, venous compliance increases by a direct effect of local temperature, and second, transmural pressure is increased by a fall in local arteriolar resistance. As a result, while the veins of the skin are a source of augmented blood volume at the onset of exercise in a cool environment, the cutaneous venous bed acts as a volume "sink" when hyperthermia develops (1).

Haemodynamic Changes During Pregnancy

Cardiac output

Resting cardiac output increases by approximately 40% during human pregnancy, due mainly to an increase in stroke volume. Recent echocardiographic evidence shows that the augmented stroke volume is achieved by maintenance of a constant ejection fraction from an enlarged left ventricle. There is no evidence that the left ventricular enlargement is due to diastolic elongation of myocardial fibres secondary to an increased filling pressure. Rather, the ventricle is apparently remodelled during pregnancy, so that its capacity at any given filling pressure is increased. During pregnancy in the guinea-pig, the pressure–volume relationship of the left ventricle shifts to the right; filling pressures in both ventricles are unchanged, but left ventricular capacity is increased (6,7). In humans, echocardiography shows that ventricular wall thickness changes very little, or not at all, during gestation; left ventricular weight does not increase during pregnancy in guinea-pigs, so hypertrophy apparently does not accompany the ventricular enlargement of pregnancy. We assume that sarcomere length in diastole is unchanged, an adaptation which, coupled with normal ventricular compliance, would preserve the availability of the Starling mechanism.

Ventricular enlargement, unaccompanied by an increase in wall thickness, results in an increase in the ratio of ventricular radius to wall thickness. This by itself would lead to an increase in wall stress. However, peripheral vascular resistance falls during pregnancy and aortic compliance increases. Both of these changes will act to reduce aortic impedance. Apparently the increased ratio of ventricular radius to wall thickness is counterbalanced by the fall in aortic impedance, so that fractional shortening and normalized shortening rate are unchanged during pregnancy, while the average systolic ejection rate increases from a nonpregnant value of 255 to 345 ml/s in the 3rd trimester of human pregnancy (8).

Resting heart rate increases progressively during human pregnancy. To our knowledge, studies of maximal heart rate during pregnancy have not been performed. We assume that maximal heart rate is unchanged. Because there is a progressive increase in resting heart rate, we might conclude that the heart rate reserve for exercise falls progressively as pregnancy advances and that maximal work capacity is proportionately reduced. This is supported by observations showing that mild nonweightbearing exercise is accompanied by a heart rate 10–15 beats/min faster during pregnancy than in the same women studied while performing the same exercise task postpartum. On the other hand, Rowell (1) reviewed a variety of stresses which increase heart rate during submaximal exercise but do not decrease maximal oxygen uptake.

Echocardiographic studies of left ventricular function are currently being performed in pregnant human subjects during isotonic and isometric exercise. Preliminary results suggest that left ventricular systolic performance, assessed by rate of shortening and extent of shortening, does not change. Early in pregnancy, stroke volume is augmented above nonpregnant values at a standard intensity of bicycle exercise. As pregnancy progresses, stroke volume falls to nonpregnant levels: tachycardia is increasingly evident during *and especially immediately after* exercise. As soon as the pregnant subject stops performing upright bicycle exercise, stroke volume plummets. Cardiac output is usually maintained, but hypotension and syncope can occur. The relative tachycardia seen during and following exercise near term is regarded as evidence of maintained sympathetic activity, an adaptation that attempts to maintain venous return by redistributing blood volume.

Redistribution of blood flow

Few data are available concerning the effects of pregnancy upon peripheral vascular responses to exercise. Werkö (9) measured renal plasma flow during upright exercise. In pregnant women he documented an increase in flow during exercise rather than the fall that is characteristic of nonpregnant subjects. These limited observations are supported by responses to orthostatic stress during pregnancy; these show that pregnant subjects respond to head-up tilting with a greater increase in heart rate than do nonpregnant controls (10), similar to that characteristic of patients with defined autonomic insufficiency.

Venous capacitance and effective blood volume

The observation that cardiac output at rest, during exercise and especially immediately after exercise is increasingly characterized by tachycardia as pregnancy advances suggests that the resources available to the heart to meet the demands of the periphery for blood flow are limited by problems with venous return. Venous compliance has been shown to increase during pregnancy, a change that would increase the capacity of the venous bed (11). In addition, the vascular bed in the uterus and broad ligaments is obviously increased in capacity.

The problem of venous pooling is intensified by the tendency of the enlarging uterus to obstruct the inferior vena cava. Although this tendency is most pronounced in supine recumbency, intra-abdominal pressure is increased in the sitting and standing positions as well. Therefore, despite an average increase of 40% in blood volume that occurs during pregnancy, it seems likely that venous pooling, to which humans are always liable, is a more significant problem during pregnancy. In addition, the active metabolism of the fetus and placenta increases the requirement for heat dissipation through the maternal skin. One would predict that the ability to divert blood flow, and especially blood volume, away from the skin during exercise would be partially compromised by the hypermetabolism of pregnancy.

Lotgering *et al.* (12) measured maternal blood volume in pregnant sheep before and during exercise at an intensity that increased oxygen consumption by an average of 5.6 times resting values. They found that plasma volume fell by 20% within 3 min of the onset of exercise. The change is more pronounced than that observed in nonpregnant humans, raising the possibility that pregnancy magnifies the tendency for transudation across the capillary membrane during exercise.

There may be a tendency for increased water loss and resultant dehydration with exercise during pregnancy, because of the additional heat generated by active fetal metabolism and the hyperventilation which is an important part of human pregnancy. It would appear that dehydration due to any cause negatively affects venous return (4).

All of these alterations raise appropriate concerns about the ability of the maternal heart to maintain during exercise uterine blood flow adequate for optimum fetal growth and development.

Effects of Exercise on Uterine Blood Flow and Fetal Development

Uterine blood flow and fetal oxygenation

Emmanouilides *et al.* (13) measured gas tensions and pH in maternal and fetal arterial blood before and immediately after prolonged treadmill exercise. They found that fetal arterial pH rose while the tensions of carbon dioxide and oxygen fell, and attributed these changes to reduction of uterine blood flow. Chandler and Bell (14) studied pregnant ewes near term and found an average 36% fall in uterine blood flow at the end of 60 min of mild treadmill exercise accompanied by declines in fetal arterial tensions of CO_2 and O_2. Four of 6 ewes studied by Curet *et al.* (15) showed a decrement in total uterine blood flow immediately after 40–60 min of treadmill exercise: myoendometrial blood flow fell in 5 of the 6 sheep by an average of 41%. Hohimer *et al.* (16) measured a decline in uterine blood flow during exercise in Pygmy goats. The reduction in uterine blood flow was proportional to the level of exertion. Lotgering *et al.* (12) found a similar decrease. Hohimer *et al.* (16) measured the distribution of uterine blood flow before and during exercise using labelled microspheres. They found that cotyledonary blood flow fell insignificantly while myoendometrial blood flow decreased by an average of 52%. These findings are consistent with a report by Morris *et al.* (17), who estimated uterine blood flow in human subjects by monitoring the rate of washout of radioactive saline injected assumedly into the uterine muscle.

Lotgering *et al.* (18) confirmed an earlier observation by Clapp (19), that uterine O_2 consumption is maintained during prolonged exercise at 70% of maximal O_2 consumption by pregnant ewes. Furthermore, fetal arterial PO_2 fell by only 3 torr, fetal arterial O_2 content by only 1.5 ml/dl and fetal arterial pH did not change significantly. Apparently the maternal haemoconcentration, increased O_2 extraction within the uterus and a redistribution of blood to favour cotelydonary areas protects the fetal lamb from hypoxia during maternal exercise.

With exhausting exercise, the tensions of O_2 and CO_2 in fetal arterial blood fall only slightly. The decline in uterine blood flow may be due to hyperthermia (20) or hypocarbia (21); however, Hohimer *et al.* (16) documented marked increases during exercise in blood epinephrine and norepinephrine concentrations to levels that have been shown (22) to produce significant reductions in uterine blood flow and significant increases (23) in uterine vascular resistance. Artal *et al.* (24) showed statistically significant increases in the circulating levels of epinephrine and norepinephrine associated with light exercise of brief duration in 23 healthy pregnant subjects. Other workers have shown that infusions of either epinephrine or norepinephrine cause proportionately greater decrements in myometrial than in cotyledonary blood flow (25,26). The possibility of neurally mediated uterine vasoconstriction also exists (23,27,28).

Fetal body temperature exceeds that of the mother by approximately 0.5°C when measured in resting sleep (29). Lotgering *et al.* (18) found that fetal temperature rises more slowly during maternal exercise but the fetal hyperthermia persists longer than does the elevation of maternal body temperature. The direct effect of heat upon fetal development as well as the cardiovascular effects of hyperthermia enter any consideration of fetal health related to maternal exercise.

Maternal exercise and fetal growth

Pregnant rats that were forced to perform extreme exercise showed increased fetal mortality, decreased fetal weight gain and delayed fetal bone ossification (30). Dhindsa *et al.* (31) reported that the birthweights of twin kids from goats that exercised during pregnancy were significantly decreased below those of kids from control animals. A subsequent study from the same laboratory (16) found no effect of maternal exercise upon the birthweight of kids: the difference in results was attributed to a difference in the way the goats were trained to exercise in the 2 studies. In the first, aversive conditioning was used; in the second, aversive stimuli were scrupulously avoided and positive reinforcement was used to teach the animals to exercise.

Collings *et al.* (32) studied 12 pregnant women who exercised at 65–75% of their age-predicted maximal O_2 consumption for approximately 45 min 3 times weekly, and compared these women and their infants with 8 control subjects. There was evidence of improved physical performance in the women who exercised. However, no statistically significant differences between pregnancy outcome of the two groups were found.

As would be predicted, some exercise enthusiasts have maintained extreme exercise schedules during pregnancy, some of them without apparent adverse effects (33–35).

Data from humans show that maternal work handicaps fetal growth. Naeye and Peters (36) found that women who work in the 3rd trimester of pregnancy deliver infants weighing significantly less at term than newborn infants of mothers who do not work. The handicap to fetal growth was particularly marked in women who worked at standing occupations. One hypothesis to explain that finding is that prolonged standing causes a limitation of venous return and cardiac output, and of uterine blood flow. However, because "work" may have different psychological implications from "exercise", the applicability of data obtained from working women to women who exercise for relatively short periods and for enjoyment is open to question.

On the basis of present evidence it seems likely that exercise of unaccustomed severity or duration should be avoided during pregnancy. More restriction is indicated for women with other handicaps to cardiac output or uterine blood flow or blood oxygen transport. The exercise programme should be discontinued if vaginal bleeding occurs, if there is evidence of fetal growth retardation, or if maternal heart rate does not return to its resting level within 15 min of stopping exercise. Exercise should not be performed in a hot environment: the intensity and duration of exercise should be kept below levels that result in substantial elevation of the mother's body temperature. Within these limits women should not be denied the psychological and physical benefits that derive from a sustained programme of moderate exercise.

References

1. Rowell, L. B. (1974). *Physiol. Rev.* **54**, 75–159.
2. Morad, M. and Rolett, E. L. (1972). *J. Physiol.* **224**, 537–558.
3. Rothe, C. F. (1983). *Physiol. Rev.* **63**, 1280–1342.
4. Nadel, E. R., Fortney, S. M. and Wenger, C. B. (1980). *J. Appl. Physiol.* **49**, 715–721.
5. Greenleaf, J. E., Convertino, V. A., Stremel, R. W., Bernauer, E. M., Adams, W. C., Vignau, S. R. and Brock, P. J. (1977). *J. Appl. Physiol.* **43**, 1026–1032.
6. Morton, M. J., Tsang, H., Hohimer, A. R., Ross, D., Thornburg, K., Faber, J. and Metcalfe, J. (1984). *Am. J. Physiol.* **246**, R40–R48.
7. Hart, M. V., Hosenpud, J. D., Rowles, J. R., Morton, M. J. and Hohimer, A. R. (1983). *Physiologist* **26**, A18.
8. Katz, R., Karliner, J. S. and Resnik, R. (1978). *Circulation* **58**, 434–441.
9. Werkö, L. (1954). *Acta Obstet. Gynecol. Scand.* **33**, 162–183.
10. Sandström, B. O. (1974). *Acta Obstet. Gynecol. Scand.* **53**, 1–5.
11. Fawer, R., Dettling, A., Weihs, D., Welti, H. and Schelling, J. L. (1978). *Eur. J. Clin. Pharmacol.* **13**, 251–257.
12. Lotgering, F. K., Gilbert, R. D. and Longo, L. D. (1983). *J. Appl. Physiol.* **55**, 834–841.
13. Emmanouilides, G. C., Hobel, C. J., Yashiro, K. and Klyman, G. (1972). *Am. J. Obstet. Gynecol.* **112**, 130–137.
14. Chandler, K. D. and Bell, A. W. (1981). *J. Develop. Physiol.* **3**, 161–176.
15. Curet, L. B., Orr, J. A., Ranklin, J. H. G. and Ungerer, T. (1976). *J. Appl. Physiol.* **40**, 725–728.
16. Hohimer, A. R., Bissonnette, J. M., Metcalfe, J. and McKean, T. A. (1984). *Am. J. Physiol.* **246**, H207–H212.
17. Morris, N. S., Osborn, B., Wright, H. P. and Hart, A. (1956). *Lancet* **ii**, 481–484.
18. Lotgering, F. K., Gilbert, R. D. and Longo, L. D. (1983). *J. Appl. Physiol.* **55**, 842–850.
19. Clapp, J. F. (1980). *Am. J. Obstet. Gynecol.* **136**, 489–494.
20. Hales, J. R. S. (1973). *Pflugers Arch.* **334**, 133–148.
21. Oakes, G. K., Walker, A. M., Ehrenkranz, R. A., Cefalo, R. C. and Chez, R. A. (1976). *J. Appl. Physiol.* **41**, 197–201.
22. Barton, M. D., Killam, A. P. and Meschia, G. (1974). *Proc. Soc. Exp. Biol. Med.* **145**, 996–1003.
23. Fuller, E. O., Galletti, P. M., Manning, J. W. and Fitzgerald, T. F. (1979). *J. Develop. Physiol.* **1**, 209–218.
24. Artal, R., Platt, L. D., Sperling, M., Kammula, R. K., Jilek, J. and Nakamura, R. (1981). *Am. J. Obstet. Gynecol.* **140**, 123–127.
25. Rosenfeld, C. R., Barton, M. D. and Meschia, G. (1976). *Am. J. Obstet. Gynecol.* **124**, 156–163.

26. Rosenfeld, D. P. and West, J. (1977). *Am. J. Obstet. Gynecol.* **127**, 276-383.
27. Ryan, M. J., Clark, K. E. and Brody, K. J. (1974). *Am. J. Physiol.* **227**, 547-555.
28. Zuspan, F. P., O'Shaughnessy, R. W., Vinsel, J. and Zuspan, M. (1981). *Am. J. Obstet. Gynecol.* **139**, 678-680.
29. Abrams, R., Caton, D., Clapp, J. and Barron, D. H. (1970). *Clin. Obstet. Gynecol.* **13**, 549-564.
30. Terada, M. (1974). *Teratology* **10**, 141-144.
31. Dhindsa, D. S., Metcalfe, J. and Hummels, D. H. (1978). *Resp. Physiol.* **32**, 299-311.
32. Collings, C. A., Curet, L. B. and Mullin, J. P. (1983). *Am. J. Obstet. Gynecol.* **145**, 702-707.
33. Dressendorfer, R. (1978). *Physic. Sportsmed.* **6**, 74-80.
34. Ruhling, R. O., Cameron, J., Sibley, L., Christensen, C. and Bolen, T. (1981). *Med. Sci. Sports Exer.* **13**, 93.
35. Sibley, L., Ruhling, R. O., Cameron-Foster, J., Christensen, C. and Bolen, T. (1981). *J. Nurse Midwifery* **26**, 3-12.
36. Naeye, R. L. and Peters, E. C. (1982). *Pediatrics* **69**, 724-727.

Management of the Newborn Circulation

Michael A. Heymann

Cardiovascular Research Institute and the Departments of Pediatrics, Physiology, and Obstetrics, Gynecology and Reproductive Sciences, University of California, San Francisco, California, USA

In general, transition from the fetal to the neonatal circulatory pattern at term is accomplished rapidly and in an orderly fashion. This is occasioned by the progressive maturation of several organ systems to a point which allows for appropriate function. Premature delivery or chronic intra-uterine stress may either interrupt or alter the normal pattern of maturation, thereby preventing or modifying the normal sequence of postnatal circulatory changes. Failure of normal circulatory adaptation may further compromise the circulation and lead to significant clinical pathophysiological changes. Two major areas will be considered:

1. establishment and maintenance of normal pulmonary blood flow and therefore the ability adequately to oxygenate blood,

2. closure of the ductus arteriosus with establishment and maintenance of normal systemic blood flow and therefore the ability adequately to deliver oxygen and substrates to peripheral tissues.

Pulmonary Blood Flow

Normal physiology

In the fetus, gas exchange occurs in the placenta; pulmonary blood flow is low, supplying only nutritional requirements for lung growth and perhaps also serving some metabolic function. In close-to-term fetal lambs (140–145 days gestation) pulmonary blood flow is about 50 ml/100 g of lung tissue or about 8% of the combined ventricular output of the heart (1,2). After birth with initiation of pulmonary ventilation, pulmonary vascular resistance falls rapidly and is associated with an 8-to-10-fold increase in pulmonary blood flow. In full term lambs, this is about 300–400 ml/min/kg of body weight shortly after birth (3).

The Physiological Development of the Fetus and Newborn
ISBN 0 12 389080 2
Copyright © 1985 by Academic Press, London.
All rights of reproduction in any form reserved.

Many phenomena have been shown to affect pulmonary vascular resistance and thereby modulate pulmonary blood flow in the fetus or newborn. However, the exact mechanism by which pulmonary blood flow increases so dramatically after birth are not yet fully understood. A clearer understanding of the normal physiologic mechanisms likely will lead to improved treatment of conditions in which normal changes do not occur spontaneously.

The fetal lung is fluid-filled and spontaneous fetal breathing movements do not appear to effect pulmonary vascular resistance. Ventilation with a gas that does not change the oxygen environment produces a small fall in pulmonary vascular resistance, probably related to surface tension factors that act at the alveolar air–liquid interface to reduce perivascular tissue pressure (4). This phenomenon probably has minimal direct physiologic importance; rather, mechanical stimulation of the lung may lead to the release of vasoactive substances which in turn effect the vasculature. The autonomic nervous system probably plays little role in controlling resting pulmonary vascular resistance (5). However, stimulation of the vagus nerve (5) or infusion of acetylcholine (4,6) in the fetus produces significant pulmonary vasodilatation, particularly close to term. Similarly, either direct stimulation of thoracic sympathetic nerves (5) or administration of α-adrenergic agonists (4) causes pulmonary vasoconstriction. The postnatal changes that occur could be mediated by changes in balance between adrenergic and cholinergic input, the latter having a dominant effect. This has not yet been evaluated.

Probably far more significant in controlling pulmonary circulating in the fetus and in the postnatal period is the interrelationship of oxygen and various vasoactive substances produces either locally or elsewhere in the fetus. In the latter portion of gestation, the pulmonary circulation is responsive to changes in the O_2 environment and this is even more so after birth (6–8). In the normal fetal lamb, pulmonary arterial blood PO_2 is about 17–20 torr. Reducing PO_2 to similar levels in newborn animals produces a marked increase in pulmonary vascular resistance; conversely, increasing fetal PO_2 above normal increases pulmonary blood flow. Therefore, it is likely that the low PO_2 found normally in the fetus, either alone or in concert with the release of vasoactive substances, is responsible for maintaining active pulmonary vasoconstriction and increased pulmonary vascular resistance, and thereby a low pulmonary blood flow. The exact mechanism by which low O_2 maintains pulmonary vasoconstriction in the fetus is not clearly established. Reflex-mediated chemoreceptor control has been investigated and plays essentially no major role. Direct local effects of changes in O_2 concentrations also have been studied in fetuses. When one fetal lung *in situ* was perfused or ventilated independently without changing the O_2 environment of the other lung, resistance changes in that lung could be produced by modifying the O_2 environment. The remaining lung was unaffected, strongly suggesting local mediation of the resistance changes (9). Increasing PO_2 to which the resistance vessels are exposed, either by ventilating with O_2 (10) or by exposure to hyperbaric oxygenation (7), also leads to increased pulmonary blood flow. However, none of these studies considered the possibility that changes in the O_2 environment may not only directly affect pulmonary vascular smooth muscle, but could lead to modifications in the production and/or release of locally produced vasoactive substances which could then act on the pulmonary circulation.

Many vasoactive substances have been shown to affect the fetal pulmonary circulation; whether they play a role in maintaining the high pulmonary vascular resistance in the fetus or in the perinatal changes is not clearly established. Angiotensin II has been considered important in the pulmonary vasoconstrictor response to hypoxaemia in adults (11) and therefore has been suggested as possibly maintaining the high pulmonary vascular resistance in the fetus. However, Saralasin blockade of angiotensin II activity in fetal lambs had no effect on pulmonary vascular resistance or on the response to hypoxaemia (12). Bradykinin, a potent vasoactive peptide, is released transiently either during ventilation of the fetal lungs with air or during hyperbaric oxygenation (7). Since bradykinin increases pulmonary flow, it probably plays some physiological role in the immediate postnatal pulmonary circulatory changes. More recent studies further support the rather transient role of bradykinin. One function of pulmonary vascular endothelium is conversion of angiotensin I to the active angiotensin II; this is performed by angiotensin converting enzyme (ACE) which also catabolizes bradykinin to its inactive metabolites. At normal fetal PO_2 pulmonary ACE activity is minimal; however, after exposure to O_2, ACE activity increases (13). This would result in increased metabolism and reduced circulating concentrations of bradykinin as soon as adequate postnatal pulmonary blood flow and oxygenation had occurred. There may be additional roles for angiotensin II or bradykinin, since they both induce or stimulate local production of prostacyclin (PGI_2), a pulmonary vasodilating substance (see below) (14).

The physiological role of the many naturally occurring products of arachidonic acid metabolism have recently undergone close scrutiny. In the fetus, prostaglandin E_2 (PGE_2) is a modest pulmonary vasodilator (15) and PGI_2 is a pulmonary vasodilator of somewhat greater potency (16). Neither of these is specific for the pulmonary circulation and generally affect the systemic vascular resistance to the same or even to a greater degree (17). This does not, however, exclude the possibility that local production and metabolism occurs in the normal perinatal period and there is evidence that PGI_2 plays a physiological role in causing pulmonary vasodilatation. Lung distension or mechanical stimulation of lungs leads to PGI_2 production (14,18) and ventilation of fetal lungs is associated with the net local production and release into blood of small amounts of PGI_2 (19). Further, inhibition of prostaglandin synthesis by indomethacin attenuated the progressive fall in pulmonary vascular resistance that normally occurred 30 s or so after ventilation started (20).

More recently another prostaglandin, PGD_2, has been shown to be a pulmonary vasodilator in perfused fetal lungs (21). In intact newly delivered term lambs with hypoxia-induced pulmonary hypertension, PGD_2 produced a significant and specific fall in pulmonary arterial pressure and calculated pulmonary vascular resistance with an increase in both pulmonary and systemic blood flows and little or no change in systemic arterial blood pressure (22). Beyond about 10 days of age, this effect was no longer present and PGD_2 produced

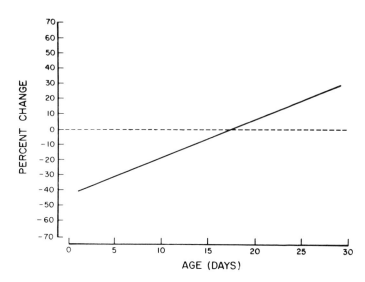

Figure 1. Age-related effects (% change from hypoxaemic baseline) on pulmonary vascular resistance of an infusion of 5 μg/kg/min PGD$_2$ in young lambs.

pulmonary vasoconstriction (23) (Fig. 1). These specific effects in the immediate newborn period strongly suggest a physiological role for PGD$_2$ in establishing a normal pulmonary circulation. Further support for this comes from studies in Rhesus monkey lungs which showed a marked increase in the number of mast cells in the latter part of gestation. Shortly after delivery there were significantly fewer mast cells in the lungs (24). Prostaglandin D$_2$ is released from mastocytoma and mast cells, so mast cell degranulation with the release of PGD$_2$ may be one important aspect of the perinatal pulmonary vascular changes. Interestingly, histamine, which is also released when mast cells are degranulated, is a pulmonary vasodilator in the perinatal period (10) whereas histamine in the adult is a pulmonary vasoconstrictor. Therefore, mast cell degranulation may be stimulated in the period of initial ventilation and both PGD$_2$ and histamine may be released. The trigger for this is unclear.

Leukotrienes, another class of substances that are derived from arachidonic acid but via the 5-lipoxygenase pathway, have generated considerable interest recently in view of their effects on smooth muscle. In adult animals, hypoxia pulmonary vasoconstriction is attenuated or abolished by agents blocking the effects of leukotrienes (25). We therefore considered that the tonic pulmonary vasoconstriction found in the fetus could, at least in part, be mediated by leukotrienes. Infusion of FPL 55712 (Fisons), a substance that blocks leukotriene effects, increases pulmonary blood flow in normal fetal lambs (26) (Fig. 2). In close-to-term fetal lambs, this increase can reach a level almost equivalent to the pulmonary blood flow found normally in the ventilated animal after birth. Therefore, we now seriously consider that control of the pulmonary circulation

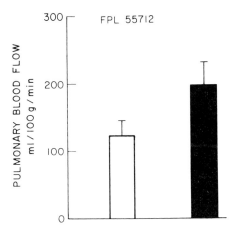

Figure 2. Effects of leukotriene blockade with FPL 55712 on fetal ($\approx$ 132 days gestation, Au: symbol? n=6) pulmonary blood flow (open bar, control; solid bar, after FPL 55712 administration). $P < 0.05$.

reflects a balance between factors producing active pulmonary vasoconstriction in the fetus and factors leading to pulmonary vasodilatation after birth. The dramatic increase in pulmonary blood flow after birth most likely reflects a shift from active pulmonary vasoconstriction to active pulmonary vasodilatation. We consider that perhaps arachidonic acid metabolism shifts from lipoxygenase products in the low oxygen environment of the fetus towards cyclo-oxygenase products in the higher oxygen environment after birth.

Pathophysiology

Failure of normal pulmonary vasodilatation to occur with the onset of spontaneous ventilation leads to a syndrome of hypoxaemia associated with pulmonary hypertension and reduced pulmonary blood flow. Right-to-left shunting at the atrial and ductus arteriosus levels (if the ductus arteriosus is patent) is invariably present (27). This diverse syndrome, currently generally called persistent pulmonary hypertension syndrome of the newborn and previously termed (inappropriately) persistent fetal circulation, has no clearly defined or as yet understood pathophysiological course. Several prenatal conditions have a high association with the development of the syndrome and have been invoked as possible causative factors. These include chronic intra-uterine stress and the use of nonsteroidal anti-inflammatory agents during pregnancy.

The major factors affecting blood flow through any organ are viscosity and the cross-sectional area of the vascular bed. Any conditions that increase viscosity or reduce cross-sectional area will lead to an increase in pulmonary arterial pressure. Any situation causing an increased haematocrit and thereby increased viscosity in an infant, e.g. maternal-to-fetal transfusion, delayed cord clamping or intra-uterine growth retardation, must therefore be considered. However, reduced cross-sectional area is likely to be a far more important cause of the syndrome, and probably the most common cause for a reduced total pulmonary vascular cross-sectional area is failure of the fetal pulmonary circulation to undergo normal postnatal vasodilatation. The exact mechanisms responsible for this failure are unknown. Perinatal hypoxaemia or asphyxia is probably causally related, but many infants in whom perinatal asphyxia occurs do not develop the syndrome. Recent pathological studies on infants dying with this syndrome have indicated an abnormal development of pulmonary vascular medial smooth muscle (28,29). The amount of smooth muscle in the walls of the resistance vessels is increased and, in addition, there is accelerated distribution of smooth muscle along the length of the resistance vessels to a degree usually seen in adult. Intra-uterine factors causing this morphologic change are not clearly established, but chronic intra-uterine stress leading to pulmonary hypertension *in utero* and the effects of pharmacological agents, administered to the mother, which constrict the ductus arteriosus and produce pulmonary hypertension have been seriously considered (30–32). Nonsteroidal anti-inflammatory agents such as salicylates, indomethacin and ibuprofen are agents falling into this latter category. Another further phenomenon that complicates the syndrome and also leads to a reduction in cross-sectional area is the development of microvascular thrombi which have been described clearly in the small pulmonary vessels in infants dying with this syndrome (33). In addition to plugging the vessels, these platelet thrombi may well release active vasoconstricting substances such as thromboxane which then aggravate the situation.

Management

Other causes of perinatal hypoxaemia must be actively excluded in these infants. The true prevalence of the syndrome is unknown but has been estimated to be approximately 1 in 1500 live births. The mortality remains high and has been estimated to vary from 20 to 50%. In general, the medical management remains mainly supportive in nature (27,34). Careful attention must be paid to maintaining normal blood glucose and calcium concentrations and to assure a normal systemic arterial blood pressure. Oxygen consumption should be kept to a minimum by maintaining the infant in a neutral thermal environment. Ventilary support is directed towards maintaining the arterial PO_2 preferably above 50–60 torr and avoiding acidaemia. This frequently is not accomplished. Current ventilatory approaches to infants with the full blown syndrome aim at producing marked respiratory alkalosis (34). In all instances the inspired oxygen concentration is 100%. Several studies have shown that maintaining the arterial PCO_2 as close to 20 torr as possible and the arterial pH greater than 7.5 improves peripheral oxygenation significantly. This usually is accomplished by moderately rapid "hyperventilation" (rates of 100–150/min). In all instances the infants are paralysed; the use of curare is suggested, initially at least, since curare releases histamine. Recent studies in lambs (35) have shown that the pH rather than PCO_2 is "critical" in improving pulmonary blood flow and thereby oxygenation. These infants are extremely brittle and, once a reasonably satisfactory ventilation pattern has been established, it generally should not be changed except in very slow movements.

A far simpler manner in which pulmonary blood flow and thereby oxygenation could be improved would be to administer a specific pulmonary vasodilating drug. Unfortunately no such agent currently exists. Several agents have been tried, including tolazoline (34) and PGI_2 (36). Both have significant systemic effects in many infants and, although somewhat useful, are not always beneficial. This is particularly true of PGI_2 which has very dramatic systemic vasodilatory effects. The more specific effects of PGD_2 in animals has led us to undertake a clinical trial with this agent (S. J. Soifer and M. A. Heymann, unpublished observations). Unfortunately, in the few infants treated so far, the responses have not been as dramatic as in the animals. The more recent findings relating to blockade of leukotrienes and the dramatic increases in pulmonary blood flow in close-to-term fetal lambs suggest that this avenue may be worth exploring more actively.

Ductus Arteriosus

Physiology

Several studies have shown the importance of an increase in oxygen tension as a stimulus for muscular closure of the ductus arteriosus after birth (37). *In vitro* experiments on isolated ductus arteriosus have suggested that oxygen constricts the ductus arteriosus by a direct action on the medial smooth muscle cells (38). However, the release of vasoactive substances such as acetylcholine, bradykinin or catecholamines also may contribute to closure of the ductus arteriosus under physiological conditions (37,38).

Since stimulation of smooth muscle contraction by prostaglandins had been shown to require oxygen, Coceani and Olley (39) investigated the possibility that prostaglandins play a role in postnatal constriction of the ductus arteriosus. *In vitro* studies using isolated ductus arteriosus strips from close-to-term fetal lambs showed that exogenous PGE_1 and PGE_2 dilate, rather than constrict, the ductus arteriosus. More recently, PGI_2 also has been shown to dilate the ductus arteriosus (40). However, the fetal ductus arteriosus is significantly more sensitive to PGE_2 than PGI_2 or its metabolites (41). Administering inhibitors of prostaglandin synthesis *in vitro* or *in vivo* to pregnant animals near term constricts the ductus arteriosus in the fetuses (42,43). Therefore, we have considered that prostaglandins play an active role in maintaining the ductus arteriosus in a relaxed and thereby dilated state during normal fetal life and that the ductus arteriosus is not merely a passive conduit as was previously thought.

The exact sites of origin of the prostaglandins responsible for maintaining the fetal ductus arteriosus dilated *in vivo* are not clearly established. Prostaglandins are formed intramurally by the ductus arteriosus (40) and therefore may exert their action locally on the muscle cells. Prostaglandins are detectable only in very low concentrations, if at all, in the plasma of adults and are not thought to act as circulating hormones (with the possible exception of PGI_2) because of their rapid clearance by catabolism in the lungs. However, the fetus has high circulating concentrations of prostaglandins, particularly PGE_2 (44). This probably results from the low fetal pulmonary blood flow and the consequently reduced prostaglandin catabolism in the lungs of the fetus, as well as placental production. Therefore, PGE_2 probably plays a hormonal role in the fetus and, since the ductus arteriosus is most sensitive to PGE_2, probably is involved in circulatory control, particularly in maintaining the ductus arteriosus in a dilated state during normal fetal life.

At birth, the placental source of PGE_2 production is removed and the increase in pulmonary blood flow from about 8% of combined ventricular output in the fetus to 100% of the cardiac output in the neonate would allow almost complete removal of any circulating PGE_2, thus enabling the ductus arteriosus to constrict in response to stimuli such as an increase in oxygen environment or the release of a vasoactive substance such as bradykinin. It thus appears that physiological patency or closure of the ductus arteriosus represents a balance between the constricting effects of oxygen and perhaps certain vasoconstrictor substances and the relaxing effects of several prostaglandins.

Pathophysiology

A major clinical problem encountered in perinatal practice is failure of the ductus arteriosus to close normally after birth in preterm infants (45,46). Several factors are involved. The constrictor response of the ductus arteriosus to increased oxygen develops over about the last third of gestation. In young fetal lambs there is little or no response and, as gestation advances, the response occurs at a progressively lower PO_2 and is progressively greater (38,47). Similarly, the sensitivity of the ductus arteriosus to the dilatating effects of PGE_2 and PGI_2 decreases with advancing gestational age (47); the ductus arteriosus in the immature infant is therefore more likely to remain patent than in the term infant. This maturational change in sensitivity can be accelerated in immature fetal animals by the administration of corticosteroids (48). Also catabolism of PGE_2 by the fetal lung varies with gestational age (49); the less mature lung is less capable of metabolizing PGE_2 than is the mature lung. All these factors acting together likely are responsible for the increased incidence of persistent patency of the ductus arteriosus in preterm infants.

Management

Knowledge of the factors responsible for controlling the state of constriction or relaxation of the ductus arteriosus has recently been applied in several clinical situations in newborn infants. Prostaglandin E_1 or E_2 has been infused in infants with a variety of congenital malformations in whom it is critical to maintain the ductus arteriosus in as dilated a state as possible (50,51). These malformations include right ventricular outflow obstructive lesions such as pulmonary atresia, left ventricular outflow obstructive lesions such as coarctation of the aorta, and transposition of the great arteries. Prostaglandin E_1 is mainly used, and generally only for short periods of time, to stabilize infants prior to surgery, either palliative or corrective.

Persistent patency of the ductus occurs in 50-80% of preterm infants, particularly those under 1000 g birthweight. In many, significant haemodynamic disturbances occur and therefore indomethacin was introduced in the management of these infants (52). Rather than treating the consequences of the left-to-right shunt through the ductus arteriosus, use of indomethacin generally leads to closure of the ductus arteriosus. Only rare significant side-effects have been reported, and more recently earlier treatment and a more aggressive approach appear to have even greater benefits (53).

Acknowledgement

This work was supported in part by a grant from the US Public Health Service, Program Project Grant HL 24056.

References

1. Rudolph, A. M. and Heymann, M. A. (1970). *Circulat. Res.* **26**, 289–299.
2. Heymann, M. A., Creasy, R. K. and Rudolph, A. M. (1973). *In:* "Proceedings of the Sir Joseph Barcroft Centenary Symposium: Fetal and Neonatal Physiology", (Comline, K. S., Cross, K. W., Dawes, G. S. and Nathanielsz, P. W., eds) pp. 129–135. Cambridge University Press, Cambridge, UK.
3. Sidi, D., Kuipers, J. R. G., Heymann, M. A. and Rudolph, A. M. (1983). *Pediat. Res.* **17**, 254–258.
4. Cassin, S., Dawes, G. S., Mott, J. C., Ross, B. B. and Strang, L. B. (1964). *J. Physiol.* **171**, 61–79.
5. Colebatch, H. J. H., Dawes, G. S., Goodwin, J. W. and Nadeau, R. A. (1965). *J. Physiol.* **178**, 544–562.
6. Lewis, A. B., Heymann, M. A. and Rudolph, A. M. (1976). *Circulat. Res.* **39**, 536–541.
7. Heymann, M. A., Rudolph, A. M., Nies, A. S. and Melmon, K. L. (1969). *Circulat. Res.* **25**, 521–534.
8. Rudolph, A. M. and Yuan, S. (1966). *J. Clin. Invest.* **45**, 399–411.
9. Campbell, A. G. M., Cockburn, F., Dawes, G. S. and Milligan, J. E. (1967). *J. Physiol.* **192**, 111–122.
10. Cassin, S., Dawes, G. S. and Ross, B. B. (1964). *J. Physiol.* **171**, 80–89.
11. Berkov, S. (1974). *Circulat. Res.* **35**, 256–261.
12. Hyman, A., Heymann, M. A., Levin, D. L. and Rudolph, A. M. (1975). *Circulation* **52**, II-132.
13. Davidson, D., Stalcup, S. A. and Mellins, R. B. (1981). *Circulat. Res.* **48**, 286–291.
14. Gryglewski, R. J. (1980). *CIBA Found. Symp.* **78**, 147–164.
15. Tyler, T. L., Leffler, C. W. and Cassin, S. (1977). *Chest* **72S**, 271S–273S.
16. Cassin, S., Winikor, I., Tod, M., Phillips, J., Frisinger, S., Jordan, J. and Gibbs, C. (1981). *Pediat. Pharmacol.* **1**, 197–207.
17. Tripp, M. E., Drummond, W. H., Heymann, M. A. and Rudolph, A. M. (1980). *Pediat. Res.* **14**, 1311–1315.
18. Gryglewski, R. J., Korbut, R. and Ocetkiewicz, A. (1978). *Nature* **273**, 765–767.

19. Leffler, C. W., Hessler, J. R. and Terrango, N. A. (1980). *Am. J. Physiol.* **238**, H282–H286.
20. Leffler, C. W., Tyler, T. L. and Cassin, S. (1978). *Am. J. Physiol.* **234**, H346–H351.
21. Cassin, S., Tod, M., Philips, J., Frisinger, J., Jordan, J. and Gibbs, C. (1981). *Am. J. Physiol.* **240**, H755–H760.
22. Soifer, S. J., Morin, F. C. III and Heymann, M. A. (1982). *J. Pediat.* **100**, 458–463.
23. Soifer, S. J., Morin, F. C. III, Kaslow, D. C. and Heymann, M. A. (1983). *J. Develop. Physiol.* **5**, 237–250.
24. Schwartz, L. W., Osburn, B. I. and Frick, O. L. (1974). *J. Allergy Clin. Immunol.* **56**, 381–386.
25. Ahmed, T. and Oliver, W., Jr. (1983). *Am. Rev. Resp. Dis.* **127**, 566–571.
26. Heymann, M. A., Soifer, S. J., Loitz, R. and Roman, C. (1984). *Pediat. Res.* **18**, 347A.
27. Levin, D. L., Heymann, M. A., Kitterman, J. A., Gregory, G. A., Phibbs, R. H. and Rudolph, A. M. (1976). *J. Pediat.* **89**, 626–630.
28. Levin, D. L., Fixler, D. E., Morriss, F. C. and Tyson, J. (1978). *J. Pediat.* **92**, 478–483.
29. Murphy, J. D., Rabinovitch, M., Goldstein, J. D. and Reid, L. M. (1981). *J. Pediat.* **98**, 962–967.
30. Goldberg, S. J., Levy, R. A., Siassi, B. and Betten, J. (1971). *Pediatrics* **48**, 528–533.
31. Levin, D. L., Hyman, A. I., Heymann, M. A. and Rudolph, A. M. (1978). *J. Pediat.* **92**, 265–269.
32. Levin, D. L., Mills, L. J. and Weinberg, A. J. (1979). *Circulation* **60**, 360–364.
33. Levin, D. L., Weinberg, A. G. and Peskin, R. M. (1983). *J. Pediat.* **102**, 299–303.
34. Drummond, W. H., Gregory, G. A., Heymann, M. A. and Phibbs, R. A. (1981). *J. Pediat.* **98**, 603–611.
35. Schreiber, M. D., Heymann, M. A. and Soifer, S. J. (1984). *Pediat. Res.* **18**, 347A.
36. Lock, J. E., Olley, P. M., Coceani, F., Swyer, P. R. and Rowe, R. D. (1979). *Lancet* **i**, 1343–1345.
37. Heymann, M. A. and Rudolph, A. M. (1975). *Physiol. Rev.* **55**, 62–78.
38. McMurphy, D. M., Heymann, M. A., Rudolph, A. M. and Melmon, K. L. (1972). *Pediat. Res.* **6**, 231–238.
39. Coceani, F. and Olley, P. M. (1973). *Can. J. Physiol. Pharmacol.* **51**, 220–225.
40. Clyman, R. I., Mauray, F., Koerper, M. A., Wiemer, F., Heymann, M. A. and Rudolph, A. M. (1978). *Prostaglandins* **16**, 633–642.
41. Clyman, R. I., Mauray, F., Roman, C. and Rudolph, A. M. (1978). *Prostaglandins* **16**, 259–264.
42. Sharpe, G. L., Larsson, K. S. and Thalme, B. (1975). *Prostaglandins* **9**, 585–596.
43. Heymann, M. A. and Rudolph, A. M. (1976). *Circulat. Res.* **38**, 418–422.
44. Challis, J. R. G., Dilley, S. R., Robinson, J. S. and Thorburn, G. D. (1976). *Prostaglandins* **11**, 1041–1052.
45. Kitterman, J. A., Edmunds, L. H. Jr., Gregory, G. A., Heymann, M. A., Tooley, W. H. and Rudolph, A. M. (1972). *N. Engl. J. Med.* **287**, 473–477.
46. Jacob, J., Gluck, L., Di Sessa, T., Edwards, D., Kulovich, M., Kurlinski, J., Merrit, T. A. and Friedman, W. F. (1980). *J. Pediat.* **96**, 79–87.
47. Clyman, R. I. (1980). *Semin. Perinatol.* **4**, 115–124.
48. Clyman, R. I., Mauray, F., Roman, C., Rudolph, A. M. and Heymann, M. A. (1981). *J. Pediat.* **98**, 126–128.
49. Clyman, R. I., Mauray, F., Heymann, M. A. and Roman, C. (1981). *Prostaglandins* **21**, 505–513.
50. Heymann, M. A. and Clyman, R. I. (1982). *Pharmacotherapy* **2**, 148–155.

51. Freed, M. D., Heymann, M. A., Lewis, A. B., Roehl, S. L. and Kensey, R. C. (1981). *Circulation* **64**, 899–905.
52. Heymann, M. A., Rudolph, A. M. and Silverman, N. H. (1976). *N. Engl. J. Med.* **295**, 530–533.
53. Mahony, L., Carnero, V., Brett, C., Heymann, M. A. and Clyman, R. I. (1982). *N. Engl. J. Med.* **306**, 506–510.

Management of Ventilation

A. C. Bryan, S. England, J. Fisher and M. H. Bryan

Respiratory Physiology, Hospital for Sick Children,
Toronto, Ontario, Canada

"Indeed there was great difficulty in inducing Oliver to take upon himself the office of respiration, a troublesome practice, but one which nature has rendered essential to our easy existence . . ." (Dickens).

We generally regard "the office of respiration to be a troublesome practice" because of either underlying parenchymal disease or abnormalities of respiratory control. The purpose of this paper is to show that these situations are seriously complicated by the unique behaviour of the infant's chest wall.

At birth infants must assume three new responsibilities: they must exchange gas with the environment, control body temperature and acquire nutrients — three responsibilities that are curiously interrelated. The term newborn generally assumes these burdens easily but the preterm does not. We have learned to cope quite well with the thermal and nutrient problems, essentially by marsupializing the infant; an incubator is but a pouch and preterm nutrients as carefully tailored as kangaroo milk. We are often less successful in managing gas exchange.

The problem starts with the first breath; the air–liquid interface has to be moved rapidly from the oropharynx to the alveolus to establish a gas exchange surface. To draw an air–liquid interface down tubes of ever decreasing cross-sections requires substantial force. Based on anatomic measurements, Avery and Mead (1) calculated that the opening pressures should be about 25–$30 \, cmH_2O$ and these have generally been confirmed by measurements by Karlberg et al. (2) and Vyas et al. (3). The pressures required are critically dependent on the surface tension at the air–liquid interface. Nilsson et al. (4) have shown that in the absence of surfactant there are epithelial lesions in the terminal airways within a few minutes. Presumably the forces required to advance the interface are greater than the force necessary to overdistend the terminal airways, disrupting the epithelium. Even when alveolar opening is successful there is a rather gradual accretion of lung volume, presumably reflecting the resorption of lung liquid and progressive

The Physiological Development of the Fetus and Newborn
ISBN 0 12 389080 2

Copyright © 1985 by Academic Press, London.
All rights of reproduction in any form reserved.

alveolar recruitment. The rise in PaO_2 is also a gradual process reflecting this change in volume and presumably also a less than instantaneous transition from fetal to adult pulmonary circulation (5). The pattern of breathing in the immediately postnatal period has been studied by Fisher *et al.* (6) and Mortola *et al.* (7) and is quite unique, consisting of deep breaths, short periods of breath-holding and great variability in both tidal volume and frequency. The breath-holding occurs at high lung volume and is of considerable interest. The pressure-volume curve of the lung has a third dimension, time, as alveolar recruitment is time-dependent. Furthermore, if the chest wall relaxes against a closed glottis, the increased alveolar pressure may assist the resorption of lung liquid. Both the variability and the breath-holding decrease substantially in the ensuing few hours. Rather surprisingly, these authors showed little differences in pattern between vaginal delivery and nonlabour caesarean section infants, except for a slightly larger V_T after vaginal delivery. We have subsequently found that in nonlabour caesarean section infants a very unusual breathing pattern persists for days. Flow volume curves reveal a markedly braked expiratory flow with a time constant sometimes approaching 2 s, compared to the normal 0.2 s. Presumably this braking is glottal and represents a subclinical grunt.

The whole problem of maintenance of a functional residual capacity (FRC) in infants is puzzling. Because the infant chest wall is highly compliant, the static passive balance of force would dictate a low FRC, while the dynamically determined end expiratory level is about 40% of total lung capacity, similar to the FRC in the adult. This has obvious advantages for the stability of terminal units and increasing the oxygen store. A number of mechanisms appear to be operating to maintain the elevated end expiratory position. Olinsky *et al.* (22) suggested that the infant did not have time to expire to passive FRC, but based this on an unrealistic estimate of airways resistance. Using a more realistic value for the passive time constant of 0.2 s and using the equation of Vinegar *et al.* (8),

$$V = \frac{V_T}{e(T_e/RC)-1},\tag{1}$$

where V is the "trapped" gas, V_T the tidal volume, T_e expiratory time, R and C resistance and compliance, this can only account for about 2 ml of "trapped" gas. But expiration in the infant is not passive. Lopes *et al.* (9) have shown, in infants, persistent activity of both the intercostals and the diaphragm throughout expiration, effectively stiffening the system. While this appears energetically costly, it is pliometric work. In addition, studies in three species of neonatal animals have shown brisk laryngeal adductor muscle activity during expiration, which is not present in adults (10–12). Laryngeal adduction will effectively increase the resistance of the system. Thus the active time constant is substantially higher than the passive time constant. This can be seen by comparing the slope of the passive flow volume curve with the slope during spontaneous expiration. A time constant of about 0.4 s would account for about 10 ml of "trapped" gas which is about the right value for the difference between the dynamic end expiratory level and the passive FRC.

However, a paradox remains: if maintaining an elevated end expiratory position is important, why is this lost during rapid eye movement (REM) sleep, the predominant behavioural state of the infant? Henderson-Smart and Read (13) showed a 30% fall in thoracic gas volume when infants went from nonrapid eye movement (NREM) to REM sleep. Following the above argument, the reduction of expiratory intercostal, diaphragmatic and laryneal adductor activity in REM sleep would shorten the time constant and T_e is shorter than in NREM sleep. The main penalty the infant pays for the low lung volume is the precipitous fall in PaO_2 during even brief apnoea as a consequence of a low oxygen store. The actual end expiratory volume in REM is characteristically very variable, presumably secondary to the variability of both the relevant muscle activity and T_e. The 30% fall reported by Henderson-Smart and Read (13) probably represents the extreme and the mean end expiratory volume in REM is substantially higher.

The plasticity of the end-expiratory level is also of significance in lung disease. A disease such as respiratory distress syndrome is characterized by a shorter time constant. From equation (1), it can be seen that this will reduce the amount of "trapped" gas and the infant's response to this is to increase the expiratory time constant by grunting. The more serious implication is the effect of mechanical ventilation on lung volume. In the acute stage it is difficult to build up lung volume because the time constant is very short. It can be done by shortening T_e either by reversing the inspiration:expiration ratio or increasing the respiratory rate. The problem, and this is particularly true after the acute phase, is that the distribution of compliances is nonuniform. The most healthy regions of the lung will have the greatest compliance and the longest time constants, which will lead to trapping, potential overdistension and rupture. It is important to note that this "occult PEEP" is not registered on the ventilator pressure gauge.

Dynamics

The highly compliant chest wall of the infant also has a profound effect on the dynamics of breathing. The caudal surface of the lung is driven by the diaphragm and the remaining surface by the intercostals and rib cage. The problem is that these two generators oppose one another. Inspiratory action of one lowers pleural pressure and has an expiratory action on the other. The magnitude of this paradoxical motion depends on the relative compliance of the rib cage and the lung, as the diaphragm acts on these in parallel and divides their displacements accordingly. In the adult, roughly half the total impedance of the respiratory system, thus about half the force generated is dissipated in moving the chest wall rather than the lung. The problem for the infant is that the passive impedance of the chest wall is very much less than the lung. Thus, it is easier for the diaphragm to reduce the volume of the rib cage than increase the volume of the lung. The flaw in this analysis is the use of a passive chest wall compliance, because in reality the system is not passive. The intercostal muscles have force–length characteristics which reduce the compliance of the rib cage progressively during distortion. Distortion of the ribs from their relaxation configuration also stiffens the system. Furthermore, as the diaphragm descends it elevates and everts the lower rib cage using the abdominal contents as a fulcrum. Thus breathing is not impossible, it is just very difficult, particularly in REM sleep when the intercostals are substantially inhibited. Estimates of the work done on the chest wall in REM sleep in infants are indirect but very impressive. The moving time average or total electromyographic power increases 50–450% (14). Calculating from wall motion and transdiaphragmatic pressure (P_{di}), Heldt *et al.* (15) estimated a 90–400% increase in work. Bellemare and Grassino (16,17) have calculated in adults a critical tension time index $TTDi$ which is the product of T_i/T_{tot} and P_{di}/P_{dimax}. Operating at a $TTDi$ above 0.15 the diaphragm inevitably fatigues. During tidal breathing in adults the $TTDi$ in about 0.03. We have made some assumptions about P_{dimax} in infants and measured P_{di}. We estimate that in NREM sleep $TTDi$ is about 0.076 and in REM 0.12 which is perilously close to the "critical" $TTDi$. If lung disease is superimposed, increasing the work that has to be done on the lung, this critical threshold is readily exceeded and fatigue may ensue.

The diagnosis of diaphragmatic fatigue is controversial (14). We have used spectral frequency analysis of the surface diaphragmatic electromyograms (EMG) in infants and to our satisfaction convinced ourselves that it is an excellent index of impending fatigue. However, it has been said that "an EMG power spectrum is something nobody understands! It is not a good measure of anything, and I don't think it ever will be because it is too complicated" (18). Despite this strong statement spectral frequency shifts correlate well with independent measures of fatigue (17). A more direct way of assessing fatigue is to examine the relationship of the electrical activity to the diaphragm (E_{di}) and the resulting trans-diaphragmatic pressure (P_{di}). In infants without chest wall distortion there is a linear increase in P_{di} as E_{di} increases. In contrast, in the presence of marked distortion increasing E_{di} produces little or no increase in P_{di}, inferring that the diaphragm is incapable of responding to increasing stimulation due to fatigue.

In response to fatigue the infant adopts several different strategies, very similar to the adult. They may alternate drive between the intercostal and the diaphragm (19). They may reduce the minute volume and let the $PaCO_2$ rise. They will shorten the T_i/T_{tot} ratio to get a longer expiratory rest. We suspect that they sometimes carry this to extremes and that some apnoeas are simply the results of a very long T_e. The strongest evidence for this is the clinical story of apnoea. Apnoea is often proportional to the respiratory load and removing the load stopps the apnoea. Substrate shortage, hypoglycaemia, hypoxia and hypocalcaemia present with apnoea. Treatment with CPAP stabilizes the chest wall and reduces diaphragmatic work. Treatment with aminophylline has been shown to alleviate muscle fatigue.

In marked contrast to this scenario, Thach and Stark (20,21) have produced evidence suggesting that most apnoeic episodes are obstructive in origin. They have shown that the "collapsing pressure" in a relaxed upper airway is quite small and that episodes are most common when the head is flexed, further narrowing the airway. We have observed "obstructive" and "mixed" apnoeas but in our experience these are rare. These differences may depend on measurement techniques or nursing practices. But the problem is not a trivial one because if "obstructive" apnoeas are as common as is claimed they will be missed by monitors which detect chest wall motion.

References

1. Avery, M. E. and Mead, J. (1959). *Am. J. Dis. Child.* **97**, 517.
2. Karlberg, P., Cherry, R. B., Escardo, F. E. and Koch, G. (1962). *Acta Paediat. Scand.* **51**, 121-136.
3. Vyas, H., Milner, A. D. and Hopkins, I. E. (1981). *J. Pediat.* **99**, 787.
4. Nilsson, R., Grossman, G. and Robertson, B. (1978). *Pediat. Res.* **12**, 249-255.
5. Koch, G. (1968). *Acta Paediat.* Suppl. **181**.
6. Fisher, J. T., Mortola, J. P., Smith, J. B., Fox, G. S. and Weeks, S. (1982). *Am. Rev. Resp. Dis.* **125**, 650-657.
7. Mortola, J. P., Fisher, J. T., Smith, J. B., Fox, G. S., Weeks, S. and Willis, D. (1982). *J. Appl. Physiol. Resp. Env. Exc. Physiol.* **52**, 716-724.
8. Vinegar, A., Sinnett, E. E. and Leith, D. E. (1979). *J. Appl. Physiol. Resp. Env. Exc. Physiol.* **46**, 867-871.
9. Lopes, J. M., Muller, N. L., Bryan, M. H. and Bryan, A. C. (1981). *J. Appl. Physiol. Resp. Env. Exc. Physiol.* **51**, 830-834.
10. Harding, R., Johnson, P. and McClellend, M. E. (1980). *Resp. Physiol.* **40**, 165-179.
11. Farber, J. P. (1978). *Resp. Physiol.* **35**, 189-201.
12. England, S. J. (1984). *Fed. Proc.* **43**, 645A.
13. Henderson-Smart, D. J. and Read, D. J. C. (1979). *J. Appl. Physiol. Resp. Env. Exc. Physiol.* **46**, 1081-1085.
14. Muller, N., Gulston, G., Cade, C., Whitton, J., Froese, A. B., Bryan, M. H. and Bryan, A. C. (1979). *J. Appl. Physiol.* **46**, 688-695.
15. Heldt, G. P., Goodrich, P. D. and McIlroy, M. B. (1981). *Pediat. Res.* **15**, 721A.
16. Bellemare, F. and Grassino, A. (1982). *J. Appl. Physiol. Resp. Env. Exc. Physiol.* **53**, 1190-1195.
17. Bellemare, F. and Grassino, A. (1982). *J. Appl. Physiol. Resp. Env. Exc. Physiol.* **53**, 1196-1206.
18. Stephens, J. A. (1980). *In:* "Muscle Fatigue: Physiological Mechanisms", CIBA Found. Symp. 82. Pitman Medical, London.
19. Lopes, J. M., Muller, N. L., Bryan, M. H. and Bryan, A. C. (1981). *J. Appl. Physiol. Resp. Env. Exc. Physiol.* **51**, 547-551.
20. Thach, B. T. and Stark, A. R. (1976). *J. Pediat.* **89**, 982-985.
21. Stark, A. R. and Thach, B. T. (1979). *J. Pediat.* **94**, 275-281.
22. Olinsky, A., Bryan, M. H. and Bryan, A. C. (1974). *J. Appl. Physiol.* **36**, 426-429.

Intra-uterine Nutrition and the Newborn

Satish C. Kalhan and Carol A. Gilfillan

Department of Pediatrics, Case Western Reserve University, School of
Medicine, Cleveland Metropolitan General Hospital, Cleveland, Ohio, USA

The process of birth, with the abrupt cessation of nutrient supply from the mother, is the single major event in life testing the ability of the human newborn for extra-uterine existence. Therefore, the newborn infant is required to mobilize his endogenous sources of fuel while at the same time developing the necessary responses for adaptation to extra-uterine life. The capacity for independent subsistence is a function both of intra-uterine nutritional endowment as well as the ability of the newborn infant to assimilate the nutrients provided either enterally or parenterally. Thus, nutrition in the newborn should be viewed in the context of the ability of the infant to mobilize endogenous substrate during periods of fasting and to utilize effectively exogenously provided nutrients. The former is a consequence of the intra-uterine environment, while the latter is the result of extra-uterine development affected in part by the intra-uterine aberrations. In this review, we will examine first the effects of intra-uterine nutrition on the ability of the infant to mobilize endogenous substrates and then briefly review the neonatal development changes which have direct bearing on assimilation of nutrients. The recent development of safe stable isotopic tracer methods and improved mass-spectrometric methods has permitted these investigations which were not previously possible.

The alterations in the intra-uterine metabolic milieu that effect fetal and newborn infants' nutrition can be described as follows:

    1. *Surfeit* of substrates as in *diabetes mellitus* in pregnancy. When maternal diabetes exists, the fetus is exposed continuously or intermittently to excessive quantities of substrates as a result of increased transport from the mother. Intermittent hyperglycaemia results in fetal hyperinsulinaemia and enhanced deposition of hepatic glycogen and adipose tissue triglycerides. The overall consequences are fetal "overnutrition" and fetal macrosomia.

The Physiological Development of the Fetus and Newborn
ISBN 0 12 389080 2

Copyright © 1985 by Academic Press, London.
All rights of reproduction in any form reserved.

2. *In utero* privation resulting in *intra-uterine growth retardation* and small for gestational age infant. Decreased delivery of substrates as a result of "placental insufficiency" in humans, or as a consequence of maternal starvation or ligation of the uterine artery in studies of animals, results in decreased hepatic glycogen accumulation, diminished corporal and head growth. Such an infant is born with reduced mobilizable depots of glycogen and adipose tissue triglycerides.

3. Prematurity: As the major accretion of nutrients and corporal growth occurs in the later part of pregnancy, preterm delivery of the infant will result in small, albeit appropriate, for gestational age infant. However, these infants are born with inadequate mobilizable fuel stores; at the same time their caloric requirements for growth are increased.

The responses to the extra-uterine environment have been examined in the context of the above three groups of newborn. In the following discussion, first the response during fasting will be presented followed by responses to alimentation in the 3 groups of newborn outlined above. The discussion in the most part will be limited to the available data in the human.

Fasting Metabolism in the Newborn

The response to fasting in the first few hours after birth has been evaluated by a number of investigators. After birth the plasma glucose declines in all infants and this is followed by a slow rise over the next few hours (1,2). There is a corresponding increase in the concentration of free fatty acids, glycerol and ketones. In the macrosomic neonate of a diabetic mother, these changes are exaggerated depending upon the extent of regulation of maternal metabolism. In recent years, we have quantified glucose turnover rates using stable isotope tracer method in normal infants, infants of diabetic mothers and infants born with intra-uterine growth retardation (IUGR) (3–5). The isotopic technique used involved infusion of a glucose tracer, labelled with a stable isotope of carbon (^{13}C) or hydrogen (^2H), into a peripheral vein at a constant rate and measurement of isotopic enrichment of plasma glucose by mass-spectrometric methods. The latter represents the magnitude of tracer dilution by the endogenously produced glucose. Initially, we used [$1\text{-}^{13}C$] glucose tracer for these studies; more recently we have utilized [$6,6\text{-}^2H_2$] glucose tracer.

Glucose Production Rate during Fasting

Results of studies on plasma glucose levels and glucose production rate in newborns are given in Table 1. Soon after birth, the plasma glucose concentration of the normal newborn infant stabilizes so that, at 4 h of age, the mean plasma glucose concentration in the normal infants is 57 ± 12.1 mg/dl (mean $\pm$ SD). In contrast, the plasma glucose concentration in the macrosomic infant of diabetic mother is 45 ± 11.4 mg/dl. The rate of glucose turnover measured by the tracer isotope dilution technique in the normal infant is 4.47 ± 0.75 mg/kg/min. Such estimate of the systemic glucose production rate expressed as oxygen equivalents

Table 1. Plasma glucose and glucose production rates (GPR) in newborn infants

	< 12 h		1 day		> 2 days	
	Glucose (mg/dl)	GPR (mg/kg/min)	Glucose (mg/dl)	GPR (mg/kg/min)	Glucose (mg/dl)	GPR (mg/kg/min)
Normal	57±12.1	4.47±0.75 (9)	52±12.1	4.55±0.72 (8)	60±6.2	4.07±1.05 (7)
Infants of diabetic mothers	45±11.4	2.94±0.75 (8)			65±12.4	5.03±1.63 (5)

Values are means±SD, ( )=n. $*P < 0.001$ when compared with normals.

would be equated to 3.4 ml O_2/kg/min. Thus, complete oxidation of endogenously produced glucose would account for 50% of the oxygen consumed (estimated as 6.4 ml/kg/min) by the normal human newborn infant. In contrast, the macrosomic infant of diabetic mother not only maintains a lower blood glucose concentration, but also has decreased rates of glucose production and utilization (Table 1) at this age. Such an infant also has lower levels of circulating alternative fuels such as free fatty acids and ketones, although there are surfeits of hepatic glycogen and adipose tissue triglycerides (1,2). Rigid antenatal regulation of maternal metabolism tends to normalize the infant's blood glucose level as well as the rates of glucose production and utilization (5). However, only very few of such observations have been made in very small groups of patients (5,6).

Over the next few days, with the introduction of feeding, the normal infant continues to maintain plasma glucose between 40 and 60 mg/dl during fasting. The endogenous rate of glucose turnover also remains either unchanged or, if at all, a small but insignificant decline is observed. In contrast, as the influence of maternal diabetes on the infant decreases, and with neonatal adaptation, the plasma glucose concentration and the systemic glucose production rate increase and reach that observed in the normal infants.

The plasma glucose concentration and glucose turnover rates during fasting in the preterm infants and infants with intra-uterine growth retardation were in the same range as in normal infants (see Table 3 later). Thus, intra-uterine malnutrition and early preterm delivery does not limit their ability to mobilize glucose. However, their capacity to maintain euglycaemia for prolonged periods of fasting may be limited.

Urea Synthesis in the Newborn Infant

As protein catabolism is an important component of total energy metabolism and provides the carbon skeleton for gluconeogenesis, we next examined the effects of fetal macrosomia as a result of maternal diabetes on rates of urea synthesis. Eight normal newborn infants and 3 infants of diabetic mothers were studied during the first 2 days of life. A nonrecycling tracer [$^{15}N_2$] urea was used at a

Table 2. Rates of urea synthesis in newborn infants

	Plasma urea (mg/dl)	Urea synthesis rate (mg/kg/h)
Normals ($n=8$)	19.0 ± 5.54	12.27 ± 3.77
Infants of diabetic mother ($n=3$)	20.7 ± 3.79	14.22 ± 1.83

Values are means ± SD.

constant infusion rate and the urea synthesis rate was calculated during isotopic steady state by tracer dilution. As shown in Table 2, both plasma urea concentration and the rates of urea synthesis were similar in the 2 groups indicating that protein catabolism does not appear to be effected by the hormonal perturbations and macrosomia caused by diabetes in pregnancy. The effects of undernutrition in IUGR infants on urea metabolism are under investigations at present.

Responses to Nutrient Supplement

Parenteral

The infant's response to parenteral administration of glucose, amino acids and fat have been studied by a number of investigators. The impetus for such studies has been not only to study normal physiology, but also to develop alternate methods of providing nutrition in infants who cannot be fed enterally. Again using stable isotopic tracer methods, we have examined the effects of intra-uterine nutrition on regulation of glucose metabolism in the newborn infants (Table 3). The responses of mammalian newborn to exogenously administered glucose has been shown to be at variance from those in adults (7–9). In part such differences depend upon the species studied, the gestational maturity and the clinical status of the infant. Clinical studies have shown a tendency towards significant hyperglycaemia particularly in low birthweight human infants and in newborn

Table 3. Effect of glucose infusion on endogenous glucose production in newborn infants

	Basal		During glucose infusion		
	Plasma glucose (mg/dl)	Ra (mg/kg/min)	Peak glucose (mg/dl)	Total Ra (mg/kg/min)	Endogenous Ra (mg/kg/min)
Normal (8)	56 ± 5.6	3.44 ± 0.08	90 ± 4.2	5.11 ± 0.18	0.97 ± 0.18
Preterm (5)	42 ± 2.9	3.22 ± 0.17	81 ± 5.1	5.25 ± 0.42	1.43 ± 0.48
IUGR (7)	52 ± 4.1	4.03 ± 0.26	71 ± 3.7	5.41 ± 0.36	2.12 ± 0.45
IDM* (5)	43 ± 3.7	3.35 ± 0.26	76 ± 8.4	5.53 ± 0.16	1.21 ± 0.09

Abbreviations: Ra = rate of appearance of glucose; IUGR = intra-uterine growth retardation; IDM = infant of diabetic mother. Values are means ± SEM.
*Data of King et al. (5).

dogs, monkey and lambs (8-10). At least in human, the hyperglycaemia could be the result of associated clinical problems which may have caused increased circulating levels of counter-regulatory hormones. However, such data are not available at present. Using tracer isotope studies, Cowett *et al.* (9,11) and Varma *et al.* (7) have shown that the hyperglycaemia in lambs, dogs and in some human newborn infants could in part be attributed to the failure to suppress endogenous glucose production.

We have examined the hepatic regulatory responses to exogenously infused glucose in the human newborn again using a $[^2H_2]$ glucose tracer. The infants were studied in the basal state and then the effects of exogenously infused glucose at 4 mg/kg/min on hepatic glucose production were examined. In each instance, an isotopic steady state was achieved prior to and following glucose infusion so that glucose turnover could be calculated assuming steady state kinetics. The data are presented in Table 3. As shown, there was significant suppression of endogenous glucose production in all groups studied, although the magnitude of suppression varied in each group. These data are somewhat in contrast to those for adults where almost complete suppression of endogenous glucose production has been observed. However, major difference in study design exist. In our studies, at least, the rate of exogenously infused glucose was barely above the endogenous glucose production rate, particularly in the IUGR infants. However, a significant increase in insulin levels was seen in all infants.

The suppression of endogenous glucose production in response to glucose infusion in normal humans and animals is the result of the autoregulatory effect of glucose and the action of insulin on the liver. In the presence of a basal insulin concentration, infusion of exogenous glucose results in a 70-90% inhibition of hepatic glucose release. However, when insulin concentration is increased, complete suppression of glucose production occurs (12-16). The release of glucose by the human fetal liver has been shown to be autoregulatory in previous studies (17). Whether glucose effects hepatic glucose release in the neonate was examined

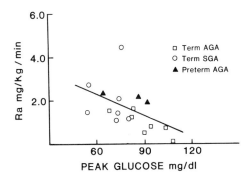

Figure 1. Relation between peak glucose concentration and endogenous glucose production rate ($r=0.51$, $P<0.05$). The values are expressed as the endogenous glucose production rate (Ra) *vs* the peak plasma glucose concentration achieved during glucose infusions of 4 mg/kg/min.

in the present study by correlating the peak glucose concentration achieved during glucose infusion with the endogenous glucose production (Fig. 1). A significant negative correlation was observed ($r = 0.51$, $P < 0.05$). Thus, glucose appears to be the major regulator of hepatic glucose production in the newborn infant. The persistent glucose release could then be due partly to the limitations of the tracer methods used. As the concentration of glycogen and glycolytic intermediates are higher in the newborn infants, the tracer will continue to be exchanged with these metabolites that are then released back into circulation as unlabelled glucose and appear as persistent glucose production. Finally, the failure of suppression observed in other studies could be due in part to the clinical status of subjects or animals studied. Thus, the human newborn can adapt to parenterally infused glucose by suppressing the production of endogenous glucose. In the most part, this phenomenon appears to be regulated by glucose in the presence of insulin, as has been observed in adults.

Fat and Amino Acids. Parenteral administration of fat and amino acids has become a routine clinical practice in neonatal units to provide calories in low birthweight infants. Administration of amino acids along with glucose has a synergistic effect on insulin secretion. Such a response has been observed in all infants irrespective of their nutritional status. Studies by a number of investigators have shown that newborn infants can tolerate the currently recommended dose of amino acids (less than 3 g/kg/day) without any problems.

Fat, administered as a 10% soybean oil emulsion (intralipid), is potentially a good source of nutrition. Administered parenterally, it can provide a greater number of calories in a small volume (1.1 cal/ml) as compared with glucose and amino acids. Because such a requirement exists primarily in low birthweight infants, the responses to administered triglycerides have been examined only in this population. Studies by Andrew et al. (18) and Gustafson et al. (19) show that intralipids are well tolerated by appropriate weight for gestational age infants who are greater than 33 weeks gestation. Premature infants of less than 33 weeks gestation had only moderate elevations of triglyceride and free fatty acids during intralipid infusion. In contrast, the infants with IUGR achieved higher peak levels of triglycerides and free fatty acids suggesting a slower rate of hydrolysis of triglycerides. The higher free fatty acid peak could be due to a decreased uptake of the free fatty acids released. However, studies by Sabel et al. (20,21) have shown that free fatty acids released are oxidized in small for age infants as evidenced by an increase in the oxygen consumption rate and a fall in the respiratory quotient. Fatty acid oxidation may be decreased in infants receiving prolonged parenteral amino acids due to the development of carnitine deficiency (22,23). As the newborn infant accumulates carnitine after birth (24), the nutrient solutions used for parenteral feeding contain no carnitine (23) and the human newborn infant does not appear to be able to synthesize carnitine from administered amino acids. The low birthweight infant in particular may develop carnitine deficiency in the absence of exogenous source of carnitine and thus limit his capacity to utilize fat as energy source.

Enteral feeding

After birth, systematic age-related changes in the gastro-intestinal hormonal responses have been observed in preterm and term infants. The presence of substrates in the gut is necessary for the adequate development of these responses. The role of these hormones in the assimilation of enterally administered nutrients is unclear. Studies in animals and humans suggest that the changes in hormonal response are associated with changes in structure and function of the gut. These data have been reviewed recently by Aynsley-Green (25).

In summary, antepartum nutritional aberrations have significant effects not only on the responses to fasting, but also upon the responses to enteral and parenteral nutrient administration in the newborn infant. An understanding of these physiological responses is required for the appropriate nutritional management of the newborn infant.

Acknowledgements

The cited work was supported by NIH grants HD 17336, HD 11089 and RR 00210. S.C.K. is the recipient of a Research Career Development Award, KO4 AM 00801 and C.A.G. is a recipient of a Clinical Associate Physician Grant from the NIH. The authors thank Ms Sandee Riedrich for her secretarial assistance.

References

1. Gentz, J., Kellum, M. and Persson, B. (1976). *Acta Paediat. Scand.* **65**, 445-454.
2. Kuhl, C., Andersen, G. E., Hertel, J. and Molsted-Pedersen, L. (1982). *Acta Paediat. Scand.* **71**, 19-25.
3. Kalhan, S. C., Savin, S. M. and Adam, P. A. J. (1976). *J. Clin. Endocrin. Metab.* **43**, 704-707.
4. Kalhan, S. C., Savin, S. M. and Adam, P. A. J. (1977). *N. Engl. J. Med.* **296**, 375-376.
5. King, K. C., Tserng, K.-Y. and Kalhan, S. C. (1982). *Pediat. Res.* **16**, 608-612.
6. Cowett, R. M., Susa, J. B., Giletti, B., Oh, W. and Schwartz, R. (1983). *Am. J. Obstet. Gynecol.* **146**, 781-786.
7. Varma, S., Nickerson, H., Cowan, J. S. and Hetenyi, Jr., G. (1973). *Metabolism* **11**, 1367-1375.
8. Sherwood, W. G., Hill, D. E. and Chance, G. W. (1977). *Pediat. Res.* **12**, 874-877.
9. Cowett, R. M., Susa, J. B., Oh, W. and Schwartz, R. (1978). *Pediat. Res.* **12**, 853-857.
10. Cowett, R. M., Oh, W., Pollak, A., Schwartz, R. and Stonestreet, B. S. (1979). *Pediat.* **63**, 389-396.
11. Cowett, R. M., Susa, J. B., Oh, W. and Schwartz, R. (1984). *Pediat. Res.* **18**, 74-79.
12. Keller, U. and Laccy, W. W. (1976). *J. Clin. Invest.* **58**, 1407-1418.
13. Bilbrey, G. L., Faloona, G. R., White, M. G. and Knochel, J. P. (1974). *J. Clin. Invest.* **53**, 841-847.
14. Sacaa, L., Hendler, R. and Sherwin, R. S. (1978). *J. Clin. Endocrin. Metab.* **47**, 1160-1163.
15. Rabinowitz, D. (1979). *J. Clin. Endocrin. Metab.* **48**, 171-175.
16. Sacca, L., Vitale, D., Cicala, M., Trimarco, B. and Ungaro, B. (1981). *Metabolism* **30**, 457-461.

17. Adam, P. A. J., Schwartz, A. L., Rahiala, E.-L. and Kekomarki, M. (1978). *Am. J. Physiol.* **234**, E560–E567.
18. Andrew, G., Chan, G. and Schiff, D. (1976). *J. Pediat.* **88**, 273–278.
19. Gustafson, A., Kjellmer, I., Olejard, R. and Victorin, L. (1972). *Acta Paediat. Scand.* **61**, 149–158.
20. Sabel, K.-G., Olegard, R., Mellander, M. and Hildingsson, K. (1982). *Acta Paediat. Scand.* **71**, 53–61.
21. Sabel, K.-G., Olegard, R., Hildingsson, K. and Karlberg, P. (1982). *Acta Paediat. Scand.* **71**, 63–69.
22. Penn, D., Schmidt-Sommerfeld, E. and Wolf, H. (1980). *Early Hum. Dev.* **4**, 23–24.
23. Schiff, D., Chan, G., Seccombe, D. and Hahn, P. (1979). *J. Pediat.* **95**, 1043–1046.
24. Schmidt-Sommerfeld, E., Novak, M., Penn, D., Wieser, P. B., Buch, M. and Hahn, P. (1978). *Paediat. Res.* **12**, 660–664.
25. Aynsley-Green, A. (1983). *J. Pediat. Gastro. Nut.* **2**, 418–427.

Blood Flow Velocity in the Fetal Aorta After β_2-Mimetic Agents

K. Vetter, S. Baer, F. Fallenstein, R. Huch and A. Huch

Department of Obstetrics and Gynaecology, University Hospital,
Zürich, Switzerland

Changes of fetal cardiovascular dynamics are used to monitor fetal condition. The study of human fetal blood flow appears to give a very sensitive image of the fetal state *in utero*. The combination of real-time and pulsed Doppler ultrasound technique permits quantitative and qualitative studies of fetal blood flow noninvasively. In addition to studies of normal and abnormal pregnancies, it is of interest to know about pharmacological effects on the fetus when the mother is treated with potent drugs.

For more than 10 years obstetricians have used β_2-mimetic drugs to inhibit premature labour. The effect of these drugs on the mother have been investigated extensively, most of which could have been foretold from their theoretical mode of action on the adrenergic receptor. Results on transfer rates of β-mimetic substances were published just recently. The direct effects on the fetus could not be studied as easily as those on the mother. Well known effects include a rise in the basal fetal heart rate (BFHR) and a postpartum hypoglycaemia, probably caused by the diabetogenic action of β_2-mimetic agents which, on the other hand, may also result in an increased gain in weight. From a theoretical point of view, other haemodynamic effects should occur in the fetus as most of these drugs do cross the placental barriers. Besides the increase in BFHR, an increase in stroke volume, an increase in blood pressure amplitude and a decrease in peripheral resistance should also be found in the fetus.

During our observations of fetal blood flow in normal and complicated pregnancies, we observed an increase in the BFHR and had the impression of an altered mean blood flow velocity in the descending aorta of the fetus under tocolytic therapy. To clarify whether this was a systematic effect of β_2-mimetic agents like fenoterol, 6 pregnant women were investigated before and during tocolytic therapy or during and after therapy.

The Physiological Development of the Fetus and Newborn
ISBN 0 12 389080 2

Copyright © 1985 by Academic Press, London.
All rights of reproduction in any form reserved.

Blood flow was investigated by means of a Kranzbuehler 8130/8105 combination
with a 3-MHz realtime scanner and a 2-MHz pulsed Doppler with pulse repetition
frequencies of 2.0 to 8.0 kHz. Blood flow could be analysed in opposite directions
simultaneously with a 2-channel spectrum analyser. The results of our
measurements in normal subjects are comparable to those of other investigators.

Six women between 31 and 37 weeks of pregnancy were included in the study,
2 of whom had measurements taken before and during oral tocolysis (1 and 2),
2 others (3 and 4) during and after oral therapy, while the last 2 (5 and 6) were
investigated before and during intravenous tocolytic therapy. The results are
summarized in Table 1.

Table 1. Mean blood flow velocities in the fetuses of 6 pregnant women
undergoing tocolytic therapy

		Fenoterol dose	Mean flow velocity (cm/s)		Difference (%)
			Without fenoterol	With fenoterol	
Before and during	1	5 × 5 mg	34.6	39.9	+ 13
po tocolysis	2	5 × 5 mg	39.5	40.2	+ 2
During and after	3	5 × 5 mg	35.7	41.0	+ 15
po tocolysis	4	5 × 5 mg	32.4	42.4	+ 31
Before and during	5	2.0 µg/min	31.0	40.0	+ 29
iv tocolysis	6	2.4 µg/min	30.5	39.7	+ 30
		Median	33.5	40.1	
		Sign-test:	$P < 0.05$		

In all fetuses, except case 2, a significant increase in mean blood flow velocity
in the descending aorta was found, as was expected, during tocolytic therapy
with fenoterol. The exception (2) with an insignificant increase of 2% was a fetus
with a pre-existing high flow velocity (39.5 cm/s) of unknown origin. His final
flow velocity of 40.2 cm/s was in the same range as that of the other 5 cases during
therapy.

These results show that β_2-mimetic drugs given to the mother to stop
premature labour have a significant effect on the fetal circulation with the well
known rise in FBHR and a rise in the mean blood flow velocity.

The clinical implications of this effect are not clear as yet. Sympathomimetic
drugs show positively inotropic, chronotropic, bathmotropic and dromotropic
effects on the heart with a consequently greater need for oxygen. In cases with
respiratory insufficiency of the placenta or in cases with fetal anaemia resulting
from blood group incompatibility, β_2-mimetic drugs might thus have a
deleterious effect on the fetal heart. This possible side-effect of tocolytic agents
should be studied in the near future.

Cross-sectional Doppler Echocardiographic Evaluation of the Fetal Cardiac Output During the Second and Third Trimesters of Pregnancy: A Longitudinal Study

E. J. Meijboom, M. C. H. De Smedt, G. H. A. Visser, W. Jager, K. K. Bossina and H. J. Huisjes

Departments of Pediatric Cardiology and Obstetrics, University Hospital, Groningen, Netherlands

In the human fetus flow has been measured in the descending aorta and in the umbilical artery and vein. We measured fetal flow over the mitral and tricuspid orifices in a longitudinal study in 34 uncomplicated pregnancies. These pregnancies were followed from 16 to 40 weeks of gestation by cross-sectional Doppler echocardiography. Serial echo studies were performed every 4 weeks until delivery and one final study was done within 3 days after birth. Estimates of gestational age and fetal weight were obtained from a 256-element 3.5-MHz linear array system. A 3- or 5-MHz pulsed Doppler sector scanner provided cardiac cross-sectional images; mitral and tricuspid velocities were obtained from apical 4-chamber views. Angle-corrected maximal and mean temporal velocities were calculated. The angle between the Doppler interrogation beam and the direction of flow was kept as small as possible. Tracings obtained using an angle larger than 30° were rejected.

Blood flow over both ostia was calculated with the formula: blood flow = $(\bar{v} \times A)/\cos\theta$; in which $\bar{v}$ is mean temporal velocity in cm/s, A is the area of the atrioventricular ostium measured by the diameter on the 4-chamber view in cm², and τ is the angle between the Doppler interrogation beam and the bloodstream. The figures obtained from the mitral and tricuspid valves are given in Table 1.

The Physiological Development of the Fetus and Newborn
ISBN 0 12 389080 2

Copyright © 1985 by Academic Press, London.
All rights of reproduction in any form reserved.

Table 1. Blood flow data

Valve	Maximum velocity (cm/sec)	$\bar{v}$ (cm/s)	Flow (ml/min)	Index flow (ml/min/kg)
Mitral	41.9 (36–54)	12 (6.5–15.8)	147 (43–383)	198
Tricuspid	48.8 (32–63)	13.2 (7.5–18.4)	180 (54–469)	260

Velocities and ventricular output increased linearly during pregnancy (at least until 36 weeks) while right-sided velocities and output calculations are consistently higher than those of the left heart side (Fig. 1). The relationship between right and left-sided cardiac output is 1.3:1 in this study.

Flow velocity curves obtained at the atrioventricular valves differ considerably from those of the great arteries. During diastole, the curves have a biphasic character with an early passive part and a late atrial contraction part. After birth, the early passive part dominates a much smaller atrial contraction part. In the fetus a reverse pattern is shown with a small early part as compared to the late part (Fig. 2). However, with progressing gestation the early part increases, whereby the ratio between early and late velocity (E/A) in the left heart changes from 0.60 ± 0.09 at 23 weeks to 0.93 ± 0.16 at 39 weeks (Fig. 3). For the right ventricle these values are 0.68 ± 0.07 and 0.92 ± 0.07, respectively (Fig. 4). Heart rate plays a major part in the balance of early and late diastolic flow as was found in recordings with a relative bradycardia and tachycardia: a large passive inflow is present in the former, whereas in the latter this flow is strongly reduced. Other factors influencing this flow pattern include preload, contractility of the atrium and

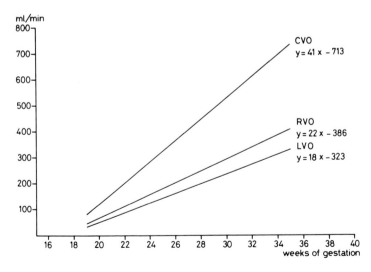

Figure 1. Left, right and combined ventricular output during pregnancy.

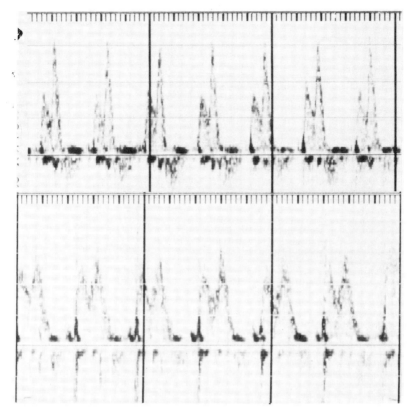

Figure 2. Left ventricular flow velocity waveforms at 18 weeks gestation (upper tracing) and 39 weeks (lower tracing).

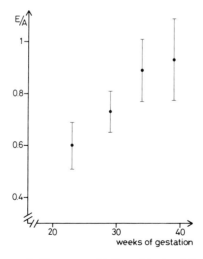

Figure 3. Changes of left ventricular *E/A* ratio.

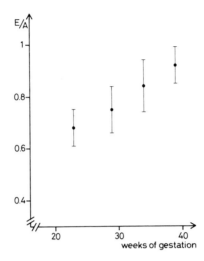

Figure 4. Changes of right ventricular *E/A* ratio.

afterload consisting of ventricular compliance and peripheral resistance. In the case where preload is dominated by placental return flow, there might be a relationship between relative increase of the passive flow and the simultaneously decreasing pulsatility index of the umbilical artery, the latter reflecting placental resistance.

   Our study suggests that measurement of flow over the fetal mitral and tricuspid orifices and the calculation of the left and right ventricular fetal cardiac output is possible. Left and right ventricular cardiac output increase linearly during the 2nd and 3rd trimesters of pregnancy and right ventricular output is consistently greater than left ventricular output. However, the combined ventricular output, related to estimated fetal weight, stays at a constant level. The meaning of the waveform changes during pregnancy is still unknown.

Fetal Heart Rate Changes in Hypertensive Pregnancies

K. J. Dalton, A. J. Dawson* and R. G. Newcombe**

Department of Obstetrics and Gynaecology, University of Cambridge, Cambridge, UK, *Department of Obstetrics and Gynaecology, and **Department of Medical Computing and Statistics, Welsh National School of Medicine, Cardiff, UK

Introduction

In order to determine whether the fetal heart behaves differently in normotensive and hypertensive pregnancies, we have prospectively investigated changes in baseline fetal heart rate from 11 weeks gestation to term in 32 women who were normotensive at the time of booking in at the antenatal clinic, and in 11 women who were hypertensive at booking. We have also studied baseline fetal heart rate in 40 women who were admitted to hospital in the 3rd trimester for assessment of pregnancy hypertension.

This has been part of our ongoing study into the effects of maternal hypertension on the fetal cardiovascular system.

Methods

Initially normotensive women

Thirty-two nulliparous women were selected randomly at their first antenatal clinic visit. They had booking blood pressures of less than 140/90 mmHg, and no previous history of hypertension. They were all in good health and gestational ages were confirmed by ultrasound scan.

Fetal heart rate recordings of 30 min duration were made at 3–4-weekly intervals from the first visit until delivery, with the mother lying in the left lateral semirecumbent position. Abdominal palpation was *not* performed. Maternal blood pressure was taken using a conventional mercury manometer and diastolic pressures were taken at Korotkoff IV.

The Physiological Development of the Fetus and Newborn
ISBN 0 12 389080 2

Copyright © 1985 by Academic Press, London.
All rights of reproduction in any form reserved.

The fetal heart beat was detected ultrasonically, using either a Sonicaid D205 fetal heart detector (up to 27 weeks) or a Hewlett Packard 8030 fetal heart monitor (from 28 weeks onwards), and the signals were fed into an HP 9825 or HP 9826 computer running the HPL programmes TELEPLOT (1) and BASELINE (2).

After delivery, the mothers were classified as sustained normotensives or eventual hypertensives, depending on their blood pressures recorded at any time during the pregnancy, in labour or in the first 24 h after delivery. Hypertensives were defined as those with blood pressures of either 140/90 mmHg on at least 2 occasions 24 h apart, or 160/110 mmHg on at least 2 occasions 15 min apart.

Statistical analysis of the results was performed using SPSS (the Statistical Package for the Social Sciences) and analysis of variance was performed using epochs of 4 weeks gestational age.

Initially hypertensive women

At the booking visit 11 women were selected because their blood pressures were found to be 140/90 mmHg or more, 4 were on treatment with hypotensive agents, and 7 were not.

They were followed through as described above, and their recordings were analysed in a similar way.

Inpatient hypertensives

We also studied 40 women who were admitted to hospital in the 3rd trimester for assessment of hypertension in pregnancy. All had blood pressures of 140/90 mmHg or more on at least 2 occasions.

Here we analysed the blood pressures recorded at the booking visit, as well as those later recorded (4 times daily) by the midwives. We analysed all those fetal heart rate recordings made (usually on alternate days) for clinical reasons.

Results

Initially normotensive women

All delivered live healthy babies, with weights within the normal range. Twenty-one women remained normotensive and 11 became hypertensive. In total, 272 recordings were made: 173 in the sustained normotensives and 99 in the eventual hypertensives.

Figure 1 shows the mean fetal heart rates at each gestational age in those pregnancies which remained normotensive or became hypertensive. In the sustained normotensives there was a clear and highly significant fall in the average fetal heart rate of around 0.3 beats/min/week over the period 15–38 weeks ($P < 0.005$). In the eventual hypertensives, on the other hand, there was no significant change in the average fetal heart rate over this period. In both groups there was a significantly more rapid fall in fetal heart rate from 11–14 weeks to 15–18 weeks ($P < 0.05$). Conversely, there appeared to be a rapid increase in fetal heart rate from 35–38 weeks to 39–42 weeks, but this did not quite reach statistical significance.

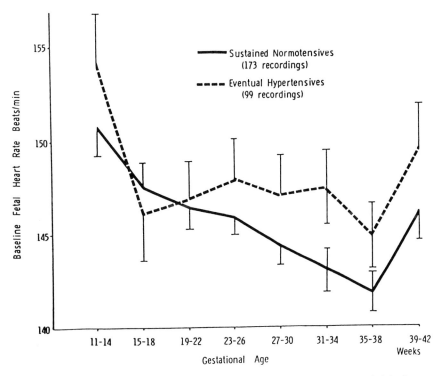

Figure 1. Averaged baseline fetal heart rates throughout pregnancy (a) in those pregnancies which remained normotensive (n = 173); and (b) in those which eventually became hypertensive (n = 99). Standard error bars are shown.

There was a highly significant correlation between fetal heart rate and the mother's mean arterial pressure ($P < 0.002$), though this correlation was not particularly strong ($r = 0.122$).

Initially hypertensive women

All delivered live healthy babies. In total, 92 fetal heart rate recordings were made. There was no significant fall in fetal heart rate between 15 and 38 weeks gestation, as was also found in those initially normotensive women who became hypertensive. There were no significant differences between those on and those off treatment.

Inpatient hypertensives

The average gestational age at booking was 14 weeks, and that at admission was 35 weeks. Overall, 164 fetal heart rate recordings were made.

We found that although there was no relationship with diastolic or mean blood pressure at booking, there was a highly significant relationship between fetal heart rate in the third trimester and the mother's systolic blood pressure at booking.

In those women who booked at or above 150 mmHg systolic pressure, the fetal heart rate was faster by 10 beats/min than if their systolic pressure was below 150 mmHg at booking ($P<0.001$). There was no immediate relationship between fetal heart rate and maternal blood pressure.

Conclusions

1. The fetal heart behaves differently in normotensive and hypertensive pregnancies.
2. Although it is frequently stated that the fetal heart rate decreases with advancing gestational age, between 15 and 38 weeks we find that this is true only in normotensive pregnancies.
3. If either early or late hypertension complicates pregnancy, we find no decrease in fetal heart rate from 15 to 38 weeks gestation.
4. However, there is always a steep fall in fetal heart rate from 11 to 15 weeks gestation, and always a rise from 38 to 42 weeks gestation.
5. If the systolic blood pressure is at or above 150 mmHg at booking, the fetal heart rate in the 3rd trimester is faster by 10 beats/min.
6. These findings suggest that the fetus adapts to maternal hypertension by making changes in its own cardiovascular system.

References

1. Dalton, K. J., Hemp, J., Dawson, A. J. and Gough, N. A. J. (1984). *Int. J. Bio-Med. Comput.* **15**, 23–24.
2. Dalton, K. J. and Dawson, A. J. (1985). *Int. J. Bio-Med. Comput.* (in press).

Characterization of Uterine Activity for the Prediction of Preterm Birth

R. L. TambyRaja and C. J. Hobel

Department of Obstetrics and Gynaecology, National University of Singapore, Singapore, and University of California (Los Angeles), Los Angeles, California, USA

Little is known about uterine activity patterns in human pregnancies prior to term. In our programme for the prevention of prematurity, we recognized that pregnancies at risk of recurrent preterm birth often experienced increased uterine activity. Since studies in the monkey (1) identified a circadian pattern of uterine activity, we set to assess whether or not normal human pregnancies at various gestational ages exhibited a uterine activity pattern in a 24 h period.

Although antenatal contractions have been known since Hicks (2) first described them in 1871, only now is their importance being recognized. Wood *et al.* (3) first suggested that increased uterine activity may be associated with preterm birth. However, Anderson and Turnbull (4) could not substantiate this. Recently, Suranyi and Szomlya (5) recorded the frequency of major contractions once in pregnancy and correlated activity to preterm birth. Bell (6) has reported that recording contractions of more than 15 mmHg is useful for the prediction of preterm labour.

Materials and Methods

An important restriction to the study of the antenatal course of patients who subsequently have preterm labour is that these patients are difficult to identify. It would be impractical to attempt such a study in the general obstetric population, in which the incidence of preterm labour is between 5 and 8% of live births. However, it would be feasible to study a group of patients known to be at increased risk of preterm labour. Intra-uterine pressure changes occurring during spontaneous antenatal contractions were measured with a modified corometrics external guardring type tocodynometer (7). Regular contractions resulting from

The Physiological Development of the Fetus and Newborn
ISBN 0 12 389080 2

Copyright © 1985 by Academic Press, London.
All rights of reproduction in any form reserved.

increasing synchronization of uterine activity with $P > 5$ mmHg and lasting at least 30 s were noted.

As antenatal uterine activity has been reported to be abnormal for periods of weeks to months before preterm labour (3,8,9), recordings between 20 weeks gestation and delivery were considered to be sufficiently frequent to detect a change in antenatal uterine activity before labour.

Normal pregnancies between 23 and 40 weeks were monitored during a 24 h period (daytime 0700–1200 h (Period 1) and 1300–1800 h (Period 2); in the evening 1900–2300 (Period 3) and at night 0000–0600 (Period 4)). Uterine activity was monitored using a modified corometrics antepartum fetal monitor.

In this study, uterine activity and maternal estradiol and progesterone levels were assessed in a group of patients considered to be at increased risk of preterm labour on the basis of their past obstetric history. The results were compared with the findings in a group of optimal obstetric patients. In the high risk group, uterine activity was recorded for 1 h every 2 weeks from 20 weeks gestation until delivery. Blood was collected for hormone analysis at the end of each recording period. Estradiol 17B and progesterone were measured as described previously (10).

Results

Normal pregnancy

Table 1 illustrates the results of these observations. Between 23 and 30 weeks, only 1 of 8 patients had daytime (Period 2) uterine activity. Between 31 and 36 weeks, all the 9 patients showed daytime activity (Periods 1 and 2) but none at night. Between 36 and 40 weeks in addition to the daytime activity, 9 of 12 patients showed a nocturnal period of activity (Period 3) but again no activity between midnight and morning (Period 4). When a group of high risk patients who had previously had a preterm birth were compared with the normal 8 patients (Table 2), a significant increase in activity was seen during all periods before the 30th week. All such patients had significant uterine activity during Period 1 compared to the normal group.

Table 1. Patterns of 24 h uterine activity at varying gestations

Gest. age	Time period 0700–1200	Uterine activity (normal patients) 1300–1800	1900–2300	2400–0600
23–30 weeks ($n=8$)	0/8	1/8	0/8	0/8
31–36 weeks ($n=9$)	9/9	7/9	0/9	0/9
37–40 weeks ($n=12$)	12/12	11/12	9/12	0/12
Sig.	0.001	0.01	0.001	NS

Table 2. Comparison of uterine activity in low and high risk patients before 30 weeks

Time period Risk status	Uterine activity (patients < 30 weeks)			
	0700–1200	1300–1800	1900–2300	2400–0500
Low risk patients (n = 8)	0/8	1/8	0/8	0/8
High risk patients (n = 9) Preterm Lab. No. 5 Preterm Del. No. 4	8/9	6/9	7/9	5/9
Sig.	0.004	0.049	0.002	0.029

Maternal antenatal estradiol and progesterone concentrations

Antenatal estradiol and progesterone concentrations of high risk patients going on to have preterm labour were within the range of the optimal group. Diurnal variations of the hormones are being studied and suggest that the highest number of "contractures" during daytime seem to correspond to the lowest progesterone levels.

Conclusion

1. Regular uterine activity is very unusual for normal pregnancies prior to 30 weeks during any phase of a 24 h period.
2. Beginning at 30 weeks and up to 36 weeks, regular uterine activity is common during daylight hours (0700–1900 h).
3. At 36 weeks a nocturnal phase of uterine activity appears (1900–2400 h).
4. Between 20 and 36 weeks from 0000 to 0700 h, regular uterine activity is unusual in normal pregnancies.
5. Regular uterine activity is common to patients at risk for preterm labour prior to 30 weeks.

Based on our preliminary findings, the following speculations seem tenable:

1. Uterine activity prior to 30 weeks gestational age is abnormal and it could increase the risk of preterm delivery.
2. Uterine activity during daylight hours after 30 weeks could represent a uterine response to distention secondary to fetal growth.
3. The nocturnal component of uterine activity which appears at 36 weeks could be secondary to fetal maturation.

This study substantiates the work of several other researchers (3,6,8,9) in this field. Increased antenatal uterine activity should be included in risk scoring programmes for preterm labour.

References

1. Taylor, N. F., Nathanielsz, P. W. and Serron Ferre, M. (1984). *Am. J. Obstet. Gynecol.* (in press).
2. Braxton Hicks contractions, quoted by Caldeyo Barcia, R. and Alvarez, H. (1953). Proc. 1st World Congress Fertility and Sterility, New York, p. 217.
3. Wood, C., Bannerman, R. H. O., Booth, R. T. and Pinkerton, J. H. M. (1965). *Am. J. Obstet. Gynecol.* **19**, 396–402.
4. Anderson, A. B. M. and Turnbull, A. C. (1969). *Am. J. Obstet. Gynecol.* **105**, 1207–1214.
5. Suranyi, S. and Szomolya, M. (1981). *J. Perinat. Med.* **9** (Suppl. 1), 140–141.
6. Bell, R. (1983). *Br. J. Obstet. Gynaec.* **90**, 884–887.
7. Smyth, C. N. (1957). *J. Obstet. Gynaec. Brit. Empire.* **64**, 59–66.
8. Bruns, P. D., Taylor, E. S., Anker, R. M. and Dose, V. E. (1957). *Am. J. Obstet. Gynecol.* **73**, 579–588.
9. Aubry, R. H. and Pennington, J. C. (1973). *Clin. Obstet. Gynecol.* **15**, 3–27.
10. TambyRaja, R. L., Anderson, A. B. M. and Turnbull, A. C. (1974). *Brit. Med. J.* **4**, 67–69.

Does Maternal Glucose Homeostasis Really Deteriorate in Pregnancy?

R. B. Fraser, F. A. Ford and G. F. Lawrence

Department of Obstetrics and Gynaecology, University of Sheffield,
Jessop Hospital for Women, Sheffield, UK

Introduction

In late pregnancy, nondiabetic, Western women show a deterioration of oral and intravenous glucose tolerance in a "diabetic" direction (1,2). This occurs despite a fall in fasting plasma glucose and an increase in plasma insulin levels. It has been suggested that pregnancy is associated with increased peripheral insulin resistance (1,3). Studies with liquid formula test meals in pregnant and nonpregnant volunteers have shown raised postprandial peaks of glucose, and delayed return to fasting levels in the pregnant subjects (4). Longitudinal studies with mixed meal feeding showed a similar delay in return to fasting levels after meals during pregnancy but the mean diurnal plasma glucose was lower in pregnancy than in the nonpregnant state. These authors interpreted their findings as showing "significant nocturnal hypoglycaemia without a concomitant decrease in absolute immuno-reactive insulin levels" (5).

In contrast, our own studies have shown improved glucose tolerance response in late pregnancy in African women (6) and improved glucose homeostasis in the third compared to the 2nd trimester of pregnancy in European women habituated to high fibre diets (7).

We have now compared plasma glucose and insulin responses in normal weight, pregnant and nonpregnant subjects fed identical low fibre diets.

Patients and Methods

Fifteen nonpregnant subjects (Group A) aged between 20 and 45 who weighed between 90 and 110% of average weight for height were compared with 14 pregnant subjects (Group B) selected using the same criteria. The pregnant group

The Physiological Development of the Fetus and Newborn
ISBN 0 12 389080 2
Copyright © 1985 by Academic Press, London.
All rights of reproduction in any form reserved.

were studied between 32 and 36 weeks gestation by dates and/or ultrasound assessment. After an overnight fast they ate the meals detailed in Table 1, and venous blood was sampled hourly. Plasma glucose and insulin levels were measured at each time point and the results compared statistically by the Wilcoxon Rank Sum Test.

Table 1. Contents of meal eaten during study, and proportions of carbohydrates, protein and fat

Breakfast (0830 h)	Rice krispies, boiled egg, white bread, butter
	Tea or coffee, milk (half-skimmed), sugar
Midmorning (1030 h)	Tea or coffee, milk, sugar
Midday meal (1230 h)	Chicken, carrots, boiled potatoes
	Meringue, cream, tea or coffee, milk, sugar
Midafternoon (1515 h)	Milk chocolate
	Sugar-free lemonade
Evening meal (1730 h)	Oxtail soup, cheese and ham salad
	White bread and butter, jelly, ice cream
	Tea or coffee, milk, sugar

Total energy = 1910 kcal

Source	Energy content (g)
Carbohydrate	202 (40%)*
Protein	96.5 (20%)
Fat	85.4 (40%)
Dietary fibre	9.7

*Figures in brackets refer to proportion of energy from each food source.

Results

The results are illustrated in Fig. 1. The postprandial glucose peaks were higher after meals for group A. The plasma glucose levels in group B were only higher than those for group A in the second hour after breakfast and the evening meal. It can be assumed that the plasma glucose levels were lower in Group B during overnight fasting. There was a trend to higher insulin levels in Group B but the differences were rarely statistically significant.

The possibility that the postprandial peak was being missed because of infrequent sampling was tested by extra sampling at 0930, 1330 and 1830 h in 2 pregnant and 2 nonpregnant subjects. The 3 averaged postprandial glucose peaks were 7.4, 6.3 and 7.2 mmol/l in the nonpregnant and 7.1, 6.2 and 7.6 mmol/l respectively in the pregnant subjects.

Discussion

There remains much to learn about the physiological relationships of glucose and insulin in normal human pregnancy. The apparent paradox of increased insulin secretion accompanying a deterioration in glucose homeostasis may be

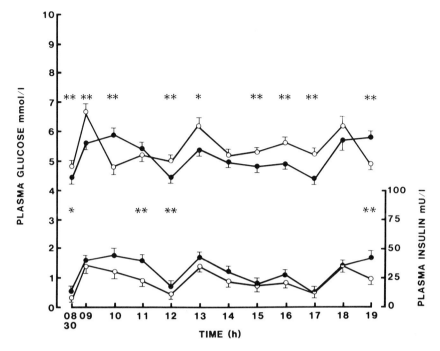

Figure 1. Plasma glucose and insulin profiles in nonpregnant (Group A, ○) and pregnant (Group B, ●) subjects, studied on diet shown in table. All values are means±SEM. Statistical significance: $P<0.05$; **$P<0.01$.

an artefact introduced by unphysiological testing with glucose solutions and liquid formula diets. It is possible that the increased insulin secretion of the third trimester of pregnancy is intended to reduce mean plasma glucose and thus reduce placental transfer of glucose and protect the fetus from the unwanted effects of an excess of this nutrient.

References

1. Lind, T. (1980). *In:* "Clinical Physiology in Obstetrics", (Hytten, F. E. and Chamberlain, G., eds) pp. 234–256. Blackwell, Oxford.
2. Fisher, P. M., Hamilton, P. M., Sutherland, H. W. and Stowers, J. M. (1974). *J. Obstet. Gynaecol. Brit. Commonwealth* **81**, 285–290.
3. Hornnes, P. J., Kühl, C. and Lauritsen, K. B. (1981). *Diabetes* **30**, 504–509.
4. Phelps, R. L., Metzger, B. E. and Freinkel, N. (1981). *Am. J. Obstet. Gynecol.* **140**, 730–736.
5. Cousins, L., Rigg, L., Hollingsworth, D., Brink, G., Aurand, J. and Yen, S. S. C. (1980). *Am. J. Obstet. Gynecol.* **136**, 483–488.
6. Fraser, R. B. (1981). *E. Afr. Med. J.* **58**, 90–94.
7. Fraser, R. B. (1983). *In:* "Nutrition in Pregnancy" (Campbell, D. M. and Gillmer, M. D. G., eds) pp. 269–277. Royal College of Obstetricians and Gynaecologists, London.

Adenosine: A Possible Mediator of the "Hypoxic Depression" of Respiration in Neonates?

H. Lagercrantz, M. Runold and B. B. Fredholm

Nobel Institute for Neurophysiology and Department of Pharmacology, Karolinska Institute and Department of Pediatrics, Karolinska Hospital, Stockholm, Sweden

Hypoxia causes rapid depression of ventilation in fetal sheep (1). Hypoxia also causes ventilatory depression in the newborn infant after a transient stimulation (2). In particular, preterm infants hypoventilate and become apnoeic even when exposed to moderate hypoxia (3). The mechanism of this hypoxic depression has not yet been elucidated. It does not seem to be due to inhibition of carotid body chemoreceptors, since the depression was seen in spite of increased firing in the sinus nerve (4). However, the hypoxic respiratory depression in the fetus can be abolished by decerebration at a mid-collicular level (5).

Various hypotheses explaining this hypoxic depression have been put forward, e.g. a direct effect on neurons (6) or increased medullary blood flow with subsequent increase of pH leading to ventilatory depression (7). An alternative explanation is that a neurohormone is mediating the hypoxic response. Naloxone was found to diminish the hypoxic respiratory depression in newborn rabbits, suggesting that endorphine may be involved (8,9). Gamma-amino-butyric acid (GABA) has been demonstrated to be released in the cerebrospinal fluid in apnoeic infants (10) and to depress ventilation (see 11). Another putative neuromodulator mediating the hypoxic depression is adenosine. It is released by hypoxia (12), particularly during perinatal asphyxia (13). It has been found to depress ventilation substantially in various animal preparations (14–16).

The effect of adenosine is antagonized by theophylline, a respiratory stimulant widely used in neonatal medicine (see 17). The possible role of adenosine as the mediator of the hypoxic depression of respiration, particularly in neonates, will be discussed in more detail in this Chapter.

The Physiological Development of the Fetus and Newborn
ISBN 0 12 389080 2

Copyright © 1985 by Academic Press, London.
All rights of reproduction in any form reserved.

Release of Adenosine

Adenosine is probably released primarily as such and high neural activity and hypoxia increase the formation of adenosine (18,19). Perinatal asphyxia might lead to an even more extensive release of adenosine. In a number of studies, high concentrations of the adenosine metabolite hypoxanthine has been found in umbilical cord blood of asphyxiated newborn infants (13,20). In preliminary studies we have found very high adenosine concentration in umbilical arterial blood in asphyxiated infants (Irestedt, Lagercrantz, Sollevi; to be published).

Respiratory Effects of Adenosine and an Adenosine Analogue

Already in 1929, Drury and Scent-Györgyi (21) reported that adenosine depresses respiration. The adenosine analogue L-N-phenyl-isopropyladenosine (L-PIA), which is more stable than adenosine, has also been found to depress ventilation markedly in adult (14) and neonatal rabbits (16), cats (15) and newborn piglets (23). The effect could be reversed or prevented by theophylline. However, all these studies were performed on anaesthetized animals. Therefore, we were interested to investigate the effects of L-PIA on animals in natural sleep. Furthermore, we wanted to see to what extent the effect is age-dependent.

We monitored the respiration of kittens and rabbit pups with the barometric method (24). This method is based on recording volume changes due to the warming of inhaled air and allows monitoring of nonanaesthetized subjects. L-PIA was given through an indwelling intraperitoneal catheter.

The marked respiratory depressive effect of L-PIA in a kitten is shown in Fig. 1. This effect could be blocked by pretreatment with theophylline. A linear dose-response relationship was observed. In particular the respiratory rate was decreased while the effect on tidal volume was more variable.

The effect of L-PIA was found to be age-dependent in both the kittens and rabbit pups. A dose of 1 μmol/kg of L-PIA caused severe apnoea and a marked decrease of ventilatory minute volume in the 1- to 2-day-old rabbit pups (maximal effect after about 15 min was $-65.2 \pm 3.0\%$, SEM, $n=4$) while the effect was more moderate in the older pups (3 days: $-43.7 \pm 3.4\%$, $n=4$; 8 days: $-31.0 \pm 7.8\%$, $n=3$). A similar pattern was observed in the kittens (unpublished observations). In older animals, even a slight stimulation of the respiration after L-PIA could be observed.

Adenosine Receptors

Most if not all cell types possess adenosine receptors. The classification of adenosine receptors is based on the relative potency of various adenosine analogues.

We have determined adenosine receptors (A1) in rabbit pup brains at the ages of 1–2, 3–4, 5–6 and 8–10 days. Specific binding of ^{3}H-L-PIA was determined (22). Minor differences in the number of L-PIA binding sites were found between

Control

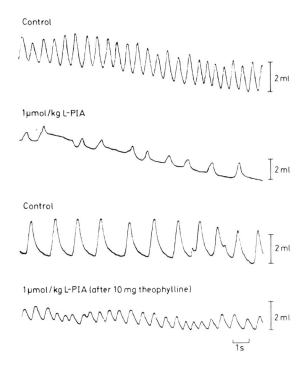

1 μmol/kg L-PIA

Control

1 μmol/kg L-PIA (after 10 mg theophylline)

Figure 1. Respiratory recordings with the barometric method from 2 1-day-old kittens. The upper two recordings show the respiration before and 15 min after injection of only L-PIA in 1 kitten. The lower 2 recordings show the effect of L-PIA in the presence of theophylline in another kitten.

the 4 age groups. However, K_D was significantly lower in the brains from the very youngest pups (Fredholm *et al.*, to be published). This could possibly be related to the higher activity of L-PIA in these very young animals.

Other Functional Effects
of Adenosine Analogues

After administration of the adenosine analogue, the animals generally became drowsy and hypotonic. Furthermore, body temperature decreased substantially. However, this decrease developed more slowly than the respiratory depression, why decrease of ventilation was probably not caused by the decreased metabolic rate. The mechanism for the hypothermia has not yet been clarified. Adenosine certainly causes vasodilatation and thus heat loss, but a central mechanism might also be involved.

Site of Action

The effect of L-PIA on respiration is assumed to be due to a direct action on central respiratory control mechanisms rather than secondary to systemic effects. L-PIA easily penetrates the blood–brain barrier. Administered in the 3rd ventricle (15) or at the exposed dorsal surface (16) of the medulla, much lower concentrations of L-PIA caused similar respiratory effects with minor circulatory effects. The effect of L-PIA was found to be similar in rabbit pups decerebrated at a mid-collicular level (16), suggesting that it acts in the lower brain stem.

Adenosine has been found to stimulate the peripheral chemoreceptors (25). This might explain why LPIA in some of the older animals caused a transient stimulation of breathing, particularly when given in a low dose.

Conclusions

Hypoxic depression of respiration is probably mediated by a neurotransmitter/ modulator rather than by a direct effect of hypoxia. This is indicated in studies on glomectomized cats where the inhibition of respiration following acute hypoxia was prolonged (26). A number of neurohormones have been shown to be released during hypoxia and to inhibit respiration (see above) and could be responsible for the "hypoxic depression". Adenosine seems to be a strong candidate:

    1. the adenosine antagonist theophylline prevents the hypoxic depression;
    2. adenosine and its analogue L-PIA have been shown to depress breathing in various animal models;
    3. adenosine is present in fairly high concentrations during hypoxia.

Adenosine might be of particular interest as a mediator of perinatal asphyxia:

    1. the adenosine metabolite hypoxanthine is found in high concentrations in asphyxiated infants;
    2. an adenosine analogue was found to depress ventilation in rabbit pups in an age-related way;
    3. adenosine receptors are present at an early stage and K_D was in fact lowest in brain material from the youngest animals;
    4. a number of other effects of perinatal asphyxia like the marked hypotonia and hypothermia might also be attributed to adenosine effects.

Finally, it is also possible that adenosine induces release of other neurohormones (see 18) like the endorphines which might act synergistically on respiration.

Acknowledgement

Supported by the Swedish Medical Research Council (grant no. 5234), National Association against Heart and Lung Disease and Majblommans Stiftelse.

References

1. Boddy, K., Dawes, G. S., Fisher, R., Pinter, S. and Robinson, J. (1974). *J. Physiol.* **243**, 599–618.

2. Cross, K. W. and Warner, P. (1951). *J. Physiol.* **114**, 283-295.
3. Rigatto, H., Brady, J. and Verduzco, R. D. (1975). *Pediatrics* **55**, 604.
4. Schwieler, G. (1968). *Acta Physiol. Scand. (suppl.)* **304**, 10-85.
5. Dawes, G. S., Gardner, W. N., Johnston, B. M. and Walker, D. W. 61983). *J. Physiol.* **335**, 535-553.
6. Cherniack, N. S., Edelman, N. H. and Lahiri, S. (1970/71). *Resp. Physiol.* **11**, 113-126.
7. Lee, L.-Y. and Millhorne, H. T. (1975). *Resp. Physiol.* **25**, 319-333.
8. Chernick, V., Madansky, D. L. and Lawson, E. E. (1980). *Pediat. Res.* **14**, 357-359.
9. Grundstein, M. M., Hazinski, T. A. and Schleuter, M. A. (1981). *J. Appl. PHysiol.* **53**, 1063-1070.
10. Hedner, T., Iversen, K. and Lundberg, P. (1982). *Early Hum. Dev.* **7**, 53-58.
11. Hedner, J., Hedner, T., Bergman, B. and Lundberg, D. (1980). *J. Develop. Physiol.* **2**, 401-407.
12. Winn, H. R., Rubio, R. and Berne, R. M. (1981). *Am. J. Physiol.* **241**, H235-H242.
13. Saugstad, O. D. (1975). *Pediat. Res.* **9**, 158-161.
14. Hedner, T., Hedner, J., Wessberg, P. and Jonason, J. (1982). *Neurosci. Lett.* **33**, 147-151.
15. Eldridge, F. L., Millhorn, E. D. and Waldrop, T. G. (1982). *Fed. Proc.* **41**, 1690.
16. Lagercrantz, H., Yamamoto, Y., Fredholm, B. B., Prabhakar, N. R. and von Euler, C. (1984). *Pediat. Res.* **18**, 387-390.
17. Aranda, J. V. and Turmen, T. (1979). *Clin. Perinatol.* **6**, 87-108.
18. Phillis, J. W. and Wu, P. H. (1981). *Progr. Neurobiol.* **16**, 187-239.
19. Zetterström, T., Vernet, L., Ungerstedt, U., Tossman, U., Jonzon, B. and Fredholm, B. B. (1982). *Neurosci. Lett.* **29**, 111-115.
20. Thiringer, K. (1982). "Hypoxanthine as Measure of Foetal Asphyxia". Academic Thesis, Gothenburg.
21. Drury, A. N. and Scent-Györgyi, A. (1929). *J. Physiol.* **68**, 213-237.
22. Fredholm, B. B. (1982). *Med. Biol.* **60**, 288-293.
23. Kattwinkel, J. and Darnall, R. (1982). *Pediat. Res.* **16**, 352A.
24. Drorbaugh, J. E. and Fenn, W. O. (1955). *Pediatrics* **16**, 81-87.
25. McQueen, D. S. and Ribeiro, J. A. (1982). *J. Physiol.* **315**, 38P-39P.

The Metabolic and Endocrine Milieu of the Human Fetus at 16-20 Weeks of Gestation

A. Aynsley-Green[1], I. Z. Mackenzie[2], P. A. Jenkins[3], G. Soltesz[3] and S. R. Bloom[4]

[1]Department of Child Health, New Medical School, Newcastle upon Tyne, UK; [2]Department of Obstetrics and [3]Department of Paediatrics, John Radcliffe Hospital, Oxford, UK; [4]Department of Medicine, Hammersmith Hospital, London, UK

Introduction

One of the most important challenges the newborn infant has to face as a result of the cutting of the umbilical cord at birth is the need to adapt to a totally new form of nutrition, namely, enteral feeding with large volumes of milk. The normal infant born at term accomplishes this transition from intra-uterine to extra-uterine nutrition with remarkably little external evidence of the dramatic changes which are occurring in the function of several physiological systems. Until recently, little has been known of the mechanisms which control and integrate the structural and functional adaptation of the gut, endocrine pancreas and liver (1). We have examined previously in an extensive series of publications (2) a hypothesis suggesting that enteral feeding itself at birth is a key trigger that stimulates the secretion of gut hormones and regulatory peptides, and it is they that control the development of the gut mucosa, increase intestinal secretions and, through adaptations of the entero-insular axis, influence postnatal hepatic metabolism.

However, it is apparent that in order to accomplish satisfactory postnatal transition to enteral feeding the gut has to be prepared for its new stimulus before birth. Several facets of prenatal gut development have been examined previously (3) but in view of our work on postnatal adaptation it seemed reasonable to find a means to investigate the prenatal milieu of the human fetus. This paper reports results from a collaborative study made possible by Mr Ian Mackenzie, who has perfected the techniques of fetoscopy.

The Physiological Development of the Fetus and Newborn
ISBN 0 12 389080 2

Copyright © 1985 by Academic Press, London.
All rights of reproduction in any form reserved.

Patients and Methods

Ten mothers of 18–21 weeks of gestation were submitted to fetoscopy and fetal blood sampling immediately before termination of pregnancy for social reasons and within the realms of the 1967 Abortion Act. The study was approved by the Hospital Ethics Committee and informed content was obtained from the mothers. Blood samples were withdrawn from the umbilical artery and vein under direct vision, the mothers remaining conscious although sedated throughout the procedure. Simultaneous maternal antecubital blood samples were also collected, as were amniotic fluid samples from 16 other mothers of equivalent gestation.

Metabolic fuels, amino acids and regulatory peptides and hormones were measured by methods previously reported (4).

Results and Discussion

The concentrations of plasma gastrin, gastric inhibition polypeptide (GIP) and pancreatic polypeptide (PP) in maternal vein, fetal artery, fetal vein and amniotic fluid shown in Fig. 1 demonstrate that substantial concentrations of immunoreactivity can be detected for the three peptides. Three patterns of profile can be determined. In the case of gastrin, fetal levels are lower than maternal vein concentrations, whereas fetal GIP levels are higher than maternal levels with the highest value being found in amniotic fluid. In the case of PP, highest levels are found in the maternal circulation. No significant vein/artery differences could be found for any of these substances in fetal circulation.

Both plasma pancreatic glucagon and gut glucagon-like immunoreactivity can

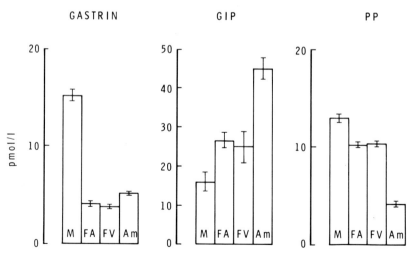

Figure 1. Maternal, fetal and amniotic fluid concentrations (means ± SEM) of gastrin, GIP and PP. M represents maternal vein concentration; FA, fetal artery; FV, fetal vein; Am, amniotic fluid concentration.

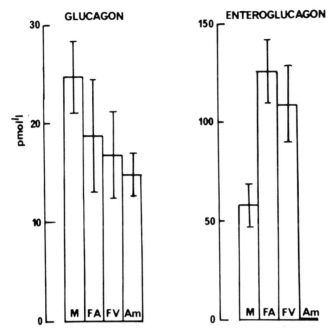

Figure 2. Maternal, fetal and amniotic fluid concentrations (means ± SEM) of glucagon and entero-glucagon. M, maternal vein; FA, fetal artery; FV, fetal vein; Am, amniotic fluid concentration.

be detected in fetal plasma, concentrations of the latter being much higher than those in the maternal circulation. Interestingly, this peptide could not be detected in amniotic fluid (Fig. 2).

No significant differences could be found between maternal and fetal circulation with reference to blood glucose or plasma insulin, nor were fetal vein/artery differences noted for these substances in this study. However, there is a materno-fetal gradient for ketone body concentrations, although not for lactate and pyruvate (maternal hydroxybutyrate (0.38 ± 0.8 mmol/l, fetal vein 0.16 ± 0.03 mmol/l, $P < 0.05$).

Finally, the total molar concentration of the 17 amino acids measured was 2.4 times greater in fetal than in maternal plasma. The mean concentrations of all amino acids were significantly higher in fetal circulation than in maternal circulation, but there was quite a marked difference in the profile as can be seen from Fig. 3, with the greatest difference between fetal and maternal circulations occurring with lysine.

There are very few data relating to the metabolic and endocrine milieu of the human fetus at this stage of gestation. Most of the data which are available have been obtained from studies which are grossly unphysiological in the sense that the blood samples were drawn after maternal anaesthesia and after fetal manipulation and disturbance at hysterotomy. This study is the first to report

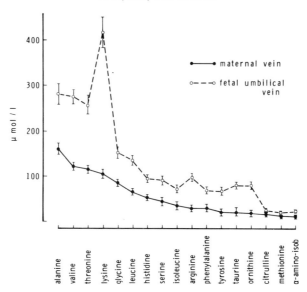

Figure 3. Plasma concentrations amino acids in maternal vein and fetal umbilical vein ($n = 10 \pm$ SEM; all values significantly different $P < 0.005$).

the interrelations of a wide range of peptides, hormones and metabolic fuels with the fetoscopy model where the mother is conscious and where there is minimal disturbance to the fetus.

The significance of the differences in maternal and fetal amniotic fluid concentrations of hormones and regulatory peptides remain to be clarified. However, it is of interest that most of these substances can be detected in amniotic fluid, a substance which is swallowed by the fetus, thus raising the possibility that they could be acting locally in the gut and, possibly, in the lung. Further work is needed to identify the molecular species of peptide present in the fetal fluids, and to determine the site of origin. However, the presence of amniotic fluid concentrations of regulatory peptides is relevant in the context of the nutritional management of the infant born with extreme prematurity. These infants are often deprived entirely of enteral fluid, being maintained totally on parental nutrition. It could be argued that instillation of amniotic fluid into the alimentary tract of these neonates could be of benefit in protecting the gut development and this is an area for future research.

The study also identifies the concentrations of metabolic fuels and amino acids at this stage of gestation; further work is needed to clarify the functional significance of the data, particularly with respect to fuel turnover rate. We conclude, however, that fetal blood sampling at fetoscopy opens up a new area of investigation in the interrelations of fetal and maternal physiology.

References

1. Lebenthal, E. (ed.) (1983). *J. Pediat. Gastroenterol. Nut.* (suppl. 1), S1–S342.
2. Aynsley-Green, A. (1982). *In:* "Metabolic-endocrine Responses to Food Intake in Infancy", (Zoppi, G., ed.) pp. 59–87. Karger, Basel.
3. Lebenthal, E. (1982). *In:* "Metabolic-endocrine Responses to Food Intake in Infancy", (Zoppi, G., ed.) pp. 17–38. Karger, Basel.
4. Aynsley-Green, A., Jenkins, P. A., Mackenzie, I. and Soltesz, G. (1985). *Biol. Neonate* **47**, 19–25.
5. Bloom, S. R. and Long, R. G. (eds) (1982). "Radioimmunoassay of Gut Regulatory Peptides". W. B. Saunders, London.

Severe Cerebral Haemorrhage in Preterm Infants: Impact on Mortality and Neurologic Status

Arthur Kopelman[1], John Wimmer[1], Steve Engelke[1], Rita Saldanha[1], Grant Somes[2] and Thomas Louis[3]

[1]Department of Pediatrics, [2]Division of Epidemiology and Biostatistics and [3]Department of Anatomy, East Carolina University School of Medicine, Greenville, North Carolina, USA

Intracranial haemorrhage occurs in 40% of preterm infants (1). While many of these infants do well, two forms of intracranial haemorrhage are associated with an increased chance of neonatal death or poor neurologic outcome (2). These are, first, the intraparenchymal cerebral haemorrhages and, second, large intraventricular haemorrhages which fill and acutely distend the cerebral ventricles. In this prospective study, we evaluated how 115 preterm infants were affected by these two forms of intracranial haemorrhage which I will refer to collectively as severe cerebral haemorrhage (SCH).

Study Design

We studied all premature infants admitted to our neonatal unit between February 1982 and October 1983 if they were 32 weeks gestation or less by Ballard exam. A cranial ultrasound study was performed at 72 ± 12 h of age using an ATL sector scanner with a 5-MHz transducer. Two of the authors independently evaluated the cranial ultrasounds for the presence or absence of SCH. We then sought correlations between the occurrence of SCH and the presence of preceding risk factors including gestational age, birthweight and perinatal asphyxia, as well as with short-term outcomes such as neonatal seizures and mortality. These were abstracted from the patient charts by one of us who had not seen the ultrasound exams. Groups were compared by χ^2 or Fisher's exact test.

The Physiological Development of the Fetus and Newborn
ISBN 0 12 389080 2

Copyright © 1985 by Academic Press, London.
All rights of reproduction in any form reserved.

Patient Population

During this study, 131 infants of ≤ 32 weeks gestation were admitted to our unit and 115 of them were entered in the study. The mean gestational age and weight were 30 weeks and 1247 g respectively: 70% were born at our hospital.

Results

Risk factors for development of SCH

Seventeen infants, 15% of those in the study, were diagnosed as having SCH. As expected, SCH occurred with increasing frequency at lower gestational age ($P=0.008$, Fig. 1), and at lower birthweight ($P=0.004$).

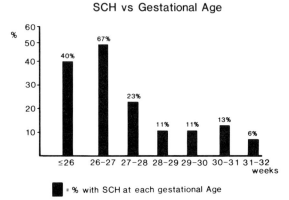

= % with SCH at each gestational Age

Figure 1. The incidence of SCH is greater at lower gestational age.

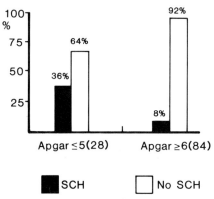

■ SCH   □ No SCH

Figure 2. The solid bar indicates the percentage of infants with SCH by ultrasound exam. The open bar shows the percentage without SCH. The number in parenthesis is the total number of infants in each group. The differences are significant ($P=0.002$).

U/S vs Acute Tubular Necrosis(ATN)

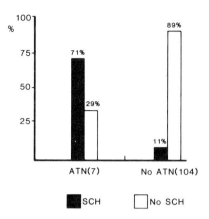

Figure 3. SCH occurred in 71% of infants with acute tubular necrosis, but in just 11% of other infants. The difference is significant ($P=0.0001$).

% SCH vs Gestational Age and Apgar Score

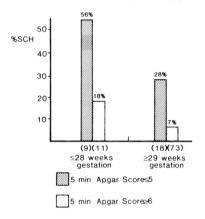

Figure 4. The figure shows the incidence of SCH in each of 4 groups defined by gestational age and 5-min Apgar scores. The bars on the left represent infants ≤28 weeks gestation, and those on the right infants ≥29 weeks gestation. The hatched bars represent infants with 5-min Apgar scores ≤5, and the stippled bars those with Apgar scores ≥6. The number in parenthesis is the number of infants in each group. The highest incidence of SCH, 56%, was in infants ≤28 weeks gestation with Apgars ≤5, while the lowest incidence, 7%, was infants ≥29 weeks gestation with Apgars ≥6. The independent effects of low gestational age and low Apgar scores on occurrence of SCH are clearly shown.

Severe cerebral haemorrhage was also seen more frequently in infants who had experienced perinatal asphyxia (Fig. 2). Occurrence of SCH was strongly correlated with a 5-min Apgar score of 5 or less, $P=0.002$. SCH was also highly associated with the development of acute tubular necrosis ($P=0.0001$, Fig. 3). Acute tubular necrosis, of course, also results from severe perinatal asphyxia. Low Apgar scores are more frequent at low gestational age; however, we found that low Apgar score correlated with SCH *independently* of gestational age, ($P \le 0.05$, Fig. 4).

In addition, SCH was more likely to occur when there was respiratory distress syndrome ($P=0.04$) or when positive pressure ventilation was required ($P=0.055$). Furthermore, occurrence of SCH was much more common following the development of a tension pneumothorax ($P=0.0002$, Fig. 5).

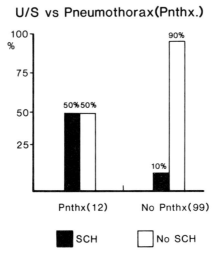

Figure 5. SCH occurred in half of the infant with pneumothorax but in only 10% of all other infants ($P=0.0002$).

Short-term clinical correlate of SCH

Neonatal seizures occurred much more frequently among infants with SCH ($P=0.0001$). Infants with SCH were also more likely to be abnormal on daily neurologic assessments in the first week. That is, they were more frequently scored abnormal for presence of stupor, coma or seizures ($P<0.015$). Finally, if SCH occurred by Day 3, the infant was more likely to die in the neonatal period, $P=0.0001$ (Fig. 6).

Discussion

The devastating consequences of SCH in preterm infants are, once again, clearly shown in this study. One-third of the infants with SCH died in the neonatal period,

Mortality vs U/S

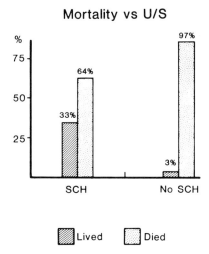

Figure 6. One-third of the infants with SCH died in the neonatal period, while only 3% of other infants died ($P=0.0001$).

a mortality rate 10-fold higher than for preterm infants without SCH. Although SCH occurred in just 15% of our patients, it was present and felt to be a major factor in 60% (9 out of 15) of all deaths.

Two-thirds of the infants with SCH survived and, as shown, many of them were abnormal neurologically or had neonatal seizures. These infants are being followed as recent reports indicate that many will have abnormal development (3).

We believe that infants with SCH do poorly because they have cerebral ischaemia or infarction and that SCH is, in fact, a marker of cerebral infarction. Using positron emission tomography, Volpe *et al.* (4) showed that cerebral intraparenchymal haemorrhage occurs within a much larger region of brain infarction. The second form of SCH, large intraventricular haemorrhages with dilated ventricles, is often associated with increased intracranial pressure. In addition we have found, as have others, that these infants have reduced cerebral blood flow velocity (5), possibly resulting in cerebral ischaemia.

The clinical conditions, which were shown to correlate with the development of SCH, are also associated with reduced cardiac output and perfusion. This is particularly true for acute tubular necrosis which results from inadequate renal perfusion, and for tension pneumothorax which results in reduced venous return and cardiac output. Acutely increased intracranial venous pressure associated with pneumothorax may also lead to a reduction in cerebral blood flow. These correlations support the hypothesis that cerebral injury in premature infants results primarily from cerebral ischaemia (6). It may be possible to reduce the occurrence of brain damage in these infants with better methods to evaluate and support their cerebral circulation, particularly in the presence of these associated conditions.

References

1. Thorburn, R. J., Lipscomb, A. P., Stewart, A. L., Reynolds, E. O., Hope, P. L. and Pape, K. E. (1981). *Lancet* **i**, 1119–1121.
2. Shankarin, S., Slovis, T. L., Bedard, M. P. and Poland, R. L. (1982). *J. Pediat.* **100**, 469–475.
3. Papile, L., Munsick-Bruno, G. and Schaefer, A. (1983). *J. Pediat.* **103**, 273–277.
4. Volpe, J. J., Herscovitch, P., Perlman, J. M. and Raichle, M. E. (1983). *Pediatrics* **72**, 589–601.
5. Bada, H. S., Hajjar, W., Chua, C. and Sumner, D. S. (1979). *J. Pediat.* **95**, 775–779.
6. McMenamin, J. B., Shackelford, G. D. and Volpe, J. J. (1984). *Ann. Neurol.* **15**, 285–290.

Evidence of Fetal Behavioural Cycles in Spontaneous and Induced Labour from Changes in Fetal Heart Rate Variability

J. A. D. Spencer and P. Johnson

Nuffield Department of Obstetrics and Gynaecology, John Radcliffe Hospital, Oxford, UK

Introduction

Heart rate variability changes have been used to identify behavioural state changes in the newborn infant [1,2]. Consecutive episodes or cycles of high and low heart rate variability are a normal feature of the continuous fetal heart rate (FHR) antepartum, and occur in association with fetal body and eye movements by 38 weeks [3]. The duration of such cycles of heart rate variability in the fetus compares favourably with similar cycles in the newborn [4,5].

FHR variability is modified by, but not dependent on, both fetal movements and fetal breathing [6,7]. Cyclical changes in variability continue after induction of labour, whilst fetal movements and fetal breathing are reduced or even absent. Therefore cycles of FHR variability may be the best guide to fetal behaviour during labour. Little has been reported concerning changes in the fetal behavioural state during labour, although the possibility of fetal "sleep" producing a "smooth" baseline during labour has been mentioned [8]. It has also been shown that decreased or absent intrapartum baseline variability occurs with equal frequency in fetuses with and without metabolic acidosis [9]. We decided to quantify fetal behavioural state changes in labour using cycles of FHR variability in a preliminary study to see how often and for how long a questionable reduction in variability might occur. We also hypothesized that such cycles of FHR variability might be more likely after the interruption of late pregnancy by induction of labour than after the onset of spontaneous labour.

The Physiological Development of the Fetus and Newborn
ISBN 0 12 389080 2

Copyright © 1985 by Academic Press, London.
All rights of reproduction in any form reserved.

Methods

Over a 19-week period between March and July 1983, all first-stage cardiotocograph (CTG) recordings of 6 h duration or longer from labours of 37 weeks gestation or more were analysed visually for consecutive episodes of low and high FHR variability. Episodes were identified by working backwards from the end of the first stage recording, and the last epoch was not included as part of a cycle. Each episode thereafter was identified by a change of at least 5 beats/min (long-term variability) sustained for at least 5 min. A complete cycle required consecutive episodes of high and low FHR variability with changes before and after. Two complete cycles were necessary before a CTG was considered to show evidence of active and quiet fetal behavioural state changes. The analysis was performed without knowledge of the details of labour, and 30% of the traces were assessed independently by a second observer. Relevant details concerning the labours were subsequently collected from the hospital records. Only the first twin of twin labours was included.

Results

The study population of 301 cases, amounting to 15% of the total deliveries and 29% of all monitored labours, comprised 94 spontaneous labours (16% of monitored spontaneous labours) and 207 induced labours (45% of monitored induced labours). The mean duration of the CTGs was 549 min (range 360–1320 minutes) and the induced labours had significantly longer CTGs (mean ± SEM: 568 ± 195 min) than the spontaneous labours (508 ± 157 min) ($P = 0.005$).

Table 1 shows that the incidence of fetal behavioural cycles was significantly greater in induced labours (68%) compared with spontaneous labours (38%). The significance was confined to CTGs of 6–9 h duration. The mean length of CTGs with cycles (594 ± 203 min) were significantly longer than the mean length of CTGs without cycles (487 ± 134 min) ($P = 0.001$), and this difference was maintained within both spontaneous labours (585 ± 182 vs 460 ± 118 min, $P = 0.001$) and induced labours (596 ± 209 vs 510 ± 144 min, $P = 0.001$). No circadian influence on the incidence of cycles in spontaneous and induced labours was found.

Table 1. Incidence of cycles of FHR variability in spontaneous and induced labour

	All CTGs (n)		CTGs 6-9 h		CTGs >9 h	
	+	−	+	−	+	−
Spontaneous labour (n=94)	36	58	15	45	21	13
Induced labour (n=207)	140	67	62	39	78	28
χ^2 test:	$P<0.0001$		$P<0.0001$		ns	

+/− indicates presence or absence of cycles.

There were no differences between labours with and without cycles in the incidence of prostaglandin and/or syntocinon used, whether membranes ruptured spontaneously or were ruptured artificially, and the use of pethidine and/or epidural for analgesia. Similarly there were no differences in the mode of delivery, or the 1- and 5-min Apgar scores at delivery between labours with and without cycles.

Table 2 describes the cycles of FHR variability and the quite and active episodes. Of the spontaneous and induced labours with cycles present, there were no differences in any aspect of the cycle characteristics. Figure 1 plots the cumulative

Table 2. Durations (in min) of FHR variability cycles in labour

	Total labours (n = 176)				Spontaneous (n = 36)		Induced (n = 140)		
	mean	SD	min.	max.	mean	SD	mean	SD	t-test
No. cycles	3.7	1.7	2	11	3.7	1.5	3.7	1.7	ns
Complete cycles	92	32	47	202	95	36	91	31	ns
Quiet episodes	25	11	12	93	28	11	25	11	ns
Active episodes	66	31	22	180	67	35	66	29	ns
First quiet	25	13	7	90	27	15	24	12	ns
First active	64	39	12	250	63	39	64	40	ns

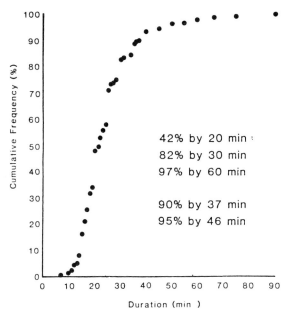

42% by 20 min

82% by 30 min

97% by 60 min

90% by 37 min

95% by 46 min

Figure 1. The cumulative distribution of first episodes of low FHR variability in labour (n = 176).

distribution of first episodes of low FHR variability against duration and shows that only 5% lasted longer than 46 min.

Of the CTGs with cycles present, the long-term variability was less than 5 beats/min in 48% of all quiet episodes (low FHR variability episodes). Of the CTGs without cycles, 24% had 1 or more periods of 20 min or longer with FHR variability less than 5 beats/min. Eight of the 16 caesarian sections said to be performed for fetal distress had CTGs with variability less than 5 beats/min and half of these were cyclers. One of these was a spontaneous labour. Seven babies had a 5-min Apgar score of 6 or less, of which 4 were cyclers and 3 had episodes of FHR variability of less than 5 beats/min. The agreement between the two assessments of 30% of the CTGs was 88%.

Discussion

Cycles of episodes of FHR variability are readily appreciated by visual assessment in the majority of cases in which they are present. Our findings of mean cycle length (92 min) and mean duration of quiet episode (25 min) are similar to previously reported values for behavioural cycles both antepartum and postpartum and strongly suggest that fetal behavioural cycles continue in many labours, particularly in induced labours.

More induced labours showed cycles than spontaneous labours particularly in 6–9-h CTGs. Labours of 6 h or longer were selected in an attempt to equate the durations of spontaneous and induced labours. Nevertheless, induced labours were longer, and after 9 h a greater proportion of both spontaneous and induced labours were cyclers, with no significant difference between them. Of these longer labours, 71% showed cycling compared with 48% of 6–9-hour labours.

Although episodes of low FHR variability may well relate to periods of quiet fetal behaviour or fetal sleep, high FHR variability cannot distinguish between active fetal sleep and awake states. In this study of 301 intrapartum CTGs longer than 6 h duration, 58% of labours showed evidence of fetal behavioural state cycles. Five per cent of first quiet episodes lasted 46–90 min and nearly half of all quiet episodes had an FHR variability of less than 5 beats/min.

Acknowledgements

We thank Mrs P. Molloy for assistance, Mrs P. Yudkin for statistical advice and Dr C. Redman and Mrs P. Yudkin for access to the computerized records held in the Oxford Obstetric Data System. We thank the DHSS and the MRC for financial support.

References

1. DeHaan, R., Patrick, J., Chess, G. F. and Jaco, N. T. (1977). *Am. J. Obstet. Gynecol.* **127**, 753–758.
2. Van Geijn, H. P., Jongsma, H. W., deHaan, J., Eskes, T. K. A. B. and Prechtl, H. F. R. (1980). *Am. J. Obstet. Gynecol.* **136**, 1061–1066.

3. Nijhuis, J. G., Prechtl, H. F. R., Martin, C. B. and Bots, R. S. G. M. (1982). *Early Hum. Dev.* **6**, 177–195.
4. Junge, H. D. (1979). *J. Perinat. Med.* **7**, 85–148.
5. Visser, G. H. A., Carse, E. A., Goodman, J. D. S. and Johnson, P. (1982). *Br. J. Obstet. Gynaec.* **89**, 50–55.
6. Greene, K. R., Natale, R. and Harrison, C. Y. (1980). *In:* "Fetal and Neonatal Physiological Measurements", (Rolfe, P., ed.) pp. 250–255. Pitman Medical, London.
7. Richardson, B., Natale, R. and Patrick, J. (1979). *Am. J. Obstet. Gynecol.* **133**, 247–255.
8. Paul, R. H., Snidan, A. K., Yeh, S.-Y., Schifrin, B. S. and Hon, E. H. (1975). *Am. J. Obstet. Gynecol.* **123**, 206–210.
9. Low, J. A., Cox, M. J., Marchmar, E. J., Panchani, S. R. and Piercy, W. N. (1981). *Am. J. Obstet. Gynecol.* **139**, 299–305.

Quantitative Two-dimensional Echocardiographic Study of Left Ventricular Shape in Normal Newborns: Early *vs* Late Umbilical Cord Clamping

Annabelle Azancot, Thomas Caudell, Joel Crequat, Georgio Toscani, J. H. Ravina and Hugh D. Allen

Hôpital Bretonneau-Bichat, INSERM U 120, Paris, France and University of Arizona Health Sciences Center, Tucson, Arizona, USA

Placental transfusion has been demonstrated to be an important factor in the cardiovascular adaptation of the newborn to early extra-uterine life (1). In a previous two-dimensional echocardiographic study of normal fetuses, newborns and infants, serial changes in left ventricular shape could be quantified (2). In normal fetuses and newborns, the septal portion of the left ventricle was flattened and distorted, resembling patterns of right ventricular volume or pressure overload, and tended towards roundness in infants. These left ventricular septal changes could be expected because of the dramatic cardiovascular adjustments that occur at birth and affect interdependent left and right ventricular geometries. Our present study was undertaken to quantify the magnitude of the effects of early and late cord clamping on left ventricular shape in normal newborns.

Patient Population

Studies were performed on 12 women having normal pregnancies after informed consent. They were randomly divided into late cord (Group I, 3 min) early cord clamping (Group II, 5 s). Fetal gestational age was evaluated by standard echographic measurements of biparietal diameter and abdominal circumference and fetal cardiac anatomy was simultaneously studied. Normalcy of pregnancy

The Physiological Development of the Fetus and Newborn
ISBN 0 12 389080 2

Copyright © 1985 by Academic Press, London.
All rights of reproduction in any form reserved.

Table 1. Clinical data and individual shape factors in late cord clamping group (IA and IB) and early cord clamping group (IIA and IIB).

Patient no.	Weight (kg)	Gestational age (weeks)	Apgar score	Sex	Haematocrit (%)	Group A			Group B		
						Time of examination (min)	Shape factor D	S	Time of examination (h)	Shape factor D	S
Group I											
1	3.5	41	9	M	63.5	20	4.95	2.60	27	5.14	2.40
2	3.0	39	10	F	63.2	5	6.00	3.60	9	4.10	3.10
3	3.6	41	10	F	51.4	35	5.30	2.73	41	3.95	3.00
4	2.8	40	9	M	55.6	50	3.70	3.65	—	—	—
5	3.2	38	10	F	55.0	40	5.45	3.01	18	5.00	2.65
6	3.1	38	10	M	61.0	—	—	—	{ 4.7 / 72	5.00 / 3.98	2.50 / 2.01
mean±SD	3.2±0.3	39.5±1.4			58.3±5.0	30±18			28.5±25		
Group II											
7	3.1	40	10	M	50.0	10	3.68	3.04	4.17	2.45	2.00
8	2.9	39	10	F	46.0	—	—	—	9.25	3.12	1.99
9	2.9	39	10	M	50.0	10	2.02	1.90	50	2.20	1.80
10	3.2	40	9	F	50.4	25	3.09	1.89	5.3	2.75	—
11	3.9	40	10	F	43.6	15	2.85	1.87	{ 5.25 / 25.25	3.00 / 2.20	1.95 / 2.15
mean±SD	3.2±0.4	39.6±0.5			48.0±3.0	15±7			16.5±18		

D = early diastolic frame; S = end-systolic frame.

and labour was confirmed by their course. No anaesthetics or analgesics were used. Vaginal delivery was timed as soon as the buttock was delivered and newborns were placed at 10 cm below a zero reference point, according to a technique utilized by Yao and Lind (2). Physical examination of the newborns was undertaken by one of the investigators. Clinical data are shown in Table 1. No significant differences were noted between Groups I and II for gestational age, weight and all Apgar scores were greater than 8. Haematocrits were obtained by venous puncture in all newborns within less than 2 h after birth and were found to differ significantly between the two groups ($P < 0.02$). Twenty-three echocardiographic examinations were performed; 1 patient from Group I was excluded because of poor imaging quality. Newborns were serially examined and each group was subdivided into subgroups A and B, according to the time of examination after birth (Table 1).

Echocardiographic Examinations and Methodology

Newborns were studied with a mechanical sector scanner (ATL Mark 300C) using a 5-MHz transducer. Although complete two-dimensional examinations were performed, only short axis views of the left ventricle at the mitral valve level were analysed. Real-time recordings on video tape allowed frame-by-frame analysis and selection of the 2 images utilized:

    1. early diastole (D), maximal opening of the mitral valve,
    2. end-systole (S), frame just before mitral valve opening.

The short axis left ventricular inner contour was traced on Polaroid photographs using a Micrographics tablet interfaced to an Apple II. The resulting co-ordinates were submitted to an Apple II shape analysis programme. The details of Fourier shape analysis have been previously reported (3). A least squares linear mapping technique places the input shape within a continuous sequence of model shapes generated from the 7 discrete samples given in Fig. 1. This model was selected

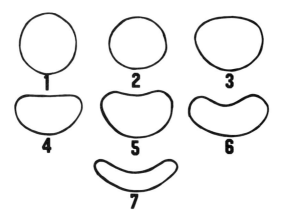

Figure 1. Seven discrete shapes which form the model sequence used in the quantitative analysis.

to match the range and type of distortion observed in the normal population (3). The shape factor is a pointer into the sequence of shapes displayed in Fig. 1 and the algorithm places the data shape in the sequence where it best fits. Data were statistically analysed by an unpaired Student t test for intergroup comparison. Normal means and variances from the previous study (3) were also compared to these groups using one sample t statistic.

Results and Discussion

The shape factor means and standard deviations for each of the subgroups and normals are presented in Table 2. Quantitative shape analysis showed significantly greater diastolic and systolic shape factors ($P < 0.01$) in late cord clamping group as opposed to the early group. A practically complete placental transfusion enhances septal flattening and distortion and produces diastolic patterns of right volume or pressure overload (Fig. 2) differing from normals ($P < 0.01$). Left ventricular configuration in newborns, who received a minimal placental transfusion, was either consistent with the normals or tended to be rounder ($P < 0.01$). In the overall population systolic shapes were all rounder than diastolic shapes as previously described (3).

Table 2. Shape factor means and standard deviations for diastolic (D) and systolic (S) frames for each of the 4 subgroups and normals

	Group A		Group B	
	D	S	D	S
Group I	5.08±0.86	3.16±0.45	4.54±0.57	2.61±0.40
Group II	2.91±0.69	2.18±0.58	2.62±0.40	1.98±0.13
Normal	3.7±0.8	2.4±0.6	3.5±0.8	2.3±0.6

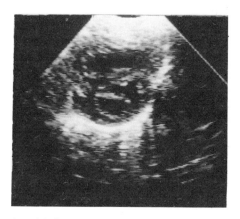

Figure 2. Two-dimensional left ventricular short axis frame in late cord clamping newborns.

Placental transfusion yields an abrupt increase in blood volume at birth. Furthermore, pulmonary artery pressure has been reported to remain near systemic level for the first hours of life in late cord clamping newborns (2). Although the buffer adjustment due to the liver capacity and plasma transudation mitigates the hypervolaemic state, our study demonstrates that placental transfusion distorts left ventricular geometry and thus affects the adaptation and interrelationship of right and left ventricles to extra-uterine life. These effects on left ventricular shape and function must be taken into account in situations with potentially high risk for the newborn.

References

1. Yao, A. C. and Lind, J. (1974). *Am. J. Dis. Child.* **127**, 128–141.
2. Yao, A. C. and Lind, J. (1969). *Lancet*, **ii**, 505–508.
3. Azancot, A., Caudell, T. P., Allen, H. D., Horowitz, S., Sahn, D. J., Stoll, C., Thies, C., Valdez-Cruz, L. M. and Goldberg, S. J. (1983). *Circulation* **68**, 1201–1211.

The Continuous Measurement of Maternal-fetal Transfer Using Mass Spectrometry: Possible Noninvasive Intrapartum Placental Function Testing

J. A. D. Spencer*, D. C. Andrews*, J. C. Wollner*,
R. S. Wolton**, P. Rolfe** and P. Johnson*

*Nuffield Department of Obstetrics and Gynaecology, **Bio-Engineering
Unit, Department of Paediatrics, John Radcliffe Hospital, Oxford, UK

Introduction

The clinical assessment of fetal respiratory status in early labour depends largely upon the interpretation of changes in the fetal heart rate (FHR), and an NIH Task Force has recommended research into new methods of fetal monitoring (1). We have developed a fetal scalp skin-surface mass spectrometer probe (2) which has been used with a modified industrial magnetic sector mass spectrometer to make continuous noninvasive measurements of fetal transcutaneous oxygen and carbon dioxide during labour (3). In the experimental animal we are developing a short repeatable test using argon inhalation, attempting to assess the basis for such a test of maternal–fetal transfer suitable for use with the skin surface mass spectrometry probes in early labour. We describe our preliminary results of the effects of uterine artery and umbilical cord occlusion on the maternal–fetal transfer of argon in the pregnant ewe.

Methods

We have modified an industrial mass spectrometer (MM 8-80, VG Medical Systems, Cheshire, UK) to accept two inlets maintained at operational vacuum. Measurements can therefore be obtained from two probes by alternating between the two inlets. For intra-arterial mass spectrometry in animals we used 18-inch

The Physiological Development of the Fetus and Newborn
ISBN 0 12 389080 2

Copyright © 1985 by Academic Press, London.
All rights of reproduction in any form reserved.

steel catheters, OD 0.028 inches, covered by a silicone rubber membrane (Silastic, Dow Corning) 0.022 inches thick and sealed at the tip with adhesive. *In vitro* testing was performed with the intravascular probes in a closed system water bath with controlled flow and temperature using saturated saline solutions. The response of these probes was linear and the 95% response time approximately 60 s. The probes were calibrated for respiratory gases *in vivo* by comparison with conventional blood gas analysis on a calibrated blood gas analyser (ABL-3, Radiometer).

One ewe in late pregnancy was studied acutely under barbiturate anaesthesia, and 4 ewes in late pregnancy were studied as chronic preparations following placement of catheters at operation under general anaesthesia. The maternal mass spectrometer probe was placed in the right carotid or femoral artery, and an arterial sampling line was placed in the left carotid. The fetal mass spectrometer probe was placed in the left femoral artery and a sampling catheter placed in the right femoral artery. Inflatable occlusion cuffs were placed around the common uterine artery and umbilical cord. Gases were administered to the mother via a tracheostomy and recordings of respiratory gas concentrations, maternal and fetal blood pressures, fetal heart rate and amniotic pressure were also made.

The ratio of fetal : maternal levels following 2 min inhalation of argon was compared with longer periods of inhalation. Subsequently, a 2-min inhalational "bolus" was used. After 3 control inhalations, the uterine arterial supply was progressively occluded in steps whilst repeating the 2-min argon inhalation tests. Three argon tests were repeated after each experiment. In the acute animal, the test was repeated following complete occlusion of the umbilical cord.

A calibration factor was calculated for each probe from the *in vivo* calibrations of oxygen and carbon dioxide. The argon readings of each probe were then adjusted by this factor and changes from normal expressed as a percentage.

Results

To be of practical value in labour it is essential that any test be of short duration. We found that 2 min inhalation of 75% argon in oxygen produced a maternal peak that was 90% of the steady-state level by 135 s and a fetal peak by 175 s that was 45% of the level achieved after 20 min inhalation. One derivative of this relationship was a fetal to maternal peak ratio of 0.31 (Fig. 1). Clearance of argon from the fetus took approximately 15–20 min following which the test was repeated.

Partial uterine artery occlusion rapidly produced a stable situation with a raised fetal pulse pressure and reduced FHR variability. The fetal carbon dioxide remained slightly elevated and fetal oxygen was slightly reduced. However, the fetal maternal argon peak ratio was reduced by up to 50% (Fig. 2). Complete uterine artery occlusion resulted in an immediate fetal bradycardia and onset of hypertension which occurred before the sharp rise in PCO_2 and fall in PO_2. The fetal : maternal argon peak ratio was reduced to one-sixth but rose again immediately after release of the occlusion. There was a rebound rise in PO_2 and pulse pressure, and a mild tachycardia following release of the uterine artery

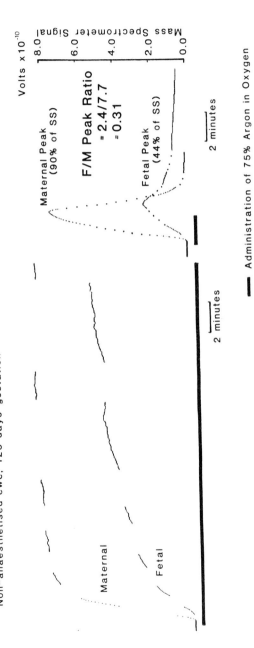

Figure 1. The maternal-fetal transfer of argon, comparing 20 min (maternal steady state) with 2 min administration and illustrating the calculation of the fetal : maternal peak ratio.

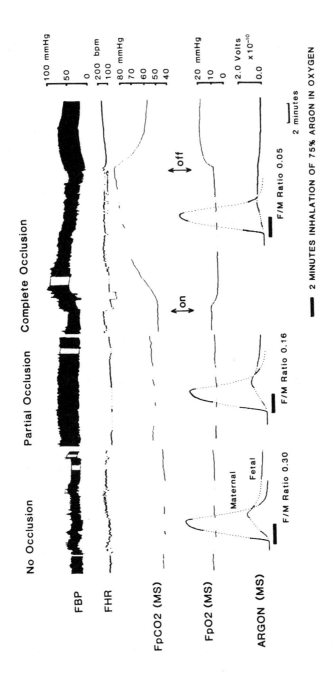

Figure 2. The effects of partial and complete uterine artery occlusion in a nonanaesthetized pregnant ewe of 130 days gestation.

occlusion. The fetal : maternal argon ratio was also raised in one experiment following release of the uterine artery occlusion and returned to normal by 2 h.

Complete umbilical cord occlusion resulted in no fetal argon being recorded, a situation which was also seen following fetal death.

Discussion

Some of the factors involved in maternal–fetal transfer have been determined previously by invasive, intermittent sampling in experimental animals (4). Because of this limitation, theories on the regulation of placental transfer have remained semiquantitative (5). Some investigators have assumed that measuring changes in oxygen transfer across the placenta would be a means of quantifying placental transfer. We feel this is unlikely since both oxygen and carbon dioxide are actively involved in fetal and placental metabolism and both of which may change independently of each other.

Experiments of chronic fetal growth retardation have shown that only the PO_2 is slightly altered from control levels (6). There is good reason to believe that measurement of FHR changes which are influenced by a variety of reflexes, or blood gas status are unlikely to relate to an initial reduction in "placental reserve" whereas maternal–fetal transfer of argon (or helium), despite its complex components, may be a useful investigative clinical test.

It has only recently been appreciated from chronic fetal studies that a reduction in uterine blood flow to 50% results in isocapnic hypoxaemia with no change in pH (7). In a similar situation, seen with partial uterine artery occlusion, the maternal–fetal transfer of argon was greatly (50%) reduced, providing an immediate index of a reduction of "placental reserve".

We have described a method of measuring placental transfer using continuous simultaneous mass spectrometer measurements in mother and fetus. It has the advantage that the measurements are immediately available and are easily repeatable. Preliminary results in ewes indicate that such measurements, reflecting both utero–placental flow and placental transfer, may well be a more reliable indication of "reserve" than observations of FHR alone as assessed in early labour.

Acknowledgements

This work is supported by grants from the Medical Research Council, the Department of Health and Social Security, the National Fund for Research into Crippling Diseases and the Oxford Medical Research Fund.

References

1. Zuspan, F. D., Quilligan, E. J., Iams, J. D. and Van Geijn, H. P. (1979). *Am. J. Obstet. Gynecol.* **135**, 287–291.
2. Rolfe, P., Burton, P. J., Crowe, J. A., Basarab-Howath, I., Goddard, P. J., Woolfson, J., Slevin, P. and Johnson, P. (1982). *Med. Biol. Eng. Comput.* **20**, 375–382.

3. Sykes, G. S., Molloy, P., Johnson, P., Turnbull, A. C., Rolfe, P., Burton, P. and Goddard, P. (1983). *Europ. J. Obstet. Gynaec. Reprod. Biol.* **14**, 438–441.
4. Barron, D. H. (1969). *Am. J. Obstet. Gynecol.* **105**, 368–373.
5. Dawes, G. S. (1973). *In:* "Fetal Pharmacology", (Boreus, L., ed.) pp. 381–399. Raven Press, New York.
6. Clapp, J. F., Szeto, H. H., Larrow, R., Hewitt, J. and Mann, L. I. (1980). *Am. J. Obstet. Gynecol.* **138**, 60–67.
7. Gu, W., Parer, J. T. and Jones, C. T. (1982). Presented at the Tenth World Congress of Obstetrics and Gynecology.

Chronic Villitis of Unknown Aetiology and Maternal Vascular Lesions in Placentae of Idiopathic Small for Gestational Age Infants

Carlos Labarrere, Omar Althabe* and Margarita Telenta

Departments of Pathology and *Obstetrics, Gascón 450 (1181),
Hospital Italiano, Buenos Aires, Argentina

Fetal growth retardation is known to be associated with a variety of adverse maternal and uterine factors, but there is a group where growth retardation occurs in the absence of any known cause. Chronic inflammatory lesions of villi have been described in placentae from small for gestational age (SGA) infants (1–4). Recently a correlation between the severity of chronic villitis and the degree of growth retardation has been reported (2,4). We report here a study of the incidence of chronic villitis of unknown aetiology (CVUE) and maternal vascular lesions in placentae from SGA infants in the absence of any known cause.

Material and Methods

Placentae from 215 uncomplicated singleton full-term pregnancies were studied. Of these, 142 corresponded to infants with normal birthweight and so served as the control group. The control group was divided into two subgroups, one which included placentae from infants with birthweight between the 10th and 25th centiles of the ponderal curve and another one which comprised those with birthweight over the 25th centile. The remaining 73 placentae were from SGA infants (under the 10th centile of the normal ponderal curve (5)).

There were no statistical differences between the groups with respect to age, parity or smoking habits (all mothers smoking fewer than 5 cigarettes/day). Neither the mothers nor infants had clinical or serological evidence of infection and all newborns, both from the control and SGA groups were physically and neurologically normal.

The Physiological Development of the Fetus and Newborn
ISBN 0 12 389080 2

Copyright © 1985 by Academic Press, London.
All rights of reproduction in any form reserved.

The placentae were fixed whole in 10% formalin for several days and they were weighed after the membranes and cord were trimmed off. After external examination the placentae were then cut into slices and standardized blocks were taken, using the technique described by Fox. A roll of membranes was prepared using the technique described by Benirschke (7). All histological sections were stained with haematoxylin and eosin: in selected cases sections were also stained with PAS or Masson's trichrome.

In all cases in which the percentage of villi showing abnormalities is quoted the counts were made on villi in the maternal zone of the central portion (6).

For statistical analysis, the following tests were used: Student's *t* for independent samples, Wilcoxon's two samples test and the χ^2 test.

Results

Chronic villitis was a common finding in placentae from all groups (Fig. 1). The lesion was present in 78% of placentae of the SGA group while in the control group this proportion was 34% ($P<0.0005$) (Table 1). A striking feature is the very high incidence of villitis found not only in the SGa group but also in the placentae of control group. Nevertheless analysing the relationship between the incidence of chronic villitis and infants birthweight in control group we found that its incidence in placentae from infants with birthweight over the 25th

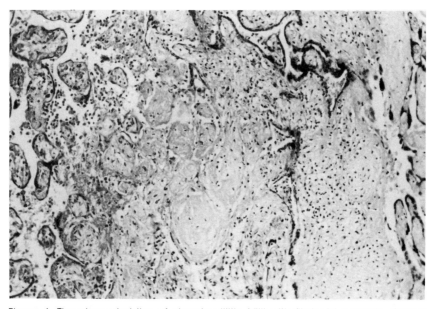

Figure 1. The characteristics of chronic villitis. Villi with fibrinoid necrosis, stromal mononuclear cell infiltration and trophoblastic necrosis are present. Surrounding the villi, there is a maternal component of lymphocytes, monocytes and macrophages. Stained with H and E. Multiplication × 100.

Table 1. Histopathological findings in the studied groups

| | | Normal birthweight | | |
	SGA	10–25 centile	25th centile	Total
Chronic villitis (%)	78	47	25	34
Inflamed villi* (%)	8.5	2.9	1.8	2.4
Anchoring villitis (%)	79	57	54	55
Placentae with maternal vascular lesions	8	2	2	4

*This value corresponds to the mean proportion of inflamed villi within each subgroup.
Chronic villitus and anchoring villitis are expressed as percent of cases with these lesions.
SGA: small for gestational age infants.

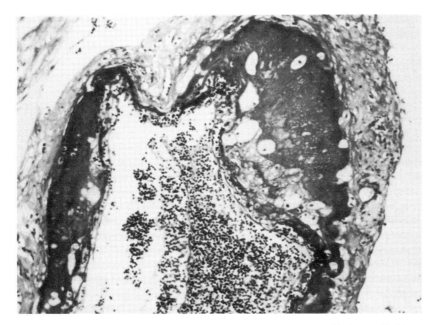

Figure 2. A spiral artery of the basal plate with acute atherosis. Stained with H and E. Multiplication × 100.

percentile was 25%, while in placentae from infants with birthweights between the 10th and 25th percentiles this incidence was 47% ($P < 0.02$) (Table 1).

In those placentae of the control group with chronic villitis, the mean proportion of inflamed villi was 2.4%, while in the SGA group a mean of 8.5% of terminal villi were inflamed ($P < 0.01$) (Table 1). Also in the control group, those placentae corresponding to infants with lower birthweights (between the 10th and 25th centiles) showed a higher incidence of inflamed villi than those from newborns with higher weights (over the 25th centile).

Another interesting finding was a lymphocytic infiltrate observed in anchoring villi within the basal plate (anchoring villitis) in 136 out of the 215 studied placentae. In the control group 55% of the placentae showed the lesion, while in the SGA group 79% of the placentae were affected ($P<0.005$) (Table 1).

Maternal vascular lesions, consisting of absence of normal trophoblastic invasion of spiral arteries in the placental bed, acute atherosis (Fig. 2) and chronic vasculitis-like lesions, were more frequently found in SGA group than in controls (Table 1).

Discussion

The results here described confirm our previous observations (3,4). We have postulated that CVUE and anchoring villitis may be the morphological expression of a maternal reaction against the fetal hemiallograft. In favour of this are:

1. absence of clinical and serological evidences of infection in mothers and their infants;
2. morphological of placental lesions different from those described for specific infections;
3. fibrinoid and trophoblastic necrosis surrounded by an intense chronic inflammatory infiltrate, probably of maternal origin;
4. chronic inflammatory infiltrate in basal plate surrounding anchoring villi exclusively;
5. lesions in maternal spiral arteries similar to those described in pre-eclampsia with or without intra-uterine growth retardation (8,9), systemic lupus erythematosus (10), and rejected renal transplants (11);
6. deposits of IgM and C_3 in acute atherosis-like lesions (12), similar to those described in pre-eclampsia (13,14) and systemic erythematosus (10).

Chronic villitis was present in a very high incidence in our material. An explanation for this may be that we considered the lesion was present with a proportion of inflamed villi as low as 0.1% or even less. An incidence of 6–10% of CVUE has been found in Australia, Canada and USA (2,15; W. A. Blanc, pers. comm.), but the exact frequency in other countries remains unknown. So, it may be possible that different populations have different incidences of this lesion.

CVUE, anchoring villitis and maternal vascular lesions in placentae may be related to a deficit in placentation. The extension and severity of this deficit may determine infants' birthweight.

References

1. Altshuler, G., Russell, P. and Ermocilla, R. (1975). *Am. J. Obstet. Gynecol.* **121**, 351–359.
2. Russell, P. (1980). *Placenta* **1**, 227–244.
3. Labarrere, C., Althabe, O. and Telenta, M. (1982). *Placenta* **3**, 309–318.

4. Althabe, O. and Labarrere, C. (1982). *In:* "Prog. Clin. Biol. Res. Vol. 112B, Recent Advances in Fertility Research—Part B: Developments in the Management of Reproductive Disorders", (Muldoon, T. G., Mahesh, V. B. and Perez-Ballester, B., eds) pp. 227–238. Alan R. Liss, New York.

5. Guayasamin, O., Benedetti, W. L., Althabe, O., Nieto, E. and Tenzer, S. (1976). *Bol. Sanit. Panam.* **81**, 481–488.

6. Fox, H. (1978). *In:* "Pathology of the Placenta", pp. 473–476. W. B. Saunders, London.

7. Benirschke, K. (1961). *Obstet. Gynecol.* **18**, 309–333.

8. Robertson, W. B., Brosens, I. and Dixon, G. (1975). *Europ. J. Obstet. Gynaec. Reprod. Biol.* **5**, 47–65.

9. Sheppard, B. L. and Bonnar, J. (1981). *Br. J. Obstet. Gynaec.* **88**, 695–705.

10. Abramowsky, C. R., Vegas, M. E., Swinehart, G. and Gyves, M. T. (1980). *N. Engl. J. Med.* **303**, 668–672.

11. Dempster, W. J., Harrison, C. V. and Shackman, R. (1964). *Br. Med. J.* **2**, 969–976.

12. Labarrere, C., Manni, J., Salas, P. and Althabe, O. (1985). Submitted for publication.

13. Kitzmiller, J. L. and Benirschke, K. (1973). *Am. J. Obstet. Gynecol.* **115**, 248–251.

14. Kitzmiller, J. L., Watt, N. and Driscoll, S. G. (1981). *Am. J. Obstet. Gynecol.* **141**, 773–779.

15. Altshuler, G. and Russell, P. (1975). *In:* "Current Topics in Pathology", (Grundmann, E. and Kirsten, W. H., eds) Vol. 60, pp. 63–112. Springer-Verlag, Berlin.

Intravenous Use of IgG in the Treatment of Neonatal Passive Immune Thrombocytopenia

F. Ciccimarra, M. De Curtis, R. Paludetto,
G. Romano and R. Troncone*

Patologia Neonatale and *Clinica Pediatrica, 2nd School of Medicine,
University of Naples, Naples, Italy

Intravenously administered gammaglobulin is an effective treatment for immune thrombocytopenic purpura in children and adults (1,2). An immediate increase in platelet count is usually seen, even if this effect is often temporary. We report a successful similar treatment in a newborn infant affected by passive immune thrombocytopenia.

Case Report

The mother, a 16-year old woman, developed acute immune thrombocytopenic purpura during the 7th month of pregnancy; despite steroid treatment her platelet count was consistently lower than $40\,000/mm^3$. A normal infant girl was delivered at 37 weeks (birthweight: 2900 g). The baby's platelet count was $48\,000/mm^3$ at birth and rapidly fell to $18\,000/mm^3$ during the first 2 days, notwithstanding the absence of detectable serum platelet antibody. On the 2nd day, diffuse petechiae and microscopic haematuria appeared. Five consecutive daily infusions of IgG (Sandoglobulin, 0.4 g/kg of body weight) resulted in an immediate increase in platelet count and remission of symptoms (Fig. 1). No relapse of the bleeding manifestations or thrombocytopenia was observed up to 6 months after discharge and no other IgG infusions were necessary.

Discussion

Passively acquired immune neonatal thrombocytopenia secondary to maternal immune thrombocytopenic purpura is a transient disorder that may persist for

The Physiological Development of the Fetus and Newborn
ISBN 0 12 389080 2

Copyright © 1985 by Academic Press, London.
All rights of reproduction in any form reserved.

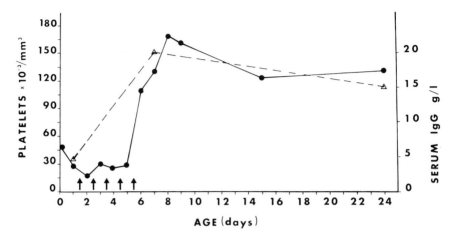

Figure 1. Platelet count (●———●) and serum IgG concentrations (▵ – – – ▵) following high-dose intravenous IgG infusions (↑) in a newborn affected by passive immune thrombocytopenia.

1–4 months. The clinical picture ranges from a lack of symptoms to severe clinical manifestations such as intracranial bleeding. Among current therapies, the use of prednisone is controversial and exchange transfusion, often followed by platelet transfusion, is reserved for cases with moderate/severe clinical signs. Nevertheless all these therapies carry inherent complications. Asymptomatic thrombocytopenic newborns do not usually receive any therapy. However, it is not justifiable to "wait and see"; all the thrombocytopenic newborns should be considered at high risk of intracranial bleeding, whatever the platelet count, platelet antibody titre or clinical course. In contrast to other therapies, no side-effects have been observed in our case, nor in the other 2 thrombocytopenic newborns similarly treated (3,4), nor in high-risk newborns also treated with high doses of intact intravenous gammaglobulin for prophylaxis or therapy of infections (5). Immune suppression has been reported in adults to follow IgG infusions (6), but increased suppressive activity is difficult to evaluate in newborns, as their lymphocytes usually strongly inhibit *in-vitro* IgG synthesis (7); pokeweed mitogen-induced *in-vitro* IgG synthesis from adult mononuclear cells was almost completely suppressed by T cells from our patient both before and 1 day after the last IgG infusion (82 and 79% inhibition, respectively).

In conclusion, in view of the transient character of neonatal passive immune thrombocytopenia and its dramatic reversal following IgG transfusions without any documented side-effects, this treatment may be a sound alternative to exchange transfusions in symptomatic patients and an effective first-choice therapy to maintain asymptomatic patients safely, until maternal antibody disappears. Furthermore, it seems worth exploring the prophylactic value of antenatal administration of gammaglobulin to the mother with auto-immune thrombocytopenia.

References

1. Imbach, P., d'Apuzzo, V., Hirt, A., Rossi, E., Vest, M., Barandun, S., Baumgartner, C., Morell, A., Schöni, M. and Wagner, H. P. (1981). *Lancet* **i**, 1228-1330.
2. Fehr, J., Hofman, V. and Kappler, U. (1982). *N. Engl. J. Med.* **306**, 1254-1258.
3. Chirico, G., Duse, M., Ugazio, A. G. and Rondini, G. (1983). *J. Pediat.* **103**, 654-655.
4. Newland, A. C., Boots, M. A. and Patterson, K. G. (1984). *N. Engl. J. Med.* **310**, 261-262.
5. Chirico, G., Duse, M., Chiara, A., Rondini, G. and Ugazio, A. G. (1983). "XVII International Congress of Pediatrics, Manila, Abstracts of Symposia", Vol. 2, p. 579.
6. Tsubakio, T., Kurata, Y., Katagiri, S., Kamakira, Y., Tamaki, T., Kuyama, J., Kamayama, Y., Yonezawa, T. and Tarui, S. (1983). *Clin. Exp. Immunol.* **53**, 697-702.
7. Morito, T., Bankhurst, A. D. and Williams, R. C. (1979). *J. Clin. Invest.* **64**, 990-995.

The Endocrine and Metabolic Response to Surgery in the Human Neonate

K. J. S. Anand*, M. J. Brown,
S. R. Bloom and A. Aynsley-Green

*Department of Paediatrics, John Radcliffe Hospital, Oxford, UK, Royal Post-graduate Medical School, Hammersmith Hospital, London, UK, **Department of Child Health, Royal Victoria Infirmary, Newcastle-upon-Tyne, UK

Introduction

Adult patients respond to surgical stress by changes in the endocrine milieu which lead to catabolism and substrate mobilization in the postoperative period (1,2). This endocrine–metabolic response is not entirely beneficial and may precipitate a number of undesirable effects (3,4).

The catabolic stress reaction to surgery assumes greater significance in the context of newborn infants. The normal neonate exists in a precarious metabolic milieu as it adapts to the postnatal environment and to postnatal nutrition (5), and has limited body reserves of carbohydrate, fat and protein (6,7). Therefore, it would seem to be particularly disadvantageous, if not life-threatening, for a seriously ill or premature neonate to experience a severe and prolonged catabolic reaction to surgery.

Little is known of the endocrine and metabolic response to surgery in the human neonate and this has led to empirical anaesthetic practice. Indeed, the need for anaesthesia at all has been questioned (8,9), and in some centres even major surgery is performed on sick and premature neonates under the influence of muscle relaxants alone (10). We have designed a study to define the ability of newborn infants to mount an endocrine and metabolic response to surgical trauma.

Methods

A total of 33 neonates undergoing surgery were studied with a mean postnatal age of 18 ± 3 days ($\pm$SEM). Venous blood samples (1.0–2.0 ml) were drawn

The Physiological Development of the Fetus and Newborn
ISBN 0 12 389080 2

Copyright © 1985 by Academic Press, London.
All rights of reproduction in any form reserved.

immediately before the induction of anaesthesia, at the end of surgery and at 6, 12 and 24 h following surgery. Blood levels of glucose, lactate, pyruvate, alanine, β-hydroxybutyrate, acetoacetate, free fatty acids and glycerol were measured by specific enzymatic methods; radio-immunoassay methods were used to measure plasma levels of insulin and glucagon; adrenaline and noradrenaline were measured by a double-isotope radio-enzymatic assay.

The infants were premedicated with atropine alone (0.02–0.04 mg/kg). Anaesthetic agents were limited to the use of thiopentone, halothane, D-tubocurarine and nitrous oxide. Intravenous fluids were adjusted to administer dextrose at a standard infusion rate of 3–7 mg/kg/min during the surgical procedure and postoperatively.

Results

The overall metabolic and hormonal data from all 33 infants are listed in Table 1. Blood glucose concentrations increased significantly during surgery ($P \ll 0.0001$) and remained elevated at 6 h ($P < 0.001$) and 12 h ($P < 0.001$) postoperatively.

Table 1. Metabolic and hormonal changes (means ± SEM) in the infants studied

	n	Preop	Endop	6 h	12 h	24 h
Metabolites						
Glucose	33	4.8±0.2	11.1±1.0	7.0±0.9	7.6±1.4	5.5±0.5
(mmol/l)			$P \ll 0.001$*	$P < 0.001$	$P < 0.001$	NS
Lactate	33	1.6±0.1	2.9±0.3	2.1±0.3	2.0±0.2	1.8±0.2
(mmol/l)			$P \ll 0.001$	$P < 0.05$	$P < 0.01$	NS
Pyruvate	33	0.10±0.01	0.16±0.02	0.13±0.01	0.13±0.01	0.11±0.01
(mmol/l)			$P \ll 0.001$	NS	NS	NS
Alanine	33	0.22±0.01	0.24±0.02	0.24±0.02	0.25±0.03	0.22±0.01
(mmol/l)			NS	NS	NS	NS
Total ketones	33	0.18±0.02	0.30±0.05	0.17±0.02	0.17±0.03	0.16±0.02
(mmol/l)			$P < 0.005$	NS	NS	NS
Glycerol	33	0.17±0.02	0.25±0.03	0.17±0.02	0.19±0.02	0.16±0.02
(mmol/l)			$P < 0.005$	NS	NS	NS
Free fatty acids	5	0.38±0.10	0.63±0.07	0.51±0.18	0.35±0.08	0.27±0.04
(mmol/l)			$P < 0.05$	NS	NS	NS
Hormones						
Adrenaline	14	0.08±0.02	0.44±0.17	0.08±0.02	0.05±0.01	0.08±0.04
(ng/ml)			$P < 0.001$	NS	NS	NS
Noradrenaline	14	0.81±0.14	1.62±0.41	1.23±0.32	1.35±0.42	0.87±0.12
(ng/ml)			$P < 0.005$	NS	NS	NS
Insulin	27	12±2	15±3	21±4	17±4	22±4
(mU/l)			NS	NS	$P < 0.025$	$P < 0.025$
Glucagon	7	29±6	31±7	23±5	16±5	16±5
(pmol/l)			NS	NS	NS	$P < 0.025$

*Wilcoxon's matched-pairs signed-ranks test from preoperative values.

There was a significant increase in blood concentrations of lactate ($P<0.001$), pyruvate ($P<0.001$), total ketone bodies (acetoacetate and β-hydroxybutyrate) ($P<0.005$), free fatty acids ($P<0.05$) and glycerol ($P<0.005$) during surgery. Levels of blood lactate remained elevated until 12 h after surgery ($P<0.01$), whereas all other metabolites reverted to preoperative levels by 6 h postoperatively. No significant changes were seen in blood alanine concentration during or after surgery.

Plasma concentrations of adrenaline ($P<0.001$) and noradrenaline ($P<0.005$) were significantly increased at the end of surgery, but levels of plasma insulin and glucagon did not change in the immediate perioperative period. By 12 h postoperatively a significant increase was recorded in plasma insulin levels ($P<0.025$) which was maintained up to 24 h after surgery ($P<0.025$), whereas plasma glucagon levels had decreased significantly by 24 h postoperatively.

Blood glucose concentrations were correlated strongly with plasma adrenaline at the end of surgery ($r/s=0.95$, $n=14$, $P<0.0001$) and with plasma glucagon at 6 h postoperatively ($r/s=0.86$, $n=7$, $P<0.05$). Levels of blood lactate were correlated with plasma adrenaline concentrations at the end of surgery ($r/s=0.61$, $n=14$, $P<0.025$) and at 6 h postoperatively ($r/s=0.70$, $n=11$, $P<0.01$). A significant correlation was also present between blood glycerol levels and plasma adrenaline ($r/s=0.76$, $n=14$, $P<0.005$) and noradrenaline ($r/s=0.63$, $n=14$, $P<0.01$) at the end of surgery.

Discussion

Remarkably little is known of the metabolic and endocrine responses of human neonates subjected to surgery (11–17). In this study, various factors which could affect perioperative metabolism were standardized as far as possible for all neonates investigated. The duration of preoperative starvation was limited to 4 h, perioperative fluid therapy was adjusted in order to deliver dextrose at a rate of 3–7 mg/kg/min, parenteral nutrition solutions containing amino acids or soluble fats were not given from 6 h preoperatively until 24 h after surgery, and the timing of postoperative analgesia was adjusted so as to have no effect on the hormonal or metabolic variables measured in this study.

The most important metabolic effect we have documented is the postoperative hyperglycaemia which was invariably present in all neonates studied. At the end of surgery, the excellent correlation between blood glucose and plasma adrenaline values implies that the hyperglycaemic response may be precipitated by adrenaline release during surgery. Six hours postoperatively, blood glucose concentrations were closely related to plasma glucagon, a correlation which achieved statistical significance even though glucagon was measured in only a small number of patients ($n=7$). Therefore, according to these data, it may be proposed that postsurgical hyperglycaemia in neonates is initiated by adrenaline release and is maintained into the early postoperative period as a result of glucagon secretion (18–20). Of greater importance, however, is the lack of insulin secretion during surgery and in the early postoperative period, probably due to a direct inhibition of insulin secretion by adrenaline release during surgery (21). Consequently, the insulin : glucose molar ratio decreased significantly at the end of surgery, reflecting inappropriately low insulin levels for the circulating glucose concentrations. However, insulin levels were found to be significantly elevated at 12 and 24 h postoperatively thereby bringing blood glucose to normal levels again. The substantial hyperglycaemic response, particularly in the severe surgical stress group has important clinical implications due to its effect on plasma osmolality (22).

Concurrent with postoperative hyperglycaemia, marked increases in blood lactate and pyruvate concentrations were seen immediately after surgery. Levels of blood lactate and plasma adrenaline were correlated significantly at the end of surgery and 6 h postoperatively. Recent studies have shown that the release of adrenaline during surgery causes an increased production of lactate and pyruvate in skeletal muscles (23). The levels of free fatty acids, glycerol and total ketone bodies increased significantly during surgery, probably due to lipolysis and ketogenesis stimulated by intra-operative catecholamine release (24). Evidence for catecholamine-dependent lipolysis is further provided by the strong correlation of blood glycerol concentrations with plasma adrenaline and noradrenaline levels at the end of surgery.

Thus, the main features of the neonatal stress response are hyperglycaemia and hyperlactataemia associated with the release of catecholamines and inhibition of insulin secretion.

References

1. Elliot, M. and Alberti, K. G. M. M. (1983). *In:* "New Aspects of Clinical Nutrition", pp. 247–270. Karger, Basel.
2. Traynor, C. and Hall, G. M. (1981). *Brit. J. Anaesth.* **53**, 153–160.
3. Kehlet, H. (1979). *Acta Anaesth. Scand.* **23**, 503–504.
4. Rose, E. A. and King, T. C. (1978). *Surg. Gynecol. Obstet.* **147**, 97–102.
5. Aynsley-Green, A. (1982). *Monogr. Paediat.* **16**, 59–87.
6. Widdowson, E. M. (1981). *In:* "Scientific Foundations of Paediatrics", (Davis, J. A., Dobbing, J., eds) pp. 330–342. Heinemann, London.
7. Widdowson, E. M. and Spray, C. M. (1951). *Arch. Dis. Childh.* **26**, 205–214.
8. Shaw, E. A. (1982). *Hosp. Update* **8**, 423–434.
9. Downes, J. J. and Betts, E. K. (1977). *Am. Soc. Anesthesiol, Refresher Courses Anesthesiol.* **5**, 47–69.
10. Lipmann, M., Nelson, R. J., Emmanoulides, G. C. *et al.* (1976). *Brit. J. Anaesth.* **48**, 365–369.
11. Elphick, M. C. and Wilkinson, A. W. (1968). *Lancet* **ii**, 539–540.
12. Elphick, M. C. (1972). Ph.D. Thesis, University of London.
13. Elphick, M. C. and Wilkinson, A. W. (1981). *Pediat. Res.* **15**, 313–318.
14. Pinter, A. (1973). *Z. Kinderchir. und Grenz* **12**, 149–162.
15. Pinter, A. (1974). *Bruns. Beit. Klin. Chir.* **221**, 234–238.
16. Pinter, A. (1975). *Acta Paediat. Acad. Scient. Hung.* **16**, 171–180.
17. Pinter, A. (1975). *Acta Paediat. Acad. Scient. Hung.* **16**, 181–188.
18. De Fronzo, R. A., Sherwin, R. S. and Felig, P. (1980). *Acta Chir. Scand.* Suppl. **498**, 33–42.

19. Exton, J. H. and Park, C. R. (1966). *Pharmac. Rev.* **18**, 181–188.
20. Deibert, D. C. and De Fronzo, R. A. (1980). *J. Clin. Invest.* **65**, 717–721.
21. Bagdade, J. D., Bierman, E. L. and Porte, D. (1967). *J. Clin. Invest.* **46**, 1549–1557.
22. Finberg, L. (1967). *Pediat.* **40**, 1031–1034.
23. Stjernstrom, H., Jorfeldt, L. and Wiklund, L. (1981). *J. Parent. Ent. Nutr.* **5**, 207–214.
24. Williamson, D. H. (1982). *In:* "Biochemical Development of the Fetus and Neonate", (Jones, C. T., ed.) pp. 621–650. Elsevier, Amsterdam.

Body Motility According to Sleep States in Normal Newborn Infants: A Preliminary Study

L. Curzi-Dascalova, P. Peirano and G. Vicente

INSERM U-29, Hôpital de Port Royal,
Paris, France

Differences in central nervous system control of many physiological variables according to sleep states in premature infants have previously been described. Dreyfus-Brisac and Monod (5) pointed out the differences in electroencephalogram (EEG) patterns. They and other authors (4,8,10) used polygraphic and behavioural parameters to describe the emergence of sleep state organization. Differences in respiratory control according to sleep states was confirmed in prematures of less than 35 weeks conceptional age (CA) (1,3). During the last few years, many authors have shown that differentiation between active and quiet sleep in prematures is possible using EEG and rapid eye movement (REM) criteria (2,7,13). However, some authors pointed out that the presence of body motility during many nonrapid eye movement (NREM) periods prevents definition of sleep state organization in human prematures (4,11).

The aim of the present study was to detect whether some finer quantitative differences in body motility, occurring in quiet and active sleep, exist before the normal term. For that we used a real-time quantification of recorded body movements. Our method also enables movements of the upper and lower limbs to be compared and analysed separately.

Subjects and Methods

The study was carried out on 26 normal infants of 31–38 weeks CA, recorded during the neonatal period up to 10 days of postnatal age. Polygraphic methods, age criteria and normality definition have previously been described (2). Movements of the upper and lower limbs were recorded with a piezo-electric

The Physiological Development of the Fetus and Newborn
ISBN 0 12 389080 2

Copyright © 1985 by Academic Press, London.
All rights of reproduction in any form reserved.

quartz accelerometer attached to the back of hands and feet. Movements of the left and right upper limbs were summed and recorded on one channel, those of the lower limbs on another channel. Infants were continuously observed by two independent observers; all events were carefully noted. Some polygraphic data, including movements, were recorded on magnetic tape. The duration of movements recorded on the upper and on the lower limbs was automatically measured with 0.01 s accuracy, and the percentage of time in which movements occurred was calculated for every sleep state. Sleep states were coded according to EEG and REM criteria.

Statistical analysis was performed using the Wilcoxon matched-pairs signed rank test and the Mann–Whitney U-test.

Results

The durations of tracings and means of the percentages of the duration of movements of the upper and lower limbs, according to age and sleep states, are presented on Table 1.

Table 1. Mean duration (per 100 min) of movements recorded on the upper and lower limbs according to sleep states and age

CA (weeks)	Total (and mean) duration of tracing (min)	Limbs	Mean % of time with movements ± SEM					
			In AS	In QS	AS/QS	In IS	AS/IS	QS/IS
31–34	708	upper	20.2±5.4	5.2±1.5	*	21.5±4.1	NS	*
(n=6)	(118)	lower	14.2±3.3	4.4±1.5	*	15.0±2.9	NS	*
35–36	1356	upper	22.4±2.9	7.0±2.4	***	12.6±1.8	***	*
(n=10)	(136)	lower	17.8±1.8	5.6±1.3	***	11.8±2.4	**	***
37–38	1141	upper	18.6±3.3	7.3±2.1	***	23.2±7.3	NS	*
(n=10)	(114)	lower	22.2±4.8	9.5±2.0	***	21.4±4.6	NS	***

Abbreviations: CA, conceptional age; n, number of infants; AS, active sleep; QS, quiet sleep; IS, indeterminate sleep; level of between-state differences; NS, not significant; *$P<0.025$; **$P<0.01$; ***$P<0.005$.

Movements of upper and lower limbs

We did not find significant differences between movements recorded on the upper and lower limbs, except for quiet sleep at 37–38 weeks CA (lower limbs > upper limbs, $P<0.025$, Table 1). In spite of the absence of statistically significant differences, at 31–34 weeks CA we noted less movements in the upper limbs than in the lower limbs. With age, duration of lower limb movements approached and subsequently exceeded that of upper limbs (Table 1).

Body movements according to sleep states

In all infants studied, the percentage of time with movements was higher in active sleep compared to quiet sleep. This prevalence was found for movements recorded both on the upper and on the lower limbs (Table 1). At all ages, the duration of movement was higher in indeterminate sleep than in quiet sleep. The duration of movements in indeterminate sleep was similar to that in active sleep, except at 35–36 weeks CA; at this age we found significantly less movements in indeterminate than in active sleep.

Discussion

The present study shows that from 31–34 to 37–38 weeks CA, movements predominate in active sleep compared to quiet sleep. This prevalence is significant for movements recorded on both upper and lower limbs.

Our results agree with the observation of Karch et al. (7) and show some difference with those of Dreyfus-Brisac (4) and Prechtl et al. (11), who did not describe clear differences between body movements in REM and NREM periods until 37–38 weeks CA and sometimes later. We think that our results cannot be compared to the results of the last authors and that apparent disagreements are due to differences in the methodology and in the aim of the studies. Dreyfus-Brisac (4) and Prechtl et al. (11) used visual observation of body motility; they made excellent descriptions of different movement patterns (startles, gross body movements etc.) at different stages. Dreyfus-Brisac (4) counted numbers of movements/20 s in prematures recorded at various postnatal ages. Prechtl et al. (11) did not quantify the duration of movements; they studied 1-min epochs without movements from the point of view of sleep state stability. Our results were based on real-time duration of movements recorded in prematures during the neonatal period. In addition, we have to take into account the improvement of perinatal care during the last 15 years; it might modify motor behaviour of prematures. Our results and those of Karch et al. (7) contrast with the findings in fetal lambs (9,12): body movements in fetal lambs seem to predominate in NREM compared to REM periods.

In active and in quiet sleep, the duration of upper limb movements does not vary between 31 and 38 weeks CA. On the other hand, duration of lower limb movements increases with age and reaches values obtained by upper limbs. These observations might be related to the cranio-caudal maturation of the nervous system. The problem has to be elucidated with a larger number of infants.

We did not observe a decrease in motility between 31 and 38 weeks CA. Prechtl et al. (11) found a decrease after 36 weeks CA, Dreyfus-Brisac (4) after 38 weeks CA and Fukumoto et al. (6) much later, at 4–8 months of postterm age. All these works and our study note large between-subject variability.

The prevalence of body motility during active, REM sleep periods, compared to quiet, NREM periods is an additional fact, testifying to the existence of differences in control of physiological variables according to sleep states as early as 31–34 weeks CA, the lower limit of our study.

820   L. Curzi-Dascalova *et al.*

References

1. Curzi-Dascalova, L. (1983). *Biol. Neonate* **44**, 325–332.
2. Curzi-Dascalova, L., Lebrun, F. and Korn, G. (1983). *Pediat. Res.* **17**, 152–156.
3. Curzi-Dascalova, L., Relier, J. P., Vasseur, O. and Castex, M. (1983). *Biol. Neonate* **43**, 298.
4. Dreyfus-Brisac, C. (1970). *Develop. Psychobiol.* **3**, 91–121.
5. Dreyfus-Brisac, C. and Monod, N. (1975). *In:* "Handbook of Electroencephalography and Clinical Neurophysiology", (Lairy, G. C., ed.) Vol. 6, Part B, pp. 7–23. Elsevier, Amsterdam.
6. Fukumoto, M., Mochizuki, N., Takeishi, M., Nomura, Y. and Segawa, M. (1981). *Brain Develop.* **3**, 37–43.
7. Karch, D., Rothe, R., Jurisch, R., Heldt-Hildebrandt, R., Lubbesmeier, A. and Lemburg, P. (1982). *Develop. Med. Child Neurol.* **24**, 30–47.
8. Monod, N. and Garma, L. (1971). *Biol. Neonate* **17**, 292–316.
9. Natale, R., Clewlow, P. and Dawes, G. S. (1981). *Am. J. Obstet. Gynecol.* **140**, 545–551.
10. Parmelee, A. H. and Stern, E. (1972). *In:* "Sleep and the Maturing Nervous System", pp. 199–228. Academic Press, New York.
11. Prechtl, H. F. R., Fargel, J. W., Weinmann, H. M. and Bakker, H. H. (1979). *Develop. Med. Child Neurol.* **21**, 3–27.
12. Ruckebusch, Y., Gaujoux, M. and Eghbali, B. (1977). *Electroenceph. Clin. Neurophysiol.* **42**, 226–237.
13. Stefanski, M., Schulze, K., Bateman, D., Kairam, R., Pedley, T. A., Masterson, J. and James, L. S. (1984). *Pediat. Res.* **18**, 58–62.

The Maturation of the Ambient Thermal Stimulus to Breathing during Sleep in Lambs

D. C. Andrews, L. Fedorko, P. Johnson and J. C. Wollner

Nuffield Department of Obstetrics and Gynaecology, University of Oxford, Oxford, UK

Maintenance of efficient breathing after birth is decisive for survival. Most investigators concentrated on chemoreception—central or peripheral—as the main factor responsible for the effective control of respiration. Other factors such as mechano-reflexes from the lung stretch receptors or the influence of ambient temperature on respiratory activity are usually regarded as modulating and adjusting the respiratory output. However, the peripheral chemoreceptors are not active in the first days of life as was found in newborn lambs (1). There is no available data about central chemosensitivity in the early neonatal period. It is now known that the biphasic response to hypoxia in the newborn is not one of the depression (2) and probably does not differ from that in the adult when oxygen consumption falls. On the other hand cooling ovine fetuses *in utero* below body temperature triggers fetal breathing during the normally apnoeic high voltage EEG periods (3). Is then the chemical regulation of breathing solely responsible for maintaining gas exchange in postnatal life?

It is known that in the sheep the minimal oxygen consumption increases in first 24 h to about 3 times that found in fetus (4). This high metabolic rate then decreases during the first month of life, as thermal efficiency of the lambs improves. The heart-rate also increases transitionally in the first days after birth to fall again over the following weeks (5). Breathing frequency also decreases during this period (5).

Previous studies (6) showed that the lambs from 2 to 6 weeks of age, in quiet sleep when breathing frequency was lowest, used their laryngeal constrictor (thyroarytenoid muscle, TA) during expiration. These studies also showed a marked irregularity of the breathing pattern when lambs at this age were

The Physiological Development of the Fetus and Newborn
ISBN 0 12 389080 2

Copyright © 1985 by Academic Press, London.
All rights of reproduction in any form reserved.

tracheostomized (laryngeal and upper airway by-pass). The changes of the breathing pattern were vagally mediated and probably evoked by a reduction of expiratory lung volume. This dysrrhythmic breathing in response to laryngeal by-pass was uncommon in younger lambs (less than 12 days) and in lambs older than 6 weeks. Furthermore experimental hypoxemia induced greater irregularity and led to respiratory failure in this age group which did not occur with an intact upper airway or the application of positive expiratory distending pressure (7).

This all suggested that the relative contribution of different mechanisms sustaining breathing underwent developmental changes during the first month of life.

The influence of the ambient temperature (Ta) on breathing frequency in lambs during the first month of life has therefore been studied.

Methods

The lambs used during this study were separated from their ewes during the first 24 h after birth. They were bottle-fed with callostrum and trained to feed themselves ad-lib using rubber teats connected with a milk supply.

The experiments were performed on 18 unanaesthetized lambs during quiet sleep. Breathing frequency and the activity of the laryngeal constrictor activity were measured using inductance plethysmography (Respitrace). The characteristics of the plethysmographic recordings allowed assessment of the presence of thyroarytenoid (TA) activity (Fig. 1).

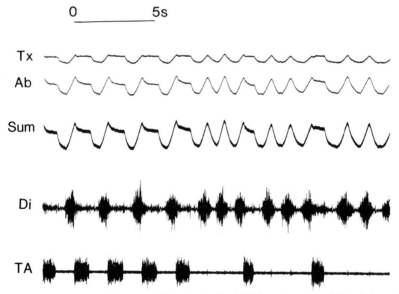

Figure 1. Upper traces: Thoracic (Tx), abdominal (Ab) and summed (Sum) signal of the inductance plethysmograph recording. Di: diaphragmatic EMG; TA: thyroarytenoid EMG.

The studies were conducted at 3, 6, 12 and 28 days of age at three different ambient temperatures 10, 15 and 20 degrees centigrade (sometimes 5°, 25° and 30°C were also studied) for at least 2 h each. In excess of 200 consecutive breaths in SWS were analysed.

In 2 animals chronic recording of the diaphragm and TA activity were also performed (Fig. 1). These animals had fenestrated tracheal tubes (Shiley) implanted which enabled a reversible by-pass of the upper airways and/or application of positive expiratory pressure during the experiments.

Implantation of the electrodes and the tracheostomy were done under halothane and N_2O anaesthesia.

A temperature-controlled room was used during the study, and the sleep state of the lambs was monitored by an infra-red closed circuit TV system.

Results

In 3- and 6-day-old lambs changes of Ta did not cause consistent changes in breathing frequency (bf) (mean bf = 39.7 breaths/min, SD = 9.0; mean bf = 37.4, SD = 11 for 3- and 6-day-old animals respectively) (Fig. 2).

Young lambs (3 days old) were observed to shiver at 10°C and their breathing frequency increased rapidly above 25°C Ta.

In 12- and 28-day-old lambs there was a significant difference in breathing frequencies at 20°C and 10°C Ta. Breathing frequency was lowest at 10°C both at 12 ($P < 0.01$) and at 28 days of age ($P < 0.05$).

There was a fall in breathing frequency between the 3rd day and 28th day of life (mean bf = 27.5; SD = 6.1) independent of the Ta between 10 and 20°C.

Laryngeal expiratory activity was present in the youngest animals in 22.7% of breaths and decreased in 6-day-old animals to 5.8%. TA activity increase as breathing frequency decreased in older lambs: 38% at 12 days of age; 53.9% at 28 days of age (Fig. 2).

Breaths in which the activity of TA during expiration occurred were significantly longer ($P < 0.001$) than breaths with no TA activity (Fig. 1).

Discussion

Breathing frequencies of lambs during the 1st week of life are largely independent of ambient temperature (within the studied range 10 to 20°C). This was observed even when the Ta was below the thermoneutral zone for youngest animals which shivered at 10°C. It is evident from studies (8) in which oxygen consumption was measured that a lamb aged 30 h, below 27°C is in a cold environment and is thus subject to a thermogenic metabolic stimulus which directly affects breathing.

In older lambs the thermal environmental changes within the presumptive thermoneutral range influenced breathing frequency. The reason for the lack of responsiveness to ambient temperature changes only during the 1st week of life is probably due to high metabolic demand of this period (4,8) associated also with the poor thermal efficiency which improves later (4).

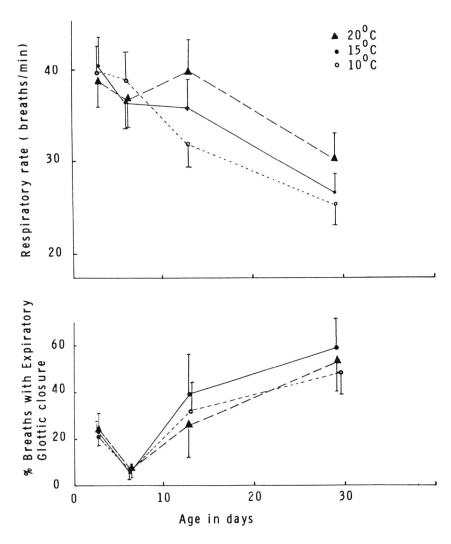

Figure 2. Upper panel: respiratory frequency between 3rd and 28th day at three ambient temperatures. Lower panel: TA activity expressed as percent of breaths with TA activity during expiration.

Breathing frequencies of the lambs in this study were lower than those previously reported in ewe-reared lambs (5). This finding may suggest that the presence of a ewe contributes significantly to the thermal environment of lambs as an additional heat source.

The laryngeal constrictor activity during expiration in lambs which was observed mainly from the 2nd week of life seems to be correlated with basic breathing frequency in a reciprocal manner. It appears when breathing frequency is low and affects the rate of deflation during the expiratory period by increasing the upper airways resistance. Thus in the absence of a thermal drive to breathing, and at lower basal breathing frequencies, the reflex laryngeal constriction—by preserving expiratory lung volume—supports effective gas exchange. However, due to reduced expiratory flow and expiratory lung distension the onset of the next inspiration is also delayed.

It may be concluded that the thermal environment within a presumative thermoneutral zone and laryngeal constrictor function constitute important factors affecting rhythmogenesis and gas exchange in lambs between 2 and 4 weeks old.

References

1. Blanco, C. E., Dawes, G. S., Hanson, M. A. and McCooke, H. B. (1984). *J. Physiol.* **351**, 25–38.
2. Blanco, C. E., Hanson, M. A., Johnston, P. and Rigato, H. (1984). *J. Appl. Physiol.* **56**(1), 12–17.
3. Gluckman, P. D., Gunn, T. R. and Johnston, B. M. (1983). *J. Physiol.* **343**, 495–506.
4. Dawes, G. S. and Mott, J. C. (1959). *J. Physiol.* **146**, 295–315.
5. Johnson, P. (1978). In: "Central Nervous Control Mechanisms in Breathing", (von Euler, C. and Lagercrantz, H., eds) pp. 337–351. Pergamon Press, Oxford.
6. Harding, R., Johnson, P. and McClelland, M. E. (1980). *Resp. Physiol.* **40**, 165–180.
7. Andrews, J. F., Mercer, J. B., Ryan, E. M. and Székely, M. (1974). *J. Physiol.* **236**, 35–36.

Perinatal Physiology, the Past, Present and Future

G. S. Dawes

The Nuffield Institute for Medical Research, University of Oxford, Oxford, UK

The start of fetal physiology goes back to the days of Professor A. St G. Huggett at St Mary's Hospital Medical School, London, who as a young man in 1927 first measured the relatively low PaO_2 of the fetus (1), and of Sir Joseph Barcroft (2) who laid the foundations of our knowledge of the fetal circulation and respiration before the Second World War. Shortly thereafter, Alfred Jost found that decapitation of the fetus hardly affected the growth of its body (3) and thus gave an astounding start to fetal endocrinology. I have commented elsewhere (4) on many of the major discoveries in perinatal physiology from 1954 onwards.

They include the identification of pulmonary surfactant, of brown adipose tissue as the major source of neonatal nonshivering thermogenesis, and of the importance of prostaglandins in the determination of uterine contractions and the closure of the ductus arteriosus. Fetal autonomy in the onset of ovine parturition, with the participation of the fetal pituitary and adrenal cortex, was proved by Mont Liggins in the late 1960s. Then there was the recognition of the development of behavioural patterns, related to sleep states prenatally, in sheep and man; the importance of the placenta in lactate metabolism; the proof that in fetal lambs the outputs of the two sides of the heart differ quantitatively under normal conditions. By the time of the Barcroft Symposium in 1973 a large range of physiological studies had provided new interesting directions for further research.

During the past 10 years there has been much further progress. The privacy of the fetus has been invaded to such an extent that the uterine environment seems no longer a barrier to research, at least in sheep and goats. Henrique Rigatto and his colleagues in Winnipeg (5) have enabled us to see the fetus directly through a plexiglass window in the wall of the uterus and maternal abdomen. We can record from a variety of fetal spinal or cranial reflexes *in utero*. Peter Gluckman in Auckland, New Zealand, has made the first stereotaxic atlases for localized

The Physiological Development of the Fetus and Newborn
ISBN 0 12 389080 2

Copyright © 1985 by Academic Press, London.
All rights of reproduction in any form reserved.

lesions in the hypothalamus or brain stem, and Vic Chernick has improved accessibility for neuronal recording. The cerebrospinal fluid space has been perfused and sampled in the unanaesthetized fetus *in utero* by Koos (6) and by Hohimer *et al.* (7). The use of twisted stainless steel (Cooner) wire has prolonged electrode life in spite of fetal movements. Computerized analysis of large quantities of data has thoroughly changed experimental design. Ultrasound transit measurements in fetal lambs have made possible the quantitative measurement of growth and movements of the limbs, the chest and the head. Real-time ultrasound observations and measurements on the human fetus *in utero* have revolutionized our understanding of human fetal development and the practice of perinatal medicine. In addition, the range of hormone assays on small samples of plasma has been immensely extended. So we have much less restriction on experimental investigations of the fetus than even 10 years ago.

When Barron and his colleagues in New Haven (8) pioneered the study of the unanaesthetized fetus *in utero*, they could not have foreseen the complications in interpretation that we have now come to appreciate. Weak contractions of the uterus, each lasting about 6 min and repeated 2–3 times/h (i.e. 12–18 min/h), are intermingled with episodic changes in electrocortical activity in the sheep fetus near term (9). The association between these events is statistically significant, but the correlation is low. Less than a quarter of the changes from low to high voltage electrocortical activity are associated with uterine contractions. They are therefore almost independent variables. There are also changes in maternal activity and posture. The problem we have to face is that they all may indirectly affect different aspects of fetal physiology to different degrees at different gestational ages. We are not dealing with a steady state *in utero* near term. It is perturbed at regular intervals by uterine contractions and less regularly by changes in fetal electrocortical activity. The transition from high to low voltage activity is associated with an increase in blood flow to some parts of the brain, the gut and the pancreas and with changes in the activity of spinal and cranial reflexes, not necessarily in the same direction. While there is no evidence of a systematic change in fetal O_2 uptake (10) there may be transient changes in umbilical blood flow. Gluckman (11) has suggested that the release of fetal growth hormone, thyrotrophin and gonadotrophin is pulsatile in the lamb. Large variations in plasma growth hormone and thyrotrophin concentrations were present at 93 days gestation, before the differentiation of fetal electrocortical activity into high/low voltage. Whether there is association between the hormonal and electrocortical rhythms later in gestation does not seem to have been reported. And there may be further complications, in that insulin release is pulsatile in adult sheep as in man (J. Bassett, personal communication). We do not yet know whether these rhythms (if their existence is confirmed) are linked during development, whether they are regular or show diurnal fluctuations, nor whether their amplitudes change with age. Clearly, the range of these unsteady states requires more detailed exploration. Gluckman (11), as an endocrinologist, naturally postulated immaturity of the negative feedback loop to explain the relatively high amplitude of the hormonal oscillations. There may be other explanations. For example, we can recall the large increases in plasma catecholamines in response to fetal hypoxia, much higher in the adult. Is this excessive secretion due to the small number of receptors, or to the relative lack of nonspecific uptake or to immaturity of other clearance mechanisms (in the lung or liver, enzymically or otherwise).

We should also reconsider the procedures commonly used to test fetal physiological behaviour. One such test is to produce isocapnic hypoxia by altering the maternal inspired gas concentrations, usually to 9% O_2 with 3% CO_2 in N_2. We have to note two points. First, this produces an unsteady state, in which the distribution of systemic blood flow changes progressively (between 15 and 30 min) and arterial pH falls over a period of hours. Secondly, the fetal heart rate usually recovers after the initial bradycardia. The usual explanation offered is that this recovery coincides with a large rise in plasma catecholamines. Another, not necessarily alternative, explanation is adaptation of the systemic arterial chemo- and baroreceptors. In adults the baroreceptors reset rapidly, allegedly in 20–30 min. When Joan Mott produced hypertension by bilateral nephrectomy in some fetal lambs (12), she found that although the arterial pressure rose from 45 to nearly 90 mmHg in 5–6 days, the heart rate rose slightly. In newborn lambs, there is evidence that the peripheral chemoreceptors also reset (13). So perhaps we should not be surprised to find a very sick fetus whose mean heart range is within the normal range. That adaptation may occur, few would doubt, but to measure the adaptation of a population of fetal sense organs *in utero* is not easy.

Another important area of fetal physiology, which is developing rapidly, concerns the identification of the areas responsible for the integration of behaviour in the brain stem, and of the possible neurotransmitters (e.g. 14,15). What we have learnt within the last few years is that control over many functions that we regarded in the past as simple (e.g. the ventilatory response to hypoxia) is complex. The models we derive to explain the results have become more sophisticated. We now recognize the multiple sites of action of drugs (such as pentobarbitone, ethanol or opiates) on areas above the pons, in the medulla and spinal cord, all to produce the same end result. Possibly, the lamb may offer the opportunity to analyse these mechanisms more readily before birth than afterwards.

Sir Joseph Barcroft wrote another classic book (as well as that entitled "Researches in Perinatal Life"), on the "Integration of Physiological Function", which had a profound influence on those students of my generation interested in systems physiology. Most of us here today have a continuing interest in this aspect of fetal physiology. I am sure we recognize its territorial limits and the need to understand effects on single cells, on membranes and the internal organization of organs. It now seems unlikely that we can approach the physiology of growth profitably in any other way. The search for general regulators of growth seems to have run into blind alleys.

Finally let me make it clear that Colin Jones, not I, chose the title of this chapter. To discuss the past too long is neither profitable nor interesting. To discuss the present is not easy: I have only touched on a few favourite themes and made no reference to many of the burning issues raised elsewhere in this book. To discuss the future is another matter altogether. If one could see far ahead, the word discovery would be inappropriate. We see through a glass, darkly. We have consistently underestimated the complexities of life before birth.

Life before birth appears to be restrained. The behaviour of the fetus is limited. It seems difficult to arouse and breathing is discontinuous; and the usual stimulants of carotid body function behave unreliably. Yet it responds vigorously when cold is applied, either to the exposed fetus (16) or *in utero* (17). So maybe rather than a specific inhibition the failure is a consequence of limited afferent input, into a system ready to respond to premature delivery. This hypothesis is not new. The problem has been to design an experiment by which it can be tested. Can we test it in the future?

References

1. Huggett, A. St G. (1927). *J. Physiol.* **330**, 50–51P.
2. Barcroft, J. (1946). *In:* "Researches in Prenatal Life". Blackwell Scientific Publications, Oxford.
3. Jost, A. (1947). *C. R. Acad. Sci. Paris* **225**, 322–324.
4. Dawes, G. S. (1984). *J. Develop. Physiol.* **6**, 259–266.
5. Rigatto, H., Moore, M., Horvath, L., Winter, A., Luz, J. and Cates, D. (1982). *In:* "Proc. IXth Int. Symp. Fetal Breathing", University of Western Ontario, Canada.
6. Koos, B. J. (1982). *J. Physiol.* **330**, 50–51P.
7. Hohimer, A. R., Bissonette, J. M., Richardson, B. S. and Machida, C. M. (1983). *Resp. Physiol.* **52**, 88–111.
8. Meschia, G., Cotter, J. R., Breathnach, C. S. and Barron, D. H. (1965). *Q. J. Exp. Physiol.* **50**, 466–480.
9. Nathanielsz, P. W., Bailey, A., Poore, E. R., Thorburn, G. D. and Harding, R. (1980). *Am. J. Obstet. Gynecol.* **138**, 653–659.
10. Walker, A. M., Fleming, J., Sunolich, J., Stunden, R., Horne, R. and Maloney, J. (1984). *J. Develop. Physiol.* **6**, 267–274.
11. Gluckman, P. D. (1984). *J. Develop. Physiol.* **6**, 301–312.
12. Mott, J. C. (1980). *Adv. Physiol. Sci., 28th Int. Congress, Budapest* **8**, 299–307.
13. Blanco, C. E., Dawes, G. S., Hanson, M. A. and McCooke, H. B. (1984). *J. Physiol.* **351**, 25–37.
14. Dawes, G. S. (1968). *J. Physiol.* **346**, 1–18.
15. Walker, D. (1984). *J. Develop. Physiol.* **6**, 225–236.
16. Dawes, G. S. (1968). *In:* "Fetal and Neonatal Physiology". Yearbook Medical Publishers, Chicago.
17. Gluckman, P. D., Gunn, T. R. and Johnston, B. M. (1983). *J. Physiol.* **343**, 496–506.

Subject Index